Photodermatology

This book has been provided to you
through an Educational Grant from

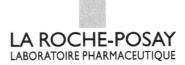

LA ROCHE-POSAY
LABORATOIRE PHARMACEUTIQUE

BASIC AND CLINICAL DERMATOLOGY

Series Editors

ALAN R. SHALITA, M.D.
Distinguished Teaching Professor and Chairman
Department of Dermatology
SUNY Downstate Medical Center
Brooklyn, New York

DAVID A. NORRIS, M.D.
Director of Research
Professor of Dermatology
The University of Colorado
Health Sciences Center
Denver, Colorado

1. Cutaneous Investigation in Health and Disease: Noninvasive Methods and Instrumentation, *edited by Jean-Luc Lévêque*
2. Irritant Contact Dermatitis, *edited by Edward M. Jackson and Ronald Goldner*
3. Fundamentals of Dermatology: A Study Guide, *Franklin S. Glickman and Alan R. Shalita*
4. Aging Skin: Properties and Functional Changes, *edited by Jean-Luc Lévêque and Pierre G. Agache*
5. Retinoids: Progress in Research and Clinical Applications, *edited by Maria A. Livrea and Lester Packer*
6. Clinical Photomedicine, *edited by Henry W. Lim and Nicholas A. Soter*
7. Cutaneous Antifungal Agents: Selected Compounds in Clinical Practice and Development, *edited by John W. Rippon and Robert A. Fromtling*
8. Oxidative Stress in Dermatology, *edited by Jürgen Fuchs and Lester Packer*
9. Connective Tissue Diseases of the Skin, *edited by Charles M. Lapière and Thomas Krieg*
10. Epidermal Growth Factors and Cytokines, *edited by Thomas A. Luger and Thomas Schwarz*
11. Skin Changes and Diseases in Pregnancy, *edited by Marwali Harahap and Robert C. Wallach*
12. Fungal Disease: Biology, Immunology, and Diagnosis, *edited by Paul H. Jacobs and Lexie Nall*
13. Immunomodulatory and Cytotoxic Agents in Dermatology, *edited by Charles J. McDonald*
14. Cutaneous Infection and Therapy, *edited by Raza Aly, Karl R. Beutner, and Howard I. Maibach*

15. Tissue Augmentation in Clinical Practice: Procedures and Techniques, *edited by Arnold William Klein*

16. Psoriasis: Third Edition, Revised and Expanded, *edited by Henry H. Roenigk, Jr., and Howard I. Maibach*

17. Surgical Techniques for Cutaneous Scar Revision, *edited by Marwali Harahap*

18. Drug Therapy in Dermatology, *edited by Larry E. Millikan*

19. Scarless Wound Healing, *edited by Hari G. Garg and Michael T. Longaker*

20. Cosmetic Surgery: An Interdisciplinary Approach, *edited by Rhoda S. Narins*

21. Topical Absorption of Dermatological Products, *edited by Robert L. Bronaugh and Howard I. Maibach*

22. Glycolic Acid Peels, *edited by Ronald Moy, Debra Luftman, and Lenore S. Kakita*

23. Innovative Techniques in Skin Surgery, *edited by Marwali Harahap*

24. Safe Liposuction and Fat Transfer, *edited by Rhoda S. Narins*

25. Pyschocutaneous Medicine, *edited by John Y. M. Koo and Chai Sue Lee*

26. Skin, Hair, and Nails: Structure and Function, *edited Bo Forslind and Magnus Lindberg*

27. Itch: Basic Mechanisms and Therapy, *edited Gil Yosipovitch, Malcolm W. Greaves, Alan B. Fleischer, and Francis McGlone*

28. Photoaging, *edited by Darrell S. Rigel, Robert A. Weiss, Henry W. Lim, and Jeffrey S. Dover*

29. Vitiligo: Problems and Solutions, *edited by Torello Lotti and Jana Hercogova*

30. Photodamaged Skin, *edited by David J. Goldberg*

31. Ambulatory Phlebectomy, Second Edition, *edited by Mitchel P. Goldman, Mihael Georgiev, and Stefano Ricci*

32. Cutaneous Lymphomas, *edited by Gunter Burg and Werner Kempf*

33. Wound Healing, *edited by Anna Falabella and Robert Kirsner*

34. Phototherapy and Photochemotherapy for Skin Disease, Third Edition, *Warwick L. Morison*

35. Advanced Techniques in Dermatologic Surgery, *edited by Mitchel P. Goldman and Robert A. Weiss*

36. Tissue Augmentation in Clinical Practice, Second Edition, *edited by Arnold W. Klein*

37. Cellulite: Pathophysiology and Treatment, *edited by Mitchel P. Goldman, Pier Antonio Bacci, Gustavo Leibaschoff, Doris Hexsel, and Fabrizio Angelini*

38. Photodermatology, *edited by Henry W. Lim, Herbert Hönigsmann, and John L. M. Hawk*

39. Retinoids and Carotenoids in Dermatology, *Edited by Anders Vahlquist and Madeleine Duvic*

40. Acne and Its Therapy, *Edited by Guy F. Webster; Anthony V. Rawlings*

Photodermatology

edited by

Henry W. Lim
Henry Ford Hospital
Detroit, Michigan, U.S.A.

Herbert Hönigsmann
Medical University of Vienna
Vienna, Austria

John L. M. Hawk
St. John's Institute of Dermatology
London, U.K.

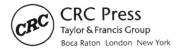

CRC Press
Taylor & Francis Group
Boca Raton London New York

CRC Press is an imprint of the
Taylor & Francis Group, an **informa** business

First published 2007 by Informa Healthcare USA, Inc.

Published 2019 by CRC Press
Taylor & Francis Group
6000 Broken Sound Parkway NW, Suite 300
Boca Raton, FL 33487-2742

© 2007 by Taylor & Francis Group, LLC
CRC Press is an imprint of Taylor & Francis Group, an Informa business

First issued in paperback 2019

No claim to original U.S. Government works

ISBN-13: 978-0-367-45319-0 (pbk)
ISBN-13: 978-0-8493-7496-8 (hbk)

Visit the Taylor & Francis Web site at
http://www.taylorandfrancis.com

and the CRC Press Web site at
http://www.crcpress.com

Series Introduction

During the past 25 years there has been a vast explosion of new information relating to the art and science of dermatology, as well as fundamental cutaneous biology. Furthermore, this information is no longer of interest to only the small but growing specialty of dermatology. Clinicians and scientists from a wide variety of disciplines have come to recognize both the importance of skin in fundamental biological processes and the broad implications of understanding the pathogenesis of skin disease. As a result, there is now a multidisciplinary and worldwide interest in the progress of dermatology.

With these factors in mind, we have undertaken this series of books specifically oriented to dermatology. The scope of this series is purposely broad, with books ranging from pure basic science to practical, applied clinical dermatology. Thus, while there is something for everyone, all volumes in this series will ultimately prove to be valuable additions to the dermatologist's library.

The latest volume in the series (No. 38), by Lim, Hönigsmann, and Hawk, presents a comprehensive and current review of photomedicine by world renowned authorities. The role of photobiology in medicine has received increased emphasis in the past decade as a result of considerable new information regarding the molecular biological effects of ultraviolet light, its effect on the immune system, its role in the promotion of skin cancer, and its abuse by profiteers who market suntan parlors. It is, therefore, critically important that dermatologists, physicians in general, biologists, and public health scientists remain current in photomedicine. I believe that Dr. Lim and his coeditors have produced a timely and critically important addition to our series, which is both timely and comprehensive.

Alan R. Shalita, MD
Distinguished Teaching Professor and Chairman
Department of Dermatology
SUNY Downstate Medical Center
Brooklyn, New York, U.S.A.

Preface

Within the past 30 years photomedicine has developed from empiricism into one of the most exciting fields in biomedical research. Studies on the effects of visible and ultraviolet radiation on skin have led to a fruitful collaboration between basic scientists and clinicians. The successful use of the new ultraviolet techniques for the treatment of skin disease, along with a rapidly increasing understanding of the pathogenesis of photodermatoses, thereby markedly improving their treatment, have been the driving force for the development of a new subspecialty of photodermatology. This now encompasses the diagnosis and treatment of sunlight-induced disorders; all aspects of phototherapy, including the use of such new modalities as photodynamic therapy for skin tumors and other diseases; as well as photoprotection, which continues to evolve with the development of new generations of ultraviolet filters. In the past decade, therefore, very significant advances have occurred throughout this novel subspecialty, particularly in photoimmunology, molecular biology, and genetics. In more detail, these include better recognition and understanding of:

- Acute and chronic effects of ultraviolet radiation on the skin: in vitro studies, animal models, photoaging, and epidemiology of skin cancers;
- Clinical manifestation of photodermatoses: actinic prurigo, pin-head papule form of polymorphous light eruption, novel genetic mutations in porphyrias, and so on;
- Pathophysiology and treatment of photodermatoses: polymorphous light eruption, actinic prurigo, chronic actinic dermatitis, xeroderma pigmentatosum, photo-exacerbated dermatoses, and so on;
- The science of photoprotection: new ultraviolet filters, photoprotection by clothing, photoprotection by oral agents, and so on;
- Phototherapy: narrowband ultraviolet B, ultraviolet A1, visible light;
- Topical photodynamic therapy;
- Medical and cosmetic applications of laser and similar radiation sources; and
- New insight on the use of laser and radiation sources on people of color.

In planning for this book, our vision as editors was to create a book that is comprehensive and up-to-date, yet is user-friendly to its intended readers who are busy, practicing dermatologists, photodermatologists, and trainees in dermatology. The editors are pleased that recognized experts from many parts of the world willingly put in the effort and contributed most informative chapters for this book.

The book consists of six sections. Section I is on history and basic principles, followed by the effects of ultraviolet radiation on normal skin in Section II. Section III covers all the photodermatoses, while Section IV and V discuss photoprotection and ultraviolet and visible radiation therapy. Section VI is a practical description of testing methods used in photodermatology and guidelines of setting up a phototherapy and laser center.

The three of us work in the United States, Europe, and the United Kingdom. We have taken great care to make sure that materials covered in this book reflect an international point of view. For example, international coverage is done on actinic prurigo (commonly seen in Central and South America), photoprotection (different ultraviolet filters available in different parts of the world), light sources and laser, and many other topics. It is our hope that the readers will find that this book provides a good perspective on the worldwide scope of photodermatology.

On a personal note, the three of us have been colleagues and friends for many years; all of us have separately published books in photodermatology in the early and late 1990s. It has been a real pleasure to combine our experience and to work on editing this book together. We do hope that the readers will enjoy this book as much as we have enjoyed writing and editing it.

Henry W. Lim, MD
Herbert Hönigsmann, MD
John L. M. Hawk, MD

Acknowledgments

Henry W. Lim would like to thank his parents, for providing him the opportunity to succeed, and his wife Mamie, for her unending patience and support.

Hebert Hönigsmann would like to thank his wife Xandi, for tolerating the lack of care and attention to the family during the preparation of this book.

John L. M. Hawk would like to thank his wife, Lorna, for her continuing tolerance and support, as ever previously, throughout the preparation of this book.

The editors would like to thank Sandra Beberman and her team at Informa Healthcare for working with us to produce this book.

Contents

Series Introduction   Alan R. Shalita, MD   *iii*
Preface   v
Acknowledgments   vii
Contributors   xiii

Section I: History and Basic Principles

1. **History of Human Photobiology   1**
   Rik Roelandts

2. **Basic Principles of Photobiology   15**
   Brian L. Diffey and Irene E. Kochevar

3. **Radiation Sources and Interaction with Skin   29**
   Harvey Lui and R. Rox Anderson

Section II: Effects of Ultraviolet Radiation on Normal Skin

4. **The Molecular and Genetic Effects of Ultraviolet Radiation
   Exposure on Skin Cells   41**
   Marjan Garmyn and Daniel B. Yarosh

5. **Photoimmunology   55**
   Thomas Schwarz and Gary M. Halliday

6. **The Acute Effects of Ultraviolet Radiation on the Skin   75**
   Lesley E. Rhodes and Henry W. Lim

7. **The Chronic Effects of Ultraviolet Radiation on the Skin: Photoaging   91**
   Mina Yaar

8. **The Chronic Effects of Ultraviolet Radiation on
   the Skin: Photocarcinogenesis   107**
   Antony R. Young and Norbert M. Wikonkál

9. **The Epidemiology of Skin Cancer   119**
   Luigi Naldi and Thomas Diepgen

Section III: Photodermatoses
Part A: Basic Principles

10. **Evaluation of the Photosensitive Patient   139**
    Henry W. Lim and John L. M. Hawk

Part B: Immunologically-Mediated Photodermatoses

11. **Polymorphous Light Eruption, Hydroa Vacciniforme, and Actinic Prurigo** *149*

Herbert Hönigsmann and Maria Teresa Hojyo-Tomoka

12. **Chronic Actinic Dermatitis** *169*

John L. M. Hawk and Henry W. Lim

13. **Solar Urticaria** *185*

Takeshi Horio and Erhard Hölzle

Part C: Drug and Chemical-Induced Photosensitivity

14. **Drug and Chemical Photosensitivity: Exogenous** *199*

James Ferguson and Vincent A. DeLeo

15. **Cutaneous Porphyrias** *219*

Gillian M. Murphy and Karl E. Anderson

Part D: DNA Repair-Deficient Photodermatoses

16. **Xeroderma Pigmentosum and Other DNA Repair-Deficient Photodermatoses** *239*

Mark Berneburg and Kenneth H. Kraemer

Part E: Photoaggravated Dermatoses

17. **Photoaggravated Dermatoses** *251*

Victoria P. Werth and Herbert Hönigsmann

Section IV: Photoprotection

18. **Photoprotection** *267*

Henry W. Lim and Herbert Hönigsmann

19. **Novel Developments in Photoprotection: Part I** *279*

Uli Osterwalder and Henry W. Lim

20. **Novel Developments in Photoprotection: Part II** *297*

André Rougier, Sophie Seite, and Henry W. Lim

21. **Public Education in Photoprotection** *311*

Cheryl Rosen and Mark Naylor

Section V: Ultraviolet and Visible Radiation Therapy

22. **Phototherapy with UVB: Broadband and Narrowband** *319*

Michael Zanolli and Peter M. Farr

23. **Ultraviolet-A1 and Visible Light Therapy** *335*

Jean Krutmann and Akimichi Morita

24. **Psoralen Photochemotherapy** *347*

Warwick L. Morison and Herbert Hönigsmann

25. **Extracorporeal Photochemotherapy (Photopheresis)** *359*

Robert Knobler and Peter W. Heald

26. **Photodynamic Therapy** *369*
    Sally H. Ibbotson and Rolf-Markus Szeimies

27. **The Principles and Medical Applications of Lasers and Intense-Pulsed Light in Dermatology** *389*
    Iltefat Hamzavi and Harvey Lui

28. **Lasers and Energy Sources for Skin Rejuvenation and Epilation** *401*
    Robert A. Weiss and Michael Landthaler

29. **Laser Treatment on Ethnic Skin** *417*
    Henry Hin Lee Chan and Brooke Jackson

Section VI: Appendices
Appendix A. **Phototesting** *433*
    Peter M. Farr and Robert S. Dawe

Appendix B. **Photopatch Testing** *441*
    Percy Lehmann, Frank C. Victor, and David E. Cohen

Appendix C. **Guidelines for Setting Up a Phototherapy Referral Center or an Office-Based Phototherapy Unit** *449*
    Michael Zanolli and Roy Palmer

Appendix D. **Guidelines for Setting Up a Laser Center** *457*
    Macrene R. Alexiades-Armenakas and Jeffrey S. Dover

Index *463*

Photodermatology

Photodermatology

Sponsored by Ciba Specialty Chemicals

Makers of the Sunscreen Actives
CIBA® TINOSORB® M and TINOSORB® S

Ciba

Contributors

Macrene R. Alexiades-Armenakas Department of Dermatology, Yale University School of Medicine, New Haven, Connecticut, U.S.A.

Karl E. Anderson Department of Internal Medicine, Division of Gastroenterology and Hepatology, University of Texas Medical Branch, Galveston, Texas, U.S.A.

R. Rox Anderson Wellman Center for Photomedicine and Department of Dermatology, Harvard Medical School, and Massachusetts General Hospital, Boston, Massachusetts, U.S.A.

Mark Berneburg Department of Dermatology, Eberhard Karls University, Tuebingen, Germany

Henry Hin Lee Chan Division of Dermatology, Department of Medicine, University of Hong Kong, and Department of Medicine and Therapeutics, Chinese University of Hong Kong, Hong Kong, China

David E. Cohen Ronald O. Perelman Department of Dermatology, New York University School of Medicine, New York, New York, U.S.A.

Robert S. Dawe Department of Dermatology, Ninewells Hospital and Medical School, Dundee University, Dundee, Scotland, U.K.

Vincent A. DeLeo Columbia University, St. Luke's–Roosevelt Hospital Center, New York, New York, U.S.A.

Thomas Diepgen Department of Clinical Social Medicine, Occupational and Environmental Dermatology, Heidelberg, Germany

Brian L. Diffey Department of Regional Medical Physics, Newcastle General Hospital, Newcastle, England, U.K.

Jeffrey S. Dover Department of Dermatology, Yale University School of Medicine, New Haven, Connecticut, and Dartmouth Medical School, Hanover, New Hampshire, U.S.A.

Peter M. Farr Department of Dermatology, Royal Victoria Infirmary, Newcastle upon Tyne, England, U.K.

James Ferguson Photobiology Unit, Ninewells Hospital, Dundee, Scotland, U.K.

Marjan Garmyn Department of Dermatology, University of Leuven, Leuven, Belgium

Gary M. Halliday Dermatology Research Laboratories, Melanoma and Skin Cancer Research Institute, University of Sydney, Sydney, Australia

Iltefat Hamzavi Department of Dermatology, Henry Ford Hospital, Detroit, and Hamzavi Dermatology, Port Huron, Michigan, U.S.A.

John L. M. Hawk Photobiology Unit, St. John's Institute of Dermatology, St. Thomas' Hospital, King's College of London, London, England, U.K.

Peter W. Heald   Department of Dermatology, West Haven VA Medical Center, Yale University School of Medicine, New Haven, Connecticut, U.S.A.

Maria Teresa Hojyo-Tomoka   Departamento de Dermatologia del Hospital General Dr. Manuel Gea González, Tlalpan, Mexico City, Mexico

Erhard Hölzle   Department of Dermatology and Allergology, Klinikum Oldenburg, Oldenburg, Germany

Herbert Hönigsmann   Department of Dermatology, Medical University of Vienna, Vienna, Austria

Takeshi Horio   Department of Dermatology, Kansai Medical University, Osaka, Japan

Sally H. Ibbotson   Department of Dermatology, Ninewells Hospital and Medical School, University of Dundee, Dundee, Scotland, U.K.

Brooke Jackson   Skin and Wellness Center of Chicago, Chicago, Illinois, U.S.A.

Robert Knobler   Division of Special and Environmental Dermatology, Department of Dermatology, Medical University of Vienna, Vienna, Austria, and Department of Dermatology, College of Physicians and Surgeons, Columbia University, New York, New York, U.S.A.

Irene E. Kochevar   Wellman Center for Photomedicine, Massachusetts General Hospital, Harvard Medical School, Boston, Massachusetts, U.S.A.

Kenneth H. Kraemer   Basic Research Laboratory, Center for Cancer Research, National Cancer Institute, Bethesda, Maryland, U.S.A.

Jean Krutmann   Department of Dermatology and Environmental Medicine, Institut für Umweltmedizinische Forschung (IUF), Heinrich-Heine University, Düsseldorf, Germany

Michael Landthaler   Department of Dermatology, University Clinic Regensburg, Regensburg, Germany

Percy Lehmann   Klinik für Dermatologie, Allergologie und Umweltmedizin, HELIOS-Klinikum Wuppertal, Universitätsklinikum der Universität Witten-Herdecke, Wuppertal, Germany

Henry W. Lim   Department of Dermatology, Henry Ford Hospital, Detroit, Michigan, U.S.A.

Harvey Lui   Department of Dermatology and Skin Science, Vancouver Coastal Health Research Institute, University of British Columbia, Vancouver, British Columbia, Canada.

Warwick L. Morison   Department of Dermatology, Johns Hopkins University, Baltimore, Maryland, U.S.A.

Akimichi Morita   Department of Geriatric and Environmental Dermatology, Nagoya City University Graduate School of Medical Sciences, Nagoya, Japan

Gillian M. Murphy   Department of Dermatology, Beaumont Hospital, Dublin, Ireland

Luigi Naldi   Centro Studi GISED, Ospedali Riuniti, Bergamo, Italy

Mark Naylor   University of Oklahoma, Tulsa, Oklahoma, U.S.A.

Uli Osterwalder   Ciba Specialty Chemicals, Basel, Switzerland

Roy Palmer   Photobiology Unit, St. John's Institute of Dermatology, St. Thomas' Hospital, London, England, U.K.

Rik Roelandts   Photodermatology Unit, University Hospital, Leuven, Belgium

Lesley E. Rhodes   Department of Dermatological Sciences, Photobiology Unit, University of Manchester, Salford Royal Foundation Hospital, Manchester, England, U.K.

Cheryl Rosen   Division of Dermatology, Toronto Western Hospital, University of Toronto, Toronto, Ontario, Canada

André Rougier   La Roche-Posay Pharmaceutical Laboratories, Asnières, France

Thomas Schwarz   Department of Dermatology, University of Kiel, Kiel, Germany

Sophie Seite   La Roche-Posay Pharmaceutical Laboratories, Asnières, France

Rolf-Markus Szeimies   Department of Dermatology, Regensburg University Hospital, Regensburg, Germany

Frank C. Victor   Ronald O. Perelman Department of Dermatology, New York University School of Medicine, New York, New York, U.S.A.

Robert A. Weiss   Department of Dermatology, Johns Hopkins University School of Medicine, Baltimore, and Maryland Laser Skin & Vein Institute, Hunt Valley, Maryland, U.S.A.

Victoria P. Werth   Department of Dermatology, University of Pennsylvania, and Philadelphia V.A. Medical Center, Philadelphia, Pennsylvania, U.S.A.

Norbert M. Wikonkál   Department of Dermatology, Semmelweis University, School of Medicine, Budapest, Hungary

Mina Yaar   Department of Dermatology, Boston University School of Medicine, Boston, Massachusetts, U.S.A.

Daniel B. Yarosh   Applied Genetics Incorporated Dermatics, Freeport, New York, U.S.A.

Antony R. Young   Division of Genetics and Molecular Medicine, St. John's Institute of Dermatology, King's College London, London, England, U.K.

Michael Zanolli   Division of Dermatology, Vanderbilt University Medical Center, Vanderbilt University, Nashville, Tennessee, U.S.A.

1 | History of Human Photobiology

Rik Roelandts
Photodermatology Unit, University Hospital, Leuven, Belgium

- Study on visible light was first published by Newton in 1672, and study on action spectrum of ultraviolet light was published by Hausser and Vahle in 1922.

- Relationship between sunlight and skin aging was first published by Unna in 1894, and relationship between sunlight and skin cancer was published by Dubreuilh in 1907.

- First description of a photodermatosis (eczema solare) was in 1798 by Wilan.

- First commercially available sunscreen (benzyl salicylate and benzyl cinnamate) was in 1928 in the United States. The concept of SPF was developed by Greiter in 1974, and adopted by the United States Food and Drug Administration in 1978.

- Modern day phototherapy started with Goeckerman in 1925 and PUVA with Parrish in 1974.

THE BEGINNING OF A SCIENTIFIC INTEREST

The endless chain of days and nights since life began must have been an important source of imagination during history. This may explain why the Egyptians saw the Sun God Re sailing the heaven in a boat and why the Greeks saw Apollo driving a chariot through the sky. The Aztecs even offered beating human hearts to the Sun God, to give him enough strength to reappear the next day. In nearly every civilization, people have adored the sun. It was not only a question of religion but also of necessity. The sun is the universal source of light and heat, and without the sun it would be dark and cold forever. This has nothing to do with science. However, from early humankind on, people realized that the sun is extremely important for life and it was, therefore, a topic of major concern. Stimulating people's interest is the beginning of science. Apart from this, there is also human experience. In many civilizations, people realized that the sun could have a beneficial effect on certain diseases and this, of course, had a stimulating effect on people's imagination. It can take a very long time before imagination evolves into a critical and structured approach, and in many cases this is a step-by-step process.

The beginning of a real scientific interest in the solar spectrum dates from the 17th century. One of the most important steps forward was the discovery of the visible spectrum of the sun by Isaac Newton in England. He published the results of his experiments in 1672, whereby the visible spectrum of the sun was fractionated by a prism into the different colors of the rainbow (1). When Newton projected green plus red light on a wall, no green or red light appeared, but only yellow light. When he added blue light, no green, red, or blue light appeared, but only white light. To make white light, Newton did not need all colors, but only red, green, and blue—the three basic colors.

In 1800, William Herschel, again in England, did some experiments with a thermometer to evaluate which colors of the visible solar spectrum had the highest temperature. He noted that the thermometer registered a higher temperature above the red visible light and, thus, discovered the infrared spectrum of the sun (2).

The discovery of ultraviolet rays came a year later and can be attributed to the German Johann Wilhelm Ritter. This discovery was partly based on previous experiments, by Carl Wilhelm Scheele in Sweden, which had already been published in 1777 (3). Scheele could show that paper strips dipped in a silver chloride solution became black after exposure to the sun, because of a reduction of the silver, and that silver chloride did not become black in the dark. Later on, this became the principle of analogous photography. Scheele could also show that this was more pronounced with blue light than with red light. Ritter, a young scientist, was convinced that invisible rays not only existed beyond the red end of the visible spectrum, as Herschel had demonstrated, but he also believed a similar invisible spectrum must exist below the visible blue end of the spectrum. He first started his experiments with a thermometer as Herschel did. Because he could not find a further decrease in temperature below the visible blue as compared to the blue, he changed to Scheele's method of using paper strips dipped in silver chloride. He started measuring below the visible blue, where Scheele had ended, and noted that the paper strips became even darker when exposed to invisible wavelengths shorter than the visible blue light. He, thus, discovered in 1801 the ultraviolet spectrum of the sun, which he called "infraviolet" (4,5). Ritter died, unhappy, at the age of 33, without ever realizing the importance of his discovery (6).

It took many years before the importance of ultraviolet rays became clear. After Ritter's death it was still a common belief that sunburn was due to heat damage. This changed with the experiments of Everard Home in England in 1820 (7). Home wondered why the skin of black people living in a hot climate was better protected than white skin, although black was absorbing more heat. Therefore he exposed one of his own hands to the sun and covered the other one with a black cloth. He developed sunburn on the exposed hand although a thermometer registered a higher temperature on the hand under the black cloth (8). Information at that time was not so easily available as it is nowadays, which is illustrated by the fact that Moriz Kaposi, as late as 1891, still believed that solar-induced erythema, and also pigmentation, were due to the heat of the sun (9). Another illustration is the fact that Niels Finsen in Denmark, as late as 1900, repeated Home's experiment, independently, unaware of the previous experiment.

Although the damaging effects of ultraviolet radiation became gradually better known, it took a few more years before real action-spectrum studies were undertaken. During Word War I, Karl Hausser was the chief radiation physicist for Siemens AG in Germany. While working near the battlefields, he got pulmonary tuberculosis and was sent to Davos in Switzerland for heliotherapy. He took long walks in the mountains and noted that sunburn occurred easier at noontime than in the afternoon hours (10). As a result, he and Vahle made the first detailed action-spectrum studies for erythema and pigmentation of human skin. They could show that erythema and pigmentation depend upon the wavelengths of the ultraviolet radiation and that the effect is mainly due to wavelengths shorter than 320 nm (11). In 1922, they published the action spectra for the induction of erythema and pigmentation in human skin using a monochromator and an artificial mercury lamp.

During the Second International Congress on Light in 1932 in Copenhagen, Denmark, William Coblentz proposed to divide the ultraviolet spectrum of the sun into three spectral regions: UVA (315–400 nm), UVB (280–315 nm), and UVC (<280 nm) (9).

Measuring the intensity of solar irradiation was another problem. Many different systems were available (12). Although cadmium cathodes were already used in Potsdam in Germany and in Davos in Switzerland as early as 1910, the first integrating analog meter was developed by Rentschler in the mid-1930s, using a zirconium photodiode (11). However, these photodiodes showed great individual variability and temperature sensitivity. In addition, good amplifiers were not available at that time. In the mid-1950s, Robertson developed a UVB detector with a stable cold cathode thyratron to amplify the weak detector output (11). This detector was later redesigned and became the popular Robertson-Berger meter.

ERYTHEMA, PIGMENTATION, AND NATURAL PHOTOPROTECTION

The concept that sun exposure is responsible for sunburn is known since early humankind. In 1799, Johan Christoph Ebermaier in Germany noticed different degrees of sunburn depending on the time of exposure, whereby paler skin types reacted more severely than darker skin types (13). However, until the experiments of Home in 1820 and even much later, it was commonly believed that the heat of the sun was responsible for sunburn. The first to show that solar-induced erythema is really induced by ultraviolet rays was Jean Martin Charcot in France in 1858. He noticed severe sunburn and keratitis in two scientists working with electric arcs (9,14). This is also the first medical publication about accidental UV exposure. In 1877, Arthur Henry Downes and Thomas Porter Blunt in England could show that sunlight also may have a bactericidal action (15).

For a long time, it was a common belief that the heat of the sun was also responsible for tanning, induced by sun exposure. In 1808, the German Placidus Heinrich noticed that the light and not the heat of the sun was responsible for tanning (16). In 1829, John Davy from Scotland first described immediate pigment darkening (9). It was only in 1885 that Paul Unna of Germany suggested that the violet end of the solar spectrum, and thus the ultraviolet radiation, was responsible for the pigmentation of the skin (17). A few years later, in 1889, Erik Johan Widmark proved experimentally in Sweden that sunburn and tanning were due to the ultraviolet rays and had nothing to do with heat (9,18). As soon as this was generally accepted, research started into the mechanism of pigmentation. In 1917, Bloch published his experiments on the mechanism of melanin formation in human skin and discovered dopa-oxidase (19). Around the same time, Riehl reported a particular form of hyperpigmentation on both cheeks and on the lateral parts of the neck after chronic sun exposure (20).

In 1928, Jean Saidman of France, published an interesting textbook, *Les rayons ultra-violets en thérapeutique*, in which he describes how the minimal erythema dose (MED) may vary according to the individual pigmentation, the site of the body, and age. He also describes variations in the MED in the case of certain skin disorders and in the case of oral intake of certain drugs (12). He even made a device with a timer and several diaphragms to determine the MED, automatically.

That sun exposure could induce an increase in skin thickness was already reported in 1799 by Ebermaier in Germany (13). In 1900, Magnus Möller reported that sun exposure could induce a double protection mechanism in the epidermis, an increase of the stratum corneum thickness, and an increase in pigmentation (21). In 1931, Guido Miescher of Switzerland noticed an increase in thickness of all layers of the epidermis after sun exposure, thus reducing the intensity of the penetrating radiation (22).

SKIN AGING AND SKIN CANCER

Gradually, it became clear that sun exposure could not only induce short-term but also long-term skin changes. In 1893, Robert Bowles of England had already suggested that sunlight could be responsible for skin cancers: "If the sun's rays will produce sunburn, erythema, eczema solare, inflammation, and blistering, it is clearly capable of producing deep and intractable ulcerations of a low and chronic nature" (23). One year later, in 1894, Paul Unna in Germany discovered the relationship between sun exposure and skin aging, by studying sailor's skin (24). He also associated the severe degenerative changes on the exposed areas of sailors' skin with the development of skin cancer (11). Around the same time, in France, Dubreuilh noticed that people working in the vineyards around Bordeaux had more skin cancers than people living in the city (25). He was the first to establish a clear-cut relationship in 1906–1907 between skin cancer and solar exposure (26). Both conditions were dose-dependent. Skin aging was, therefore, more pronounced in the neck of people working outside, which resulted in the description of cutis rhomboidalis nuchae by Jadassohn and Nikolsky in 1925 (27).

In 1928, George Findlay reported that daily irradiation of mice with ultraviolet light from a mercury arc could induce skin cancer (28) and that the interval time was reduced if tar were used before the ultraviolet exposure. The first action-spectrum studies of skin photocarcinogenesis were published by Angel Roffo from Argentina in 1939 (29), where he showed that window glass can prevent the induction of skin cancer by both mercury arc radiation and by natural sunlight. Shortly afterward, Harold Blum, Kirkby-Smith, and Grady, in the United States, conducted a comprehensive series of experiments on photocarcinogenesis in mice and were able to obtain highly reproducible ultraviolet-induced skin cancers (30). These experiments were the beginning of a large number of experiments on animal photocarcinogenesis during the following decades.

PHOTODERMATOSES

Probably the first to describe a photodermatosis was Robert Willan in 1798. He called the disease eczema solare (31). The same condition was again described in 1887 by Veiel. What they called eczema solare was, most likely, what we currently consider as polymorphous or polymorphic light eruption. The name polymorphous light eruption was first used by Rasch in Copenhagen, in 1900 (8). The same condition had also been described as prurigo aestivalis, by Jonathan Hutchinson in 1878 (32). In 1919, Haxthausen used the term polymorphous light eruption as a collective name for eczema solare and prurigo aestivalis, because it was not possible to differentiate between the two conditions (33).

Hydroa vacciniforme was first described by Bazin in 1860 (8). Later on, this term became more confusing because it was not only used to describe hydroa vacciniforme, as it is known currently. Some authors used the same terminology to describe what is, presently, called congenital erythropoietic porphyria.

Moriz Kaposi was the first to describe xeroderma pigmentosum in 1870 (8), but he did not make the relationship with solar exposure or light, which was only done many years later by Paul Unna (24).

The symptoms of congenital erythropoietic porphyria have been described under different names such as pemphigus leprosus by Schultz in 1874 (34), xeroderma pigmentosum by Gagey in 1896 (35), hydroa vacciniforme by M'Call Anderson in 1898 (36), hereditary syphilis by Vollmer in 1903 (37), hydroa aestivale by Ehrmann in 1905 (38) and Linser in 1906 (39), until Günther described the condition, in 1911, as a porphyria (40). One of the first symptoms of this disease is the dark coloration of the urine, which was already noticed in the first description by Schultz in 1874 (34), whereas M'Call Anderson was the first to recognize in his description of 1898 that the disease was caused by light (36). That the lesions resulted from the sensitization of the skin to light exposure by porphyrins, was first suggested by Ehrmann, in 1909 (41). The name Günther's disease, to describe congenital erythropoietic porphyria, dates from a later period. Even in 1926, Rasch still proposed to call the disease M'Call Anderson's disease (8).

The same year the same author published a case report of a patient with porphyrinuria and blisters on the back of both hands (8). Rasch did not make use of the terminology porphyria cutanea tarda, till that time, but he clearly made the link with alcoholism. The name porphyria cutanea tarda was first used in 1937 by Waldenström, who also extensively studied acute intermittent porphyria (42). The other porphyrias were described later, even after World War II.

While the previous photodermatoses have mainly been described for the first time in the 19th century, solar urticaria has been described at the beginning of the 20th century. Probably the first report of the induction of urticaria by sunlight is the one reported by Merklen, in 1904 (43). He was the first to consider urticaria, caused by light, to be a distinct clinical entity. A year later in 1905, Ward, for the first time, provoked urticaria by means of sun exposure under controlled conditions (44). The name "solar urticaria" was suggested by Duke in 1923 (45), and in 1928, Wucherpfennig could quantify the urticarial response by phototesting with increasing doses of different wavelengths (46). In 1942, Rajka reported the passive transfer to normal volunteers by an intradermal injection of serum from a person with solar urticaria (47).

The history of topically or systemically-induced photosensibilization starts earlier. The first reports of systemically-induced photosensibilization were mainly due to occasional intake of plant extracts. Already, in the 16th century, skin reactions have been observed in animals after eating buckwheat followed by sun exposure (48). Similar observations have been made in the 18th century in Sicily and in Napels in Italy, where white sheep showed severe skin reactions after eating Hypericum, while the black sheep did not (49).

Between 1908 and 1910 Hausmann discovered that hematoporphyrin can photosensitize animal skin and that the responsible wavelengths are in the green visible light around 500 nm (50). The first clinical proof that some substances can photosensitize human skin in combination with sun exposure dates from 1912, when our colleague Meyer-Betz injected himself with hematoporphyrin and exposed himself to the sun (51). By doing this he could demonstrate that the combination of a photosensitizing substance and sun exposure can induce a skin reaction that each of these two components separately would not induce, which is the definition of a photosensibilization. Another example of a systemic photosensibilization in human skin is the "eosin disease," which was seen in patients treated with oral eosin for epilepsy or for other reasons (50).

In 1939, Stephen Epstein could demonstrate in human volunteers, using sulfanilamide as the photosensitizer, that two mechanisms are involved: a dose-dependent phototoxic reaction and a nondose-dependent photoallergic reaction (52).

It was first reported in 1913 by Louis Lewin, that topically applied agents can photosensitize in workers using coal tar pitch (53). In 1916, Emanuel Freund reported phototoxic reactions to eau de cologne, which was the first description of a berloque dermatitis, and he concluded that oil of bergamot was most probably the photosensitizing substance (54). The first description of a phytophotodermatitis dates from 1920 by Moritz Oppenheim (55). Hans Kuske could show that the photosensitizing substances in these plants were furocoumarins, and that their action spectrum was mainly between 334 and 366 nm, which was the first determination of an action spectrum for the furocoumarins (56). The photopatch test was introduced in 1941 by Burckhardt (57).

PHOTOPROTECTION

It has always been part of human nature to protect the skin against sunburn by avoiding sun exposure or by wearing appropriate clothes. During history, many substances have probably been tried out as photoprotectors. As far as we know, the first scientific reports date from the end of the 19th century. In 1878, Veiel reported the use of tannin as a photoprotector, but its use was limited because of its staining potential (58). In 1891, Friedrich Hammer of Germany even published a monograph, probably the first large monograph on photobiology, discussing photoprotection and experimenting with different topical agents, to prevent sunburn (9,59).

When Hausser and Vahle, in 1922, reported that sunburn in human skin is caused by a specific part of ultraviolet spectrum between 280 and 315 nm (60), one realized that the skin could be protected by filtering out these specific wavelengths. This resulted in a growing interest in sunscreen agents. The first commercially available sunscreen appeared on the market in 1928, in the United States, as an emulsion containing benzyl salicylate and benzyl cinnamate (61). During the subsequent years, sunscreens were not widely available and were not used on a large scale. In Germany the first commercial sunscreen became available in 1933 (62) and in France, in 1936 (63). The German product was an ointment. The French one was an oil preparation and became a great success, because it was launched the same year that paid holidays were granted.

During World War II, there was a real need for good sun protection for soldiers engaged in tropical warfare. One of the most practical and effective agents for sun protection turned out to be Red veterinary petrolatum, and was used as standard equipment (64). After the war, styles were changing in many countries and a number of filters were synthesized, tested, and marketed. In many cases these were less effective oil preparations, apparently with the sole purpose of promoting tanning. During the 1970s, holiday travel to sunny areas steadily became more popular, resulting in an increasing demand for sunscreens with better and broader protection. This became possible by incorporating UVB filters into milks and creams instead of oils. In 1979, real UVA filters became available and a further advance was the introduction of micronized inorganic powders such as titanium dioxide since 1989, and zinc oxide since 1992 (65).

With the increasing use of sunscreens, there was also an increasing need to find a good method to evaluate their protection. In the early years, the usual way was to determine the absorption spectrum of the sunscreen. In 1934, Friedrich Ellinger in Berlin proposed to use a biological method by determining the MED in protected and unprotected skin, using both forearms and a mercury lamp (66). He concluded that the method of choice was the way in which the MED could be decreased. He was right, but the right irradiation source was not yet used. In 1956, Rudolf Schulze in Germany proposed to test commercially available sunscreens by giving them a protection factor (67). The idea was to divide the exposure time needed to induce erythema with sunscreen by the exposure time needed without sunscreen. He used a series of Osram-Ultra-Vitalux lamps to apply a series of increasing ultraviolet doses (40% increases), in both protected and unprotected skin. The light source he used was more similar to the solar spectrum than the light source used by Ellinger. The method was further improved in 1974 in Austria by Franz Greiter, who developed the concept of the sun protection factor (SPF) (68). In 1978, this method was adopted by the Food and Drug Administration (FDA), in the United States (69) and became internationally accepted. At that time sunscreens were mainly used to prolong the exposure time in order to tan, and at the same time to avoid sunburn.

THE BEGINNING OF A THERAPEUTIC INTEREST

Over the centuries, sunlight has been used in the treatment of many diseases in different countries such as ancient Egypt, Greece, and Rome, but the records are mostly anecdotal. In addition, many believed that the therapeutic effect was due to red light and the heat of the sun, because there was no notion of ultraviolet rays.

Gradually, and especially in the second half of the 19th century, more and more people became interested in heliotherapy. In 1855, Arnold Rikli from Switzerland opened a thermal station in Veldes Slovenia for the provision of heliotherapy (70). In 1856, Florence Nightingale in the United Kingdom protested against the orientation of the Royal Victoria Hospital in Netley, near Southampton, observing that no sunlight could enter its wards (71). In 1877 Downes and Blunt showed that sunlight could kill anthrax bacilli and, thus, had a bactericidal action (15). In 1890, Palm from Edinburgh suggested that the sun could play a therapeutic role in rachitis (72).

At the end of the 19th century, many people started to realize that ultraviolet rays of the sun were the most important wavelengths for its therapeutic effects. This resulted in the use of filtered solar radiation and of artificial light sources. In 1893, Niels Finsen in Denmark used filtered sunlight in the treatment of lupus vulgaris. At a time when no antibiotics or anti-inflammatory agents were available, Finsen's phototherapy was more than welcome. Because a treatment session with filtered natural sunlight could take several hours, and because natural sunlight was not always available in Denmark, Finsen became logically interested in more powerful artificial irradiation sources. In 1894, Heinrich Lahmann in Germany was probably the first to use an artificial light source in the treatment of skin diseases (70), although he was not the first to construct such a lamp. The first to make a (mercury) lamp was, probably, Way around 1856 to 1860 (12).

In April 1896, Finsen founded the "Lysinstitut" or Medical Light Institute (later Finsen Institute), in Copenhagen, where he continued to use filtered natural sunlight; but from 1897 onward he also used a new carbon arc lamp in combination with quartz filters (73). Around the same time, in 1898, Willibald Gebhardt published what is probably the first book on phototherapy, *Die Heilkraft des Lichtes* (74). A major problem when using a carbon arc lamp to irradiate human skin was the high temperature. Finsen et al. developed a water-cooling system and an irradiation unit where four patients were irradiated at the same time. This irradiation source became internationally known as the Finsen lamp. After Finsen in 1901 published his therapeutic results with lupus vulgaris, treated by concentrated UV doses from a carbon arc lamp, he received the Nobel Prize for Medicine in 1903, the only Nobel Prize ever to be awarded for dermatology (73). From this time on the Finsen lamp was used in all major dermatology departments inside and also outside Europe in the treatment of lupus vulgaris. Finsen also wrote the foreword in the first French textbook on phototherapy, *Photothérapie et Photobiologie*, written by Leredde and Pautrier and published in 1903 (75). In 1904, a smaller lamp was constructed by Finsen and Reyn, the Finsen-Reyn lamp, which allowed therapist to irradiate one single patient and which was more convenient in smaller treatment centers. All these lamps were used only for localized irradiations. In the same year, 1904, the Schott Company in Jena, Germany, was able to construct an ultraviolet tube (9), using the low-pressure mercury lamp developed by the American Peter Hewitt in 1902 (76), and using a new type of glass containing barium sulfate.

About the same time, the first experiments started with the use of photosensitizers and visible light in the treatment of skin cancer that became the principle of photodynamic therapy, nearly a century later. During the winter of 1897 and 1898, Oscar Raab, in Munich, had already noticed that the death of the paramecia, which he was studying, not only depended upon the concentration of the dye acridine but also on the intensity of the light in the laboratory (77). In 1905, Albert Jesionek and Hermann von Tappeiner could cure three out of five basal cell carcinomas they had treated with intralesional eosin and light exposure (78).

A lot of research was done in the construction of new phototherapy equipment. In 1906, Hans Axmann in Germany constructed a horizontal treatment cabin equipped with a series of low-pressure mercury tubes, allowing total body irradiations (9,79). Unfortunately, the output of these lamps was not high enough to obtain a sufficient therapeutic effect in lupus vulgaris and, therefore, could not compete with the Finsen-Reyn lamp. In 1906 also, Richard Küch in Hanau, Germany, made the first quartz lamp. By using quartz instead of lead glass, he was able to develop a high-pressure mercury lamp with a higher output (80). In the beginning these lamps were only used to illuminate streets and warehouses, where they gradually replaced the carbon arc lamps, which had a lower output and higher running costs (9). Soon after, the high-pressure mercury lamp was also used for therapeutic purposes, because of the same reasons. In 1908, Carl Franz Nagelschmidt made a table model of the high-pressure mercury lamp for total body irradiation, but this was nothing more than a prototype. After Hugo Bach constructed his own quartz lamp in 1911, this "Höhensonne" lamp was modified many times and was used for almost 50 years for total body irradiations (9). When in 1912 Ernst Kromayer in Berlin made a quartz lamp with a high UV output, and improved the lamp by using a water cooling system, it became possible to treat different skin diseases (81,82). Kromayer commercialized his lamp in 1906, and it became one of the most popular treatment lamps in dermatology for decades. It was not only used in Europe but also in Asia and the United States, although it could only be used for localized irradiations.

In 1919, the pediatrician Kurt Huldschinsky published his therapeutic results with high-pressure mercury lamps in the treatment of rachitis (83). This again was a very interesting indication for the use of phototherapy in medicine. Its success was greatly due to the use of the new radiography technique as a way to control the evolution of the disease.

Lupus vulgaris was not the only indication for the use of phototherapy in dermatology. William Henry Goeckerman, in the United States, started testing different photosensitizers in the treatment of psoriasis in order to improve the therapeutic effect of the sun. In 1925, he published his results using coal tar in combination with ultraviolet exposure from a high-pressure mercury lamp (84). This treatment became very popular worldwide and was used for decades to treat psoriasis. Later on, John Ingram in the United Kingdom combined this treatment with dithranol (85).

In 1927, Erich Uhlmann could induce repigmentation in vitiligo patients combining bergamot oil and exposure to natural sunlight or to a Kromayer lamp (86).

In 1947, a new type of lamp was born, the high-pressure xenon lamp. In contrast to the high-pressure mercury lamp, this lamp had a continuous spectrum ranging from the ultraviolet to the infrared spectrum, similar to the natural solar spectrum. Because this lamp was more costly to use it did not become popular for therapeutic purposes but was only used for research and phototesting.

In 1958, the use of blue light phototherapy (420–480 nm) was reported for the treatment of newborns with jaundice, after a nurse noticed that the yellow pigmentation in jaundiced babies faded away after sun exposure (87). Apart from its use in pediatrics to treat jaundice in newborns, heliotherapy and phototherapy were done on an organized scale to treat tuberculosis, leg ulcers, and skin diseases.

HELIOTHERAPY FOR TUBERCULOSIS

In 1903, Rollier in Leysin, Switzerland, opened the first hospital to treat lung tuberculosis and rachitis by sun exposure. In 1914, he published his therapeutic results in a book, *La Cure du Soleil*, which unfortunately was published in French at the start of World War I and therefore had no great effect outside Switzerland (88). When in 1923 his book was translated and published in English under the title *Heliotherapy*, the use of sun exposure in the treatment of tuberculosis became increasingly popular (82). It was only when the first tuberculostatics became available, in 1946, that the use of sun exposure in the treatment of lung tuberculosis and the use of phototherapy in the treatment of lupus vulgaris became part of history.

HELIOTHERAPY AND PHOTOTHERAPY FOR LEG ULCERS

Another application of an organized use of sun exposure and phototherapy was in the treatment of leg ulcers. The first to report a therapeutic effect of sun exposure in the treatment of ulcers was Larrey, Napoleon's private physician. He noted, during Napoleon's campaign in Egypt, in 1798 and 1799, that the soldiers' traumatic ulcers healed more quickly after sun exposure (89). In 1904, Bernhard in Switzerland described heliotherapy as a treatment for skin ulcers (89,90). Later on, this was confirmed by other authors (91,92) whereafter the treatment of wounds with sunlight gradually gained ground, especially in Switzerland, Germany, and France. During World War I from 1914 to 1918, ulcers were treated by exposure to natural sunlight or to quartz lamps in Germany, the United Kingdom, France, and Italy. During World War II from 1940 to 1945, this "open-air treatment" with sunlight or with quartz lamps was still being used. When the first antibiotics became available, however, interest in using phototherapy for wound healing faded.

PHOTOTHERAPY FOR SKIN DISEASES

Heliotherapy with natural sunlight was mainly used in thermal stations to treat tuberculosis and in wartime to treat leg ulcers. However, both indications became part of history. This was not the case with the use of phototherapy in the treatment of skin disorders. During history and up to the present, several skin disorders have been treated with heliotherapy or phototherapy.

Before the end of the 19th century its use was more anecdotal. Probably the first report of the use of sunlight in the treatment of skin disorders dates from about 1400 BC, when plant extracts followed by sun exposure to treat vitiligo was used in India (93). The same treatment was also used in ancient Egypt. The anecdotal use of heliotherapy during the centuries changed at the end of the 19th century with Niels Finsen. He was the first to use sun exposure in a more standardized way on a large scale for a specific indication, with a detailed account of its therapeutic results. He was also the first to switch from heliotherapy with natural sunlight to phototherapy with artificial lamps, making it more practical. The Nobel Prize he won in 1903 had a booster effect on phototherapy. Probably a similar effect happened at the end of the last century with the development of phototherapeutic UVA (PUVA) treatment or photochemotherapy.

Photochemotherapy has a long history (94). It started with the use of plant extracts and sun exposure to treat vitiligo and resulted in the use of oral 8-methoxypsoralen (8-MOP) and total body UVA-irradiation cabins to treat psoriasis. Many different steps have been involved. The first step was the use of certain plant extracts to treat vitiligo (95). The next step was the isolation of the active ingredients in these plants as 8-MOP and 5-methoxypsoralen (5-MOP), in 1947, and the first trials with 8-MOP and sun exposure in vitiligo patients (96–99). Later, the action-spectrum studies were introduced (100,101). These were followed by the topical use of 8-MOP in combination with UV irradiation to treat psoriasis (102) and in 1967 by the oral use of 8-MOP to treat psoriasis (103). The next step was the use of "blacklight" UVA tubes in combination with topical 8-MOP in the treatment of vitiligo (104). One year later, in 1970, Mortazawi used the same type of UVA tubes in a total body irradiation cabin, using topical 8-MOP to treat psoriasis (105,106). The use of UVA tubes in a total body irradiation cabin was new. Although the UVA output of these tubes was effective when the 8-MOP was used topically, it was insufficient when administered orally. In 1974, Parrish et al. reported the use of a new type of a high-intensity UVA tube in combination with oral 8-MOP in the treatment of psoriasis (107). This approach was more effective and was the real start of PUVA therapy, which revolutionized dermatological treatment.

The history of UVB phototherapy is not as old as the history of photochemotherapy, and was started at the end of the 19th century with the work of Niels Finsen on lupus vulgaris. In 1923, Alderson recommended the use of a mercury quartz lamp to treat psoriasis. In 1925, Goeckerman associated tar with UV irradiations in the treatment of psoriasis, and this remained for about half a century as the most popular form of phototherapy in dermatology (84). The main drawback of this treatment was the low output of the lamps. In 1958, Zimmerman in the United States described an irradiation cabin, using fluorescent UVB tubes (108). Later, several other total body irradiation sources were described (109,110). After a successful start of PUVA treatment, Wiskemann suggested, in 1978, using an irradiation cabin with broadband UVB tubes (111). During the subsequent years, broadband UVB phototherapy became an alternative for PUVA treatment. Because broadband UVB phototherapy was less efficient for psoriasis than PUVA therapy, it never achieved its popularity. This changed in 1988 when narrowband UVB phototherapy was introduced in the treatment of psoriasis by van Weelden et al. (112) and Green et al. (113). This was more efficient than broadband UVB phototherapy.

In the meantime, other types of phototherapy have been developed such as extracorporeal photopheresis for cutaneous T-cell lymphoma (114), high-dose UVA1 phototherapy for atopic dermatitis and localized scleroderma (115), and topical photodynamic therapy with visible light for actinic keratoses and superficial basal cell carcinoma (116).

JOURNALS, SOCIETIES, AND MEETINGS

The first real journal dealing exclusively with photobiology and photodermatology was probably the Transactions from Finsen's Medical Light Institute, which were published in Danish and German. The journal appeared from 1900 until 1904, when Finsen died. In 1912, Hans Meyer in Germany started the new journal *Strahlentherapie*, dealing not only with phototherapy but also with radiotherapy. Because phototherapy became less important after World War II, this journal is no longer a photobiological or photodermatological journal.

In 1927, the *Deutsche Gesellschaft für Lichtforschung* (German Society for Research on Light) was founded (9). The first president was Hans Meyer, editor of the journal *Strahlentherapie*. One year later, in 1928, the first international society was founded by a group of French colleagues, called *Comité International de la Lumière*, with Axel Reyn as the first president. Reyn was Danish and a pupil of Finsen. The First International Congress on Light was held in 1929 in Paris, France, with Jean Saidman as its president. The second congress was in Copenhagen, Denmark, in 1932 and the third one took place in Wiesbaden, Germany, in 1936. In 1937, the decision was made to attribute a prize—the Finsen medal—during each congress to an outstanding cutaneous photobiologist. The next congress was again held in Paris, France, in 1951. At that time, the name of the society became the *Comité International de Photobiologie* and the name of the congress changed to the "International Congress on Photobiology" (9).

In 1962, Douglas McLaren started the first journal in English, named "Photochemistry and Photobiology: An International Journal." The American Society of Photobiology was founded in 1972 (11) and the Japanese Society for Photomedicine and Photobiology in 1978. In 1984, Christer Jansén from Finland and Göran Wennersten from Sweden started another international journal in English, named "Photodermatology clinical and experimental," the name (and size) of which changed in 1990 to "Photodermatology, Photoimmunology & Photomedicine." The Photomedicine Society in the United States was founded in 1991 and the European Society for Photodermatology in 1999.

In 2004, another journal was launched, named "Photodiagnosis and Photodynamic Therapy." Apart from these journals several other journals are available dealing only partly with cutaneous photobiology and photomedicine, such as the "Journal of Photochemistry and Photobiology. B: Biology," which started in 1987 as part of the "Journal of Photochemistry."

BUILDING ON THE PAST

The history of human photobiology is as old as humankind. During the centuries a lot of people were involved. Some of them had the bright ideas and others had the merit of putting them into practice. The result is a beautiful example of how science is built up stone by stone. In this period, when we have the idea that we can realize everything, we often forget that we are just building on the foundations laid out by others before us. History therefore is a good lesson in modesty.

REFERENCES

1. Newton I. New theory about light and colours. Philosophical transactions 1672; I:3075–3087.
2. Herschel W. Investigation of the powers of the prismatic colours to heat and illuminate objects. Philos Trans R Soc Lond 1800; I:255–283.
3. Scheele CW. Chemische Abhandlung von der Luft und dem Feuer. Upsala, Leipzig: Swederus, Crusius, 1777.
4. Ritter JW. Physisch-chemische Abhandlungen in chronologischer Folge. Band II. Leipzig 1806; 81–107.
5. Ritter JW. Entdeckungen zur Elektrochemie, Bioelektrochemie und Photochemie. Ostwalds Klassiker der exakten Wissenschaften. Band 271. Leipzig: Akademische Verlagsgesellschaft Geest & Portig K.-G., 1986.
6. Roelandts R. Bicentenary of the discovery of the ultraviolet rays. Photochem Photoimmunol Photomed 2002; 18:208.
7. Home E. On the black rete mucosum of the Negro, being a defense against the scorching effect of the sun's rays. Philos Trans R Soc London 1820; 111:1.
8. Rasch C. Some historical and clinical remarks on the effect of light on the skin and skin diseases. Proc R Soc Med 1926; 20:11–20.
9. Lentner A. Geschichte der Lichttherapie. Aachen: Foto-Druck Mainz, 1992.
10. Hausser KW, Vahle W. Sonnenbrand und Sonnenbräunung. Wiss Veröff Siemens-Konzern 1927; 6:101.

11. Urbach F, Forbes PD, Davies RE, Berger D. Cutaneous photobiology: past, present, and future. J Invest Dermatol 1976; 67:209–224.
12. Saidman J. Les rayons ultra-violets en thérapeutique. Paris: Gaston Doin & Cie, 1928.
13. Ebermaier JC. Versuch einer Geschichte des Lichtes in Rücksicht seines Einflusses auf die gesamte Natur, und auf den menschlichen Körper, ausser dem Gesichte, besonders. Osnabrück: Karl und Comp, 1799.
14. Charcot P. Erythème produit par l'action de la lumière électrique. C R Soc Biol (Paris) 1858; 5: 63–65.
15. Downes AH, Blunt TP. Researches on the effect of light upon bacteria and other organisms. Proc R Soc Lond 1877; 26:488–500.
16. Heinrich P. Von der Natur und den Eigenschaften des Lichts. St. Petersburg: Veröffentl d kaiserlichen Akademie der Wissenschaften, 1808.
17. Unna PG. Uber das Pigment der menschlichen Haut nebst einem Vorschlag für wanderlustige Kollegen. Med prakt Derm 1885; 4:277–294.
18. Widmark EJ. Ueber den Einfluss des Lichtes auf die Haut. Hygiea Festband 1889; 3:1–23.
19. Bloch B. Das Problem der Pigmentbildung in der Haut. Arch f Derm u Syph 1917; 124:129–208.
20. Riehl. Uber eine eigenartige Melanose. Wien klin Wochenschr 1917; 780.
21. Möller M. Der Einfluss des Lichtes auf die Haut in gesundem und krankhaften Haut. Stuttgart: Nägele, 1900.
22. Miescher G. Die Schutzfunktionen der Haut gegenüber Lichtstrahlen. Strahlentherapie 1931; 39: 601–618.
23. Bowles RL. On the influence of solar rays on the skin. Br J Dermatol 1893; 237.
24. Unna PG. Die Histopathologie der Hautkrankheiten. Berlin: Hirschwald, 1894.
25. Dubreuilh W. Des hyperkeratoses circonscrites. Ann Derm Syph 1896; 7:1158–1204.
26. Dubreuilh W. Epithéliomatose d'origine solaire. Annales de Derm et Syph 1907; 387.
27. Jadassohn. Cutis rhomboidalis nuchä mit colloider Degeneration. Zentr f Haut u Geschlechtskrankh 1925; XVII:272.
28. Findlay GM. Ultraviolet light and skin cancer. Lancet 1928; 2:1070–1073.
29. Roffo AH. Uber die physikalische Aetiologie der Krebskrankheit mit besonderer Betonung des Zusammenhangs mit Sonnenbestrahlungen. Strahlentherapie 1939; 66:328–350.
30. Blum HF, Kirkby-Smith S, Grady HG. Quantitative induction of tumors in mice with ultraviolet radiation. J Natl Cancer Inst 1941; 2:259–268.
31. Willan R. On cutaneous diseases. London: Johnson, 1808.
32. Hutchinson J. Lectures on clinical surgery. Vol 1. London: Churchill, 1878.
33. Brodthagen H. Polymorphous light eruption. In: Urbach F, ed. The Biological Effects of Ultraviolet Radiation. New York: Pergamon Press 1969:479–486.
34. Schultz JH. Ein Fall von Pemphigus leprosus, kompliciert durch Lepra visceralis. Inaug. Diss. Greisswald, 1874.
35. Gagey. Cas d'hémoglobinurie au cours d'un xeroderma pigmentosum. Thèse de Paris, 1896.
36. M'Call Anderson T. Hydroa vacciniforme. Br J Dermatol 1898; 1.
37. Vollmer. Uber hereditäre Syphilis und Hämatoporphyrinuria. Archiv f Derm u Syph 1903; 1XV:221.
38. Ehrmann. Arch f Derm u Syph 1905; 1XXVII:163.
39. Linser. Hydroa aestivale und Hämatoporphyrinuria. Archiv f Derm u Syph 1906; 1XXIX:251.
40. Günther. Die Hämatoporphyrie. Dtsch Arch f klin Med 1911; 105:89–146.
41. Ehrmann S. Weitere Untersuchungen über Lichtwirkung bei Hydroa aestivalis (Bazin), Summereruption (nach Hutchinson). Arch f Derm u Syph 1909; 97:75–86.
42. Waldenström J. Studien über porphyrie. Acta Med Scand 1937; suppl. 82:133.
43. Merklen P. Urticaria. In: Besnier E, Brocq L, Jacquet L, eds. La Pratique Dermatologique: Trait de Dermatologie Appliquée. Paris: Masson et Cie, 1904:728–771.
44. Ward SB. Erythema and urticaria with a condition resembling angioneurotic edema caused by exposure to sun's rays. NY Med J 1905; 81:742–743.
45. Duke WW. Urticaria caused by light. JAMA 1923; 80:1835–1838.
46. Wucherpfennig V. Pathologische Lichtüberempfindlichkeit in qualitativer und quantitativer Hinsicht, nebst Untersuchungen zur Pathogenese der Lichtquaddel. Arch Dermatol Syph (Berl.) 1928; 156:520–544.
47. Rajka E. Passive transfer in light urticaria. J Allergy Clin Immunol 1942; 13:327–345.
48. Merian L. Experimentelle Beiträge zur Buchweizenerkrankung (Fagopyrismus) der Tiere. Arch Anat Physiol, Physiol Abt 1915; 161:188.
49. Barth J. Historisch und aktuelle Aspekte der Fotosensibilisierung. Derm Mschr 1976; 162: 961–973.
50. Lipschitz W. Im Blut kreisende Substanzen als Grundlage für Lichtdermatosen. Strahlentherapie 1928; 29:9–19.
51. Meyer-Betz F. Untersuchungen über die biologische (photodynamische) Wirkung des Hämatoporphyrins und anderer Derivate des Blut- und Gallenfarbstoffs. Dtsch Arch klin Med 1913; 112:476–503.

52. Epstein S. Photoallergy and primary photosensitivity to sulfanilamide. J invest Derm 1939; 2:43–51.
53. Lewin L. Uber die photodynamische Wirkungen von Inhaltsstoffen des Steinkohlenteerpechs am Menschen. Münch Med Wochenschr 1913; 60:1529–1530.
54. Freund E. Uber bisher noch nicht beschreibende künstliche Hautverfärbungen. Dermatol Wochenschr 1916; 63:931.
55. Oppenheim M, Fessler A. Über eine streifenförmige bullöse Dermatitis (Freibad- und Wiesendermatitis). Derm Wschr 1928; 86:183–187.
56. Kuske H. Perkutane Photosensibilisierung durch pflanzliche Wirkstoffe. Dermatologica 1940; 82: 274–338.
57. Burckhardt W. Untersuchungen über die Photoaktivität einiger Sulfanilamide. Dermatologica 1941; 83:63–68.
58. Henschke U. Untersuchungen an Lichtschutzmitteln. Strahlentherapie 1940; 67:639–668.
59. Hammer F. Uber den Einfluss des Lichtes auf die Haut. Stuttgart: F. Enke, 1891.
60. Hausser KW, Vahle W. Die Abhängigkeit des Lichterythems und der Pigmentbildung von der Schwingungszahl (Wellenlänge) der erregenden Strahlung. Strahlentherapie 1922; 13:47–71.
61. Jass HE. Cosmetic suntan products. Cutis 1979; 23:554–561.
62. Finkel P. Lichtschutzmittel. In: Umbach W, ed. Kosmetik. Stuttgart, New York: Georg Thieme Verlag, 1995:147–163.
63. Rebut D. The sunscreen industry in Europe: past, present and future. In: Lowe NJ, Shaath NA, eds. Sunscreens, Development, Evaluation, and Regulatory Aspects. New York: Marcel Dekker, Inc, 1990:161–171.
64. MacEachern WN, Jillson OF. A practical sunscreen "Red Vet Pet." Arch Dermatol 1946; 89:147–150.
65. Roelandts R. Advances in sunscreen technology: choosing the sunscreen to suit. Current Opinion in Dermatology 1995:173–177.
66. Ellinger F. Zur Frage der Wertbestimmung von Lichtschutzmitteln. Arch exp Path u Pharmakologie 1934; 175:481–488.
67. Schulze R. Einige Versuche und Bemerkungen zum Problem der handelsüblichen Lichtschutzmittel. Parf u Kosmet 1956; 37:310–315.
68. Greiter F. Sonnenschutzfaktor – Entstehung, Methodik. Parf u Kosmet 1974; 55:70–75.
69. Dept of Health, Education and Welfare, Food and Drug Administration. Sunscreen drug products for over-the-counter human use. Federal Register, August 25 1978; 43:38206–38269.
70. Barth J, Köhler U. Photodermatologie in Dresden-ein historischer Abriss. Festschrift anlässlich des 75. Geburtstages von Prof. Dr. h.c. H.-E. Kleine-Natrop (1917–1985). Dresden 1992.
71. From a special correspondent. Royal Victoria Hospital, Netley. Br Med J 1966; 5484:412–413.
72. Palm TA. The geographical distribution and aetiology of rickets. The Practitioner October and November 1890.
73. Roelandts R. A new light on Niels Finsen, a century after his nobel prize. Photodermatol Photoimmunol Photomed 2005; 21:115–117.
74. Meffert H, Bahr T. Willibald Gebhardt (1861–1921). Sein Leben und seine Verdienste um die Photomedizin. Dermatol Monatsschr 1989; 175:699–705.
75. Leredde, Pautrier. Photothérapie et Photobiologie. Paris: Naud, 1903.
76. Heusner HL. Zum zehnjährigen Jubiläum der medizinischen Quarzlampe. Strahlentherapie 1916; 7:628–638.
77. Raab O. Untersuchungen über die Wirkung fluorezierende Stoffe. Z Biol 1899; 39:16.
78. Jesionek A, Tappeiner HV. Zur Behandlung der Hautcarcinome mit fluorescierenden Stoffen. Dtsch Arch Klin Med 1905; 82:223–227.
79. Axmann H. Weitere Erfahrungen über die Uviolbehandlung, sowie einen neuen Apparat zur Bestrahlung des ganzen Körpers mittels ultravioletten Lichtes (Uviolbad). Dtsch Med Wochenschr 1906; 32:583–584.
80. Küch R, Retschinsky T. Photometrische und spektralphotometrische Messungen am Quecksilberbogen bei hohem Dampfdruck. Ann Physik 1906; 20:563–583.
81. Kromayer E. Quecksilber-Wasserlampen zur Behandlung von Haut und Schleimhaut. Dtsch med Wochenschr 1906; 32:377–380.
82. Rollier A. Heliotherapy. Oxford: Oxford Medical Publications, 1923.
83. Huldschinsky K. Heilung von Rachitis durch künstliche Höhensonne. Dtsch med Wochenschr 1919; 45:712–713.
84. Goeckerman WH. Treatment of psoriasis. Northwest Med 1925; 24:229–231.
85. Ingram JT. The approach to psoriasis. Br Med J 1953; II:591–594.
86. Uhlmann E. Pigmentbildung bei Vitiligo. Med Klin 1927; 23:279–280.
87. Cremer RJ, Perryman PW, Richards DH. Influence of light on the hyperbilirubinaemia of infants. Lancet 1958; I:1094–1097.
88. Saleeby CW. Sunlight and Health. London: Nisbet & Co:1923–1926.
89. Bernhard O. Light treatment in surgery. London: Edward Arnold & Co, 1926.

90. Bernhard O. Über offene Wundbehandlung durch Insolation und Eintrocknung. Münch med Wochenschr 1904:Nr 1.
91. Haeberlin. Zur Behandlung granulierender Wunden. Münch med Wochenschr 1907:Nr 8.
92. Dosquet W. Offene Wundbehandlung und Freiluftbehandlung. Leipzig: Georg Thieme, 1916.
93. Fitzpatrick TB, Pathak MA. Historical aspects of methoxsalen and other furocoumarins. J Invest Dermatol 1959; 31:229–331.
94. Roelandts R. The history of photochemotherapy. Photodermatol Photoimmunol Photomed 1991; 8:184–189.
95. Marquis L. Arabian contributors to Dermatology. Int J Dermatol 1985; 24:60–64.
96. Fahmy IR, Abu-Shady H. Ammi majus Linn: pharmacognostical study and isolation of a crystalline constituent, ammoidin. Q J Pharmacol 1947; 20:281–291.
97. Fahmy IR, Abu-Shady H, Schönberg A, et al. A crystalline principle from Ammi majus L. Nature 1947; 160:468–469.
98. Fahmy IR, Abu-Shady H. Ammi majus Linn: the isolation and properties of ammoidin, ammidin and majudin, and their effect in the treatment of leukoderma. Q J Pharmacol 1948; 21:499–503.
99. El-Mofty AM. A preliminary clinical report on the treatment of leukoderma with Ammi majus Linn. J Egypt Med Assoc 1948; 31:651–665.
100. Buck HW, Magnus IA, Porter AD. The action spectrum of 8-methoxypsoralen for erythema in human skin. Br J Dermatol 1960; 72:249–255.
101. Pathak MA, Fellman JH. Activating and fluorescent wavelengths of furocoumarins: psoralens. Nature 1960; 185:382–383.
102. Allyn B. Studies on phototoxicity in man and laboratory animals. Paper presented at the Twenty-First Annual Meeting of the American Academy of Dermatology. Chicago, December 1962.
103. Oddoze L, Témime P, Marchand JP, et al. L'association "meladinine" per os et rayons U.V. dans le traitement du psoriasis. Bull Soc Fr Dermatol Syph 1967; 74:609–610.
104. Fulton JE, Leyden J, Papa C. Treatment of vitiligo with topical methoxsalen and blacklite. Arch Dermatol 1969; 100:224–229.
105. Mortazawi SMA. Meladinine und UVA bei Vitiligo, Psoriasis, Parapsoriasis und Akne vulgaris. Dermatol Monatsschr 1972; 158:908–909.
106. Mortazawi SMA, Oberste-Lehn H. Lichtsensibilisatoren und ihre therapeutischen Fähigkeiten. Z Haut-Geschl Kr 1973; 48:1–9.
107. Parrish JA, Fitzpatrick TB, Tanenbaum L, et al. Photochemotherapy of psoriasis with oral methoxsalen and longwave ultraviolet light. N Engl J Med 1974; 291:1207–1211.
108. Zimmerman MC. Ultraviolet light therapy. Arch Dermatol 1958; 78:646–652.
109. Wiskemann A. Die neuere Entwicklung der Lichttherapie. Dermatol Wochenschr 1963; 147:377–383.
110. Forck G. Ganzkörperbestrahlung mit UV-Licht. Aufbau einer neuartigen Anlage. Dermatol Wochenschr 1964; 150:290–294.
111. Wiskemann A. UVB-Phototherapie der Psoriasis mit einer fur die PUVA-Therapie entwickelten Stehbox. Z Hautkr 1978; 53:633–636.
112. van Weelden H, De La Faille HB, Young E, et al. A new development in UVB phototherapy of psoriasis. Br J Dermatol 1988; 119:11–19.
113. Green C, Ferguson J, Lakshmipathi T, et al. 311 nm UVB phototherapy—an effective treatment for psoriasis. Br J Dermatol 1988; 119:691–696.
114. Edelson R, Berger C, Gasparro F, et al. Treatment of cutaneous T-cell lymphoma by extracorporeal photochemotherapy. Preliminary results. N Engl J Med 1987; 316:297–303.
115. Krutmann J, Schopf E. High-dose-UVA1 phototherapy: a novel and highly effective approach for the treatment of acute exacerbation of atopic dermatitis. Acta Derm Venereol Suppl (Stockh). 1992; 176:120–122.
116. Kennedy JC, Pottier RH. Endogenous protoporphyrin IX, a clinically useful photosensitizer for photodynamic therapy. J Photochem Photobiol B Biol 1992; 14:275–292.

2 | Basic Principles of Photobiology

Brian L. Diffey
Department of Regional Medical Physics, Newcastle General Hospital, Newcastle, England, U.K.

Irene E. Kochevar
Wellman Center for Photomedicine, Massachusetts General Hospital, Harvard Medical School, Boston, Massachusetts, U.S.A.

- Application of photobiology to dermatology relies on knowledge from a wide range of areas, including climatology, optical physics, photochemistry, cellular and molecular biology, and pathology.

- Ultraviolet, visible, and infrared radiations are all ranges of optical radiation and are part of the electromagnetic spectrum.

- Ultraviolet radiation is divided into UVA, UVB, and UVC wavelength ranges.

- The energy of a photon is inversely related to the wavelength of the radiation.

- The exposure dose, rather than the rate of delivery of the radiation (dose rate), is responsible for the photobiological response.

- Only photons that are absorbed by molecules in skin can initiate a response.

- Each chromophore (light-absorbing molecule) in skin absorbs a unique combination of wavelengths; this is termed the absorption spectrum.

- Photochemical reactions convert chromophores into new molecules called photoproducts.

- Photoproducts stimulate processes in cells that lead to observed clinical responses.

INTRODUCTION

From entering the skin to causing biological and clinical effects, optical radiation has to initiate a number of processes as shown in Figure 1. These pathways encompass a variety of seemingly unconnected areas of knowledge ranging from climatology, optical physics, photochemistry, cellular and molecular biology through to clinical medicine and pathology (1).

The observable clinical effects that result from the interaction of optical radiation, especially ultraviolet radiation (UVR), with the skin can be both beneficial and detrimental. The effects can be either acute, which is of rapid onset and generally short duration, or chronic, which is of gradual onset and long duration. Examples of acute effects include sunburn, tanning, and vitamin D production, whereas photoaging and skin cancer are the results of chronic exposure over many years. These effects are discussed in more detail elsewhere.

ULTRAVIOLET AND VISIBLE RADIATION

In 1666, Isaac Newton wrote: "*. . . procured me a Triangular glass-Prisme, to try therewith the celebrated Phaenomena of Colours*" and opened up a new era into the scientific investigation of light (2). It was not until 1801 that Johann Ritter discovered the ultraviolet (UV) region of the solar spectrum by showing that chemical action was caused by some form of energy in the dark portion beyond the violet (3). In 1800, Sir William Herschel had demonstrated the existence of radiation beyond the red end of the visible spectrum, a component now known as infrared radiation (4).

These three components of the solar spectrum—UV, visible, and infrared—are referred to collectively as optical radiation. But it is the UV rays, comprising about 5% of terrestrial sunlight, which hold the greatest interest in photodermatology.

WAVELENGTH RANGES
Ultraviolet Radiation

UV radiation covers a small part of the electromagnetic spectrum. Other regions of this spectrum include radio waves, microwaves, infrared radiation (heat), visible light, X-rays, and gamma radiation. The feature that characterizes the properties of any particular region of the spectrum is the wavelength of the radiation. UV radiation spans the wavelength region from 400 to 100 nm. Even in the UV portion of the spectrum the biological effects of the radiation vary enormously with wavelength, and for this reason the UV spectrum is further subdivided into three regions. The notion to divide the UV spectrum into different spectral regions was first put forward at the Copenhagen meeting of the Second International Congress on Light held during August 1932 by Coblentz (5), using the transmission properties of three

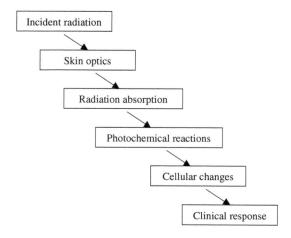

FIGURE 1 Pathways in skin photobiology.

TABLE 1 Wavelength Ranges and Perception of Color

Color	Wavelength range (nm)
Red	700–610
Orange	610–590
Yellow	590–570
Green	570–500
Blue	500–440
Violet	440–400

common glass filters. A barium-flint filter defined the UVA (315–400 nm); a barium-flint-pyrex filter the UVB (280–315 nm); and a pyrex filter defined the UVC (wavelengths shorter than 280 nm). So, the basis of these divisions has its grounding in physics, and not biology. Although these are the official designations of the Commission Internationale de l'Éclairage (CIE), other authorities, especially in the biological and clinical sciences, use different definitions such as UVA (320–400 nm), UVB (290–320 nm), and UVC (200–290 nm).

The division between UVB and UVC is chosen as 290 nm since UV radiation at shorter wavelengths is unlikely to be present in terrestrial sunlight, except at high altitudes. The choice of 320 nm as the division between UVB and UVA is perhaps more arbitrary. Although radiation at wavelengths shorter than 320 nm is generally more photobiologically active than longer wavelength UV, advances in molecular photobiology indicate that a subdivision at 330–340 nm may be more appropriate and for this reason the UVA region has, more recently, been divided into UVA-1 (340–400 nm) and UVA-2 (320–340 nm).

Visible Radiation

Visible radiation, or light, is increasingly used in phototherapy as illustrated in section V of this book. The visible spectrum is the portion of the optical radiation spectrum that is visible to the human eye. A typical human eye will respond to wavelengths from 400 to 700 nm, although some people may be able to perceive wavelengths from 380 to 780 nm. A light-adapted eye typically has its maximum sensitivity at around 555 nm, in the green region of the optical spectrum. The wavelength ranges associated with the perception of different colors of visible light are listed in Table 1.

It has been common practice in photomedicine to talk of ultraviolet light (UVL). This is incorrect; the term "light" should be reserved for those wavelengths of radiation that reach the retina and result in a sensation of vision. The correct term is UVR.

ENERGY AND WAVELENGTH

Electromagnetic radiation is so named due to the electric and magnetic properties of the wave. These two properties propagate at right angles to one another in a sinusoidal manner at the velocity of light, usually represented by the symbol c and equal to 3×10^8 ms^{-1}. The waves obey the general form:

$$c = \nu\lambda$$

where ν is the frequency of the radiation (in s^{-1}) and λ is the wavelength of the radiation (in m), that is the distance between successive troughs or peaks on the wave.

Although it is most often useful to think of electromagnetic radiation as a wave, the radiation can also demonstrate particulate nature as well. By using a particle theory, electromagnetic radiation can be examined as if it were composed of small particles of energy called quanta or photons. The energy (Q Joules) of each quanta or photon is expressed by Planck's law and is given by:

$$Q = h\nu$$

where h is Planck's constant (6.63×10^{-34} Js). By combining the two equations it becomes clear how the principles apply to one another.

$$Q = hc/\lambda$$

It can clearly be seen that the energy of each quanta of radiation is inversely proportional to the wavelength; the longer the wavelength the smaller the energy content.

Planck's law is applied if we need to know, for example, how many photons cause mild erythema in whole body narrow-band UVB (TL01) phototherapy. These lamps emit an approximate monochromatic spectrum at a wavelength of 311 nm. The UV dose to result in mild erythema from the lamps is typically 0.7 Jcm^{-2}, and the body surface area of a "standard" adult male is 1.73 m^2. Hence, the total energy incident over the body surface when mild erythema results is:

$$0.7 \text{ Jcm}^{-2} \times 17{,}300 \text{ cm}^2 = 1.21 \times 10^4 \text{ J}$$

From Planck's law we calculate that the energy of one photon having a wavelength of 311 nm is:

$$[6.63 \times 10^{-34} \times 3 \times 10^8]/[311 \times 10^{-9}] = 6.4 \times 10^{-19} \text{ J}$$

So the number of photons over the body surface is simply:

$1.21 \times 10^4/6.4 \times 10^{-19}$, which equals 2×10^{22}.

.   Approximately 10% of radiation of wavelength 311 nm incident on the skin will be transmitted to the dermis, so more than 1000 million, million, million photons reach the dermis during a single session of narrow-band UVB phototherapy.

PRODUCTION OF OPTICAL RADIATION

Artificial sources of incoherent (i.e., nonlaser) optical radiation may be produced either by heating a body to an incandescent temperature or by the excitation of a gas discharge. The most common source of incandescent optical radiation is the sun, and although there are artificial incandescent sources such as the quartz halogen lamps, in general, they are not efficient emitters of the UV component of optical radiation. For this reason, the most usual way to produce UVR artificially is by the passage of an electric current through a gas, usually vaporized mercury. Examples of lamps that emit incoherent UVR include low- and high-pressure mercury arc lamps, fluorescent lamps, metal halide lamps, and xenon arc lamps. Further details of optical radiation sources are given in Chapter 3.

Spectral Power Distribution

It is common practice to talk loosely of "UVA lamps" or "UVB lamps." However, such a label does not characterize adequately the UV sources since nearly all lamps (as well as the sun) used in photobiology will emit both UVA and UVB, and sometimes even UVC, visible light, and infrared radiation. The only correct way to specify the nature of the emitted radiation is by reference to the spectral power distribution. This is a graph (or table) that indicates the radiated power as a function of wavelength. An example of the spectrum of European summer daylight is shown in Figure 2.

QUANTITIES AND UNITS

The two most common dosimetric terms found in photodermatology are irradiance and dose. Irradiance refers to the intensity of radiation incident on a patient and is normally expressed in units of milliwatts per square centimeter (mWcm^{-2}). Dose is the time integral of the irradiance and is normally expressed in Joules per square centimeter (Jcm^{-2}). The term dose, commonly

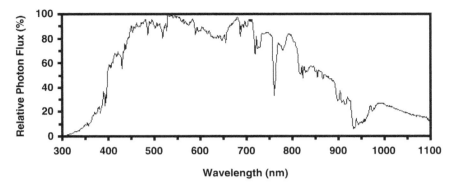

FIGURE 2 The spectrum of European summer daylight. *Source*: Adapted from Ref. 35.

found in the dermatological literature, is rather loose and more strictly should be termed radiant exposure or exposure dose.

The most frequent radiometric calculation is to determine the time for which a patient (or other object), who is prescribed a certain dose (in Jcm^{-2}), should be exposed when the dosimeter indicates irradiance in $mWcm^{-2}$. The relationship between these three quantities (time, dose, and irradiance) is simply:

$$\text{Exposure time (min)} = \frac{1000 \times \text{Prescribed dose (Jcm}^{-2})}{60 \times \text{Measured irradiance (mWcm}^{-2})}$$

Although radiometric terminology is widely used in photobiology, the units chosen vary throughout the literature. For example, exposure doses may be quoted in $mJcm^{-2}$ or kJm^{-2}. Table 2 summarizes the equivalence of these units.

Standard Erythema Dose and Minimal Erythema Dose

The problem of dosimetry in photodermatology lies in the fact that the ability of UV radiation to elicit erythema (and other clinical end-points) in human skin depends strongly on wavelength, encompassing a range of four orders of magnitude between 250 and 400 nm (see section "Action Spectra") . Thus, a statement that a subject received an exposure dose of 1 Jcm^{-2} of UV radiation conveys nothing about the consequences of that exposure in terms of erythema. If the radiation source were a UVA fluorescent lamp, no erythemal response would be seen apart from in people exhibiting severe, abnormal pathological photosensitivity. The same dose delivered from an unfiltered mercury arc lamp or fluorescent sunlamp would result in marked erythema in most white-skinned individuals. Consequently, there is often a need to express the exposure as an erythemal weighted quantity.

It has been common practice for many years to use the term minimal erythema dose (MED) as a "measure" of erythemal radiation. This is absurd because the MED is not a standard measure of anything but, on the contrary, encompasses the variable nature of individual sensitivity to UV radiation.

TABLE 2 Equivalent Radiometric Quantities

To convert from	To	Multiply by
Jcm^{-2}	$mJcm^{-2}$	10^3
Jcm^{-2}	Jm^{-2}	10^4
Jm^{-2}	$mJcm^{-2}$	10^7
kJm^{-2}	Jcm^{-2}	10^7
kJm^{-2}	$mJcm^{-2}$	10^{10}

TABLE 3 A Classification of Skin Phototypes Based on Susceptibility to Sunburn in Sunlight, Together with Indicative Minimal Erythema Doses That Might be Expected Following UV Exposure on Unacclimatized Skin

Skin phototype	Sunburn susceptibility	Tanning ability	Classes of individuals	UV exposure (in SED) that results in a minimal erythema (i.e., 1 MED)
I	Always burn	No tan	Melano-compromised	1–3
II	High	Light tan		
III	Moderate	Medium tan	Melano-competent	3–7
IV	Low	Dark tan		
V	Very low	Natural brown skin	Melano-protected	7–>12
VI	Extremely low	Natural black skin		

Abbreviations: SED, standard erythema dose; MED, minimal erythema dose.

The MED is generally determined by exposing adjacent areas of skin to increasing doses of radiation (usually employing a geometrical series of dose increments) and recording the lowest dose of radiation to achieve minimal erythema at a specified time, usually 24 hours, after irradiation. The difficulty in judging a minimal erythema response accurately is reflected by the varying definitions proposed for this value; these range from the dose required to initiate a just perceptible erythema (6), to that dose which will just produce a uniform redness with sharp borders (7). The former end-point has been shown to be more reproducible and less prone to interobserver differences (8).

To avoid further confusing abuse of the term MED, it has been proposed (9) that this term be reserved solely for observational studies in humans and other animals. The term standard erythema dose (SED) should be used to refer to erythemal effective exposure doses from natural and artificial sources of UV radiation; 1 SED is equivalent to an erythemal effective exposure dose of 100 Jm^{-2} (10).

A classification of skin phototypes based on susceptibility to sunburn in sunlight (11), together with indicative MEDs (expressed in SEDs) that might be expected following exposure on unacclimatized skin, is given in Table 3.

DOSE AND DOSE RATE EFFECTS

Experiments in which the photoresponse of a material is investigated as a function of irradiance (or dose rate) are commonly called reciprocity law experiments. Bunsen and Roscoe (12) are credited with conducting the first reciprocity law experiments. Reciprocity holds in photobiology when the observable response depends only on the total administered dose and is independent of the two factors that determine total dose, that is, irradiance and exposure time.

Since the reciprocity law depends only on total dose, its validation for a particular end-point can have many experimental manifestations. Assuming that the reciprocity law is valid, then each manifestation should be equivalent to the others as long as the integrated total dose is the same. Thus, when the reciprocity law is obeyed, the same photobiological response is observed when specimens receive the same integrated total dose regardless as to whether the exposure is performed.

These exposure regimes, as shown in Figure 3, are adapted from a similar representation given by Forbes et al. (13).

A summary of reciprocity experiments carried out in human and mouse skin are reviewed by Martin et al. (14). In every case, reciprocity for erythema was shown to hold. Of particular relevance to phototherapy, where exposure times will vary from a few minutes up to half-an-hour or so depending on the power and spectral output of the lamps, Meanwell and Diffey (15) showed that exposure to polychromatic radiation for time periods ranging from 1 second to 1 hour induced degrees of delayed erythema ranging from minimal to marked that depended only on dose and not dose rate. These findings both support and extend those of previous studies in which the end point was confined to minimal erythema.

On the other hand, reciprocity has been shown not to hold in UV-induced carcinogenesis where, in general, for a fixed dose of UV radiation the carcinogenic effectiveness increases as the irradiance decreases or is fractionated (16–18).

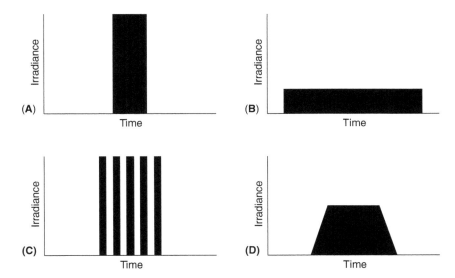

FIGURE 3 A selection of irradiance versus exposure time regimes for testing the law of reciprocity in which the integrated areas (i.e., dose) for each exposure regime are identical. When the reciprocity law is obeyed, the photoresponse for each of these exposure regimes is the same. (**A**) At a high irradiance for a short period of time. (**B**) At a low irradiance for a long period of time. (**C**) By repeatedly switching a radiation source on-or-off and controlling both the on-off frequency of the radiation and the length of time that the radiation remains in the on and the off state. Experiments in which the radiation is turned on-and-off at an extremely high frequency are called flash photolysis experiments, whereas experiments in which the radiation is turned on-and-off at a low frequency are called intermittency experiments. (**D**) By ramping the irradiance to a high level, holding the irradiance for a specified period of time, and then ramping it back down to a lower level or any variant of these stress regimes.

ABSORPTION OF UV AND VISIBLE RADIATION BY MOLECULES IN SKIN

UV and visible photons enter the skin where they may be absorbed by molecules in the epidermis and dermis or scattered by structures, such as collagen fiber bundles. The first process, absorption, initiates acute and chronic responses in skin because the photon energy is transferred to molecules in cells, which then undergo chemical changes (Fig. 1). Only photons that are absorbed can initiate biological and clinical responses. The second process, scattering, influences the depth that photons of different wavelengths penetrate into the epidermis and dermis. These effects are discussed under the topic of "Skin Optics" in chapter 3.

Absorption Spectra

Each type of molecule in skin, for example, an amino acid, a nucleotide, or a porphyrin, absorbs a unique combination of wavelengths and is generally referred to as a chromophore. Some chromophores absorb only UVB, some absorb both UVB and UVA, and others absorb throughout the UV and visible wavebands. These differences in absorption characteristics between biomolecules underlie the diverse effects produced when skin is exposed to different wavebands. In addition, information about the absorption spectra of chromophores is needed to identify the wavelengths and radiation sources that are most appropriate for UV phototherapy or photodynamic therapy (PDT). Thus, it is important to learn more about the relationship between molecules and the wavelengths they absorb.

The structure of a molecule, that is, the arrangement of the atoms and the distribution of electrons around this framework, strongly influence which wavelengths of UV or visible radiation are absorbed. The chemical structure also determines the probability of absorption of photons at each wavelength, that is, how much radiation is absorbed as a function of wavelength. A plot of the probability of absorption of photons against the wavelength is called an absorption spectrum. The wavelengths that are absorbed with the highest probability are called absorption maxima.

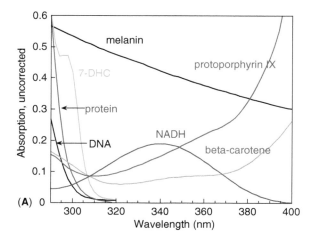

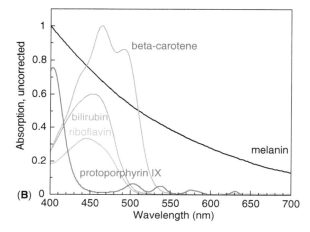

FIGURE 4 Absorption spectra of chromophores in skin. (**A**) Spectra of molecules in skin absorbing in the UVB and UVA ranges. (**B**) Spectra of molecules in skin absorbing in the visible range. Note that many molecules absorb in more than one wavelength range. The relative heights of the absorption peaks in this figure do not indicate the relative amounts of radiation absorbed by these chromophores in skin. The actual amount of radiation absorbed by each chromophore is related to the amount of the present in skin.

Examples of absorption spectra for some of the chromophores in skin are shown in Figure 4. The aromatic amino acids in proteins, in particular tryptophan and tyrosine, absorb UVB radiation. The purine and pyrimidine bases in DNA and RNA are also important UVB-absorbing chromophores for cutaneous responses. The 7-dehydrocholesterol (7-DHC) absorbs UVB and is one of the few chromophores that initiate the beneficial effects of sunlight on skin. The absorption maxima for these UVB-absorbing chromophores are actually in the UVC range and consequently are not shown in Figure 4A. In fact, most chromophores absorb in more than one spectral range. Some examples are NADH that has an absorption maximum at about 340 nm, but also absorbs UVB radiation (Fig. 4A), β-carotene that has absorption maxima at about 465 and 490 nm in the visible, but also absorbs in the UV range (Fig. 4B), and protoporphyrin IX that has an absorption maximum at about 405 nm, but also absorbs UVA strongly (Fig. 4B). The NADH is shown as an example of a UVA chromophore, but many others are also present in cells. Certain drugs causing phototoxicity, such as tetracyclines and fluorinated quinolones, also absorb UVA radiation. Other endogenous chromophores absorbing visible light include riboflavin, hemoglobin, and bilirubin. The photosensitizing dyes used in PDT generally absorb at longer visible wavelengths (>650 nm) (see chap. 25). Melanin is unique since it absorbs throughout the UVB, UVA, and visible wavebands without an absorption maximum.

The spectra in Figure 4 are intended to show only the distribution of wavelengths absorbed by various chromophores and not their relative absorption of UVR and visible light in skin. The amount of radiation actually absorbed by these molecules in skin is related to the amount of each chromophore present. For example, DNA absorbs much more of the UVB radiation incident on skin than 7-DHC because it is present at a much greater concentration than 7-DHC.

Excited States of Biomolecules

When a molecule absorbs the energy of a UV or visible photon, it becomes an "excited state," a higher energy state of the molecule. Originally, the molecule was in the so-called "ground state," where the electrons have a certain distribution around the framework of nuclei that make up the structure of the molecule. The electron distribution, but not the nuclear framework, changes when the molecule absorbs the photon energy. The principles of quantum mechanics allow only certain energy gaps between the ground state and the excited state. Consequently, each molecule can only absorb photons with certain energies. Since the photon energy is inversely related to the wavelength, each unique chromophore has a unique absorption spectrum. A signature property of excited states is their brief lifetime. Each excited state exists for only a very short period before returning to the ground state by giving off light or heat or by undergoing chemical reactions.

The first excited state formed is called a singlet-excited state. It typically exists for only a few nanoseconds (ns, 10^{-9} s). Most singlet-excited states return to the ground state by emitting the excess energy as fluorescence or releasing the energy as heat, a process called internal conversion (Fig. 5). Fluorescence is used in diagnosis, for example, for the presence of porphyrins in the urine of certain porphyria patients. Another example is the emission observed when using a Wood's lamp to examine skin pigmentation. The blue light observed is fluorescence from components in the dermal collagen. The heat generated by the return of singlet-excited states to the ground state is not usually apparent. The exception is when a laser with short, intense pulses is used. In this case, many chromophores are excited to the singlet state at the same time and give off their energy as heat when returning to the ground state almost simultaneously. This is the basis for the thermal effects produced during laser treatments as discussed in chapter 26.

The singlet-excited state of a chromophore in skin can undergo photochemical reactions, thereby initiating responses in cells as discussed subsequently (Fig. 5). Alternatively, the singlet-excited state may convert into a triplet-excited state, which is more stable and exists for a somewhat longer period, that is, a few microseconds (μs, 10^{-6} s). Singlet- and triplet-excited states differ by the "spins" of a pair of electrons. Spin is a quantum mechanical property of electrons in molecules. If the spins of the pair of electrons are opposite, the molecule is a singlet state. If the spins are the same, the molecule is a triplet state. Similar to the singlet-excited state, the triplet-excited state can give off excess energy as optical radiation (phosphorescence), as heat

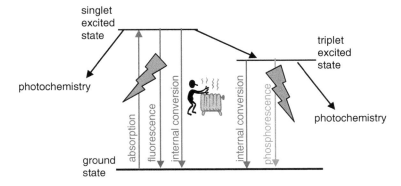

FIGURE 5 Energy levels and photoprocesses of a molecule (modified Jablonski diagram). The ground state molecule absorbs the energy of a photon to form the excited singlet state (*red arrow*). The excited singlet state then either releases the energy as light (fluorescence; *blue*) or as heat (internal conversion; *purple*), undergoes a chemical reaction, or converts into a triplet excited state. The triplet excited state releases energy as light (phosphorescence; *orange*) or heat (internal conversion; *purple*) or undergoes a chemical reaction (including energy transfer).

(internal conversion), or can undergo photochemical reactions, including energy transfer to oxygen as described subsequently (Fig. 5).

Photochemical reactions of excited-state molecules are the processes of greatest interest in photodermatology because the products formed initiate cellular changes that subsequently lead to clinical responses (Fig. 1). However, some molecules that absorb in the UVR and visible wavelength ranges very rarely undergo photochemical reactions. Hemoglobin and β-carotene are two examples.

The efficiency of any of the processes of excited states is described in terms of a quantum yield. The quantum yield is simply the ratio of the number of events, for example, number of photons of fluorescence emitted, to the number of photons absorbed.

PHOTOCHEMICAL REACTIONS LEADING TO CELL RESPONSES

A photochemical reaction converts the chromophore into a new molecule with a different structure called a photoproduct. In some cases, the photochemical reaction only changes the structure of the chromophore (unimolecular reaction) and in other cases an additional molecule is changed (bimolecular reaction). An example of the former type is the photochemistry of 7-DHC. After absorbing a photon of UVB radiation, 7-DHC is transformed into previtamin D_3 by a rearrangement of some of the carbon–carbon bonds in its structure. Previtamin D_3 then undergoes another bond-switching rearrangement in the dark to form vitamin D_3, which is transported from the skin bound to vitamin D-binding protein (19). Further biochemical modifications produce the active forms of vitamin D. Thus, in contrast to other UVR-induced clinical effects, the responses to 7-DHC photochemistry in the skin occurs at a distant body sites.

DNA Photochemistry

Most photoproducts that initiate clinical responses arise from bimolecular reactions. A very important example is the formation of photoproducts along the DNA strands after absorption of UVB radiation in keratinocytes. These photoproducts are responsible for the mutations that initiate skin cancer as well as being involved in UVB-induced immune suppression, tanning, and sunburn. The excited-singlet states of purine and pyrimidine bases in DNA are extremely short-lived (<0.1 ns). Even in this short time however, the excited singlet state of a pyrimidine base (thymine or cytosine) can react with another pyrimidine base adjacent to it on a strand of DNA. Covalent bonds are formed between two carbons on each of the pyrimidines and the photoproduct is a cyclobutyl pyrimidine dimer (CPD). The CPD is stable and, unless accurately repaired by specific repair enzymes, leads to a change in the sequence of DNA bases and, consequently, a mutation. Another product, called a 6-4 photoproduct, is also formed between two adjacent pyrimidine bases and is similarly mutagenic. Specific mutations that are signatures for CPD and six to four photoproducts are found in most nonmelanoma skin cancers. The skin responses to these DNA photoproducts are discussed in detail in section II.

Bimolecular photoreactions between a psoralen and pyrimidine nucleotides initiate the phototoxic and phototherapeutic effects of psoralens. In this case, psoralen molecules that are intercalated into double-stranded DNA absorb UVB and UVA radiation. The psoralen excited state molecules react with thymine and cytosine to form cyclobutyl ring structures, not unlike those in CPD. When the psoralen is positioned in the appropriate DNA sequences, two cyclobutyl structures may form after two photons are absorbed resulting in a psoralen crosslink between the two strands of DNA. Chapters 23 and 24 discuss the responses of skin to the formation of psoralen photoproducts.

Photosensitization

In skin responses initiated by photosensitization reactions, the mechanism frequently involves transfer of energy from the excited triplet state of the chromophore molecular oxygen that is dissolved in the cell. The chromophore is referred to as a photosensitizer. The oxygen molecule that has accepted the energy becomes an excited singlet state, "singlet oxygen." Notice that the ground state photosensitizer is regenerated after the energy transfer to oxygen.

$$\text{Photosensitizer} + O_2 \longrightarrow \text{Photosensitizer} + {}^1O_2$$

| Excited triplet state | | Ground state | Singlet oxygen |

Consequently, the same photosensitizer can recycle many times, typically >1000 times, generating a singlet oxygen with each cycle. This cycle is at least partially responsible for the high efficiency of photosensitization involving a singlet oxygen mechanism. Protoporphyrin IX is the photosensitizer for the photosensitivity associated with EPP. When cells containing protoporphyrin IX are exposed to blue light, singlet oxygen is produced that causes lipid peroxidation. A subsequent series of biochemical steps leads to the immediate smarting, erythema and whealing produced by sunlight on skin of EPP patients (see chap. 15). Singlet oxygen is also formed after PDT agents absorb longer wavelengths, for example, red light, and is believed to initiate oxidation reactions that cause cytotoxicity to tumor cells (see chap. 25). In addition, UVA-induced responses, such as apoptosis of lymphocytes in certain inflammatory skin diseases, are believed to be initiated by formation of singlet oxygen, although the UVA-absorbing chromophores have not been identified (20).

Singlet oxygen exists for less than 4 µs in cells, which limits the distance it can move to less 200 nm (21). Consequently, it oxidizes nearby cellular molecules. For example, protoporphyrin IX, many PDT dyes and other photosensitizers localize at least partially in cell membranes and oxidize unsaturated lipids in the membranes to form hydroperoxides. These oxidized lipids react further in the dark, often in chain reactions, to amplify the oxidizing effect initiated by singlet oxygen. Similarly, PDT dyes that localize in mitochondria photosensitize damage to mitochondrial components and initiate apoptosis (22). Oxidation of guanine in DNA forms specific oxidation products that are mutagenic. Certain amino acid side chains in proteins (histidine, tyrosine, tryptophan, cysteine, and methionine) and other peptides, for example, glutathione, are also highly susceptible to oxidation by singlet oxygen. Formation of oxidation products in these molecules by photosensitization with UVA or visible radiation generates oxidative stress in cells. Oxidative stress produces many responses by initiating signal transduction pathways, leading to activation of transcription factors and enhanced gene expression. For example, the oxidative stress induced by singlet oxygen after UVA irradiation initiates a signaling pathway, leading to production of IL-1 and IL-6 and subsequently to production of interstitial collagenase by dermal fibroblasts (23).

ACTION SPECTRA

The wavelength dependency of a given photobiological effect is demonstrated by its action spectrum, which depends principally on the absorption spectrum of the chromophore and

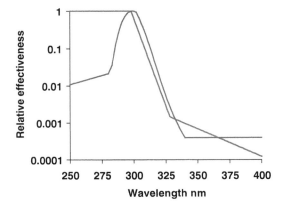

FIGURE 6 The Commission Internationale de l'Éclairage (CIE) (1987) reference action spectrum for erythema in human skin (*red*), and the CIE (2000) action spectrum for photocarcinogenesis (*blue*).

the optical properties of the skin (24). Conventionally in dermatology, the reciprocal of the dose required to produce a given end-point is plotted against wavelength to obtain an action spectrum. Action spectroscopy and studies with different broad-spectrum sources show that UVB is much more effective than UVA for most endpoints studied in human skin. These include erythema (25–27), delayed pigmentation (28), DNA photodamage (29), urocanic acid photoisomerization (30), and nonmelanoma skin cancer (31,32). An example of two of these action spectra is given in Figure 6.

In general, UVB is three to four orders of magnitude more effective per unit physical dose (Jcm^{-2}) than UVA, but one exception is the action spectrum for immediate pigment darkening (IPD) where UVA is more effective than UVB (33).

Knowing the action spectrum of a patient's photosensitivity can be helpful in determining their management. This can be especially useful in drug-induced photosensitivity (34). In addition, phototherapy will be most efficient when the emission of the lamp most closely matches the action spectrum for the beneficial response.

REFERENCES

1. Magnus IA. Dermatological Photobiology. Oxford: Blackwell Scientific Publications, 1976:3.
2. Newton I. A new theory about light and colours. Phil Trans R Soc Lond 1672; 6:3075–3087.
3. Ritter JW. Physisch-Chemische Abhandlungen, Vol. 2. Leipzig: 1801.
4. Herschel W. Experiments on the refrangibility of invisible rays of the sun. Phil Trans R Soc Lond 1800; 90:255–326.
5. Coblentz WW. The Copenhagen meeting of the Second International Congress on Light. Science 1932; 76:412.
6. Epstein JH. Polymorphous light eruptions. Wavelength dependency and energy studies. Arch Dermatol 1962; 85:82–88.
7. Willis I, Kliginan AM. Aminobenzoic acid and its esters. Arch. Dermatol 1970; 102:405-417.
8. Quinn AG, Diffey BL, Craig PS, Farr PM. Definition of the minimal erythema dose used for diagnostic phototesting. Br J Dermatol 1994; 131:56.
9. Diffey BL, Jansen CT, Urbach F, Wulf HC. The standard erythema dose: a new photobiological concept. Photodermatol Photoimmunol Photomed 1997; 13:64–66.
10. CIE Standard. Erythema reference action spectrum and standard erythema dose. CIE S 007/E-1998. Vienna: Commission Internationale de l'Éclairage, 1998.
11. WHO World Health Organization. Artificial tanning sunbeds—risks and guidance. Geneva, 2003.
12. Bunsen RW, Roscoe HE. The laws of photochemical action. Phil Trans R Soc Lond 1859; 149:876–926.
13. Forbes PD, Davies RE, Urbach F. Aging, environmental influences, and photocarcinogenesis. J Invest Dermatol 1979; 73:131–134.
14. Martin JW, Chin JW, Nguyen T. Reciprocity law experiments in polymeric photodegradation: a critical review. Prog Org Coat 2003; 47:292–311.
15. Meanwell EF, Diffey BL. Reciprocity of ultraviolet erythema in human skin. Photodermatology 1989; 6:146-148.
16. Forbes PD, Blum HF, Davies RE. Photocarcinogenesis in hairless mice: dose–response and the influence of dose–delivery. Photochem Photobiol 1981; 34:361–365.
17. de Gruijl FR, van der Leun JC. Effect of chronic UV exposure on epidermal transmission in mice. Photochem Photobiol 1982; 36:433–438.
18. Kelfkens G, van Weelden H, de Gruijl FR, van der Leun JC. The influence of dose rate on ultraviolet tumorigenesis. J Photoch Photobio B 1991; 10:41–50.
19. Holick MF. Environmental factors that influence the cutaneous production of vitamin D. Am J Clin Nutr 1995; 61 (suppl. 3):638–645S.
20. Morita A, Werfel T, Stege H, et al. Evidence that singlet oxygen-induced human T helper cell apoptosis is the basic mechanism of ultraviolet-A radiation phototherapy. J Exp Med 1997; 186:1763–1768.
21. Snyder JW, Skovsen E, Lambert JD, et al. Subcellular, time-resolved studies of singlet oxygen in single cells. J Am Chem Soc 2005; 127:14,558–14,559.
22. Xue LY, Chiu SM, Fiebig A, et al. Photodamage to multiple Bcl-xL isoforms by photodynamic therapy with the phthalocyanine photosensitizer Pc 4. Oncogene 2003; 22:9197–9204.
23. Wlaschek M, Wenk J, Brenneisen P, et al. Singlet oxygen is an early intermediate in cytokine-dependent ultraviolet-A induction of interstitial collagense in human dermal fibroblasts in vitro. FEBS Lett 1997; 413:239–242.
24. Young AR. Chromophores in human skin. Phys Med Biol 1997; 42:789–802.
25. Anders A, Altheide H.-J, Knälmann M, Tronnier H. Action spectrum for erythema in humans investigated with dye lasers. Photochem Photobiol 1995; 61:200–205.

26. Diffey BL. Observed and predicted minimal erythema doses: a comparative study. Photochem Photobiol 1994; 60:380–381.
27. CIE Standard. Erythema reference action spectrum and standard erythema dose. CIE S 007/E-1998. Vienna: Commission Internationale de l'Éclairage, 1998.
28. Parrish JA, Jaenicke KF, Anderson RR. Erythema and melanogenesis action spectra of normal human skin. Photochem Photobiol 1982; 36:187–191.
29. Young AR, Chadwick CA, Harrison GI, Nikaido O, Ramsden J, Potten CS. The similarity of action spectra for thymine dimers in human epidermis and erythema suggests that DNA is the chromophore for erythema. J Invest Dermatol 1998; 111:982–988.
30. McLoone P, Simics E, Barton A, Norval M, Gibbs NK. An action spectrum for the production of cis-urocanic acid in human skin in vivo. J Invest Dermatol 2005; 124:1071–1074.
31. de Gruijl FR. Action spectrum for photocarcinogenesis. Recent Results Cancer Res 1995; 139:21–30.
32. Commission Internationale de l'É clairage, Vienna. CIE 132/2; TC 6-32 report: action spectrum for photocarcinogenesis (non-melanoma skin cancers) 2000.
33. Irwin C, Barnes A, Veres D, Kaidbey K. An ultraviolet radiation action spectrum for immediate pigment darkening. Photochem Photobiol 1993; 57:504–507.
34. Diffey BL, Farr PM. The action spectrum in drug induced photosensitivity. Photochem Photobiol 1988; 47:49–54.
35. Ensminger PA. Life Under the Sun. Yale University Press, 2001.

3 | Radiation Sources and Interaction with Skin

Harvey Lui
Department of Dermatology and Skin Science, Vancouver Coastal Health Research Institute, University of British Columbia, Vancouver, British Columbia, Canada

R. Rox Anderson
Wellman Center for Photomedicine and Department of Dermatology, Harvard Medical School, and Massachusetts General Hospital, Boston, Massachusetts, U.S.A.

- Radiation refers to the transfer of energy as waves and particles, and can be depicted on an electromagnetic spectrum.

- Quantum theory forms the basis for explaining why each photobiologic event can be energized by only certain forms of light; this in turn, dictates the need for many different types of radiation sources.

- Radiation sources encountered in dermatology include the sun and medical devices that transform electrical power into specific forms of light.

- Incandescent light is produced by heating tungsten filaments with electricity.

- Fluorescent lamps produce radiation through low-pressure mercury vapor lamps that are coated with fluorescing phosphors.

- Lasers generate intense, monochromatic, coherent light by amplifying stimulated emission of radiation within specially configured optical cavities.

- Light emitting diodes generate radiation by passing current through semiconductor bilayers.

- The output spectrum of the radiation source should closely match the absorption or action spectrum in order to have an efficient photobiologic event.

RADIATION AS A FORM OF ENERGY: THE ELECTROMAGNETIC SPECTRUM

Radiation refers to the transfer of energy in the form of both electromagnetic oscillations and particles. According to wave theory, radiation is propagated through space as oscillations that have frequency and wavelength. Radiation waves can be further characterized as being electromagnetic since they are composed of two orthogonal oscillatory waves carrying electric and magnetic components. When electromagnetic radiation interacts with matter, it exhibits particle-like behavior since its interactions with molecules are restricted to discrete packets of energy called photons. The energy of a photon is directly proportional to the frequency and inversely proportional to the wavelength of its simultaneous existence as a wave.

Electromagnetic radiation exists on a continuum that can be depicted as a spectrum (Fig. 1). While radiation can be characterized in terms of its physical properties (i.e., wavelength, frequency, photon energy), it is more relevant to parse it according to its biologic effects. Also keep in mind that even though radiation basically represents energy, by convention, the various forms of radiation are numerically distinguished and categorized according to wavelength rather than by frequency or even photon energy. The ultraviolet (UV), visible, and infrared (IR) regions of the electromagnetic spectrum are the most relevant for human photobiology, and the photon energy from these wavebands is sufficient to induce electronic and vibrational energy transitions within molecules. Radiation sources that emit these wavebands are therefore capable of driving covalent chemical reactions and/or producing heat. The individual subdivisions of the electromagnetic spectrum are so named on the basis of their biologic effects. The term "light" is sometimes restricted to electromagnetic radiation that is visible to the human eye (i.e., 400 ~ 700 nm), but it is not uncommon for the entire region from UV through IR to be referred to interchangeably as either light or radiation, as in this chapter. The UV region is further subdivided into UVC, UVB, and UVA. The 290 mm cut off between UVC and UVB defines the lower limit of UV light that reaches the earth's surface, while the 320 nm boundary between UVB and UVA separates terrestrial UV light that is either more (UVB) or less (UVA) efficient at inducing cutaneous erythema.

Within molecules, energy transformations can occur only between discontinuous levels known as quanta; these levels are, to some extent, like the individual steps of a staircase. The interaction between matter and a photon is a phenomenon that is either all or none, and absorption will occur only if a photon's energy exactly matches the quantum difference or step that corresponds to a specified molecular transition. The requirement that energy be transferred only through the absorption of specific photons is dictated by quantum mechanics, and this principle explains why only certain wavelengths of light can induce any given photobiologic skin reaction, even though all light sources serve as sources of energy. Thus, in photodermatology it is the quantum laws of physics that fundamentally drive the need for a wide array of different radiation sources.

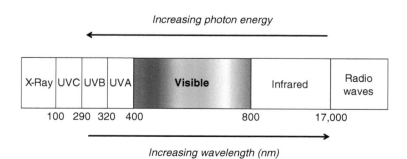

FIGURE 1   The electromagnetic spectrum.

RADIATION SOURCES

There is one natural radiation source, which sustains all life on our planet, and multiple artificial devices that generate radiation to either mimic the output of the sun or isolate only certain specific wavebands.

NATURAL LIGHT FROM THE SUN

Sunlight represents the ultimate source of life and energy on this planet, yet excessive exposure to solar energy is clearly deleterious to biologic systems. For humans the correct balance of light exposure necessary for health maintenance varies dramatically between individuals based on skin phenotype, presence of pathologic photosensitivity, and genetic factors. For otherwise normal and healthy individuals, sunlight is necessary for promoting a psychological sense of well being as well as providing the energy for endogenous vitamin D synthesis. On the other hand, excessive sunlight leads to photoaging, immunosuppression, and photocarcinogenesis. For certain dermatologic patients, sunlight can represent either the key pathogen that precipitates a dermatosis (e.g., solar urticaria) or the means by which a skin condition can be ameliorated or treated (e.g., psoriasis). Furthermore, as exemplified by polymorphous light eruption, sunlight can also, paradoxically, serve as the inciting factor and also a means for relief (i.e., natural hardening with repeated sunlight exposure).

Solar radiation reaching the earth's surface includes UV, visible, and IR radiation between 290 and 4000 nm (Fig. 2). Terrestrial sunlight fluctuates dramatically not only in terms of overall intensity but also in its spectral composition by time of day, elevation, and latitude. These effects on spectral irradiance predominantly affect the UV component of the solar spectrum. The quality and quantity of solar radiation vary depending on geography and time. In certain locations and climates sunlight is sufficiently uniform and predictable to be an inexpensive and readily available radiation source that may be sufficient for diagnostic or therapeutic use. Judicious and controlled exposure to outdoor sunlight may be helpful for confirming suspected cases of clinical photosensitivity. For treatment, natural light dosimetry is empiric, since providing light meters to patients is impractical. Nevertheless, with natural sunlight, exposure guidelines can be individualized to some extent by considering a person's light tolerance in terms of his/her sunburn propensity and the rate at which photoadaptation occurs.

ARTIFICIAL RADIATION

Artificial light can be made to closely mimic the sun or to isolate only certain parts of the UV to IR spectrum (Table 1). Solar simulators fall in the former category and are used primarily in investigational settings for diagnostic evaluation of suspected photosensitivity or sunscreen evaluation (1).

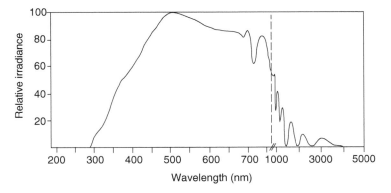

FIGURE 2 Terrestrial solar light spectral irradiance.

TABLE 1 Important Wavebands and Therapeutic Radiation Sources in Dermatology[a]

Waveband		Arc (gas discharge)[b]	Fluorescent	Laser	IPL	LED
		Radiation source				
UV	UVB broadband	X	X			
	UVB narrowband		X	X		
	UVA	X	X			
	UVA-1	X	X			
Visible	Blue		X			
	Green			X	X	
	Yellow			X	X	
	Red	X		X	X	X
IR				X	X	

[a]Incandescent lamps are not included in this table since their use as therapeutic devices is relatively uncommon in dermatology.
[b]Metal halide lamps are the most common form of arc-type radiator now in use.
Abbreviations: IPL, intense pulsed light; LED, light emitting diode.

All devices that produce artificial radiation feature a means for generating light, then modifying the light in terms of its spectral properties, and finally delivering the light to the skin over a uniform exposure field. Virtually all medical light devices generate radiation by converting electrical energy into photon energy. Optical filters or specific fluorophores are used to shape the desired spectral output of the source, while mirrors, lenses, and fibers are used to direct the light to the target. There are a multitude of radiation sources available and the choice of device depends on the specific clinical application, photobiologic mechanism, and region of the skin that needs to be exposed. Cost and practicality must also be factored in. Light sources in dermatologic use include incandescent lamps, arc lamps, fluorescent lamps, lasers, and intense pulsed light; with the latter three now being the most commonly used devices for irradiating the skin.

Incandescent Lamps

When a metallic object is heated it will glow and release light energy by a process known as incandescence. In an incandescent light bulb, electric current is passed through a thin tungsten filament, which generates heat and light due to electrical resistance. The spectral output and intensity of the light bulb is dependent on the temperature that the filament achieves, with a more luminous and whiter beam being produced at higher temperatures. Incandescent lamps are relatively inefficient visible light sources, since much of the electrical energy is used to generate heat, which in turn leads to filament evaporation and eventual bulb burn out. The potential for filament failure thus limits the operating temperature, intensity, and spectral quality of incandescent lamps. The life of a tungsten bulb can be extended by sealing the filament in a quartz envelope that contains a halogen, such as bromine or iodine. This allows the filament to be electrically driven to a higher temperature where there is a spectral shift towards more energetic photons in the UV range without reducing the bulb's lifetime. These so-called quartz halogen lamps can emit a significant amount of UV, in addition to visible and IR light. The final desired spectral output of a quartz halogen lamp is achieved with optical filters that allow only certain wavebands to pass. For example, quartz halogen bulbs that are used for general illumination are fitted with a glass covering over the bulb in order to block UV. In clinical dermatology incandescent lamps have been primarily used in situations where visible light is required including photodynamic therapy, photo-testing, and noninvasive optical diagnosis, such as reflectance spectroscopy. For example, conventional slide projector lamps provide a convenient and uniform beam of visible light that can be used in diagnostic phototesting (2).

Arc Lamps

An arc lamp discharges light when high voltage is applied across two electrodes that are sealed in a transparent envelope containing a gas, such as mercury or xenon. The electric current will excite electrons within the gas, which then emits light as the gas returns to its physical ground state. The "arc" refers to the plasma between the electrodes from which light radiates. The specific gas determines the spectral output of the lamp. These lamps are also referred to as gas discharge lamps. The output spectrum of a gas discharge lamp can be further modulated by varying the gas pressure within the glass envelope. At higher pressures the spectral emission peaks broaden and start to approach an output that is more continuous (or "spectrally neutral") throughout its output range.

Historically, the first effective artificial light sources were arc lamps. Finsen, the father of modern photomedicine who received the 1903 Nobel prize in medicine, used carbon arc lamps for treating lupus vulgaris (3). The carbon electrodes would be heated by the arc and actually emit light by incandescence. Because these electrodes would burn out with use, this form of "electric light," eventually, gave way to mercury vapor lamps, which were equipped with quartz envelopes in order to allow UV transmission.

In a mercury vapor lamp, mercury is first ionized and vaporized to a gas by electrically igniting an arc. As the lamp heats up more mercury vapor builds up to sustain the arc. The spectral output corresponds to mercury's quantum transitions as the excited electrons in the arc return to their ground state. At low operating pressures of mercury, the spectral emission is predominantly at the UV end of the spectrum with sharp lines corresponding to mercury's characteristic quantum transitions, especially 254 nm. When mercury arc lamps are operated at progressively higher pressures and temperatures, the output shifts towards UVB and UVA with some broadening of the spectral maxima that are centered around the mercury lines at 297, 302, 313, 334, and 365 nm. Both low and high ("cold" and "hot" quartz) pressure mercury vapor lamps were used in dermatology prior to the widespread adoption of fluorescent tube technology. Although hot quartz lamps have a limited field size, they can probably be considered as the first practical form of targeted phototherapy. More recently a "short arc maximum pressure" mercury lamp has been developed for clinical use. This is a relatively compact light source and because the arc is small, its output can be coupled to a UV transmitting fiber or light guide, which then directs light to a specific skin-target area. Due to the very high pressure within a short arc mercury lamp, the UV output is spectrally more broad and continuous than a hot quartz lamp.

If a metal halide is added to mercury in a high pressure gas discharge lamp, additional emissions between the mercury spectral lines are filled such that the output becomes virtually continuous throughout the UV spectrum. These lamps can be equipped with specific long pass optical filters to restrict the output to UVB plus UVA, UVA (broad spectrum), or UVA-1 (4). Metal halide lamps are more expensive and cumbersome to operate than fluorescent lamp-based phototherapy units, but the higher output with metal halide allows for shorter treatment times.

For simulating solar radiation, xenon is used in arc lamps because its output spectrum provides the best match to that of terrestrial sunlight. Xenon discharge lamps are the same type of light source used for projecting movies in cinemas. Recently, a xenon chloride-based excimer device (*excimer = exci*ted di*mer*) with very narrow-band incoherent emission (308 ± 2 nm) centered at the XeCl spectral line has been introduced for delivering targeted UV phototherapy. The therapeutic effect of this device would be expected to be similar to the XeCl excimer laser. Technical details as to how light is generated from XeCl in this "monochromatic excimer light" device have not yet been published, although nominally, it also has 15% of its output as UVA (5).

Fluorescent Lamps

Fluorescent radiation represents the re-emission of photons following light absorption by a chromophore. The photons that are emitted by the chromophore are usually of a lower energy than the incident photons that were initially absorbed, and thus are of a longer wavelength. In the context of fluorescence, chromophores are more specifically referred to as "fluorophores."

Fluorescent light is most commonly produced within sealed cylindrical glass tubes containing mercury. The primary radiation that is initially produced within a fluorescent lamp is analogous to that emitted by a low-pressure mercury lamp. When electric current is applied to the ends of a fluorescent tube, the mercury is vaporized and excited to a higher energy level. Upon relaxation of the mercury to its ground state, radiation is released at emission peaks characteristic for mercury. This primary output is then transformed by fluorescence to higher wavelengths. The inside of the tubes is coated with special fluorophores called phosphors. The radiation that is generated from the primary mercury emissions is absorbed by the phosphors that coat the fluorescent tube. These phosphors will, in turn, re-emit light at longer wavelengths than the main mercury emission of 254 nm. The fluorescence properties of the specific phosphor coating determine the final output of the fluorescent lamp.

In dermatology, fluorescent lamps are by far the most common source of therapeutic UV light. Different phosphors are used to produce light that is predominantly UVB or UVA. Fluorescent lamps for general illumination will have phosphors that generate visible light, and for safety reasons, be constructed with glass to minimize UV transmission. The most recent important advance in UVB fluorescent technology was the development of the narrowband lamp, which has a prominent emission band centered at 311 nm (Phillips TL-01) (6). The impetus for developing this lamp came from the classic psoriasis action spectrum studies, showing that longer wavelength UVB was more effective while being less erythemogenic than shorter UVB wavelengths (7). A subdivision of the UVA spectrum has also been demonstrated to have specific therapeutic advantages, and fluorescent lamps are now available to provide UVA-1 light (340–400 nm). Fluorescent technology in dermatology is not limited to UV phototherapy; "U-shaped" blue-light-emitting fluorescent lamps provide the energy to activate protoporphyrin IX in topical aminolevulinic acid-based photodynamic therapy (8).

Other essential components of fluorescent lamps include electric ballasts, which stabilize the lamp's output and lifetime by regulating current flow within specific limits. Longitudinal reflective mirrors are also configured to maximize the light reaching the skin. Fluorescent lamps are available in a range of lengths and housings to treat smaller areas such as the palms and soles, or the whole body at once.

Lasers

Laser is an acronym for "light amplification by the stimulated emission of radiation," which aptly defines this technology. Fundamental to understanding how lasers work is the concept of stimulated emission. Excited molecules can emit radiation as they return to their lower energy ground state. This process can occur in the absence of external factors in which case the emission is said to be spontaneous. In contrast, stimulated emission occurs when an excited molecule is struck by a photon whose energy exactly matches the quantal-energy transition between the excited and ground states for those molecules. In stimulated emission, the incident and emitted photons are of identical wavelength, phase, and direction which gives rise to the properties of monochromaticity, coherence, and collimation.

In a laser, light is amplified through a special optical configuration that is designed to dramatically increase the probability of stimulated emission. The essential components of a laser include (*i*) a lasing medium within which stimulated emission occurs, (*ii*) a longitudinal optical cavity (also known as an optical resonator) with mirrors at each end, one of which is only partially reflecting, and (*iii*) an external energy source (Fig. 3). The lasing medium is contained within the laser cavity and the external energy source serves to excite the molecules of the medium. Energy is "pumped" into the lasing medium to create a population inversion in which more molecules are present in an excited, rather than ground state. Spontaneous emission will generate photons that will, in turn, lead to the stimulated emission of additional radiation within the population inversion; a photon cascade ensues, all the while generating coherent monochromatic light. Amplification is further enhanced because the two mirrors reflect photons back and forth within the lasing medium. Laser light is released from the laser cavity through the partially reflecting mirror, which transmits some of the light generated within the lasing medium to a laser delivery component, which then directs the light to the skin.

Laser radiation is spectrally very pure, because it is produced by stimulated radiation. The spectral output of a laser is considered monochromatic and in practical terms is usually specified by a single wavelength. The wavelength will be determined by the specific discrete energy transitions of the lasing medium. The lasing medium can exist as a gas, liquid, or

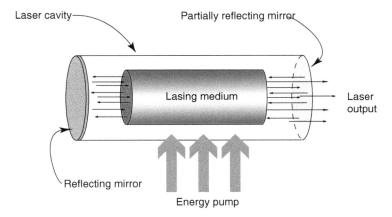

FIGURE 3 Laser components and stimulated emission.

solid; lasers are named according to their lasing medium (i.e., ruby, carbon dioxide, excimer). The laser-pumping source that provides the energy to generate and maintain the population inversion within the lasing medium is most often a radiofrequency generator or an intense light source such as a flashlamp.

Lasers produce light in either continuous or pulsed modes, and this is mostly determined by the nature of the pumping source that is used. For example, flashlamps emit brief, intense flashes of broadband incoherent light; lasers that are pumped by flashlamps will therefore deliver pulsed radiation. By far, the most common use of lasers in dermatology is to generate heat within the skin. Specific structures within the skin can be targeted for permanent photothermal alteration by choosing the appropriate wavelength and pulse duration. This concept is known as selective photothermolysis, and lasers are, arguably, the best light source available for this technique because it is possible to match a laser with the required wavelength and pulse duration. The laser wavelength used for a given application is chosen according to the absorption characteristics and depth of the target chromophore, whereas the desired pulse duration is largely a function of the physical size of the target. Smaller targets require a correspondingly shorter laser pulse in order to achieve selectivity. Targets such as melanosomes or tattoo particles may require a sub-microsecond laser exposure. So-called Q-switched lasers provide ultra high intensity and fast pulses, which last for less than 100 nanoseconds. The Q-switch is an optical device that enhances the Q- or "quality" factor within the laser's optical cavity by allowing the population inversion to be maximally saturated before stimulated emission is allowed to occur. In an optical cavity with a high Q factor, the laser will build to a very intense level and be discharged very quickly as soon as the Q-switch is triggered.

There are now myriad lasers available for treating the skin, all within a complex matrix of seemingly complicated parameters and competing medical claims. Lasers can be classified in a number of ways according to the nature of the lasing medium (gas, liquid, or solid), wavelength, or mode of operation (pulsed or continuous). Perhaps the most useful approach to organizing lasers used in practice is to consider first the specific clinical applications (i.e., vascular, hair removal, pigmented lesions, and resurfacing) and the corresponding photobiologic mechanisms. This will determine the optimum treatment parameters required. The appropriate laser is then considered from the menu of available devices. An exhaustive compilation of lasers and their applications is beyond the scope of this chapter, but the general categories are outlined in Table 2.

Intense Pulsed Light

Intense pulsed light devices, also known as IPLs, are essentially filtered xenon flashlamps that deliver intense light to the skin (9). The fundamental technology underlying an IPL is the same as that of an electronic camera flash. Flashlamps are also found as components of many medical lasers where they serve as the external power source for creating the population inversion

TABLE 2 Classification of Common Cutaneous Laser Applications

Application	Mechanism	Chromophore	Common lasers used
Vascular lesions	Photocoagulation of blood vessels	Hemoglobin	Pulsed dye laser (585–600 nm) Frequency doubled Nd:YAG (532 nm)
Pigmented lesions and tattoo removal	Photomechanical disruption of melanosomes or tattoo particles	Melanin/Tattoo ink particles	Q-switched Nd:YAG (1064 and 532 nm) Q-switched ruby (694 nm) Q-switched alexandrite (755 nm)
Hair removal	Photothermal destruction of hair follicles	Melanin within hair shafts	Alexandrite (755 nm) Diode (800 nm) Nd:YAG (1064 nm) Ruby (694 nm)
Resurfacing	Skin ablation and dermal remodeling	Water	Carbon dioxide (10,600 mm) Erbium:YAG (2940 nm)
Psoriasis	Photoimmunomodulation Photocoagulation of blood vessels	Unknown Hemoglobin	Excimer (308 nm) Pulsed dye laser (585–600 nm)
Vitiligo	Photoimmodulation and melanogenesis	Unknown	Excimer (308 nm)
PDT	Photochemical generation of singlet oxygen	PDT photosensitizer	Various

Abbreviations: PDT, photodynamic therapy; Nd:YAG, neodymium:yttrium-aluminum-garnet.

within the lasing medium. Unlike a laser, the spectral output of a flashlamp is polychromatic and incoherent. Flashlamps and lasers are both capable of emitting very intense light over a short time, which is essential for achieving selective photothermolysis. Because of this similarity, the flashlamp has been developed and promoted as a means of simulating the biologic and therapeutic effects of laser. This requires that the flashlamp's spectral output need to be modified by using appropriate optical filters.

In a flashlamp, a sealed transparent tube is filled with a mixture of gases, principally xenon. The ends of the tubes are fitted with electrodes across which very high voltage is applied. The voltage is delivered by a capacitor, which can be triggered to discharge its energy over a short period of time. This results in ionization of the gas that is now more electrically conductive. The pulse of current that then flows through the gas will excite electrons with the xenon molecules. Return of these excited molecules to their resting state will generate the broad-spectrum light characteristic of xenon. Xenon flashlamps produce very intense light for short periods of time.

IPLs can, indeed, be used for many of the same applications that were originally developed for lasers (9). Their intense broadband output, particularly, in the IR range is of unknown clinical importance, however. IPL is typically delivered to the skin via quartz crystals that are held in direct contact with the skin.

Light Emitting Diodes

Light emitting diodes or LEDs are ubiquitous in modern life and are popular because of their efficiency, low cost of operation, and compact size. LEDs generate light by passing current through semiconductor diodes. Diodes are essentially semiconducting bilayers of aluminum-gallium-arsenide (AlGaAs) that are doped with impurities. All diode bilayers consist of two types of semiconductor materials, N- and P-type, that are bonded together. The N-type material is doped in such a way that it contains an excess of electrons and, therefore, carries a net negative charge, while the P-type material is overall positively charged and, therefore, is said to contain holes into which electrons can move. In a diode's ground state, at the immediate junction between the N-type and P-type materials, some electrons from the N-type material will fill the holes of the P-type material, thereby creating a zone that has no net charge, and across which no electric current passes. If a sufficient voltage is applied across the diode by connecting the N-side of the diode to the negative end of a circuit and the P-side to the positive end, the nonconducting zone at the N-P junction will actually lessen to the point where electric current can pass through the entire diode.

As the free electrons fill the holes in the diode, they move from a higher to a lower energy state with the difference in energy being released as electromagnetic radiation. To create a diode that functions primarily to produce light (i.e., a LED), the N- and P-materials are specifically chosen so that the energy difference corresponds to that of visible or IR photons as the free electrons enter the holes. Thus the spectral output of an LED depends critically on the specific N- and P-materials used to construct the diode.

Being small and compact, individual LEDs emit light within a relatively, narrow waveband and at low overall intensities. When configured in two-dimensional arrays a collection of multiple LEDs will generate sufficient visible or IR light to drive some photobiologic reactions. Unlike lasers, LED devices are not sufficiently powerful to photothermally target specific structures via selective photothermolysis, but LEDs have been successfully used for driving photochemical reactions in photodynamic therapy (10). The role of LEDs will likely expand in dermatology as devices that emit in the UV range become practically available.

LED arrays have been advocated for use in so-called low intensity photobiologic reactions, particularly photojuvenation (11). The exact clinical and scientific basis for these claims has not yet been rigorously tested.

INTERACTIONS BETWEEN RADIATION SOURCES AND THE SKIN

In essence, exposing the skin to any radiation source is synonymous with applying energy to the skin. In order for photon energy to have any biologic and therapeutic effect on the skin, two essential processes must occur. First, the light must somehow reach the intended target structure within the skin and then, once there, the photon must be absorbed by a chromophore within or near the target. Achieving the first step, propagating light through the skin, requires an understanding of the optical properties of the skin, whereas the events that occur subsequent to photon absorption is, generally, considered under the rubric of photobiology.

TISSUE OPTICS AND THE PROPAGATION OF LIGHT THROUGH THE SKIN

Until it interacts with the skin in some way, light that passes directly through any tissue component is said to be transmitted. Most light does, eventually, interact directly with the skin in one of three ways: reflection, scattering, or absorption. Reflection occurs at the skin surface and can provide information about the topography of the skin. At any level in the skin, the direction of light propagation can be physically altered through scattering. Multiple scattering events can occur for any given photon and in any direction. The effect of scattering is greatest in the dermis where collagen is the most important light scattering material. The probability of scattering is wavelength dependent, and between the UV through near IR regions, lower wavelength photons are scattered to a greater extent, denoting that longer wavelength light penetrates more deeply in the skin. Only light that reaches the target can be absorbed and, yet, the probability of absorption will depend on the absorption spectrum of the chromophore in accordance with quantum theory. Once absorbed a photon no longer exists and its energy is transferred to the chromophore which, in turn, is promoted to an excited state. Subsequent release of the energy with return of the chromophore to the ground state will drive photobiologic reactions and phenomena.

Clinical examination of the skin in dermatology fundamentally relies on complex perceptual and cognitive processes by which the overall interplay of tissue-optical effects, as manifested in the visual appearance of skin lesions, are used to render diagnoses. Clinical morphology therefore exploits the effects that skin has on light. In contrast, phototherapeutics is focused primarily on the effects of light on the skin.

PHOTOBIOLOGY AND THE SKIN

Photobiologic reactions can result in skin disease or be used to treat the skin. Specific clinical details are described throughout this book. Although the range of light-dependent reactions is diverse, they must all be initiated by chromophore absorption of photons. Subsequent relaxation of excited chromophores to the ground state releases the stored energy to (*i*) drive chemical reactions, (*ii*) produce heat, or (*iii*) re-emit light. The vast majority of photobiologic reactions that occur in clinical dermatology are presumed to involve photochemical processes. In some instances such as photodynamic therapy, PUVA, or drug-induced photosensitivity the detailed photochemistry is very well characterized and understood, whereas for idiopathic photodermatoses and UV phototherapy the exact photochemical links between light absorption and the clinical effects or outcome are largely speculative. For example, the putative chromophore and chemical reactions that underlie UVB phototherapy have still not been resolved with any certainty.

In terms of pathologic photothermal effects, erythema ab igne is probably one of the few examples where heat produced in the skin through photon absorption (i.e., infrared) leads to a specific skin disorder. In dermatology, photothermal effects are more commonly encountered on the therapeutic side when lasers or IPLs are used to irreversibly heat specific structures in the skin through selective photothermolysis.

The re-emission of absorbed light by the skin is termed fluorescence and this is the third possible path by which excited chromophores discharge their absorbed energy. Pathologically or therapeutically, there are no clinical examples of skin diseases that result from or can be treated by cutaneous fluorescence. The importance of fluorescence in the skin primarily lies in its use for diagnosis. The Wood's lamp emits longwave UVA near 365 nm. Cutaneous fluorophores including collagen, elastin, and porphyrins will absorb the UVA, which is invisible and then re-emit fluorescent light at a longer wavelength, where it is visible to the human eye.

Photoaging and photocarcinogenesis are the result of chronic light exposure, and demonstrate that the skin has a finite capacity to repair damage resulting from repeated cycles of pathologic photobiologic reactions.

CHARACTERIZING RADIATION SOURCES: SPECTRAL IRRADIANCE

It is absolutely critical to recognize that any given light source is important only in terms of the quality and quantity of light that it delivers to the skin. Thus, when we refer to "fluorescent" or "laser" light we are really referring only to the method by which the light was produced. A photon is a photon—the skin does not truly care what particular light source a photon came from, only that the photon that it receives is of the appropriate wavelength and that a sufficient number of photons are delivered at an appropriate rate. A plethora of light sources are commercially available to meet specific photobiologic (e.g., selective photothermolysis, photochemistry), clinical (e.g., localized vs. diffuse treatment areas), and practical (e.g., cost and efficiency) needs. There is also a certain degree of redundancy amongst radiation sources since certain specific spectral regions of interest can be produced by more than one type of radiation source. For example, the 311 narrow band UVB lamp, the UV excimer laser, and the incoherent monochromatic excimer light source all function as "narrow band" UVB sources.

The correct way to accurately characterize and compare light emitted from various radiation sources is to determine their emission spectra. In an emission spectrum, the irradiance of the source is measured and plotted as a function of wavelength. Figure 4 depicts the emission spectrum of a narrowband TL-01 UVB lamp. This lamp was engineered to produce light maximally at 311 nm. It is also apparent from the emission spectrum that other UV wavebands, including UVA, are emitted by this lamp (although not shown on the spectrum, some visible light is also produced by this lamp). The same holds true for UVA and broadband UVB lamps; they are not necessarily spectrally pure, and their nominal designation as being "UVA" or "UVB" light sources only refers to the fact that their spectral emission and biologic activity is predominantly that of a certain waveband. The emission spectrum of a light source is rarely measured directly in the clinical setting, since spectroradiometers are expensive. Fortunately for regular clinical use, commerical lamp manufactures maintain relatively consistent standards for lamp operating characteristics such as spectral emission.

In the research setting, spectral irradiance is often a critical factor that is overlooked in experiments involving light. Any photobiologic phenomenon can be attributed to a specific

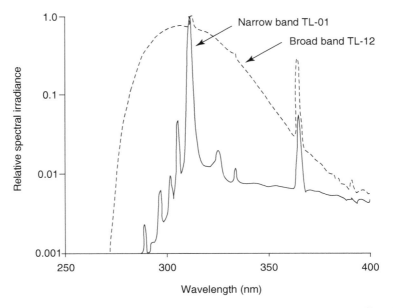

FIGURE 4 Spectral irradiance for a narrow band Phillips TL-01, 311 nm UVB fluorescent lamp. Note that the relative irradiance is shown on a logarithmic scale. *Source*: Adapted from Ref. 12.

waveband only if the spectral output of the light source used is reliably known. For example, although a certain light source may be emitting UVA, the small traces of UVB that may also be emitted may have a significant biologic effect since UVB can be more biologically active than UVA by several orders of magnitude.

Only certain wavelengths of light are efficient for inducing or producing the desired biologic or therapeutic effect and this relationship is best described through the action spectrum. Analogous to an absorption spectrum, which depicts the efficiency by which photons are absorbed by a chromophore according to wavelength, the action spectrum refers to the efficiency of a given photobiologic reaction occurring as a function of wavelength. Action spectra are usually plotted as the reciprocal photon numbers required for a photobiologic effect on the ordinate and wavelength on the abscissa. Photobiologic reactions occur most efficiently when there is a good match between the action spectrum and the spectral irradiance of the light source that is driving the reaction. Where the action spectrum is known, it is ideal for the spectral irradiance of the light source to match the action spectrum for maximal efficiency and also to prevent potential unwanted side reactions.

LIGHT DOSIMETRY AND THE SKIN

Radiation is measured in units of total energy, joules (J) or energy flux or power, watts (W). Since the skin surface is essentially two dimensional, it is customary to consider light that is incident on the skin in terms of its energy or power density per unit area. These are referred to as fluence or irradiance respectively, and in dermatology are generally measured in units of J/cm^2 or W/cm^2. Irradiance and fluence are mathematically related as follows:

Fluence = Irradiance × Light exposure duration

In the clinic, the irradiance is measured with a radiometer. For a specified delivered radiation dose, the duration of exposure can be calculated from the above formula. Each radiation source requires its own specific radiometer, since the spectral sensitivity should match the source's spectral output.

Light dosimetry is largely determined empirically in clinical practice. In general it is safest to start with subthreshold levels of light and then gradually increase the fluence with subsequent treatments. There is some degree of latitude in terms of the time duration over which the light exposure can be delivered because of the Bunsen-Roscoe law of light dose reciprocity. Basically, for any given delivered fluence there is a reciprocal relationship between the duration of exposure and the irradiance of the source. For example, if the irradiance is reduced by half, the same biologic or therapeutic effect will be achieved by doubling the exposure time. One very important exception to the law of reciprocity is the use of lasers to selectively heat the skin. Heat must be generated within a very narrow time frame otherwise selective photothermolysis will not occur.

CONCLUSIONS

Available technologies that collectively cover the photobiologically active spectrum include incandescent lamps, arc (gas discharge) lamps, fluorescent lamps, lasers, flashlamps, and light-emitting diodes. Choosing the ideal light source for therapeutic or diagnostic purposes is determined by the type of photobiologic reaction desired and by matching the action spectrum of the effect to the spectral irradiance of the light source. The area of skin that is to be irradiated as well as the cost and practicality of the radiation source are also paramount considerations.

REFERENCES

1. Food and Drug Administration. Sunscreen products for over-the-counter human use. Final monograph FR. Federal Register 1999; 64(98):27666–27693.
2. Roelandts R. The diagnosis of photosensitivity. Arch Dermatol 2000; 136:1152–1157.
3. Iversen Møller K, Kongshoj B, Philipsen PA, Thomsen VO, Wulf HC. How Finsen's light cured lupus vulgaris. Photodermatol Photoimmunol Photomed 2005; 21:118–124.
4. Mutzhas MF, Hölzle E, Hofmann C, Plewig G. A new apparatus with high radiation energy between 320–460 nm: physical description and dermatological applications. J Invest Dermatol 1981; 76:42–47.
5. DEKA M.E.L.A., Excilite Operator's Manual 2005, page II.2.
6. Van Weelden H, Baart de la Faille H, Young E, Van Der Leun JC. A new development in UVB phototherapy of psoriasis. Br J Dermatol 1988; 119:11–19.
7. Parrish JA, Jaenicke KF. Action spectrum for phototherapy of psoriasis. J Invest Dermatol 1981; 76:359–362.
8. Jeffes EW, McCullough JL, Weinstein GD, Kaplan R, Glazer SD, Taylor JR. Photodynamic therapy of actinic keratoses with topical aminolevulinic acid hydrochloride and fluorescent blue light. J Am Acad Dermatol 2001; 45:96–104.
9. Ross EV, Laser versus intense pulsed light: competing technologies in dermatology. Lasers Surg Med 2006; 38:261–272.
10. Lui H, Hobbs L, Tope WD, et al. Photodynamic therapy of multiple nonmelanoma skin cancers with verteporfin and red light-emitting diodes: two-year results evaluating tumor response and cosmetic outcomes. Arch Dermatol 2004; 140:26–32.
11. Weiss RA, McDaniel DH, Geronemus RG, et al. Clinical experience with light-emitting diode (LED) photomodulation. Dermatol Surg 2005; 31:1199–1205.
12. Das S, Lloyd JJ, Farr PM. Similar dose-response and peristence of erythema with broad-band and narrow-band ultraviolet B lamps. J Invest Dermatol 2001; 117:1318–1321.

4 | The Molecular and Genetic Effects of Ultraviolet Radiation Exposure on Skin Cells

Marjan Garmyn
Department of Dermatology, University of Leuven, Leuven, Belgium

Daniel B. Yarosh
Applied Genetics Incorporated Dermatics, Freeport, New York, U.S.A.

- Of the solar spectrum a small portion of UVB and more significant portion of UVA penetrates human skin.

- The main cellular chromophores for UV are DNA, RNA, and reactive oxygen species (ROS) generating chromophores.

- UVB mainly causes direct DNA damage, the common lesions being cyclobutane pyrimidine dimers (CPDs), while ROS production becomes more important with UVA.

- Ligand dependent or independent activation of cell surface receptors triggers of signal transduction pathways leading to transcription factor activation and modulation of gene expression.

- Cellular adaptive responses of skin against UV damage include growth arrest, DNA repair, and when damage is beyond repair, apoptosis.

INTRODUCTION

One of the greatest advances in photodermatology over the past decade is in the understanding of the molecular events that follow ultraviolet (UV) irradiation of skin. These studies have been able to trace the formation of skin cancer back to the initial absorption of a UV photon by a base in the DNA as a critical step. A range of other molecules that absorb UV are now connected to cellular responses. A vast network of intracellular signaling has been revealed, which remains an intense area of study. Communication between UV-damaged cells and both UV exposed and unexposed cells in the skin has been defined by their characteristic cytokine and growth factor proteins, and now the profiles of their concerted induction, release, and down-regulation are under investigation. The panorama of the molecular effects of UV radiation (UVR) is reviewed here.

ULTRAVIOLET DAMAGE
Ultraviolet A and Ultraviolet B: Energy and Penetration
Solar Ultraviolet

UVR from the sun reaching the earth's surface has wavelengths ranging from about 280 to about 400 nm. For convenience, this spectrum is divided into UVB (280–320 nm) and UVA wavelengths (320–400 nm). This convenience should not obscure the fact that all UVR, given in sufficient dose, can produce approximately the same biological effects in skin—whether it is DNA damage, lipid oxidation, or skin cancer. The difference between them is that the efficiency in producing one of these effects by photons at one wavelength is greater than that by photons of another wavelength. The relationship between a range of wavelengths and the efficiency for producing any biological endpoint is called an action spectrum. The shape and peak of the action spectrum give important information about chromophore(s)—the molecule(s) in skin that are responsible for absorbing the UVR and producing a biological effect. The converse is also true: for UVR to have an effect on skin, it must be absorbed by a molecule. Connecting molecules absorbing UVR to biological effects is a major goal of modern photodermatology.

UVR that strikes the skin deposits its energy as it travels into the skin. The shorter the wavelength, the more energetic the photons, and the more shallow in the skin the photons are absorbed. Thus, most UVB is absorbed in the epidermis, but some does reach the dermis. Conversely, longer wavelength UVA is partially absorbed in the epidermis, but a higher fraction than UVB penetrates deeper into the skin and reaches the dermis. However, because damaged epidermal cells release cytokines that communicate with dermal cells and damaged immune-competent cells migrate from the epidermis, it is overly simplistic to ascribe biological effects of UVB and UVA to higher or lower layers in skin simply on the basis of how far on average the wavelengths penetrate.

DNA Effects

A biologically important chromophore in skin is the DNA in living cells. DNA absorbs all wavelengths of UVR, but pure DNA has a peak of absorption at about 260 nm, and the action spectrum for DNA damage shows a logarithmic decline in absorption as the wavelengths grow longer. However, in order to reach DNA in skin, the UVR must travel to layers beneath the outermost stratum corneum, which absorbs and diffuses particularly well the shorter wavelengths of light. Therefore, the most efficient wavelengths of light for causing DNA damage in living skin is around 313 nm—shorter wavelengths are absorbed by stratum corneum and longer wavelengths are significantly less efficient in producing damage.

The part of DNA that most efficiently absorbs UV is the 5-6 double bond of the pyrimidine bases. When one of two adjacent pyrimidines absorbs a photon here, the most common result is the instantaneous formation of a cyclobutane ring linking the two pyrimidines at the 5 and 6 position—this is called a cyclobutane pyrimidine dimer (CPD). Occasionally, a bond between the adjacent pyrimidines is formed through a 6-4 linkage, which is called the pyrimidine–pyrimidone photoproduct. From experiments with cultured cells, it has been estimated that CPDs are 20 to 40 times more frequent than any other DNA photoproduct after irradiation with simulated sunlight (1).

Aside from these direct effects of UVR, DNA damage can form by indirect effects, particularly from oxidation. UVR absorbed by as yet poorly defined chromophores in skin can generate oxygen radicals that react with DNA. The most vulnerable place in DNA is oxidation of the 8 position of guanine, yielding 8-oxo-guanine (8oG). Another detectible oxidized base is the thymine glycol. UVA, which produces relatively more oxidation damage than photoproducts when compared with UVB, still produces three to six times more CPD than 8oG in DNA (2). Single- or double-stranded breaks are uncommon events resulting from UVR.

DNA is repaired by a complex of proteins and enzymes that organize together at the site of damage (3). DNA that has sustained bulky lesions or lesions that distort its structure (such as a CPD) is repaired by nucleotide excision repair (NER), in which approximately 29 bases are replaced.

DNA that has modified bases (such as 8oG) is repaired by base excision repair, which replaces only the damaged base and a few neighboring bases. In either case, the opposite undamaged strand of DNA is used as a template to resynthesize the DNA sequence. This type of DNA repair occurs at anytime nearly anywhere in the genome [global genomic repair (GGR)]. However, localized regions of transcribed DNA are repaired much faster by a group of proteins performing transcription-coupled repair (TCR). They are attracted to the site by a transcription fork that has stalled, and TCR accelerates repair of the transcribed strand. If a lesion is not repaired by the time the DNA must be replicated, damage-specific polymerases eta or zeta can insert bases to allow continued replication in a process called translesion synthesis (4). If all these measures fail and too much DNA damage remains, the cell activates a suicide pathway call apoptosis.

During the repair or replication of DNA damage, erroneous bases, additions, deletions, or rearrangements are inserted at a frequency of approximately one in a million, or more frequently if the cell relies on the very error-prone polymerase zeta for translesion synthesis. Because of the large amount of unused DNA and the redundancy of the genetic code, these mutations often make no difference. However, mutations introduced at certain sequence locations in key genes, called oncogenes or tumor-suppressor genes, can contribute to the formation of a cancer cell. The best-studied example is the p53 tumor-suppressor gene in squamous cell carcinoma. This product of this gene, which has been called the "guardian of the genome," organizes many of the cells responses to UVR, including repair, cell division, and apoptosis. Squamous cell carcinomas from sun-exposed skin frequently have mutations in the p53 gene, and these mutations are characteristic of those induced by CPDs (5). Mutations in key genes leading to both basal cell carcinoma and melanoma are also similar to these signature mutations. This is among the strongest evidence directly linking UVR-induced DNA damage to skin cancer.

Lipid Effects

The action spectrum for UV effects in skin does not correlate with the absorption spectrum of lipids. However, UVR directly and indirectly damages the free lipids in the stratum corneum and the lipid membranes of living cells by generating reactive oxygen species (ROS). Over the course of a summer, the generation of ROS depletes the endogenous antioxidant system in the stratum corneum (5). ROS oxidize lipids by directly oxidizing their double bonds or by initiating a chain reaction of one oxidized lipid reacting with another. In living cells, the damaged membranes are processed by nonenzymatic and enzymatic mechanisms. Keratinocyte membranes damaged by singlet oxygen release ceramides by a nonenzymatic reaction, and these signal activation of transcription factor activator protein-1 (AP-1), resulting in expression of many stress response genes, for example, intercellular adhesion molecule-1 and vascular endothelial growth factor (5). Oxidized lipids in the membranes of keratinocytes are cleaved by phospholipase A_2 (PLA_2) to form arachidonic acid, which is the substrate of cyclo-oxygenase-1 and the inducible form-2 (COX-1 and COX-2) (5). These enzymes convert arachidonic acid into prostaglandins, which mediate many inflammatory reactions in the skin and elsewhere.

Protein Effects

Proteins in skin may also be oxidized by ROS generated from sunlight. However, since most types of proteins occur in multiples and are constantly degraded and resynthesized, the consequences may not be as severe. Enzymes from the family of methionine sulfoxide reductases patrol the epidermis and keeps protein oxidation levels very low by degrading oxidized proteins, even in chronically UV-exposed skin (5). UVR may also directly crosslink proteins, particularly collagen and elastin in the dermis and even cause them to degrade. However, the primary cause of degradation is probably not a direct effect of UVR, but rather due to the production by fibroblasts of proteases that digest the surrounding collagen and elastin (5).

Proteins that have been proposed as chromophores for many of the effects of UVR are cell surface receptors. UVR causes these receptors to cluster even without binding ligands (5). Receptor clustering is a well-known mechanism for transfer of extracellular signals into cellular activation. For example, UVB-induced clustering of the CD95 receptors activates these death receptors and leads to apoptosis, independently of nuclear DNA damage (5). UV has also been proposed to inactivate protein tyrosine phosphatases, which results in their target proteins remaining phosphorylated (5). The persistence of phosphorylated forms of key signaling molecules may result in prolonged activation of damage response pathways, such as metalloproteinase (MMP) production or immune suppression.

ULTRAVIOLET-INDUCED SIGNALING AND GENE REGULATION
Cytokines and Soluble Factors

UV exposure changes the cytokine profile within the epidermis. Keratinocytes are the main source of these cytokines. Other epidermal cells, such as Langerhans cells (LHC) and melanocytes, together with infiltrating leukocytes are also active contributors to changed cytokine profile after UV exposure. Keratinocytes are able to secrete a wide variety of pro-inflammatory cytokines upon UV exposure, including interleukins IL-1α, IL-1β, IL-3, IL-6, IL-8, granulocytes colony stimulating factor (G-CSF), macrophage-CSF (GM-CSF), interferon gamma, (INF-γ), platelet-derived growth factor (PDGF), transforming growth factor alpha (TGF-α), TGF-β, and tumor necrosis factor alpha (TNF-α) (6–8).

The processes that regulate cytokine production by UV are complex. Nuclear factor kappa B (NFkB) is an important transcription factor regulating cytokine gene expression by UV, whereas the protein kinase p38 (a member of the MAPK family of protein kinases) is known to mediate the expression of cytokine-encoding genes by events ranging from transcriptional and translational control to mRNA stability (9). Both ROS-mediated and direct DNA damage have been implicated in the production of the primary cytokine TNF-α (10,11).

These cytokines, induced by UV, can then act in a paracrine or autocrine way to stimulate intracellular signaling and gene expression. Hence, cytokines like IL-1, TNF-α, and TGF-β can bind to their respective receptors in the cell membrane and initiate signal transduction (12).

Nitric oxide (NO) is produced by keratinocytes after UVB irradiation (13), and keratinocytes express the enzyme required to synthesize NO. Increased expression of mRNA for inducible NO synthetase has been detected in skin exposed to UV light (14). NO reacts with superoxide to form peroxynitrite, which is a potent activator of various signaling pathways, including the MAPK (15) and tyrosine kinase signaling cascades (16). Peroxynitrite can also activate transcription factors including NFkB (17). NO is also involved in the inflammatory response leading to vasodilation and erythema (13) and in the tanning response (18).

Urocanic acid (UCA) is a naturally occurring component of the superficial cornified epidermis. It is synthesized as a *trans*-isomer, which contains an acyclic carbon–carbon double bound and absorbs in the UVB range. Upon absorption of UVB light, *trans*-UCA isomerizes to *cis*-UCA, which can induce immune suppression (19). Although the mechanisms by which UCA initiates biological activity are not known, there is evidence that absorption of UV light by the chemical can generate ROS (20).

UV can also stimulate the release of lipid mediators such as the prostaglandin, PGE_2, platelet-activating factor, and sphingolipid ceramide (21). Released PGE_2 and platelet-activating factor can mediate their biological activities via highly specific membrane receptor-initiated signaling (22,23). Inhibitors of PG synthesis, including indomethacin and aspirin, have been shown to decrease (but not completely suppress) the erythemal response, providing evidence for the involvement of PG in UV-induced erythema.

Cell Surface Receptor Activation

UVB-induced cytokines and growth factors can bind to their respective receptors and by this activate downstream signal transduction pathways; however, UVB can also activate multiple cell surface receptors in a ligand-independent way, including CD95/Fas (24), the TNF-alpha receptor (TNF-αR), the interleukin-1 (IL-1) receptor, the epidermal growth factor (EGF) receptor (25), the insulin receptor (26), the PDGF receptor (27), and the KGF receptor (28).

UVB induces clustering of these membrane receptors and subsequent activation of downstream signaling pathways (24,25). Aragane showed that UVB radiation induces CD95 clustering. Rosette and Karin showed that UVB induced TNF clustering and its association with TNFR1-associated death domain. Tobin et al. (29) showed that UVB was able to functionally activate the TNF-1 receptor by activating TNF receptor associated factor-2 (TRAF-2). How UVB leads to clustering and activation of the cell surface receptors remains unclear. Physical perturbation of the plasma membrane (secondary to lipid peroxidation) or conformational changes of the receptor, caused by energy absorption or oxidation, are possible explanations.

Activation of the EGF receptor by UV light can not only be observed in human keratinocytes in vitro but also in human skin in vivo (30).

Protein Kinase-Mediated Signal Transduction

Ligand-dependent or ligand-independent activation of cell surface receptors triggers off signal transduction pathways that may result in the activation of transcription factors and ultimately modulation of gene expression. This subsequent downstream signaling triggered off by UV-induced receptor activation and leading to transcription factor activation is called the "UV response." Protein kinases, which activate their downstream targets via phosphorylation, play an important role in signal transduction. Two important groups of protein kinases are involved in the UV response: the MAPK family of protein kinases and a group directly implicated in the genome integrity checkpoint, such as ATR, Chk2, and DNA-PK.

The MAPK family of protein kinases is known to respond to stress, such as membrane damage and oxidative stress, and play an important role in the UV response. MAPK includes the extracellular signal-regulated kinases (ERKs), the c-Jun NH2-terminal kinases (JNKs) and the p38 MAPK. p38 MAPK has four isoforms (α, β, γ, and δ), JNK has three isoforms (1/2/3), and ERK has two isoforms (1/2). All three groups of MAPKs are activated by dual phosphorylation on threonine and tyrosine by one or more MAPK kinases (MAPKKs). These MAPKKs are in turn phosphorylated and activated by MAPKK kinases (MAPKKK) (31). JNKs and p38 kinases are activated by stress, including UVB. ERKs are typically activated by growth factors, and UVB is only a weak activator of ERK in keratinocytes (32).

UVB also activates the phosphoinositide 3-kinase (PI3K) pathway in an ERK and p38 kinase-dependent mechanism (33). In human keratinocytes, activation of PI3K and its downstream target, the anti-apoptotic kinase, Akt, are also thought to be dependent on the activation of EGF receptors (34). The mechanisms mediating MAPK activation by UV may occur through binding of growth factors or cytokines to their receptors or may occur through ligand-independent receptor activation, which may or may not involve UV-induced oxidative stress. Recent studies indicate that MAP kinase activation, more specifically JNK and p38 signaling, can also occur via growth factor and growth factor receptor independent mechanism, via the ribotoxic stress response (35,36).

A second group of protein kinases (ATR, Chk2, DNA-PK,) is implicated in the genome integrity checkpoint, a molecular cascade that detects and responds to several forms of DNA damage caused by genotoxic stress (37). ATR (ATM-Rad3-related kinase) is a primary DNA sensor and essential for UV-induced phosphorylation of several G1/S checkpoint proteins. ATR was also shown to bind UVB-damaged DNA, with a resulting increase in its kinase activity towards p53 (38). Activated p53 in turn is known to orchestrate DNA damage response pathways, including cell cycle arrest, DNA repair, and apoptosis, as discussed later.

Stalled DNA Replication and RNA Transcription

The UV-induced CPDs and pyrimidine (6-4) pyrimidone photoproducts cause distortions in the DNA helix and halt RNA polymerase (RNAP) elongation along DNA, thus inhibiting gene expression but also leading to recruitment of the NER complex (referred to as GGR), which repair these helix distorting DNA photoproducts.

DNA lesions on the actively transcribed strands have been shown to arrest RNA-PII, and thereby inhibit transcript cleavage. The active repression of transcription initiation occurs by phosphorylation of RNA-PII. This stalled RNAP-II would, on the one hand, lead to fast recruitment of the NER complex (referred to as TCR), but, on the other hand, interact with p53 resulting in stabilization and accumulation of the p53 protein.

TCR occurs fast, in a gene-dependent manner, and only repairs the template strand of transcriptionally active DNA. GGR occurs slower, repairing also the nontemplate strand and the nontranscribed areas. Cell survival depends more on TCR than GGR, but genomic integrity is more influenced by GGR (39,40).

Transcription Factors (p53, AP-1, and NFKB)

Three transcription factors are strongly implicated in the UV response: p53, AP-1, and NFkB. p53 is a tumor suppressor protein and is the most frequent target for mutations in human cancer. p53 is mutated in approximately 50% of all cancers, and this frequency increases to more than 90% in squamous cell carcinoma of the skin. The importance of wild-type p53 in the regulation of the response to stress, and more specifically the UVB response, is ascribed predominantly to its ability to transactivate a plethora of genes with an active role in either cell cycle arrest, global genomic DNA repair, or apoptosis. p53 becomes activated in response to a myriad of stress types, which includes but is not limited to DNA damage (induced by either UV, IR, or chemical agents). This activation is marked by two major events. First, the half-life of the p53 protein is increased drastically, leading to a quick accumulation of p53 in stressed cells. Secondly, a conformational change forces p53 to take on an active role as a transcriptional regulator in these stressed cells. The critical event leading to p53 activation is phosphorylation of its N-terminal domain, which contains a large number of phosphorylation sites and can be considered as the primary target for kinases transducing stress signals. Both the MAPK family of protein kinases and a group of kinases, directly implicated in the genome integrity checkpoint such as ATR, are known to target the transcriptional activation domain of p53 (39,41).

NFkB is a ubiquitously expressed transcription factor that belongs to the Re1 family and regulates genes involved in inflammation, immunity, cell cycle progression, apoptosis, and oncogenesis. The NFkB transcription factors are regulated through interaction with their inhibitor IkB that sequesters them in the cytoplasm. NFkB can be activated by a wide range of stimuli, including UV light. Most signals that activate NFkB stimulate directly or indirectly the phosphorylation of IkB by IkB kinase (IKK), thereby increasing their susceptibility to ubiquitin-dependent degradation (42), leading to the translocation of NFKB to the nucleus and transcriptional activation of target. The mechanism of NFkB activation by UV radiation does not exactly conform to this established pathway in that the ubiquitin dependence of degradation of IkB occurs relatively late and does not depend on its phosphorylation on the usual N-terminal serine residues nor on the activation of IKK (43).

Pathways responsible for NFkB activation by UVB in keratinocytes and skin are complex, and over the years, several molecular mechanisms have been suggested. NFkB activation by

UVB can occur independent of DNA damage (44). Adachi (45) showed that in normal human keratinocytes, UVB can activate NFkB, but the pathway does not involve IKK. It has also been shown that NFkB can be activated by UVB via NADPH oxidase and COX, which activate ROS (46). Additionally, UVB can cause a rapid association of TNF receptor 1 with its downstream partner TRAF-2, which leads to NFkB activation in keratinocytes (29). It has also been suggested that UV radiation causes the release of TNF-α in normal human keratinocytes, which can activate NFkB (47). NFkB is an important transcription factor for cytokines and can, in this way, regulate the pro-inflammatory and immunomodulatory effects of UVB. NFkB has also been ascribed a role in regulating UVB-induced apoptosis; however, both pro- and anti-apoptotic roles have been ascribed to NFkB (43,48).

AP-1 is not a single transcription factor, but instead a series of related dimeric complexes of Fos and Jun family proteins. Changes in AP-1 activity due to changes in the expression of AP-1 family members, post-translational modification, or both occur in response to a wide variety of signals including UV light. Both the ERK and JNK pathways are important signaling pathways leading to AP-1 activation; AP-1 activation by GF is at least partly regulated by ERK pathway. The JNK pathway is an important signaling pathway leading to AP-1 activation upon UV radiation (49). The transcription factor AP1 plays an important role in UVB-induced photoaging, as it regulates several ECM proteins (e.g., matrix MMPs and type I procollagen) (50) and UVB-induced skin tumor promotion (51). Both pro- and anti-apoptotic affects have been attributed to UV-induced AP-1 activation as reviewed by Assefa et al. (43).

Transcriptional Responses to UV

DNA microarrays have allowed a large-scale analysis of transcriptional response of skin cells to UV. Different factors may influence the transcriptional targets of UV, including wavelength, dose, cell type, and the time of expression after irradiation. Hence, keratinocytes, melanocytes, and fibroblasts have, in general, similar transcriptional targets involving DNA damage repair, cell cycle arrest, and/or apoptotic machinery, whereas transcriptional responses of immunomodulatory factors seem overlapping but distinct. The dose applied also affects the transcriptional response. Indeed, UV doses causing cell cycle arrest of apoptosis provoke transcriptionally highly divergent responses. Downregulation of transcription is very prominent in apoptotic cells. However, UV-induced repression of transcription is also specific, as the targets downregulated by a low dose of UV are different from those downregulated by a high apoptotic dose (40). Specifically, for p53-regulated genes, a low UVB dose resulting in survival induces genes involved in cell cycle arrest and repair, such as p21 and p53R2, whereas the same genes are downregulated after a high UVB dose (52). Genes also follow a specific time course; for example, genes involved in cell cycle arrest are first upregulated, whereas genes involved in cytoskeleton are first downregulated or unchanged, then upregulated later, reflecting the recovery of UVB-damaged cellular activities (53).

A recent study by Enk et al. found that UVB-induced gene expression profile of human epidermis in vivo is different from that of cultured keratinocytes. The expression profile in intact epidermis was geared mainly towards repair, whereas cultured keratinocytes responded predominantly by activating genes associated with cell cycle arrest and apoptosis, which may reflect differences between mature differentiating keratinocytes in the suprabasal layers and exponentially proliferating cells in culture (54).

CELLULAR RESPONSES
Cell Types in Skin (Keratinocytes, Fibroblasts, Melanocytes, and T-Cells)

The skin is composed of three layers: the epidermis, the dermis, and the subcutis. The epidermis is a stratified squamous epithelium and its prime function is to act as a skin barrier. This skin barrier function is continuously challenged by environmental hazards, the most ubiquitous of which is UV in sunlight. The three main cell populations in the epidermis are the keratinocytes, the melanocytes, and the LHC. The basal layer of the epidermis consists of keratinocytes that are either dividing or nondividing and is secured to the basement membrane by hemidesmosome. During the upward migration of keratinocytes, from the proliferative basal layer through the spinous and granular layer, keratinocytes undergo terminal differentiation ultimately leading to anuclear corneocytes, continuously desquamating into the environment.

The melanocytes make 5% to 10% of the basal cell population. These cells synthesize melanin and transfer it via the dendritic processes to the neighboring melanocytes. The epidermis has an important immunological function. The LHC are involved in the cellular immunity. They are dendritic bone marrow derived cells characterized by the Birbreck granules. They play an important role in antigen presentation. The T-lymphocytes are believed to circulate through normal skin where they are thought to mature to helper, delayed hypersensitivity, cytotoxic, and suppressor T cells. Keratinocytes are part of the innate immune system of the skin, since they can produce themselves pro-inflammatory cytokines and express on their surface immune-reactive molecules such as MHC class II antigens and intercellular adhesion molecules.

The dermis consists of an upper part, pars papillaris, which lies immediately below the epidermis, and a deeper part, the pars reticularis. The dermis contains fibroblasts (which synthesize collagen, elastin, and glycosaminoglycans), dermal dendrocytes, mast cells, macrophages, and lymphocytes.

Cell Cycle Arrest

One of the cellular responses to UVB-induced damage is the induction of cell cycle arrest, both in the G1 and G2 phases. These checkpoints allow DNA damage to be repaired before DNA replication (G1/S checkpoint) or before chromosome segregation (G2/M checkpoint). The cyclin-dependent kinase inhibitor p21/WAF1 is a direct target of p53 and an important mediator of the G1 arrest (39). The involvement of cdk inhibitor p21 in a G1 arrest upon UVB in keratinocytes has been demonstrated (55,56). p21 mediates cell cycle arrest by binding to and inactivating Cyclin D/cdk4 and Cyclin D/cdk6, thereby inhibiting phosphorylation of the retinoblastoma protein, essential for G1-S transition. C/EBPa, a p53-regulated UVB-inducible gene, has also a critical function in G1 checkpoint response (57).

Arrest in the G2 phase involves other p53-dependent factors, including 14-3-3 sigma (58) and GADD45 (growth arrest and DNA damage inducible gene) (59). GADD45 promotes G2/M arrest via nuclear export and kinase activity of Cdc2. Also p53-independent mechanisms (60) are involved in UVB-induced growth arrest.

Apoptosis

Apoptosis is a conserved, energy-requiring and highly regulated form of cell death that ensures the elimination of superfluous, infected, irreparably damaged, or transformed cells. Apoptosis is induced by various stress conditions including genotoxic damage, such as UVB.

The apoptotic process itself is characterized by stereotypical morphological changes such as cell shrinkage, membrane blebbing, chromatin condensation, and DNA fragmentation, leading to a cell with a pycnotic nucleus, and ultimately the formation of apoptotic bodies. Hence, when skin is irradiated with a sufficient high UVB dose, cells with pycnotic nucleus and eosinophilic cytoplasm, a typical apoptotic morphology, also called "the sunburn cell" (SBC), appear in the epidermis. At the biochemical level, the induction of apoptotic cell death is accomplished by specialized cellular machinery where a family of cysteine proteases, the caspases, play a central role. There are two main pathways leading to apoptotic cell death. The intrinsic pathway is activated at the mitochondria. Death-inducing signals (including DNA damage) promote BAX-dependent release of cytochrome C, which together with Apaf-1 leads to formation of the apoptosome and procaspase 9 activation. In contrast, signaling through the cell surface death receptor (e.g., CD95/Fas, TNF-alphaR) activates the extrinsic pathway, which relies on initiator caspase-8 activation at the death-inducing signaling complex. Both pathways converge into the activation of the effector caspases (caspases-3, -6, and -7) that are directly responsible for the cleavage of cellular proteins resulting in the characteristic morphology of apoptosis. Cleavage of Bid by caspase-8 allows crosstalk between both pathways.

UV-induced cell death has been proposed to involve three processes contributing independently to the activation of the intrinsic and the extrinsic apoptotic pathways. These three processes are DNA damage, membrane receptor clustering, and formation of ROS (61). Recent studies, however, indicate that irradiating keratinocytes with physiologically relevant UVB doses induce apoptosis mainly through the intrinsic pathway (62).

Molecular determinants/signalling pathways regulating cell death in UVB-irradiated keratinocytes are the p53 protein, p38, Fas/Fas-L, and the apoptosome (43). Molecular determinants counteracting UVB-induced apoptosis are Bcl-2, surviving AKT, and NFkB (63). SBC's main function is to reduce the risk of malignant transformation, following the tenet "better death than wrong." Which death route in SBC is engaged depends on the keratinocyte's state, UVB dose, and on the balanced presence of survival and death factors in the keratinocyte microenvironment. UVB-induced cell death in murine skin and cultured human keratinocytes, for example, requires p53 in the differentiating population, whereas p53 or p53-regulated proteins rather enhance DNA repair and not apoptosis in the basal layer, to maintain the proliferative potential of this cellular compartment (64). This assumption is reinforced by the observation that p53 knockdown by siRNA in normal proliferating keratinocytes does not prevent apoptosis but enhances cell sensitivity to UVB-induced cell death, whereas it delays the onset of confluence-induced senescence (65).

Vitamin D Production

The cutaneous photosynthesis of vitamin D_3 represents the main source of vitamin D in humans. It is formed from 7-dehydrocholesterol (7-DHC of provitamin D_3), which is present in large amounts in the cell membranes of keratinocytes of the basal and spinous epidermal layers. By the action of UVB light, the B ring of 7-DHC can be broken to form previtamin D_3. Previtamin D_3 has a very low affinity for vitamin D binding protein (DBP), precluding its entrance into the circulation. In the lipid bilayer of the membranes, the unstable previtamin D_3 is further isomerized to vitamin D_3 by thermal energy. The conformational change due to this isomerization can project vitamin D3 into the circulation, where it is caught by DBP and transported to the liver and kidney for further metabolization to 1,25D3 (66). Epidermal keratinocytes not only produce vitamin D_3, but also express CYP27A1, CYP2R1, and CYP27B1, enabling them to convert vitamin D_3 via 25D_3 to 1,25D_3 (67,68).

Vitamin D is a well-known antioxidant in skin, with also an important role in calcium metabolism. A growing body of evidence shows a reduction in different types of cancers after intake of vitamin D supplements. Regarding this, UV irradiation might be part of cancer therapy via elevation of vitamin D levels (69). In addition, results indicate that vitamin D_3 has photoprotective characteristics not related to its endogenous antioxidant property (70). Consequently, addition of vitamin D_3 to cell culture medium leads to heightened viability, reduced CPD, and less SBC formation after UV irradiation. This protection appears to be dependent on the dose and the duration of vitamin D exposure and is at least partially a consequence of a vitamin D-induced growth arrest (70–72).

Melanocyte Tanning Responses

Melanocytes are pigment-producing cells that are found in the basal layer of the epidermis and disperse melanosomes, containing melanin, among the surrounding keratinocytes. These melanosomes encapsulate two main classes of pigment found in human skin: eumelanin, which is brown or black, and pheomelanin, which is reddish-brown. The relative amounts of these two pigments and the size and density of the melanosomes largely determine the differences in skin color among humans. Skin color has an enormous effect on the risk of skin cancer because this constitutive melanin absorbs and reflects a broad spectrum of UVR.

Some skin types respond to UVR by increasing pigment production, what we recognize as a tanning response (73). The molecular signal-initiating tanning is not well understood, but it has been suggested to be related to DNA damage or repair (74). Binding of α-melanocyte stimulating hormone to melanocytes also stimulates increased melanin production by a pathway that includes NO, cGMP, and protein kinase G (75). NO donors or compounds that stimulate NO production also increase tanning (75).

Unfortunately, the tanning response does not contribute as much photoprotection as is generally thought. The sun protection factor of a tan is in the range of only 2 to 3 (73). This may be because the melanin produced in a tan is widely distributed throughout the epidermis and is slowly sloughed off over a week or so as the tan fades. In contrast, constitutive melanin is deposited as "caps" over the nuclei of keratinocytes, guaranteeing that the genetic material is well protected.

Wound-Healing Response

It is not possible to get a full picture of the molecular responses to UVR by studying the effects on individual cells or one cell type. Certainly, UVR directly induces responses in irradiated cells. However, damaged cells also communicate with each other, as well as with undamaged cells, by means of cytokines and growth factors. For example, UVR damages the DNA of keratinocytes as well as other chromophores, which then activates transcription factors, such as AP-1, AP-2, and NF-kappa B. These in turn increase the gene expression of many genes including those for proteolytic enzymes that degrade collagen and elastin. Some of these gene products are cytokines and growth factors that are released and travel to other cells such as IL-10 and TNFα that alter the immune response of T-cells in the epidermis (whether or not these cells have been irradiated) (76).

The emerging view is that photoaging is the result of repeated microscopic wound-healing responses, which over time coalesce into "solar scars" (77). UVR signals directly to fibroblasts, but also signals from damaged keratinocytes, causes the release of MMP-1, which selectively degrade large collagen cables (78). As part of this response, MMP-2 and -9, which are responsible for digesting small collagen fragments, are downregulated by UVR. This results in the accumulation of collagen fragments, which severs the anchorage of fibroblasts and inhibits their ability to produce new collagen. Repeated rounds of this type of imperfect wound healing produces many of the microscopic hallmarks of photoaged skin.

CONCLUSIONS

A small fraction of the high-energy UVB (280–320 nm) and a significant portion of the UVA (320–400 nm) reach the earth's surface and penetrate the human skin. Most of the UVB wavelengths are absorbed in the epidermis, whereas UVA penetrates deeper into the skin and reaches the dermis. These wavelengths cause damage to DNA, proteins, and lipids and modulate cell signaling and gene expression. The main cellular chromophores for UV are DNA, RNA, and ROS generating chromophores. The nucleic acids of DNA contain strongly absorbing chromophores for UVB, the most common result being the CPDs. Activation and synthesis of many genes are associated with the formation of DNA photoproducts as they trigger repair processes. UV light-induced damage to RNA has also been identified as a potential mediator of signaling that can lead to changes in gene expression. UV produces also ROS through interaction with endogenous photosensitizers. UVB can produce some amount of ROS; however, UV-induced ROS production becomes more important with UVA. These ROS can in turn damage proteins, membranes, and DNA and are important triggers for signaling pathways modulating gene expression.

UV-induced release of cytokines and growth factors which bind to their respective receptors are also important triggers of gene expression. UV can also directly activate these receptors in ligand-independent way. Direct or indirect activation of these GF and cytokine receptors subsequently may lead to MAPK signaling and activation of transcription factors, such as AP-1 and NFkB, known as the UV response.

Cellular adaptive responses to UV damage include growth arrest, repair, and, when damage is beyond repair, apoptosis. Hence, apoptosis can be considered as a fail-safe mechanism to avoid replication of cells with damaged DNA. The tumor suppressor p53 plays an important role in this response, which aims at safeguarding the genomic integrity of the cell. The epidermis not only photosynthesizes vitamin D_3 but is also able to convert it to 1,25 vitamin D_3. Vitamin D_3 has photoprotective characteristics related both to its endogenous antioxidant property and to its capacity to induce growth arrest. UV-induced melanogenesis is another important photoprotective response of the epidermis.

REFERENCES

1. Yoon J.-H, Lee C.-S, O'Connor TR, et al. The DNA damage spectrum produced by simulated sunlight. J Mol Biol 2000; 299:681–693.
2. Courdavault S, Baudouin C, Chreveron M, et al. Larger yield of cyclobutane dimers than 8-oxo-7,8-dihydroguanine in the DNA of UVA-irradiated human skin cells. Mutat Res 2004; 556:135–142.
3. Sancar A, Lindsey-Boltz L, Unsal-Kacmaz K, et al. Molecular mechanisms of mammalian DNA repair and the DNA damage checkpoints. Ann Rev Biochem 2004; 73:39–85.
4. Cleaver J. Common pathways for ultraviolet skin carcinogenesis in the repair and replication defective groups of xeroderma pigmentosum. J Dermatol Sci 2000; 23(1):1–11.
5. Ziegler A, Jonason AS, Leffell DJ, et al. Sunburn and p53 in the onset of skin cancer. Nature 1994; 372: 773–776.
6. Ansel J, Perry P, Brown J, et al. Cytokine modulation of keratinocyte cytokines. J Invest Dermatol 1990; 94:101S–107S.
7. Luger TA, Schwarz T. Evidence for an epidermal cytokine network. J Invest Dermatol 1990; 95:100S–104S.
8. Enk AH, Katz SI. Early molecular events in the induction phase of contact sensitivity. Proc Natl Acad Sci USA 1992, 89:1398–1402.
9. Hildesheim J, Fornace AJ Jr. Invited Mini Review: the dark side of light: the damaging effects of UV rays and the protective efforts of MAP kinase signalling in the epidermis. DNA Repair 200; 3:567–580.
10. Yarosh D, Both D, Kibital J, et al. Regulation of TNFα production and release in human and mouse keratinocytes and mouse skin after UV-B irradiation. Photodermatol Photoimmunol Photomed 2000; 16:263–270.
11. Pupe A, Degreef H, Garmyn M. Induction of tumor necrosis factor-alpha by UVB: a role for reactive oxygen intermediates and eicosanoids. Photochem Photobiol. 2003; 78(1):68–74.
12. Heck DE, Gerecke DR, Vetrano AM, et al. Solar ultraviolet radiation as a trigger of cell signal transduction. Toxicol Appl Pharmacol 2004; 195:288–297.
13. Deliconstantinos G, Villiotou V, Stavrides JC. Release by ultraviolet B (u.v.B) radiation of nitric oxide (NO) from human keratinocytes: a potential role for nitric oxide in erythema production. Br J Pharmacol 1995; 114:1257–1265.
14. Kuhn A, Fehsel K, Lehmann P, et al. Aberrant timing in epidermal expression of inducible nitric oxide synthase after UV irradiation in cutaneous Lupus erythematosus. J Invest Dermatol 1998; 111:149–153.
15. Nabeyrat E, Jones GE, Fenwick PS, et al. Mitogen-activated protein kinases mediate peroxynitrite-induced cell death in human bronchial epithelial cells. Am J Physiol Lung Cell Mol Physiol 2003; 284:L1112–L1120.
16. Klotz LO, Schroeder P, Sies H. Peroxynitrite signalling: receptor tyrosine kinases and activation of stress-responsive pathways. Free Radical Biol Med 2002; 33:737–743.
17. Cooke CL, Davidge ST. Peroxynitrite increases ions through NFkB and decreases prostacyclin synthase in endothelial cells. Am J Physiol 2002; 282:C395–C402.
18. Romero-Graillet C, Aberdam E, Clement M, et al. Nitric oxide produced by ultraviolet-irradiated keratinocytes stimulates melanogenesis. J Clin Invest 1997; 99(4):635–642.
19. De Fabo Ec, Noonan FP. Mechanism of immune suppression by ultraviolet irradiation in vivo. I. Evidence for the existence of a unique photoreceptor in skin and its role in photo-immunology. J Exp Med 1983; 158:84–98.
20. Haralampus-Grynaviski N, Ransom C, Ye T, et al. Photogeneration and quenching of reactive oxygen species by urocanic acid. J Am Chem Soc 2002; 124:3461–3468.
21. Magnoni C, Euclidi E, Benassi L, et al. Ultraviolet B radiation induces activation of neutral and acidic sphingomyelinases and ceramide generation in cultured normal human keratinocytes. Toxicol In Vitro 2002; 16:349–355.
22. Miller CC, Hale P, Pentland AP. Ultraviolet B injury increases prostaglandin synthesis through a tyrosine kinase-dependent pathway. Evidence for UVB-induced epidermal growth factor receptor activation. J Biol Chem 1994; 269:3529–3533.
23. Barber LA, Spandau DF, Rathman SC, et al. Expression of the platelet-activating factor receptor results in enhanced ultraviolet B radiation-induced apoptosis in a human epidermal cell line. J Biol Chem 1998; 273:18891–18897.
24. Aragane Y, Kulms D, Metze D, et al. Ultraviolet light induces apoptosis via direct activation of CD95 (Fas/APO-1) independently of its ligand CD95L. J Cell Biol 1998; 140:171–182.
25. Rosette C and Karin M. Ultraviolet light and osmotic stress: activation of the JNK cascade through multiple growth factor and cytokine receptors. Science 1996; 274:1194–1197.

26. Coffer PJ, Burgering BM, Peppelenbosch MP, et al. UV activation of receptor tyrosine kinase activity. Oncogene 1995; 11:561–569.

27. Gross S, Knebel A, Tenev T, et al. Inactivation of protein-tyrosine phosphatases as mechanism of UV-induced signal transduction. J Biol Chem 1999; 10:26378–26386.

28. Marchese C, Maresca V, Cardinali G, et al. UVB-induced activation and internalization of keratinocyte growth factor receptor. Oncogene 2003; 22:2422–2431.

29. Tobin D, Van Hogerlinden M, Toftgard R. UVB-induced association of tumor necrosis factor (TNF) receptor 1/TNF receptor-associated factor-2 mediates activation of Rel proteins. Proc Natl Acad Sci USA 1998; 95:565–569.

30. Fisher GJ, Talwar HS, Lin J, et al. Retinoic acid inhibits induction of c-jun protein by ultraviolet radiation that occurs subsequent to activation of mitogen-activated protein kinase pathways in human skin in vivo. J Clin Invest 1998; 101:1432–1440.

31. Bode AM, Dong Z. Mitogen-activated protein kinase activation in UV-induced signal transduction. Sci STKE 2003; 167:RE2.

32. Assefa Z, Garmyn M, Bouillon R, et al. Differential stimulation of ERK and JNK activities by ultraviolet B irradiation and epidermal growth factor in human keratinocytes. J Invest Dermatol 1997; 108:886–891.

33. Nomura M, Kaji A, Ma WY, et al. Mitogen- and stress-activated protein kinase 1 mediates activation of Akt by ultraviolet B irradiation. J Biol Chem 2001; 276:25558–25567.

34. Wang HQ, Quan T, He T, et al. EGF receptor-dependent, NF-κB independent activation of PI-3-kinase: Akt pathway inhibits ultraviolet irradiation-induced caspases 3, 8, and 9 in human keratinocytes. J Biol Chem 2003; 278:45737–45745.

35. Laskin JD, Heck DE, Laskin DL. The ribotoxic stress response as a potential mechanism for MAP kinase activation in xenobiotic toxicity. Toxicol Sci 2002; 69:289–291.

36. Iordanov MS, Choi RJ, Ryabinina OP, et al. The UV (ribotoxic) stress response of human keratinocytes involves the unexpected uncoupling of the Ras-extracellular signal-regulated kinase signaling cascade from the activated epidermal growth factor receptor. Mol Cell Biol 2002; 22:5380–5394.

37. Zhou BB, Elledge SJ. The DNA damage response: putting checkpoints in perspective. Nature 2000; 408:433–439.

38. Unsal-Kacmaz K, Makhov AM, Griffith JD, et al. Preferential binding of ATR protein to UV-damaged DNA. Proc Natl Acad Sci USA 2002; 99:6673–6678.

39. Decraene D, Agostinis P, Pupe A, et al. Acute response of human skin to solar radiation: regulation and function of the p53 protein. J Photochem Photobiol B: Biol 2001; 63:78–83.

40. Latonen L, Laiho M. Cellular UV damage responses—functions of tumor suppressor p53. Biochim Biophys Acta 2005;1755:71–89.

41. Decraene D, Smaers K, Gan D, et al. A synthetic superoxide dismutase/catalase mimetic (EUK-134 inhibits membrane-damage-induced activation of mitogen-activated protein kinase pathways and reduces p53 accumulation in ultraviolet B-exposed primary human keratinocytes. J Invest Dermatol 2004; 122(2):484–491.

42. Orlowski RZ, Baldwin AS Jr. NF-kappaB as a therapeutic target in cancer. Trends Mol Med 2002; 8:385–389.

43. Assefa Z, Van Laethem A, Garmyn M, et al. Ultraviolet radiation-induced apoptosis in keratinocytes: on the role of cytosolic factors, Biochim Biophys Acta 2005; 1755(2):90–106.

44. Simon MM, Aragane Y, Schwarz A, Luger TA, Schwarz T. UVB light induces nuclear factor kappa B (NF kappa B) activity independently from chromosomal DNA damage in cell-free cytosolic extracts. J Invest Dermatol 1994; 102:422–427.

45. Adachi M, Gazel A, Pintucci G, et al. Specificity in stress response: epidermal keratinocytes exhibit specialized UV-responsive signal transduction pathways. DNA Cell Biol 2003; 22:665–677.

46. Beak SM, Lee YS, Kim JA. NADPH oxidase and cyclooxygenase mediate the ultraviolet B-induced generation of reactive oxygen species and activation of nuclear factor-kappaB in HaCaT human keratinocytes. Biochimie 2004; 86:425–429.

47. Köck A, Schwarz T, Kirnbauer R, et al. Human keratinocytes are a source for tumor necrosis factor a. Evidence for synthesis and release upon stimulation with endotoxin or ultraviolet light. J Exp Med 1990; 172:1609–1614.

48. Claerhout S, Van Laethem A, Agostinis P. Pathways involved in sunburn cell formation: deregulation in skin cancer. Photochem Photobiol Sci 2006; 5(2):199–207.

49. Wisdom R. AP-1: one switch for many signals. Exp Cell Res 1999; 253:180–185.

50. Rittie L, Fisher GJ. UV-light induced signal cascades and skin aging. Ageing Res Rev 2002; 1(4):705–720.

51. Bowden GT. Prevention of non-melanoma skin cancer by targeting ultraviolet-B-light signalling. Nat Rev Cancer 2004; 4:23–35.

52. Decraene D, Smaers K, Maes D, Matsui M, Declercq L, Garmyn M. A low UVB dose, with the potential to trigger a protective p53-dependent gene program, increases the resilience of keratinocytes against future UVB insults. J Invest Dermatol 2005; 125(5):xviii−xix.
53. Lee KM, Lee JG, Seo EYE, et al. Analysis of genes responding to ultraviolet B irradiation of HaCaT keratinocytes using a cDNA microarray. Br J Dermatol 2005; 152:52−59.
54. Enk AD, Jacob-Hirsch J, Gal H, et al. The UVB-induced gene expression profile of human epidermis in vivo is different from that of cultured keratinocytes. Oncogene 1006:1−14.
55. Petrocelli T, Poon R, Drucker DJ, Slingerland JM, Rosen CF. UVB radiation induces p21$^{Cip1/WAF1}$ and mediates G1 and S phase checkpoints. Oncogene 1996; 12:1378−1396.
56. Courtois SJ, Segaert S, Degreef H, Bouillon R, Garmyn M. Ultraviolet B suppresses vitamin D receptor gene expression in keratinocytes. Biochem Biophys Res Commun 1998; 246:64−69.
57. Yoon K, Smart RC. C/EBPalpha is a DNA damage-inducible p53 regulated mediator of the G1 checkpoint in keratinocytes. Mol Cell Biol 2004; 24(24):10650−10660.
58. Hermeking H, Lengauer C, Polyak K, et al. 14-3-3 sigma is a p53-regulated inhibitor of G2/M progression. Mol Cell 1997; 1(1):3−11.
59. Maeda T, Hanna AN, Sim AB, Chua PP, Chong T, Tron VA. GADD45 regulates G2/M arrest, DNA repair, and cell death in keratinocytes following ultraviolet exposure. Soc Invest Dermatol 2002; 119(1):22−26.
60. Pavey S, Russell T, Gabrielli B. G2 phase cell cycle arrest in human skin following UV irradiation. Oncogene 2001; 20(43):6103−6110.
61. Kulms D, Poppelman B, Yarosh D, et al. Nuclear and cell membrane effects contribute independently to the induction of apoptosis in human cells exposed to UVB radiation. Proc Natl Acad Sci USA 1999; 96:7974−7979.
62. Van Laethem A, Van Kelst S, Lippens, et al. Activation of p38 MAPK is required for Bax translocation to mitochondria, cytochrome c release and apoptosis. FASEB J 2004; 18(15):1946−1948.
63. Van Laethem A, Claerhout S, Garmyn M. The sunburn cell: regulation of death and survival of the keratinocyte. Int J Biochem Cell Biol 2005; 37(8):1547−1558.
64. Tron VA, Trotter MJ, Tang L, et al. p53-regulated apoptosis is differentiation dependent in ultraviolet B-irradiated mouse keratinocytes. Am J Pathol 1998; 153(2):579−585.
65. Chaturvedi V, Qin JZ, Stennet D, et al; Resistance to UVB induced apoptosis in human keratinocytes during accelerated senescence in associated with functional inactivation of p53. J Cell Physiol 2004; 198:100−109.
66. Holick MF. Evolution and function of vitamin D. Recent Results Cancer Research 2003; 164:3−28.
67. Lehmann B, Tiebel O, Meurer M. Expression of vitamin D$_3$ 25-hydroxylase (CYP27) mRNA after induction by vitamin D$_3$ or UVB radiation in keratinocytes of human skin equivalents—a preliminary study. Arch Dermatol Res 1999; 291:507−510.
68. Vantieghem K, Kissmeyer AM, De Haes P, et al. UVB-induced production of 1,25-dihydroxyvitamin D3 and vitamin D activity in human keratinocytes pretreated with a sterol Delta7-reductase inhibitor. J Cell Biochem 2006; 98(1):81−92.
69. Grant WB. Ecologic studies of solar UV-B radiation and cancer mortality rates. Recent Results Cancer Res 2003; 164:371−377.
70. Lee J, Youn JI. The photoprotective effect of 1,25-dihydroxyvitamin D$_3$ on ultraviolet light B-induced damage in keratinocyte and its mechanism of action. J Dermatol Sci 1998; 18:11−18.
71. De Haes P, Garmyn M, Degreef H, et al. 1,25-Dihydroxyvitamin D$_3$ inhibits ultraviolet B-induced apoptosis, Jun kinase activation, and interleukin-6 production in primary human keratinocytes. J Cell Biochem 2003; 89:663−673.
72. De Haes P, Garmyn M, Verstuyf A, et al. 1,25-Dihydroxyvitamin D3 and analogues protect primary human keratinocytes against UVB-induced DNA damage. J Photochem Photobiol B 2005; 78(2):141−148.
73. Young A, Sheehan J. UV-induced pigmentation in human skin. In: Giacomoni P, ed. Sun Protection in Man. New York: Elsevier, 2001:357−375.
74. Eller MS, Gilchrest BA. Tanning as part of the eukaryotic SOS response. Pigment Cell Res 2000; 8:94−97.
75. Brown D. Skin pigment enhancers. In: Giacomoni P, ed. Sun Protection in Man. New York: Elsevier, 2001: 637−675.
76. Barr R, Walker S, Tsang W, et al. Suppressed alloantigen presentation, increased TNFα, IL-1, IL-rRa, IL-10 and modulation of TNF-R in UV-irradiated human skin. J Invest Dermatol 1999; 112:692−698.
77. Fisher GJ, Datta SC, Talwar HS, et al. Molecular basis of sun-induced premature skin aging and retinoid antagonism. Nature 1996; 379:335−339.
78. Brennan M, Bhatti H, Nerusu KC, et al. Matrix metalloproteinase-1 is the major collagenolytic enzyme responsible for collagen damage in UV-irradiated human skin. Photochem Photobiol 2003; 78:43−48.

BIBLIOGRAPHY

1. An KP, Athar M, Tang X, et al. Cyclooxygenase-2 expression in murine and human nonmelanoma skin cancers: implications for therapeutic approaches. Photochem Photobiol 2002; 76:73–80.
2. Grether-Beck S, Timmer A, Felsner I, et al. Ultraviolet A-induced signalling involves a ceramide-mediated autocrine loop leading to ceramide *de novo* synthesis. J Invest Dermatol 2005; 125:545–553.
3. Hellemans L, Corstjens H, Neven A, et al. Antioxidant enzyme activity in human stratum corneum shows seasonal variation with an age-dependent recovery. J Invest Dermatol 2003; 120: 434–439.
4. Ogawa F, Sander C, Hansel A, et al. The repair enzyme peptide methionine-S-sulfoxide reductase is expressed in human epidermis and upregulated by UVA radiation. J Invest Dermatol 2006; 126: 1128–1134.

5 | Photoimmunology

Thomas Schwarz
Department of Dermatology, University of Kiel, Kiel, Germany

Gary M. Halliday
Dermatology Research Laboratories, Melanoma and Skin Cancer Research Institute, University of Sydney, Sydney, Australia

- Ultraviolet radiation suppresses the immune system in a specific rather than a general fashion.

- Both UVB and UVA can affect the immune system though by different mechanisms.

- UVB can suppress the immune system both in a local and systemic fashion.

- UVB-induced immunosuppression is a complex process in which alteration of antigen-presenting cells, release of immunosuppressive cytokines, and induction of regulatory T-cells are involved.

- UV-induced immunosuppression certainly contributes to photocarcinogenesis.

- A variety of therapeutic effects of UV radiation may be due to its immunosuppressive effects.

INTRODUCTION

More than 25 years have passed since the discovery that ultraviolet (UV) radiation can affect the immune system. Since then, numerous studies in the field of photoimmunology have tried to identify the biological impact of UV-induced immunosuppression. The vast majority of photoimmunologic studies utilized UVB, although many studies have used sources contaminated with UVC that does not reach the surface of the earth, and there is also recent evidence that the long wave range (UVA, 320–400 nm) can affect the immune system. To better understand the biological impact of UV radiation on human health, great efforts have been made to identify the molecular mechanisms underlying UV-induced immunosuppression.

UV radiation is divided into three wavebands, UVC (200–290 nm), UVB (290–320 nm), and UVA (320–400 nm). Longer wavelengths make up the visible light portion of sunlight. UVC is absorbed by stratospheric ozone and the atmosphere and does not reach the surface of the earth, as can be seen in Figure 1. However, many studies in photoimmunology have used UV sources contaminated with UVC and these need to be treated with caution, as their relevance to human biology or health is unclear. A small amount of UVB is present in terrestrial sunlight, with about 20-fold greater levels of UVA. The intensity of different wavebands alone does not indicate their biological effectiveness, as this is also dependent on absorption by molecules in the skin (chromophores), and penetration of the skin. Shorter wavelength UVB does not penetrate the skin as deeply as longer wavelength UVA (1); however, the shorter wavelengths have greater energy per photon. These issues mean that the effects of different wavebands on immunity can only be determined experimentally and are complex. The immune system is an intricate organ with multiple levels of regulation at the molecular and cellular levels. It also has components that work locally in the skin, and aspects that require activation and regulation in secondary lymphoid organs, particularly skin draining lymph nodes. Considering the nature of UV, the multiple potential chromophores in the skin and the multifaceted cellular and molecular components of the immune system that are potential targets for dysregulation by UV, it is not surprising that photoimmunology is an intricate and incompletely understood topic.

THE SKIN'S IMMUNE SYSTEM

Immune responses can be divided into two arms, cellular and humoral, which are responsible for immune recognition and destruction of the invading pathogen or skin cancer. They destroy

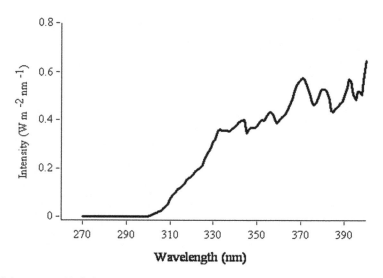

FIGURE 1   Sunlight measured in Sydney on November 18, 2004 at 3:15 PM on a cloudless afternoon at 1 nm intervals.

their target in different ways. Humoral immunity is due to B lymphocytes, which reside in secondary lymphoid organs where they secrete antibody, complex proteins that enter the blood stream and from there find their target to cause its destruction by activation of a number of mechanisms, including phagocytosis and the complement cascade. This contrasts with cellular immunity, mediated by T lymphocytes. T cells, like B cells, become activated in secondary lymphoid organs, primarily skin draining lymph nodes, but unlike T cells they destroy their target from close range, and therefore need to leave the secondary lymphoid organs and migrate to the skin where they physically interact with their target, causing its destruction via a variety of mechanisms. These include the activation of apoptosis by engaging with the Fas molecule on their target cells (2); insertion of channels into the cell membrane of the target for secretion of granzyme, which also initiates apoptosis of the target cell (3); or secretion of a variety of cytokines such as lymphotoxin and interferon (IFN)-γ that act at close range, destroying their target.

Activation of both cellular and humoral immunity has grave consequences. It utilizes large amounts of the body's reserves of energy and protein and could destroy normal tissue. Consequently, the activation of immunity has many checks and balances in the form of T-helper cells required for activation of the effector T or B cells, and T regulatory or suppressor lymphocytes that inhibit activation of the effector lymphocytes. Prior to first encounter with an antigen, there are only a few lymphocytes in the body capable of recognizing any particular antigen. During activation, these specific lymphocytes undergo massive levels of proliferation. While many of these cells arising from clonal proliferation of the original few specific lymphocytes die after the target has been eliminated, many do not, and instead differentiate into memory lymphocytes. Consequently, after resolution of the immune response there are many more specific lymphocytes in the body than there were before initial encounter with antigen. There is a major difference between these memory lymphocytes and naïve lymphocytes that have not encountered antigen in addition to their vaster numbers; they are easier to reactivate upon a subsequent encounter with the same antigen. Secondary or memory immunity occurs faster than primary immunity due to the larger number of memory lymphocytes and their reduced reliance upon receiving activation signals. Nevertheless, as will be discussed subsequently, UV suppresses both the initial activation of naïve lymphocytes and the reactivation of memory lymphocytes. These cellular interactions, which coordinate immunity, occur in the skin draining lymph nodes, and are dependent upon initiating signals from antigen-presenting cells that migrate from the skin to these lymph nodes with antigen. Before activation of immunity, the lymphocytes that cause the response reside in a different part of the body to the target. The lymphocytes are in skin-draining lymph nodes, whereas the target requiring destruction is in the skin. This problem is resolved by dendritic cells (DCs) that reside in the epidermis, called Langerhans cells (LCs), or dermis, called dermal DC (Fig. 2). These sample their environment, which may contain a target antigen to be destroyed, and then transport this to the skin-draining lymph nodes where they interact with the lymphocytes (4).

While many cell types, including B lymphocytes and macrophages, are involved in antigen presentation or can reactivate memory lymphocytes, DC are the only type of antigen-presenting cell capable of initiating activation of naïve lymphocytes upon their first encounter with antigen, and are therefore often referred to as professional antigen-presenting cells (5). While skin-derived DC carry the antigen to draining lymph nodes, it is not clear whether they are primarily responsible for presenting antigen to and activating lymphocytes, as they pass the antigen to other DC that are resident in the lymph nodes and have not arrived there from the skin (6,7). In addition to other types of antigen-presenting cells, such as B lymphocytes and macrophages within draining lymph nodes, there are many subtypes of DC within lymph nodes that are likely to have specialized functions during induction of immunity (8). Dermal DC arrive at the lymph node earlier than epidermally derived LC, at least under some circumstances (9), raising the distinct possibility that, depending upon antigen concentration and localization within the skin, different waves of DC at different times, which then pass the antigen to other antigen-presenting cells, is likely to be required for optimal T-cell activation. Elegant studies have visualized the migration of LC through the basement membrane separating the epidermis from dermis, and utilization of cytoplasmic processes to pull

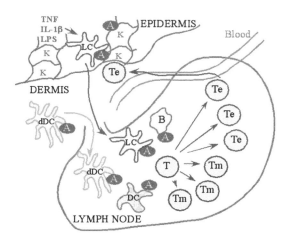

FIGURE 2   Immunology of the skin. Infection of the epidermis with bacteria or virus results in production of factors, such as LPS, that bind to toll-like receptors on Langerhans cells (LCs) inducing their migration from the epidermis. Keratinocytes (K) stressed by the infection or other stimuli produce cytokines, including tumor necrosis factor and interleukin-1β, that also induce LC migration from the epidermis. The LC and dermal dendritic cells take up antigen (A) from the infectious agent or developing tumor, and migrate via dermal lymphatics to draining lymph nodes. Here they pass the antigen to other antigen-presenting cells, such as lymph node resident dendritic cells and B lymphocytes (B). These antigen-presenting cells activate antigen-specific T lymphocytes (T) resulting in clonal expansion of these specific T cells into either long-lived memory T cells (Tm) or T effector lymphocytes (Te). The effector T cells then migrate via the blood stream to the skin where they destroy the antigen-bearing target cells. The UV interferes with this process resulting in immunosuppression. *Abbreviations*: IL-1β, interleukin-1β; LPS, lipopolysaccharide; TNF, tumor necrosis factor.

themselves along collagen fibrils within the dermis during their migration from the epidermis to draining lymph nodes (10). Additionally, LC need to disengage themselves from tight junctions with keratinocytes via E-cadherin to enable them to leave the epidermis (11,12). This is likely to explain why LC migration to draining lymph nodes takes longer than dermal DC migration.

During DC migration from the skin to draining lymph nodes, they undergo functional maturation whereby they become less able to take up and process antigen, but more capable of presenting the antigen to T cells, resulting in their activation (13,14). These changes in LC as they mature into a phenotype with greater ability to activate T lymphocytes include increased expression of major histocompatibility complex (MHC) II molecules; costimulatory molecules, such as CD86 and CD40; and increased production of T-cell activating cytokines, such as interleukin (IL)-12 (15,16).

Many factors regulate this cascade of cellular events resulting in skin immunity, including the production of certain molecules commonly produced by many infectious agents, release of cytokines from keratinocytes, nerve fibers, and other mediators. Keratinocytes and mast cells produce a wide range of cytokines and other soluble factors that regulate skin immunity, including tumor necrosis factor (TNF) and IL-1β that enhance DC migration from the skin (17,18), transforming growth factor β (TGFβ) that inhibits DC migration from the skin (19), IL-10 that inhibits skin immunity (20), and prostaglandins (PGs) such as PGE$_2$ (21,22). All of these factors regulate skin immunity at other levels in addition to DC migration or function, such as T-cell function. Nerves in the skin produce factors, such as substance P and calcitonin gene-related peptide (CGRP), that also influence skin immunity by regulating DC in addition to blood flow and T-cell migration into the skin across endothelial cells lining blood vessels (23,24). Pathogens produce a range of common molecules, such as lipopolysaccharide (LPS) and single stranded RNA, that can be recognized by toll-like receptors on DC, initiating their migration and maturation (25,26). Thus, recognition of factors, such as LPS, or altered production of regulatory factors by pathogen-induced stress on keratinocytes, mast cells, or nerves, can initiate skin immunity.

Considering the complexities of both the induction and mediation of skin immunity, the multiple cell types, and regulatory factors involved, there are multiple levels at which UVB and UVA radiation can influence this process, modulating the induction of primary or the reactivation of memory immunity. These include modulation of LC or dermal DC maturation, antigen uptake, migration from the skin, interaction with lymph node antigen-presenting cells, activation of effector, regulatory or memory lymphocytes, migration of effector lymphocytes into the skin, or the eventual function of effector lymphocytes. UV modulation of any of the cellular or molecular events that regulate skin immunity will affect the final response.

UV RADIATION SUPPRESSES THE INDUCTION OF LOCAL OR SYSTEMIC PRIMARY IMMUNITY AS WELL AS MEMORY, OR RECALL IMMUNITY

First evidence that UV radiation influences the immune system was the observation that UV radiation inhibits the immunologic rejection of transplanted tumors. Skin tumors induced by chronic UV exposure in mice are highly immunogenic since they are rejected when transplanted into naïve syngeneic hosts (27). However, when the recipient mice were given immunosuppressive drugs, the injected tumors were not rejected but grew, implying that the rejection is immunologic in nature. Rejection was also prevented when the recipient animals received an exposure to UVB radiation instead of immunosuppressive drugs. This clearly indicated that UV radiation could act in a similar manner to immunosuppressive drugs.

The same phenomenon can be observed for other immunologic in vivo models, the induction of contact hypersensitivity (CHS) or delayed type hypersensitivity (DTH) responses, induced by epicutaneous application of contact allergens or injection of antigens into the dermis, respectively. The CHS and DTH differ from each other not only due to the site of antigen exposure (epidermal or dermal), but also to the local antigen-presenting cell most likely involved. For CHS the local antigen-presenting cell that first encounters the antigen will be LC, whereas for DTH it will be the dermal DC. Exposure to UV causes a time-dependent enhancement of the differences in local antigen-presenting cells between epidermis and dermis as it induces the migration of IL-10 producing macrophages initially into the dermis and then into the epidermis at later times (28,29). Furthermore, undefined factors produced by UV-irradiated keratinocytes that suppress DTH but not CHS have been described (30), and UV-induced IL-10 appears to be involved in the suppression of DTH but not CHS (31), further highlighting the differences between these responses.

To fully develop their antigenic features, reactive, low molecular weight contact sensitizers have to bind to proteins, and thus are called haptens. Trinitrochlorobenzene (TNCB) is one such chemically reactive contact sensitizer. It conjugates the hapten trinitrophenyl (TNP) directly to lysine groups on peptides already bound in the MHC-I and MHC-II grooves on the surface of cells (32). T cells recognize the TNP group, and the peptide itself only affects T cell recognition of the hapten via its ability to anchor the TNP group into the MHC groove. Thus, TNP-specific T cells can react to TNP bound to different peptides, provided that the peptides bind strongly to the MHC molecules (33–35). It is probably for this reason that an abnormally large number of T cells respond to contact sensitizers, so that the CHS response is larger than normal immune responses. On the basis of up-regulation of T cell activation markers CD11a (LFA-1) and CD44, as well as IFNγ production, up to 15% of lymph node cells have been shown to be hapten responsive (36). In sharp contrast to this, DTH is usually to a protein or whole cells injected into the dermis. The antigen is taken up, processed, and presented conventionally on MHC Class I and II molecules so that both the epitope recognized by T cells and the MHC anchoring residues are unique to that particular antigen. The hypersensitivity, therefore, is different to CHS as it is due to hyperimmunization activating a large number of T cells or a large number of epitopes on the surface of whole cells or complex proteins. It is difficult to know which is the better model for UV suppression of immunity to skin tumors or skin infections. Skin tumors arise in the epidermis and therefore the location of the antigen is modelled by CHS; however, the chemical nature of the protein antigen is better modelled by a DTH.

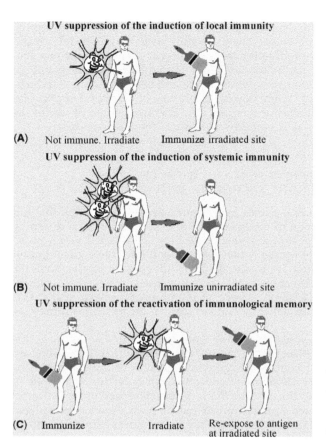

UV suppression of the induction of local immunity

(A)   Not immune. Irradiate   Immunize irradiated site

UV suppression of the induction of systemic immunity

(B)   Not immune. Irradiate   Immunize unirradiated site

UV suppression of the reactivation of immunological memory

(C)   Immunize   Irradiate   Re-expose to antigen at irradiated site

FIGURE 3 Ultraviolet (UV) radiation suppresses the induction of primary immunity, as well as reactivation of memory, or secondary immunity. The UV irradiation of a naïve individual who has not previously been exposed to the specific antigen, followed by antigen exposure at the UV-irradiated site causes what is referred to as local UV-induced immunosuppression (**A**). The UV irradiation of a naïve individual followed by antigen exposure at a skin site distal to that which was irradiated causes what is referred to as systemic UV-induced immunosuppression (**B**). The UV exposure of subjects previously immunized, suppresses reactivation of memory immunity in response to re-exposure to the same antigen (**C**).

Nevertheless, UV suppresses both CHS and DTH, but probably by different mechanisms. Local immunosuppression refers to the situation where the antigen is applied locally to the same skin site as the UV radiation. Systemic immunosuppression is when antigen is applied to a different skin site to that which was irradiated (Fig. 3). Additionally, UV can inhibit both the activation of a primary immune response in an individual not previously exposed to that antigen, and also the reactivation of memory immunity in an individual who has been previously immunized to this specific antigen. Thus, UV can locally or systemically suppress the induction of primary, or reactivation of memory immunity. UV suppression of memory immunity probably explains why UV radiation can be an effective therapy for chronic autoimmune disorders, such as psoriasis.

For local induction of immunosuppression, painting of haptens on skin areas that have been exposed to low doses of UV radiation does not induce CHS, whereas administration of the same compound to the same skin site in an unirradiated animal induces a normal CHS response (37). Inhibition of the induction of CHS by UV radiation is clearly associated with a depletion in the number of LC at the site of exposure (37,38). The LCs are the primary antigen-presenting cells in the epidermis, implying that UV radiation interferes with antigen presentation. Local inhibition of recall immunity is also associated with UV-reducing LC from human epidermis (39,40), although it is unclear whether reduced LC causes local suppression of memory immunity.

Higher UV doses also affect immune reactions induced at a distant, non-UV-exposed site. Accordingly, CHS cannot be induced in mice that are exposed to high doses of UV radiation even if contact allergen is applied at an unirradiated site (41). Similarly, UV causes systemic suppression of the reactivation of memory immunity in humans (42). This systemic immunosuppression is certainly mediated by different mechanisms than local immunosuppression.

The question how UV radiation can interfere with the induction of an immune response at a distant non-UV-exposed skin area remained unanswered for quite a long time. Nowadays it is clear that UV radiation stimulates keratinocytes to release immunosuppressive soluble mediators, including IL-10, which enter the circulation and thereby can suppress the immune system in a systemic fashion, as subsequently shown.

UVB, UVA, AND SOLAR-SIMULATED UV ARE ALL IMMUNOSUPPRESSIVE IN BOTH HUMANS AND MICE

UVB and UVA, in addition to a spectrum containing both wavebands, designed to mimic the UV portion of sunlight [solar-simulated UV (ssUV)], are immunosuppressive in humans and animal models. UVA, UVB, and ssUV have been shown to be locally and systemically immunosuppressive in humans (42–45) and mice (46–49).

While UVB is universally found by researchers to be immunosuppressive, this is not the case for UVA, with reports that UVA can even protect the immune system from the suppressive effects of UVB (50,51). Studies indicate that UVA immunosuppression is strongly regulated by unknown genes, with not all mouse strains being suppressed under defined conditions (49,52). Unlike UVB, which has a dose response showing increased levels of immunosuppression with increasing dose, UVA, at least under some circumstances, has a bell-shaped dose–response curve so that after the maximum immunosuppressive dose has been reached, higher doses cause lower levels of immunosuppression until a dose is reached that is no longer suppressive (49). This all occurs over dose ranges to which humans can be exposed during normal daily outdoor activities. While this might appear to indicate that UVB is the more important waveband in sunlight for causing immunosuppression, ssUV-induced immunosuppression dose responses have been reported to be identical to UVA. Removal of UVB from the irradiation source has no discernable effect on ssUV-induced immunosuppression (48,52). Furthermore, numerous studies using sunscreens to filter UVB from ssUV have shown the importance of UVA within the sunlight spectrum for causing immunosuppression in humans and mice (53–58).

A further complication in identification of the wavebands responsible for immunosuppression is the interactive effects between UVB and UVA and their different time courses for causing immunosuppression. Recent studies in humans have shown that UVB suppresses reactivation of memory immunity to antigen applied as early as 24 hours following exposure. In contrast, 48 hours following UVA exposure is required for antigen to cause immunosuppression. However, by 72 hours following exposure, ssUV can cause immunosuppression at doses lower than can be accounted for by either the UVB or UVA wavebands of the ssUV (59). Thus, there are interactions between pathways activated by UVA and UVB, to make the combination of these spectra in ssUV suppressive at lower doses than can be achieved by either UVA or UVB alone (Fig. 4). However, this is dependent upon the time between irradiation and antigen exposure.

Thus, even before delving into molecular or cellular mechanisms, UV has a complex suppressive effect on the immune system. It is able to suppress not only the activation of primary immunity at UV-irradiated and -unirradiated skin sites, but also the reactivation of memory immunity. Additionally, both the UVB and UVA wavebands within sunlight are suppressive, but they also interact to make sunlight more potent than either waveband alone. Only low doses of sunlight are required to suppress immunity. Doses that can be achieved with normal daily activities that are too low to cause sunburn can inhibit immunity. Considering these issues, and the complexity of skin immunity, it is not surprising that the mechanism of photoimmunosuppression is complex and incompletely understood.

UV RADIATION AFFECTS ANTIGEN PRESENTATION

Since LC are the major antigen-presenting cells in the epidermis (60), their depletion by UV seems to be largely responsible for the inhibition of the induction of CHS following UV exposure (37) and probably an important cause of UV suppression of the reactivation of

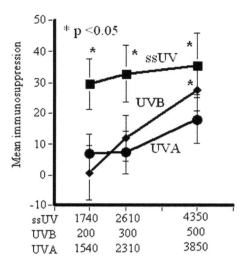

FIGURE 4 Solar-simulated UV (ssUV) is more immunosuppressive than the UVB and UVA wavebands, which make up ssUV. Groups of 15 nickel allergic volunteers were given single exposures to ssUV, UVB or UVA, the UVA and UVB doses were the relative amounts present in ssUV at each respective point. Nickel was applied 72 hrs after UV to reactivate memory immunity. While UVB was significantly immunosuppressive only at the highest dose, tested ssUV suppressed immunity at all doses and was greater than the additive effects of UVB and UVA. X axis shows the doses given in mJ/cm^2. *Abbreviation*: ssUV, solar-simulated UV. *Source*: Adapted from Ref. 59.

memory immunity (39). Depending on the UV dose applied the disappearance of LC may be due to the emigration of LC out of the epidermis since LC harbouring UV-mediated DNA damage can be detected in the draining lymph nodes (61). UV-induced LC migration from the skin has been directly observed in sheep (62) and humans (63). Higher doses of UV may also induce apoptotic death of LC (64). In addition, both UVB and UVA suppresses the expression of MHC class II surface molecules and adenosinetriphosphatase (ATPase) activity in LC and their ability to mature (38,65). Both markers, in particular MHC class II, are used to identify LC in the epidermis. Furthermore, upon UV exposure LC are impaired in their capacity to present antigens (66). Inhibition of the expression of the adhesion molecule ICAM-1 by UV radiation may be responsible for impaired clustering between LC and T cells. Accordingly, inhibition of antigen presentation by UV radiation was proven both in vitro and in vivo. Injection of antigen-loaded LC or DC exposed to UV radiation does not result in sensitization, whereas injection of antigen-pulsed unirradiated cells mounts an immune response (67).

Other antigen-presenting cells, including human peripheral blood-derived DC and splenic DC, when exposed to UV either in vitro or in vivo are also significantly impaired in their ability to stimulate allogeneic T cells. The UV radiation suppresses the expression of the costimulatory B7 surface molecules (CD80/86) that are expressed on antigen-presenting cells and crucial for interaction with T cells. Accordingly, UV radiation down-regulates the expression of CD80 and CD86 on human LC and on blood-derived DC (68,69). It was discovered recently that UVB also induces reactive oxygen species that may also contribute to impairment of the function of antigen-presenting cells by UV radiation (70). Reduced lipid peroxidation by treatment with α-tocopherol inhibits UV from reducing the number of LC from the epidermis (71). Nitric oxide (NO) is involved in UVA-induced loss of LC from the epidermis (72). Antigen presentation, however, may also be impaired indirectly by the photoproduct *cis*-urocanic acid (UCA) and by immunosuppressive cytokines or neuropeptides (see subsequently).

The UV irradiation of human and murine skin causes infiltration by IL-10 producing macrophages and other inflammatory cells into the dermis and epidermis that, along with the reduction in DC, results in activation of immune suppression (28,73,74). Thus, UV radiation results in marked changes in skin antigen-presenting cells (APC), with a reduced number of damaged DC and infiltration by macrophages.

Despite the effect of UV radiation on DC and macrophages in the skin, UV does not appear to alter the function or phenotype of DC in draining lymph nodes (75,76). UVB but not UVA radiation, however, activates B lymphocytes in draining lymph nodes so that they are larger and express higher levels of MHC Class II and B220 but not costimulatory molecules. When conjugated to antigen and injected into host mice to present the antigen to the immune system, these B cells induce immunosuppression via a mechanism that involves the inhibition of lymph node DC. Because IL-10 has this same effect it appears likely that UVB induction of IL-10 activates B lymphocytes in draining lymph nodes so that they inhibit DC activation of immunity (76,77). Thus, in summary, UV disrupts antigen presentation by reducing the number of DC and increasing the number of suppressive macrophages in the skin, and by activating B lymphocytes in draining lymph nodes so that they inhibit lymph node DC. It is likely that after UV, defective DC migrate from the skin to lymph nodes and somehow pass antigen to other antigen-presenting cells, such as B lymphocytes, and interact in a way that activates T-cell mediated immunosuppression. The molecular mechanisms by which this occurs have not been completely elucidated, but will be discussed subsequently.

UV RADIATION INDUCES IMMUNOLOGIC TOLERANCE

Painting of contact allergens onto UV-exposed skin does not result in the induction of CHS but induces tolerance, since application of the same hapten several weeks later again does not induce CHS (37). This indicates that the initial application of the hapten onto UV-exposed skin induces long-term immunologic unresponsiveness. However, immune responses against other unrelated haptens are not suppressed which excludes that the animals were generally immunosuppressed by the initial UV exposure. This also implies that the immunologic unresponsiveness induced by UV radiation is hapten-specific, a phenomenon called hapten-specific tolerance. Induction of UV-mediated tolerance is not only observed in local but also systemic immunosuppression (78). The UV-induced tolerance appears to be mediated via the generation of hapten-specific T suppressor cells, nowadays renamed regulatory T cells.

The UV-induced tolerance has been shown to occur in humans. In one investigation, which purposefully used a dose of UV too low to induce immunosuppression in all individuals, about 45% of UV immunosuppressed humans were tolerant (79). Tolerance was hapten-specific, since the individuals responded normally upon subsequent immunization with other, nonrelated haptens (79). Other studies reported a higher proportion of subjects to develop tolerance when the hapten was applied onto skin areas exposed to higher erythemogenic UV doses (80). It is unclear whether all humans can be rendered tolerant following exposure to UV radiation. This may be dependent on spectrum, dose, and timing. There are no sufficient studies to resolve this issue.

UV RADIATION INDUCES T CELLS WITH REGULATORY/SUPPRESSOR ACTIVITY

Hapten-specific tolerance induced by UV radiation appears to be mediated via the generation of T cells with inhibitory/suppressive activity. Injection of splenocytes from mice tolerized by the application of a hapten onto UV-exposed skin into naïve syngeneic mice rendered the recipients unresponsiveness to this particular antigen (81). Transfer of tolerance can be observed both in the local (81) and in the systemic model (82). The UV-induced activation of regulatory T cells has also been implicated in suppression of memory immunity (83). Although the transfer of UV-mediated suppression was subsequently shown in a convincing fashion in a variety of different immunological in vivo models, the postulated UV-induced suppressor T cells were unable to be phenotypically characterized for many years, causing many to doubt the concept of suppressor T cells in general immunology. Nowadays, the concept of active suppression is unanimously accepted in general immunology, but the term regulatory T cells is preferred to the term suppressor T cells.

For the first time, Shreedar et al. (84) succeeded in isolating T cell clones from UV-exposed mice, which were sensitized against fluoresceine isothiocyanate. Cloned cells were $CD4^+$, $CD8^-$, TCR-α/β^+, MHC restricted and specific for fluoresceine isothiocyanate. They produced

IL-10, but not IL-4 or IFN-γ. These T cells blocked antigen-presenting cell functions and IL-12 production and, even more importantly, upon injection into naïve recipients suppressed the induction of CHS against fluorescein isothiocyanate.

Because of the existence of different UV-mediated tolerance models (local, systemic, induction, memory, high dose, and low dose), different regulatory T cells with unique phenotypes appear to be involved in these systems. Currently, best characterized are the regulatory T cells involved in the low dose suppression of CHS. Cells transferring suppression in this model appear to belong to the CD4$^+$CD25$^+$ subtype (85); they express CTLA-4 (86), bind the lectin dectin-2 (87), and in contrast to the classical CD4$^+$CD25$^+$ T cells, release high amounts of IL-10 upon antigen-specific activation (86). These cells may represent a separate subtype of regulatory T cells since they exhibit characteristics of naturally occurring regulatory T cells, for example, expression of CD4 and CD25, but also of type 1 regulatory T (Tr1) cells, for example, release of IL-10 (88).

Intravenous injection of T cells from UV-tolerized mice into naïve but not sensitized recipients was found to cause unresponsiveness to the respective hapten (89). This gave rise to the speculation that regulatory T cells inhibit the induction but not the elicitation of CHS, and thus are inferior to T effector cells. However, when regulatory T cells were injected into the area of challenge of sensitized mice, the elicitation of CHS was suppressed in a hapten-specific fashion (85). But when ears of oxazolone-sensitized mice were injected with dinitrofluorobenzene-specific regulatory T cells and painted with dinitrofluorobenzene before challenge with oxazolone, CHS was suppressed. Therefore, once regulatory T cells are activated antigen-specifically, they suppress in an antigen-independent fashion. This phenomenon is named bystander suppression and has been initially described for type 1 regulatory T cells (Tr1). The UV-induced regulatory T cells express the lymph node homing receptor L-selectin but not the ligands for the skin homing receptors E- and P-selectin. Thus, UV-induced regulatory T cells are able to inhibit T effector cells, but do not suppress the elicitation of CHS upon intravenous injection due to an inability to migrate into the skin. Because of the capacity of bystander suppression, speculations exist about the therapeutic potential of regulatory T cells, which could be generated in response to antigens known to be present in the target organ that are not necessarily the precise antigen that drives the pathogenic response (90). However, these findings indicate that this strategy will be successful only if the regulatory T cells can home to the target organ. The unique migratory behavior of regulatory T cells might explain why in the vast majority of in vivo studies intravenous injection of regulatory T cells prevents but does not cure various diseases.

IL-12 has been described by several groups to be able to prevent suppression of CHS by UV and the development of regulatory T cells and even to break UV-induced tolerance by unknown mechanisms (91–93). Since the prevention of UV-induced DNA damage inhibits UV-induced immunosuppression in humans and mice, DNA damage is regarded as a major molecular trigger of UV-mediated immunosuppression (39,94–96). DNA damage has been implicated in UV suppression of the induction of primary as well as the reactivation of memory immunity and therefore is an initiator of many manifestations of the effects of UV on the immune system. The prevention of UV-induced immunosuppression by IL-12 may be due to its recently described capacity to reduce DNA damage via induction of DNA repair (97), since the preventative effect of IL-12 is not observed in DNA repair deficient mice (61). The UV-induced DNA damage appears to be also an important trigger for the induction of UV-induced regulatory T cells. This assumption is based on the observation that reduced DNA damage in LC in the regional lymph nodes by IL-12 treatment prevents the development of regulatory T cells (61). Again, in DNA repair deficient mice, IL-12 failed to prevent the development of UV-induced regulatory T cells.

The UV-induced regulatory T cells also appear to play an important role in photocarcinogenesis. Although their crucial role in supporting the development of UV-induced skin tumors had been already described in the eighties (98), these cells have been characterized only recently. They appear to belong to the natural killer T cell (NKT) lineage since they express the T cell marker CD3 and also the NK marker DX5 (99). Transfer of these UV-induced CD3$^+$DX5$^+$ cells, which produced high amounts of IL-4, into recipient mice suppressed

DTH responses and anti-tumoral immunity against highly immunogenic UV-induced skin tumors in an antigen-specific manner.

UV RADIATION INDUCES THE RELEASE OF IMMUNOSUPPRESSIVE MEDIATORS

The UV radiation causes damage to genes, proteins, and lipids either directly or via reactive oxygen or nitrogen species, disrupting antigen-presenting cells in the skin and lymph nodes, eventually leading to activation of regulatory T cells that cause immunosuppression. However, the molecular events downstream of UV that lead to these cellular alterations to the immune system are only partially understood. The finding that mice, which are exposed to higher doses of UV radiation, cannot be immunized even when the antigen is applied on a skin area that was not UV exposed (41) clearly indicated that UV radiation suppresses the immune system in a systemic fashion and that soluble mediators are likely to be involved. As UVB and UVA are immunosuppressive but can interact to increase the level of suppression, there are likely to be a number of different mediators with varying levels of importance, depending upon the conditions. Keratinocytes have been recognized as a rich source of a variety of soluble mediators, including immunostimulatory and pro-inflammatory cytokines. Cytokine release by keratinocytes can be effectively induced by UV radiation (100). The UV radiation, however, can also stimulate the secretion of immunosuppressive mediators since intravenous injection into naive mice of supernatants obtained from UV-exposed keratinocytes renders the recipients unresponsive to hapten sensitization (101). The UV-induced keratinocyte-derived immunosuppressive mediators may get into the circulation and inhibit immune reactions in the skin-draining lymph nodes, or at skin areas not directly exposed to UV radiation, explaining the phenomenon of systemic immunosuppression.

A major soluble player involved in systemic UV-induced immunosuppression appears to be IL-10. Keratinocyte-derived IL-10, released by UV radiation (102), abrogates the ability of LC to present antigens to Th1 clones and even tolerizes them. Injection of IL-10 into the skin area of hapten application prevents the induction of CHS and induces hapten-specific tolerance (103). In turn, neutralization of IL-10 with an antibody in UV-irradiated mice prevents systemic UV-induced suppression of the induction of DTH (104).

There are many other soluble mediators involved in UV-induced immunosuppression besides IL-10. The TNF secreted in response to UV appears to be a major cause of LC migration from the epidermis to draining lymph nodes where they have impaired function (105). It has even been proposed that polymorphisms in the TNF gene regulate susceptibility to UVB-induced immunosuppression (106). The neuropeptide calcitonin gene related peptide (CGRP) is decreased following UV irradiation and a topical receptor antagonist reduces UV immunosuppression, showing that CGRP is also involved in UV immunosuppression, possibly by regulation of LC (107). Another neuropeptide, α-melanocyte stimulating hormone, is secreted in response to UV radiation, where it acts as an immunomodulator (108) and contributes to UV-induced immunosuppression and tolerance, possibly by inducing the production of IL-10 and by effects on antigen-presenting cells (23,109). Inhibition of UV-induced NO production has also been shown to prevent UV-induced immunosuppression in rodents (107) and humans (110). The NO inhibition appears to act at least in part by preventing UV-induced loss of LC from the epidermis (72).

One pathway by which UV radiation causes systemic immunosuppression appears to involve lipid peroxidation and release of the phospholipid mediator platelet-activating factor (PAF), which activates cyclooxygenase-2 (COX-2) to produce prostaglandin E_2 (PGE_2) (111). The UV-induced PGE_2 then initiates a cytokine cascade of IL-4 and IL-10, leading to systemic immunosuppression (112). IL-4-deficient mice are sensitive to UV-induced local but not systemic immunosuppression, implying a role for IL-4 in systemic but not local immunosuppression (113). Lack of IL-4 caused dysfunction in dermal mast cells, which therefore appear to be involved further downstream of these events. Mast cell deficient mice are not susceptible to UV-induced systemic immunosuppression and histamine appears to be the mast cells product that then leads to immunosuppression (114,115). This suggests that a complex cascade of events initiated by UV and involving PAF, PGE_2, IL-4, and mast cell release of histamine results in changes to antigen-presenting cells in draining lymph nodes, including activation of suppressor B lymphocytes and activation of regulatory T cells, leading to systemic immunosuppression.

UROCANIC ACID IS INVOLVED IN UV-INDUCED IMMUNOSUPPRESSION

UCA has been recognized as another chromophore in the epidermis to be involved in UV-induced immunosuppression (116,117). UCA, a metabolic product of the essential amino acid histidine, accumulates in the epidermis because keratinocytes lack the enzymes required for its catabolization. There are two tautomeric forms of UCA, trans (E)- and cis (Z), and UV converts *trans*- into *cis*-UCA. Removal of UCA by tape stripping the epidermis prevents UV-induced suppression of the induction of CHS, suggesting that *cis*-UCA is involved in photoimmunosuppression (116). Furthermore, injection of *cis*-UCA partially mimics the immunoinhibitory activity of UV radiation (118) and antibodies directed against *cis*-UCA restore DTH but not CHS responses after UV exposure (119). *Cis*-UCA also inhibits the presentation of tumor antigens by LC (120), which can be reversed by IL-12 (121). In addition, injection of *cis*-UCA antibodies reduces the incidence of UV-induced skin tumors in a photocarcinogenesis model, suggesting a role of *cis*-UCA in the generation of UV-induced skin cancer (121).

BIOLOGICAL RELEVANCE OF UV-INDUCED IMMUNOSUPPRESSION

UV-induced immunosuppression is a highly complex process in which several different pathways are involved (Fig. 5). The biological implications of UV-induced immunosuppression may be several-fold. In a variety of experimental models it has been demonstrated that UV

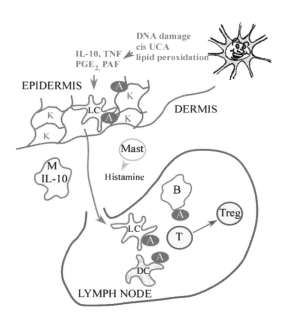

FIGURE 5   Ultraviolet (UV) radiation causes a cascade of biological events that lead to immunosuppression. UV from the sun causes DNA damage to Langerhans cells (LCs) and keratinocytes (K), causing the damaged LC to migrate to draining lymph nodes with antigen (A). UV also causes trans to cis isomerisation of urocanic acid and lipid peroxidation. These cause production of multiple immunoregulatory factors in the epidermis, including interleukin-10 (IL-10), tumor necrosis factor, platelet-activating factor, and prostaglandin E_2. These may act on the LC or at other levels. UV also causes infiltration into the dermis of IL-10 secreting macrophages (M), release of histamine from mast cells, and activation of B lymphocytes (B) into suppressor B cells in draining lymph nodes. In the lymph nodes, interactions between the antigen-presenting cells, damaged LC, lymph node DC (DC) and suppressor B lymphocytes results in the activation of regulatory T cells (Treg), which mediate immunosuppression. *Abbreviations*: PAF, platelet-activating factor; PGE_2, prostaglandin E_2; TNF, tumor necrosis factor; UCA, urocanic acid.

radiation suppresses protective immune responses against viral, bacterial, and fungal infections (122). The most frequently used infectious agents to study these phenomena are herpes simplex virus (HSV), listeria, leishmania, mycobacteria, and candida (123).

Exposure of mice previously immunized with HSV to UVB prior to epidermal challenge with HSV resulted in the development of severe lesions in 92% of mice. Only 59% of unirradiated mice developed mild lesions (124). This was associated with reduced MHC class II expression on antigen-presenting cells and therefore may have been due to UVB-induced immunosuppression. The UVB prior to infection with *Mycobacterium bovis bacillus Calmette-Guerin* (BCG) significantly delayed the development of DTH and increased the number of bacteria in the spleen and lymph nodes (125). Thus, UVB inhibited the development of immunity to BCG, enhancing infection. This inhibition of bacterial clearance could be prevented with anti-IL-10 antibodies suggesting that UVB-induced immunosuppression was mediated via production of IL-10, which then prevented bacterial clearance (126).

Other animal experiments indicating that UVB suppresses immunity to infectious agents, inhibiting resistance to the infection, include the parasite *Trichinella spiralis* (127,128), the murine malaria parasite *Plasmodium chabaudi* (129), the bacteria *Listeria monocytogenes* (130), the Lyme spirochete *Borrelia burgdorferi* (131), and the extracellular *Mycobacterium ulcerans* (132).

There is also evidence that UV exacerbates infections in humans, but it is not always clear whether this is due to immunosuppression or some other effects of UV radiation. The HSV causes a latent infection of local sensory ganglia in humans, which can be reactivated to form skin lesions. Exposure of patients with HSV or herpes labialis to UV radiation results in the development of skin lesions (133,134). A significantly higher frequency of herpes zoster infection has been reported in the summer months in north-eastern Italy (135). In a cohort of 137 renal transplant patients, a high rate of HSV infections was found in spring, and high rates of herpes zoster and fungal/yeast infections in summer, indicating an association of these infections with short-term sunlight exposure. A higher risk of bacterial infections was associated with a higher lifetime exposure (136). A transient reduction in antibody titre has been observed in subjects who received their first Hepatitis B vaccination in summer compared to winter (137). The immune response to antigens of Lepromin induces a granulomatus reaction that limits or suppresses infection and is a measure of immunological activity. It has been shown that UV irradiation significantly reduces the size of granulomatus reactions, and suppresses the number of infiltrating lymphocytes in 29 healthy, lepromin-positive contacts of leprosy patients immunized with *Mycobacterium leprae* (138). Thus, while the studies in humans are limited, they support experiments in mice, indicating that UV immunosuppression reduces immunity to a variety of infectious agents. However, based on daily clinical practice, it is obvious that acute and severe exacerbations of infectious diseases, especially bacterial infections following solar exposure, are extremely rare in humans. It is possible that the effect of UV immunosuppression on infections is subtle, or that chronic exposure is more important than acute exposure.

However, the immune system not only protects from infectious agents, but also from malignant cells. Transformed cells in particular in the early stage can be recognized as "foreign" and attacked by the immune system (tumor immunology). This may apply in particular for both nonmelanoma skin cancer and malignant melanoma. Striking evidence exists for a strong correlation between the risk of developing skin cancer and immunosuppression. Individuals who are pharmacologically immunosuppressed, such as transplant patients, exhibit a significantly increased risk of skin cancer (139). Patients with a positive history of skin cancer are more sensitive than controls without a history of skin cancer to UVB-induced suppression of CHS responses (79).

The negative impact of UV radiation on host defense against skin tumors has been convincingly demonstrated in various experimental animal models. The UV-induced immunosuppression enables the outgrowth of transplanted epithelial skin cancers and melanomas in mice (140–143). Specific T cells activated in UVB-irradiated mice by antigen exposure can transfer suppression to normal recipients, inhibiting tumor immunity and therefore enabling UV-induced skin tumors to grow (144).

Furthermore, restoration or even enhancement of an immune response by topical or systemic application of immunomodulators, such as IFNs or imiquimod, is a successful therapeutic strategy for the treatment of skin cancer (145–147). All this clearly supports the notion that the immunosuppressive impact of UV radiation may be much more relevant for carcinogenesis than for the exacerbation of infectious diseases.

CONCLUSION

Exposure to doses of UV radiation that are only 30–50% as high as what is required to cause barely detectable sunburn suppress immunity in humans. Therefore, normal daily outdoor activities during the spring and summer months are likely to cause some degree of immunosuppression in a large proportion of humans. Both the UVB and UVA wavebands contribute to sunlight-induced immunosuppression, although an interaction between them makes sunlight more suppressive than either waveband alone. It is therefore important to protect the skin from both UVB and UVA. UV suppresses immunity to antigens applied to irradiated skin and also to antigens applied to skin sites distal to the UV radiation indicating that systemic factors can be released from irradiated skin, disrupting immunity at distant sites. The UV radiation suppresses the activation of primary, and the reactivation of memory immunity. It can suppress CHS responses initiated in the epidermis and DTH responses initiated in the dermis. This is of clinical importance as it impedes immune rejection of skin cancers, and also immune-mediated destruction of skin infections.

Owing to the multiple different experimental systems suppressed by UV and the dependence on dose, timing, waveband and skin site, we currently do not have a comprehensive understanding of how UV has this potent effect on the immune system. However, many different molecular and cellular events have been implicated. The molecular mechanisms responsible for disruption to cellular immunity are initiated by DNA damage, trans to cis isomerization of UCA, and peroxidation of lipids. These alter the factors produced by keratinocytes that regulate immunity, resulting in a cascade of factors with production of PAF leading to PGE_2, IL-4, IL-10, and histamine release from mast cells. While these immunosuppressive factors could then directly effect T cell activation, migration into skin sites, or their effector function, it appears more likely that they alter antigen-presenting cells, leading to activation of suppressor lymphocytes, which then suppress skin immunity.

UV radiation has profound effects on antigen-presenting cells. It damages LC so that they migrate to lymph nodes with altered function, while causing IL-10 producing suppressor macrophages to infiltrate the skin and activating B lymphocytes in draining lymph nodes so that they have suppressor function. It is likely that interaction between these UV-altered antigen-presenting cells results in the activation of suppressor T lymphocytes. There is good evidence that these T suppressor cells are responsible for a large amount of the reduction in immunity caused by UV.

It is both obvious and striking that UV radiation at rather low doses suppresses an immune response. Thus, one may speculate that a certain degree of immunosuppression may be beneficial. The skin is an organ which is constantly exposed to potential allergens, in addition the skin is an organ which is prone to autoimmunity (148,149). Hence, it is tempting to speculate that a certain degree of constant immunosuppression by daily solar exposure may prevent the induction of these immune responses. If this is the case it remains to be clarified in the future. However, even if this turns out to be true, excessive and chronic solar exposure will remain one of the major environmental threats for human health.

ACKNOWLEDGMENTS

This work was supported by grants of the German Research Association (DFG, SCHW1177/1-1, SFB415/A16), Federal Ministry of Environmental Protection St.Sch_4491, the National Health and Medical Research Council of Australia, Cure Cancer Australia, and the CERIES Award 2004.

REFERENCES

1. Bruls WA, Slaper H, van der Leun JC, Berrens L. Transmission of human epidermis and stratum corneum as a function of thickness in the ultraviolet and visible wavelengths. Photochem Photobiol 1984; 40:485–494.
2. Satchell AC, Barnetson RS, Halliday GM. Increased Fas ligand expression by T cells and tumour cells in the progression of actinic keratosis to squamous cell carcinoma. Brit J Dermatol 2004; 151:42–49.
3. Sutton VR, Davis JE, Cancilla M, et al. Initiation of apoptosis by granzyme B requires direct cleavage of Bid, but not direct granzyme B-mediated caspase activation. J Exp Med 2000; 192:1403–1413.
4. Halliday GM. Skin immunity and melanoma development. In: Thompson JF, Morton DL, Kroon BBR, eds. Textbook of Melanoma. London: Martin Dunitz, 2004:25–42.
5. Steinman RM. Dendritic cells and the control of immunity: enhancing the efficiency of antigen presentation. Mt Sinai J Med 2001; 68:160–166.
6. Knight SC, Iqball S, Roberts MS, Macatonia S, Bedford PA. Transfer of antigen between dendritic cells in the stimulation of primary T cell proliferation. Eur J Immunol 1998; 28:1636–1644.
7. Carbone FR, Belz GT, Heath WR. Transfer of antigen between migrating and lymph node-resident DCs in peripheral T-cell tolerance and immunity. Trends Immunol 2004; 25:655–658.
8. Shortman K, Liu YJ. Mouse and human dendritic cell subtypes. Nat Rev Immunol 2002; 2:151–161.
9. Kissenpfennig A, Henri S, Dubois B, et al. Dynamics and function of Langerhans cells in vivo: dermal dendritic cells colonize lymph node areas distinct from slower migrating Langerhans cells. Immunity 2005; 22:643–654.
10. Stoitzner P, Pfaller K, Strossel H, Romani N. A close-up view of migrating Langerhans cells in the skin. J Invest Dermatol 2002; 118:117–125.
11. Tang A, Amagai M, Granger LG, Stanley JR, Udey MC. Adhesion of epidermal Langerhans cells to keratinocytes mediated by E-cadherin. Nature 1993; 361:82–85.
12. Blauvelt A, Katz SI, Udey MC. Human Langerhans cells express E-cadherin. J Invest Dermatol 1995; 104:293–296.
13. Streilein JW, Grammer SF, Yoshikawa T, Demidem A, Vermeer M. Functional dichotomy between Langerhans cells that present antigen to naive and to memory/effector T lymphocytes. Immunol Rev 1990; 117:159–183.
14. Byrne SN, Halliday GM. Dendritic cells: making progress with tumour regression? Immunol Cell Biol 2002; 80:520–530.
15. Hart DNJ. Dendritic cells—unique leukocyte populations which control the primary immune response. Blood 1997; 90:3245–3287.
16. Cumberbatch M, Gould SJ, Peters SW, Kimber I. MHC class-II expression by Langerhans cells and lymph node dendritic cells—possible evidence for maturation of Langerhans cells following contact sensitization. Immunology 1991; 74:414–419.
17. Cumberbatch M, Kimber I. Dermal tumour necrosis factor-alpha induces dendritic cell migration to draining lymph nodes, and possibly provides one stimulus for Langerhans' cell migration. Immunology 1992; 75:257–263.
18. Cumberbatch M, Dearman RJ, Kimber I. Langerhans cells require signals from both tumour necrosis factor-alpha and interleukin-1-beta for migration. Immunology 1997; 92:388–395.
19. Weber F, Byrne SN, Le S, et al. Transforming growth factor-beta(1) immobilises dendritic cells within skin tumours and facilitates tumour escape from the immune system. Cancer Immunol Immun 2005; 54:898–906.
20. Kondo S, Mckenzie RC, Sauder DN. Interleukin-10 inhibits the elicitation phase of allergic contact hypersensitivity. J Invest Dermatol 1994; 103:811–814.
21. Kanda N, Mitsui H, Watanabe S. Prostaglandin E-2 suppresses CCL27 production through EP2 and EP3 receptors in human keratinocytes. J Allergy Clin Immunol 2004; 114:1403–1409.
22. Luft T, Jefford M, Luetjens P, et al. Functionally distinct dendritic cell (DC) populations induced by physiologic stimuli: prostaglandin E-2 regulates the migratory capacity of specific DC subsets. Blood 2002; 100:1362–1372.
23. Luger TA, Bhardwaj RS, Grabbe S, Schwarz T. Regulation of the immune response by epidermal cytokines and neurohormones. J Dermatol Sci 1996; 13:5–10.
24. Asahina A, Hosoi J, Grabbe S, Granstein RD. Modulation of Langerhans cell function by epidermal nerves. J Allergy Clin Immunol 1995; 96:1178–1182.
25. Blander JM, Medzhitov R. Toll-dependent selection of microbial antigens for presentation by dendritic cells. Nature 2006; 440:808–812.
26. Suzuki H, Wang BH, Shivji GM, et al. Imiquimod, a topical immune response modifier, induces migration of Langerhans cells. J Invest Dermatol 2000; 114:135–141.
27. Kripke ML. Immunologic unresponsiveness induced by UV radiation. Immunol Rev 1984; 80: 87–102.

28. Meunier L, Batacsorgo Z, Cooper KD. In human dermis, ultraviolet radiation induces expansion of a CD36(+) CD11b(+) CD1(−) macrophage subset by infiltration and proliferation—CD1(+) Langerhans-like dendritic antigen-presenting cells are concomitantly depleted. J Invest Dermatol 1995; 105:782–788.

29. Kang KF, Gilliam AC, Chen GF, Tootell E, Cooper KD. In human skin, UVB initiates early induction of Il-10 over Il-12 preferentially in the expanding dermal monocytic/macrophagic population. J Invest Dermatol 1998; 111:31–38.

30. Kim TY, Kripke ML, Ullrich SE. Immunosuppression by factors released from UV-irradiated epidermal cells: selective effects on the generation of contact and delayed hypersensitivity after exposure to UVA or UVB radiation. J Invest Dermatol 1990; 94:26–32.

31. Rivas JM, Ullrich SE. The role of IL-4, IL-10, and TNF-alpha in the immune suppression induced by ultraviolet radiation. J Leukocyte Biol 1994; 56:769–775.

32. Martin S, Lappin MB, Kohler J, et al. Peptide immunization indicates that CD8+ T cells are the dominant effector cells in trinitrophenyl-specific contact hypersensitivity. J Invest Dermatol 2000; 115:260–266.

33. Kohler J, Martin S, Pflugfelder U, Ruh H, Vollmer J, Weltzien HU. Cross-reactive trinitrophenylated peptides as antigens for class II major histocompatibility complex-restricted T cells and inducers of contact sensitivity in mice. Limited T cell receptor repertoire. Eur J Immunol 1995; 25:92–101.

34. Martin S, von Bonin A, Fessler C, Pflugfelder U, Weltzien HU. Structural complexity of antigenic determinants for class I MHC-restricted, hapten-specific T cells. Two qualitatively differing types of H-2Kb-restricted TNP epitopes. J Immunol 1993; 151:678–687.

35. Kohler J, Martin S, Pflugfelder U, Ruh H, Vollmer J, Weltzien HU. Cross-reactive trinitrophenylated peptides as antigens for class II major histocompatibility complex-restricted T cells and inducers of contact sensitivity in mice—limited T cell receptor repertoire. Eur J Immunol 1995; 25:92–101.

36. Xu H, Banerjee A, Dilulio NA, Fairchild RL. Development of effector CD8+ T cells in contact hypersensitivity occurs independently of CD4+ T cells. J Immunol 1997; 158:4721–4728.

37. Toews GB, Bergstresser PR, and Streilein JW. Epidermal Langerhans cell density determines whether contact hypersensitivity or unresponsiveness follows skin painting with DNFB. J Immunol 1980; 124:445–453.

38. Aberer W, Schuler G, Stingl G, Honigsmann H, Wolff K. Ultraviolet light depletes surface markers of Langerhans cells. J Invest Dermatol 1981; 76:202–210.

39. Kuchel JM, Barnetson RS, Halliday GM. Cyclobutane pyrimidine dimer formation is a molecular trigger for solar-simulated ultraviolet radiation-induced suppression of memory immunity in humans. Photoch Photobio Sci 2005; 4:577–582.

40. Kuchel JM, Barnetson RSC, Zhuang L, Strickland FM, Pelley RP, Halliday GM. Tamarind inhibits solar-simulated ultraviolet radiation-induced suppression of recall responses in humans. Lett Drug Des Discov 2005; 2:165–171.

41. Noonan FP, De Fabo EC, Kripke ML. Suppression of contact hypersensitivity by ultraviolet radiation: an experimental model. Springer Semin Immun 1981; 4:293–304.

42. Moyal DD, Fourtanier AM. Broad-spectrum sunscreens provide better protection from the suppression of the elicitation phase of delayed-type hypersensitivity response in humans. J Invest Dermatol 2001; 117:1186–1192.

43. Hersey P, Bradley M, Hasic E, Haran G, Edwards A, McCarthy WH. Immunological effects of solarium exposure. Lancet 1983; 12(March):545–548.

44. LeVee GJ, Oberhelman L, Anderson T, Koren H, Cooper KD. UVA II exposure of human skin results in decreased immunization capacity, increased induction of tolerance and a unique pattern of epidermal antigen-presenting cell alteration. Photochem Photobiol 1997; 65:622–629.

45. Damian DL, Barnetson RS, Halliday GM. Low-dose UVA and UVB have different time courses for suppression of contact hypersensitivity to a recall antigen in humans. J Invest Dermatol 1999; 112:939–944.

46. Bestak R, Halliday GM. Chronic low-dose UVA irradiation induces local suppression of contact hypersensitivity, Langerhans cell depletion and suppressor cell activation in C3H/HeJ mice. Photochem Photobiol 1996; 64:969–974.

47. Halliday GM, Bestak R, Yuen KS, Cavanagh LL, Barnetson RS. UVA-induced immunosuppression. Mutat Res—Fund Mol M 1998; 422:139–145.

48. Nghiem DX, Kazimi N, Clydesdale G, Ananthaswamy HN, Kripke ML, Ullrich SE. Ultraviolet A radiation suppresses an established immune response: Implications for sunscreen design. J Invest Dermatol 2001; 117:1193–1199.

49. Byrne SN, Spinks N, Halliday GM. The induction of immunity to a protein antigen using an adjuvant is significantly compromised by ultraviolet A radiation. J Photoch Photobio B 2006; 84:128–134.

50. Reeve VE, Bosnic M, Boehm-Wilcox C, Nishimura N, Ley RD. Ultraviolet A radiation (320–400 nm) protects hairless mice from immunosuppression induced by ultraviolet B radiation (280–320 nm) or cis-urocanic acid. Int Arch Allergy Immun 1998; 115:316–322.

51. Reeve VE, Tyrrell RM. Heme oxygenase induction mediates the photoimmunoprotective activity of UVA radiation in the mouse. P Natl Acad Sci USA 1999; 96:9317–9321.

52. Byrne SN, Spinks N, Halliday GM. Ultraviolet A irradiation of C57BL/6 mice suppresses systemic contact hypersensitivity or enhances secondary immunity depending on dose. J Invest Dermatol 2002; 119:858–864.

53. Bestak R, Barnetson RSC, Nearn MR, Halliday GM. Sunscreen protection of contact hypersensitivity responses from chronic solar-simulated ultraviolet irradiation correlates with the absorption spectrum of the sunscreen. J Invest Dermatol 1995; 105:345–351.

54. Damian DL, Halliday GM, Barnetson RS. Broad-spectrum sunscreens provide greater protection against ultraviolet-radiation-induced suppression of contact hypersensitivity to a recall antigen in humans. J Invest Dermatol 1997; 109:146–151.

55. Fourtanier A, Gueniche A, Compan D, Walker SL, Young AR. Improved protection against solar-simulated radiation-induced immunosuppression by a sunscreen with enhanced ultraviolet A protection. J Invest Dermatol 2000; 114:620–627.

56. Kelly DA, Seed PT, Young AR, Walker SL. A commercial sunscreen's protection against ultraviolet radiation-induced immunosuppression is more than 50% lower than protection against sunburn in humans. J Invest Dermatol 2003; 120:65–71.

57. Poon TSC, Barnetson RS, Halliday GM. Prevention of immunosuppression by sunscreens in humans is unrelated to protection from erythema and dependent on protection from ultraviolet A in the face of constant ultraviolet B protection. J Invest Dermatol 2003; 121:184–190.

58. Wolf P, Hoffmann C, Quehenberger F, Grinschgl S, Kerl H. Immune protection factors of chemical sunscreens measured in the local contact hypersensitivity model in humans. J Invest Dermatol 2003; 121:1080–1087.

59. Poon TSC, Barnetson RSC, Halliday GM. Sunlight-induced immunosuppression in humans is initially because of UVB, then UVA, followed by interactive effects. J Invest Dermatol 2005; 125:840–846.

60. Stingl G, Tamaki K, Katz SI. Origin and function of epidermal Langerhans cells. Immunol Rev 1980; 53:149–174.

61. Schwarz A, Maeda A, Kernebeck K, van Steeg H, Beissert S, Schwarz T. Prevention of UV radiation-induced immunosuppression by IL-12 is dependent on DNA repair. J Exp Med 2005; 201:173–179.

62. Dandie GW, Clydesdale GJ, Radcliff FJ, Muller HK. Migration of Langerhans cells and gamma delta(+) dendritic cells from UV-B-irradiated sheep skin. Immunol Cell Biol 2001; 79:41–48.

63. Kolgen W, Both H, van Weelden H, et al. Epidermal Langerhans cell depletion after artificial ultraviolet B irradiation of human skin in vivo: apoptosis versus migration. J Invest Dermatol 2002; 118:812–817.

64. Rattis FM, Concha M, Dalbiezgauthier C, Courtellemont P, Peguetnavarro J. Effects of ultraviolet B radiation on human Langerhans cells—functional alteration of CD86 upregulation and induction of apoptotic cell death. J Invest Dermatol 1998; 111:373–379.

65. Furio L, Berthier-Vergnes O, Ducarre B, Schmitt D, Peguet-Navarro J. UVA radiation impairs phenotypic and functional maturation of human dermal dendritic cells. J Invest Dermatol 2005; 125:1032–1038.

66. Stingl LA, Sauder DN, Iijima M, Wolff K, Pehamberger H, Stingl G. Mechanism of UV-B-induced impairment of the antigen-presenting capacity of murine epidermal cells. J Immunol 1983; 130:1586–1591.

67. Fox IJ, Sy MS, Benacerraf B, Greene MI. Impairment of antigen-presenting cell function by ultraviolet radiation. II. Effect of in vitro ultraviolet irradiation on antigen-presenting cells. Transplantation 1981; 31:262–265.

68. Young JW, Baggers J, Soergel SA. High-dose UV-B radiation alters human dendritic cell costimulatory activity but does not allow dendritic cells to tolerize T-lymphocytes to alloantigen in vitro. Blood 1993; 81:2987–2997.

69. Weiss JM, Renkl AC, Denfeld RW, et al. Low-dose UVB radiation perturbs the functional expression of B7.1 and B7.2 co-stimulatory molecules on human Langerhans cells. Eur J Immunol 1995; 25: 2858–2862.

70. Caceresdittmar G, Ariizumi K, Xu S, Tapia FJ, Bergstresser PR, Takashima A. Hydrogen peroxide mediates UV-induced impairment of antigen presentation in a murine epidermal-derived dendritic cell line. Photochem Photobiol 1995; 62:176–183.

71. Yuen KS, Halliday GM. Alpha-tocopherol, an inhibitor of epidermal lipid peroxidation, prevents ultraviolet radiation from suppressing the skin immune system. Photochem Photobiol 1997; 65:587–592.

72. Yuen KS, Nearn MR, Halliday GM. Nitric oxide-mediated depletion of Langerhans cells from the epidermis may be involved in UVA radiation-induced immunosuppression. Nitric Oxide 2002; 6:313–318.

73. Kang KF, Hammerberg C, Meunier L, Cooper KD. CD11b(+) macrophages that infiltrate human epidermis after in vivo ultraviolet exposure potently produce IL-10 and represent the major secretory source of epidermal IL-10 protein. J Immunol 1994; 153:5256–5264.

74. Sluyter R, Halliday GM. Enhanced tumor growth in UV-irradiated skin is associated with an influx of inflammatory cells into the epidermis. Carcinogenesis 2000; 21:1801–1807.

75. Gorman S, Tan JWY, Thomas JA, et al. Primary defect in UVB-induced systemic immunomodulation does not relate to immature or funtionally impaired APCs in regional lymph nodes. J Immunol 2005; 174:6677–6685.

76. Byrne SN, Halliday GM. B cells activated in lymph nodes in response to ultraviolet irradiation or by interleukin-10 inhibit dendritic cell induction of immunity. J Invest Dermatol 2005; 124:570–578.

77. Byrne SN, Ahmed J, Halliday GM. Ultraviolet B but not A radiation activates suppressor B cells in draining lymph nodes. Photochem Photobiol 2005; 81:1366–1370.

78. Kripke ML, Morison WL. Studies on the mechanism of systemic suppression of contact hypersensitivity by ultraviolet B radiation. Photodermatol 1986; 3:4–14.

79. Yoshikawa T, Rae V, Bruins-Slot W, Van den Berg JW, Taylor JR, Streilein JW. Susceptibility to effects of UVB radiation on induction of contact hypersensitivity as a risk factor for skin cancer in humans. J Invest Dermatol 1990; 95:530–536.

80. Cooper KD, Oberhelman L, Hamilton TA, et al. UV exposure reduces immunization rates and promotes tolerance to epicutaneous antigens in humans—relationship to dose, CD1a-DR+ epidermal macrophage induction, and Langerhans cell depletion. P Natl Acad Sci USA 1992; 89:8497–8501.

81. Elmets CA, Bergstresser PR, Tigelaar RE, Wood PJ, Streilein JW. Analysis of the mechanism of unresponsiveness produced by haptens painted on skin exposed to low dose ultraviolet radiation. J Exp Med 1983; 158:781–794.

82. Noonan FP, De Fabo EC, Kripke ML. Suppression of contact hypersensitivity by UV radiation and its relationship to UV-induced suppression of tumor immunity. Photochem Photobiol 1981; 34:683–689.

83. Nghiem DX, Kazimi N, Mitchell DL, et al. Mechanisms underlying the suppression of established immune responses by ultraviolet radiation. J Invest Dermatol 2002; 119:600–608.

84. Shreedhar VK, Pride MW, Sun Y, Kripke ML, Strickland FM. Origin and characteristics of ultraviolet-B radiation-induced suppressor T lymphocytes. J Immunol 1998; 161:1327–1335.

85. Schwarz A, Maeda A, Wild MK, et al. Ultraviolet radiation-induced regulatory T cells not only inhibit the induction but can suppress the effector phase of contact hypersensitivity. J Immunol 2004; 172:1036–1043.

86. Schwarz A, Beissert S, Grosse-Heitmeyer K, et al. Evidence for functional relevance of CTLA-4 in ultraviolet-radiation-induced tolerance. J Immunol 2000; 165:1824–1831.

87. Aragane Y, Maeda A, Schwarz A, Tezuka T, Ariizumi K, Schwarz T. Involvement of dectin-2 in ultraviolet radiation-induced tolerance. J Immunol 2003; 171:3801–3807.

88. Beissert S, Schwarz A, Schwarz T. Regulatory T cells. J Invest Dermatol 2006; 126:15–24.

89. Glass MJ, Streilein JW. UVB radiation and DNFB skin painting induce suppressor cells universally in mice. J Invest Dermatol 1990; 94:273–278.

90. Maloy KJ, Powrie F. Regulatory T cells in the control of immune pathology. Nat Immunol 2001; 2: 816–822.

91. Schmitt DA, Owenschaub L, Ullrich SE. Effect of IL-12 on immune suppression and suppressor cell induction by ultraviolet radiation. J Immunol 1995; 154:5114–5120.

92. Muller G, Saloga J, Germann T, Schuler G, Knop J, Enk AH. Il-12 as mediator and adjuvant for the induction of contact sensitivity in vivo. J Immunol 1995; 155:4661–4668.

93. Schwarz A, Grabbe S, Aragane Y, et al. Interleukin-12 prevents ultraviolet B-induced local immunosuppression and overcomes UVB-induced tolerance. J Invest Dermatol 1996; 106:1187–1191.

94. Kripke ML, Cox PA, Alas LG, Yarosh DB. Pyrimidine dimers in DNA initiate systemic immunosuppression in UV-irradiated mice. P Natl Acad Sci USA 1992; 89:7516–7520.

95. Nishigori C, Yarosh DB, Ullrich SE, et al. Evidence that DNA damage triggers interleukin 10 cytokine production in UV-irradiated murine keratinocytes. P Natl Acad Sci USA 1996; 93:10,354–10,359.

96. Stege H, Roza L, Vink AA, et al. Enzyme plus light therapy to repair DNA damage in ultraviolet-B-irradiated human skin. P Natl Acad Sci USA 2000; 97:1790–1795.

97. Schwarz A, Stander S, Berneburg M, et al. Interleukin-12 suppresses ultraviolet radiation-induced apoptosis by inducing DNA repair. Nat Cell Biol 2002; 4:26–31.

98. Fisher MS, Kripke ML. Further studies on the tumor-specific suppressor cells induced by ultraviolet radiation. J Immunol 1978; 121:1139–1144.

99. Moodycliffe AM, Nghiem D, Clydesdale G, Ullrich SE. Immune suppression and skin cancer development: regulation by NKT cells. Nat Immunol 2000; 1:521–525.

100. Schwarz T, Urbanski A, Luger TA. Ultraviolet light and epidermal cell derived cytokines. In: Luger TA, Schwarz T, eds. Epidermal Growth Factors and Cytokines. New York: Marcel Dekker, 1994:303–363.

101. Schwarz T, Urbanska A, Gschnait F, Luger TA. Inhibition of the induction of contact hypersensitivity by a UV-mediated epidermal cytokine. J Invest Dermatol 1986; 87:289–291.

102. Rivas JM, Ullrich SE. Systemic suppression of delayed-type hypersensitivity by supernatants from UV-irradiated keratinocytes—an essential role for keratinocyte-derived IL-10. J Immunol 1992; 149:3865–3871.
103. Enk AH, Saloga J, Becker D, Mohamadzadeh M, Knop J. Induction of hapten-specific tolerance by interleukin-10 in vivo. J Exp Med 1994; 179:1397–1402.
104. Ullrich SE. Mechanism involved in the systemic suppression of antigen-presenting cell function by UV irradiation—keratinocyte-derived IL-10 modulates antigen-presenting cell function of splenic adherent cells. J Immunol 1994; 152:3410–3416.
105. Moodycliffe AM, Kimber I, Norval M. Role of tumour necrosis factor-alpha in ultraviolet B light-induced dendritic cell migration and suppression of contact hypersensitivity. Immunology 1994; 81:79–84.
106. Niizeki H, Inoko H, Streilein JW. Polymorphisms in the TNF region confer susceptibility to UVB-induced impairment of contact hypersensitivity induction in mice and humans. Methods 2002; 28:46–54.
107. Gillardon F, Moll I, Michel S, Benrath J, Weihe E, Zimmermann M. Calcitonin gene-related peptide and nitric oxide are involved in ultraviolet radiation-induced immunosuppression. Eur J Pharm—Environ 1995; 293:395–400.
108. Böhm M, Luger TA. Alpha-melanocyte-stimulating hormone. Its relevance for dermatology. Hautarzt 2004; 55:436–445.
109. Luger TA, Schwarz T, Kalden H, Scholzen T, Schwarz A, Brzoska T. Role of epidermal cell-derived alpha-melanocyte stimulating hormone in ultraviolet light mediated local immunosuppression. Ann NY Acad Sci 1999; 885:209–216.
110. Kuchel JM, Barnetson RS, Halliday GM. Nitric oxide appears to be a mediator of solar-simulated ultraviolet radiation-induced immunosuppression in humans. J Invest Dermatol 2003; 121:587–593.
111. Walterscheid JP, Ullrich SE, Nghiem DX. Platelet-activating factor, a molecular sensor for cellular damage, activates systemic immune suppression. J Exp Med 2002; 195:171–179.
112. Shreedhar V, Giese T, Sung VW, Ullrich SE. A cytokine cascade including prostaglandin E-2, IL-4, and IL-10 is responsible for UV-induced systemic immune suppression. J Immunol 1998; 160:3783–3789.
113. Hart PH, Grimbaldeston MA, Jaksic A, et al. Ultraviolet B-induced suppression of immune responses in interleukin-4-/-mice: Relationship to dermal mast cells. J Invest Dermatol 2000; 114:508–513.
114. Hart PH, Grimbaldeston MA, Finlay-Jones JJ. Mast cells in UV-B-induced immunosuppression. J Photoch Photobio B 2000; 55:81–87.
115. Reeve VE, Bosnic M, Boehmwilcox C, Cope RB. Pyridoxine supplementation protects mice from suppression of contact hypersensitivity induced by 2-acetyl-4-tetrahydroxybutylimidazole (THI), ultraviolet B radiation (280–320 nm), or cis-urocanic acid. Am J Clin Nutr 1995; 61:571–576.
116. De Fabo EC, Noonan FP. Mechanism of immune suppression by ultraviolet irradiation in vivo. I. Evidence for the existence of a unique photoreceptor in skin and its role in photoimmunology. J Exp Med 1983; 158:84–98.
117. Norval M, Gibbs NK, Gilmour J. The role of urocanic acid in UV-induced immunosuppression—recent advances (1992–1994). Photochem Photobiol 1995; 62:209–217.
118. Kondo S, Sauder DN, McKenzie RC, et al. The role of cis-urocanic acid in UVB-induced suppression of contact hypersensitivity. Immunol Lett 1995; 48:181–186.
119. Moodycliffe AM, Bucana CD, Kripke ML, Norval M, Ullrich SE. Differential effects of a monoclonal antibody to cis-urocanic acid on the suppression of delayed and contact hypersensitivity following ultraviolet irradiation. J Immunol 1996; 157:2891–2899.
120. Beissert S, Mohammad T, Torri H, et al. Regulation of tumor antigen presentation by urocanic acid. J Immunol 1997; 159:92–96.
121. Beissert S, Ruhlemann D, Mohammad T, et al. IL-12 prevents the inhibitory effects of cis-urocanic acid on tumor antigen presentation by Langerhans cells: implications for photocarcinogenesis. J Immunol 2001; 167:6232–6238.
122. Norval M. Effects of solar radiation on the human immune system. J Photoch Photobio B 2001; 63:28–40.
123. Chapman RS, Cooper KD, Defabo EC, et al. Solar ultraviolet radiation and the risk of infectious disease: Summary of a workshop. Photochem Photobiol 1995; 61:223–247.
124. El-Ghorr AA, Norval M. The effect of UV-B irradiation on secondary epidermal infection of mice with herpes simplex virus type 1. J Gen Virol 1996; 77:485–491.
125. Jeevan A, Kripke ML. Effect of a single exposure to ultraviolet radiation on Mycobacterium bovis Bacillus Calmette-Guerin infection in mice. J Immunol 1989; 143:2837–2843.
126. Jeevan A, Ullrich SE, Degracia M, Shah R, Sun Y. Mechanism of UVB-induced suppression of the immune response to Mycobacterium ovis Bacillus Calmette-Guerin—role of cytokines on macrophage function. Photochem Photobiol 1996; 64:259–266.
127. Goettsch W, Garssen J, Deijns A, De Gruijl FR, Van Loveren H. UV-B exposure impairs resistance to infection by Trichinella spiralis. Environ Health Perspect 1994; 102:298–301.

128. Goettsch W, Garssen J, De Gruijl FR, Van Loveren H. UVB-induced decreased resistance to Trichinella spiralis in the rat is related to impaired cellular immunity. Photochem Photobiol 1996; 64:581–585.

129. Yamamoto K, Ito R, Koura M, Kamiyama T. UV-B irradiation increases susceptibility of mice to malarial infection. Infect Immun 2000; 68:2353–2355.

130. Goettsch W, Garssen J, de Klerk A, et al. Effects of ultraviolet-B exposure on the resistance to Listeria monocytogenes in the rat. Photochem Photobiol 1996; 63:672–679.

131. Brown EL, Ullrich SE, Pride M, Kripke ML. The effect of UV irradiation on infection of mice with Borrelia burgdorferi. Photochem Photobiol 2001; 73:537–544.

132. Cope RB, Hartman JA, Morrow CK, Haschek WM, Small PL. Ultraviolet radiation enhances both the nodular and ulcerative forms of Mycobacterium ulcerans infection in a Crl:IAF(HA)-hrBR hairless guinea pig model of Buruli ulcer disease. Photodermatol Photo 2002; 18:271–279.

133. Perna JJ, Mannix ML, Rooney JF, Notkins AL, Straus SE. Reactivation of latent herpes simplex virus infection by ultraviolet light: a human model. J Am Acad Dermatol 1987; 17:473–478.

134. Rooney JF, Bryson Y, Mannix ML, et al. Prevention of ultraviolet-light-induced Herpes Labialis by sunscreen. Lancet 1991; 338:1419–1422.

135. Gallerani M, Manfredini R. Seasonal variation in herpes zoster infection. Brit J Dermatol 2000; 142:588–589.

136. Termorshuizen F, Hogewoning AA, Bavinck JNB, Goettsch WG, Fijter JW, Loveren H. Skin infections in renal transplant recipients and the relation with solar ultraviolet radiation. Clin Transplant 2003; 17:522–527.

137. Termorshuizen F, Garssen J, Norval M, et al. A review of studies on the effects of ultraviolet irradiation on the resistance to infections: evidence from rodent infection models and verification by experimental and observational humane studies. Int Immunopharmacol 2002; 2:263–275.

138. Cestari TF, Kripke ML, Baptista PL, Bakos L, Bucana CD. Ultraviolet radiation decreases the granulomatous response to lepromin in humans. J Invest Dermatol 1995; 105:8–13.

139. Euvrard S, Kanitakis J, Pouteil-Noble C, Claudy A, Touraine JL. Skin cancers in organ transplant recipients. Ann Transplant 1997; 2:28–32.

140. Kripke ML. Antigenicity of murine skin tumors induced by ultraviolet light. J Natl Cancer I 1974; 53:1333–1336.

141. Kripke ML, Fisher MS. Immunologic parameters of ultraviolet carcinogenesis. J Natl Cancer I 1976; 57:211–215.

142. Sluyter R, Halliday GM. Infiltration by inflammatory cells required for solar-simulated ultraviolet radiation enhancement of skin tumor growth. Cancer Immunol Immun 2001; 50:151–156.

143. Donawho CK, Kripke ML. Evidence that the local effect of ultraviolet radiation on the growth of murine melanomas is immunologically mediated. Cancer Research 1991; 51:4176–4181.

144. Ullrich SE, Kripke ML. Mechanisms in the suppression of tumor rejection produced in mice by repeated UV Irradiation. J Immunol 1984; 133:2786–2790.

145. Barnetson RSC, Satchell A, Zhuang L, Slade HB, Halliday GM. Imiquimod induced regression of clinically diagnosed superficial basal cell carcinoma is associated with early infiltration by CD4 T cells and dendritic cells. Clin Exp Dermatol 2004; 29:639–643.

146. Ooi T, Barnetson RS, Zhuang L, et al. Imiquimod-induced regression of actinic keratosis is associated with infiltration by T lymphocytes and dendritic cells: a randomized controlled trial. Brit J Dermatol 2006; 154:72–78.

147. Hersey P. Immunotherapy of melanoma: principles. In: Thompson JF, Morton DL, Kroon BBR, eds. Textbook of Melanoma. London and New York: Martin Dunitz, 2004:559–572.

148. Mehling A, Loser K, Varga G, et al. Overexpression of CD40 ligand in murine epidermis results in chronic skin inflammation and systemic autoimmunity. J Exp Med 2001; 194:615–628.

149. Casciola-Rosen LA, Anhalt G, Rosen A. Autoantigens targeted in systemic lupus erythematosus are clustered in two populations of surface structures on apoptotic keratinocytes. J Exp Med 1994; 179:1317–1330.

6 The Acute Effects of Ultraviolet Radiation on the Skin

Lesley E. Rhodes
Department of Dermatological Sciences, Photobiology Unit, University of Manchester, Salford Royal Foundation Hospital, Manchester, England, U.K.

Henry W. Lim
Department of Dermatology, Henry Ford Hospital, Detroit, Michigan, U.S.A.

- Exposure to UVB or UVA, can result in erythema with different time course.

- Mediators of sunburn response include reactive oxygen species (ROS), transcription factors, vasoactive mediators, proinflammatory cytokines, and adhesion molecules.

- Pigment darkening and delayed tanning are predominantly the effect of UVA; the latter is associated with melanogenesis.

- Mediators of melanogenesis include DNA repair fragments, α-melanocyte stimulating hormone, nitric oxide, and histamine.

- Other acute effects of UV radiation include epidermal hyperplasis, synthesis of vitamin D, photoimmunosuppression, exacerbation of photodermatoses, and disturbance of skin barrier function.

INTRODUCTION

The acute effects of ultraviolet radiation (UVR) on the skin comprise a range of responses, many of which are harmful in the short term or after cumulative exposure in the longer term, and others that are beneficial. The best-known short-term manifestations of UVR exposure are sunburn, pigment darkening, tanning, vitamin D synthesis, immunosuppression, and the photosensitivity disorders; and these types of manifestations form the focus of this chapter.

Ultraviolet-A (UVA, 320–400 nm) and -B (UVB, 290–320 nm) reach the earth's surface and both can cause acute effects on human skin. Ninety-five percent of UVR reaching the surface of the earth is UVA and the rest is UVB. The shorter wavelength UVB is more potent in causing several acute effects of UVR, and the action spectrum for various acute effects of UVR varies from UVB alone, to UVA alone, to a combination of both wavebands. The effects are determined by the UVR absorption spectrum of the molecule(s) initiating the specific effect; that is, the chromophore. The depth of UVR penetration in the skin also plays a role; most UVB is absorbed in the epidermis with a small proportion reaching the upper dermis (1,2), while UVA penetrates deeply into the dermis. UVB, nevertheless, produces a range of dermal effects; these may be partly attributable to UVB-induced release of mediators by epidermal cells, particularly keratinocytes (3), and partly due to direct effects of UVB on upper dermal structures and cells, including endothelial cells (4), and fibroblasts (5).

UVA is divided into UVA-1 (340–400 mm) and UVA-2 (320–340 mm); this division is made since the latter is more akin to UVB in its effects. However, the spectrum is a continuum with overlap of effects. UVR causes effects on a range of cellular structures; that is, DNA, proteins, and lipids. Whereas UVB conveys direct effects through absorption by a range of molecules, both UVB and UVA convey indirect effects through the generation of reactive oxygen species (ROS), produced when UVR is absorbed by endogenous photosensitizers in the presence of molecular oxygen. ROS mediate a range of UVR-induced effects including induction of transcription factors, modulation of signal transduction pathways, and downstream events.

THE SUNBURN RESPONSE
Nature of the Sunburn Response

Sunburn is an acute inflammatory response of the skin to the UVB radiation in sunlight (6). UVA can also cause skin erythema, requiring approximately 1000-fold higher doses than UVB. Thus, a higher risk of sunburn is seen when the UVB to UVA ratio is relatively high, as occurs between 11 AM and 3 PM in the summer months in temperate climates, and at latitudes approaching the Equator. In addition to being a UVB dose-dependent response, the risk of sunburn depends on the skin phototype of the individual, with skin types 1 and 2 showing the highest propensity to sunburn.

Time Course

As an acute inflammatory response, sunburn may manifest with features of heat, pain, swelling, and erythema. Systemic upset can also occur in cases of severe generalized sunburn. The most consistent clinical feature, however, is that of erythema. This first becomes visible between three and six hours postexposure, peaks at 12 to 24 hours, and is maintained to 48 hours, followed by resolution (Fig. 1). With the use of noninvasive reflectance instruments and laser Doppler flowimetry, it has been demonstrated that the vasodilatation, underlying sunburn, commences much earlier than the clinically visible response—changes occurring within 30 minutes of UV exposure (7). Such instrumentation has also revealed that the time course of erythema is UVB dose dependent, with the minimal erythema dose (MED, the sunburn threshold) of UVB producing an erythema that peaks earlier and resolves faster than higher doses (8). In contrast to UVB, UVA causes an immediate postexposure erythema, resolving gradually in 48 to 72 hours (Fig. 2).

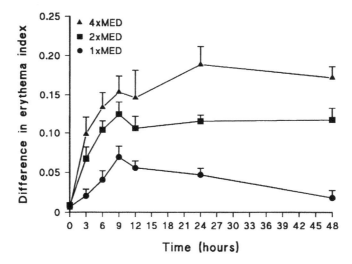

FIGURE 1   The time course of UVB-induced erythema, as determined by reflectance spectrophotometry, $n = 6$, data are mean $\pm$ SEM. *Abbreviation*: MED, minimal erythemal dose. *Source*: Adapted from Ref. 111.

Histology

Although UVB is mainly absorbed within the epidermis, a proportion certainly reaches the upper dermis (1,2), and dermal effects are also initiated indirectly via mediators released by epidermal cells. Dermal endothelial cell swelling is an early feature, evident within 30 minutes of UV exposure, reaching a maximum by 24 hours and persisting for three days. Langerhans cells show morphological changes, and depletion in cell numbers is seen within a few hours. Neutrophils quickly accumulate in the dermis with a perivascular distribution seen immediately to postirradiation, peak numbers occurring around 14 hours, and a decline at 48 hours (9). A mononuclear infiltrate occurs later, reaching a plateau at around 14 to 21 hours and decreasing by 48 hours (9).

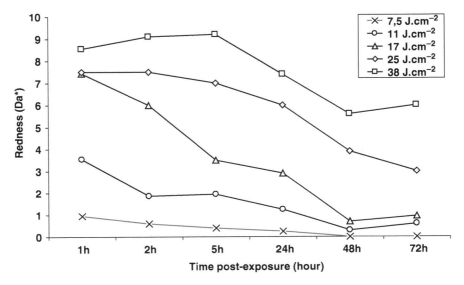

FIGURE 2   The time course of UVA-induced erythema, illustrating an immediate and sustained erythema. *Source*: Adapted from Ref. 112.

In the epidermis, "sunburn cells" may be seen within 30 minutes of UVB exposure, with a peak at 24 hours. These cells are damaged keratinocytes and show shrunken chromatin and eosinophilic cytoplasm. They are apoptotic cells, representing a protective mechanism to eliminate DNA-damaged cells, and can occur in the absence of skin inflammation, but their number increases as the sunburn response increases. Epidermal spongiosis is also evident at 24 hours post irradiation. UVA induces less epidermal damage than UVB, sunburn cells not being seen (10).

Mechanism

The sunburn response involves a concerted response of resident epidermal and dermal cells and leukocytes, induced to migrate into the skin by UVR. Keratinocytes express a wide range of cytokines and chemokines, following UVB exposure and are generally regarded as the cells that most likely initiate the UVB-induced inflammatory response (Table 1) (3). Dermal cells could be recruited to the response both via soluble mediators secreted by keratinocytes and via the direct effects of UVR.

Initiating Events

The nature of the chromophore for the sunburn response is still uncertain. There is some evidence to suggest that this may be DNA. Patients with the DNA-repair disorder xeroderma pigmentosum show an abnormally amplified and prolonged sunburn response, which can be reduced by topical application of the DNA repair enzyme endonuclease (11). Further, indirect evidence is provided by the similarity of the action spectra for UVR-induced erythema and thymidine dimer formation in human skin (12). UVR is known to damage many tissue components, including membrane phospholipids, proteins, and nucleic acids; and these may trigger a variety of proinflammatory molecular responses, which may appear in parallel as well as in sequence. It is increasingly recognized, however, that many of the cellular effects of UVR are due to alterations in signal transduction pathways leading to aberrant gene expression. The mechanisms by which UVR triggers cell signal transduction are multifactorial, and include the release of cytokines, growth factors, lipid mediators, and ROS (13).

Oxidative Stress

The contribution of oxidative stress to UVR-induced inflammation is poorly understood. However, ROS, particularly superoxide anion, hydrogen peroxide, and hydroxyl radical, are known to mediate induction of transcription factors, modulation of signal transduction pathways, and a range of downstream inflammatory events. Moreover, antioxidants are reported to be effective in reducing the sunburn response in humans (14).

TABLE 1 Mediators of Sunburn Response

Reactive oxygen species
Transcription factors
   NF-κB
   AP-1
Vaso-active mediators
   PGE$_2$
   Nitric oxide
Proinflammatory cytokines
   TNF-α
   IL-1
   IL-6
   IL-8
   IL-12
Adhesion molecules
   ICAM-1
   E-selectin

Abbreviations: AP, activator protein; ICAM, intercellular adhesion molecule; IL, interleukin; NF, nuclear factor; TNF, tumor necrosis factor.

Transcription Factors

UVR induces the activation of transcription factors, including NF-κB and AP-1, which control the expression of a wide range of genes. The transcription factors may be induced through UVR-induced ROS, growth factors, and cytokine signal transduction pathways. The activation of NF-κB, in particular, leads to the formation of a wide range of inflammatory mediators including cytokines, adhesion molecules, and inflammatory enzymes that include nitric oxide synthase and cyclooxygenase (15).

Vasoactive Mediators

There is evidence that the erythema component of the sunburn response is mediated by the vasoactive mediators prostaglandin (PG) E_2 and nitric oxide, in combination (8). UVR activates cell membrane phospholipase A_2, releasing arachidonic acid that is then used to synthesize mediators of the eicosanoid family. Prostanoids are elevated in suction blister fluid following UVB, that is, the prostaglandins PGD_2, PGI_2, PGE_2, and $PGF_{2\alpha}$, along with hydroxyeicosatetranoic acid (12-HETE) (16). It appears that PGE_2 is the most potent with regards to erythema production (17). Cyclooxygenase inhibitors applied by various routes reduce UVB-induced erythema (16,18–20), and it has recently been found that PGE_2 is more involved at higher doses of UVB, whereas nitric oxide appears to play a greater role in the mediation of erythema at lower doses around the MED (8). The latter inhibitor studies also provided evidence that both these mediators are active throughout the first 48 hours of the sunburn response. Increased expression of messenger RNA for inducible nitric oxide synthase (NOS)-2 has been detected in skin, which is exposed to UVR (21), and nitric oxide has been directly detected in the sunburn response by dermal microdialysis (8). In vitro studies have also shown upregulation of the activity and expression of NOS1 and NOS3 by UVB (22,23). The vasoactive mediator histamine is also reported to be elevated early in the course of UV-induced inflammation (24), although the overall effects may be small since antihistamines reduce the sunburn response minimally, if at all (25,26). Histamine and arachidonic acid metabolites are also released following UVA exposure of the skin (27).

Proinflammatory Cytokines

UVR induces the release of several pro-inflammatory cytokines, including TNF-α (28,29), Interleukin (IL)-1 (30), IL-6 (31), IL-8 (32,33), and IL-12 (34). These may play important roles at various stages of UV-induced inflammation, including activation of transcription factors (particularly by IL-1, TNF-α), induction of endothelial adhesion molecules, and the chemotaxis of leukocytes from the vasculature into the dermis (particularly by IL-8, TNF-α). It has been proposed from time-course studies of cytokine induction, following UVB radiation of human skin, that TNF-α is the key early cytokine involved in UV-induced inflammation (35). However, a later time course of expression has been found in an immunohistochemical study (33). IL-1 activities have been detected in human skin in vivo within 30 minutes of UVB exposure, with a biphasic time course, which may suggest the release of preformed IL-1 and subsequent IL-1 synthesis (36). Both IL-1 and IL-6 have been found in the serum following wide area UVB exposure, with IL-6 persisting longer than IL-1 and, probably, mediating the systemic features of the sunburn response (37,38).

Adhesion Molecules

UVB radiation induces ICAM-1 expression on keratinocytes (39,40) and expression of E-selectin and ICAM-1 on dermal endothelial cells (41,4). E-selectin and ICAM-1 induce chemotaxis of neutrophils and lymphocytes, respectively, and it has been shown that in human skin in vivo, the expression of E-selectin correlates with the dermal neutrophil count (33). Similarly, UVA induces E-selectin and ICAM-1 on dermal endothelial cells (42). There is evidence that the effects of UVA on adhesion molecule-expression are mediated by the generation of ROS (43). Once present in the skin, the leukocytic infiltrate, particularly the neutrophils, produce large amounts of ROS, which cause damage to the cells targeted by these inflammatory cells.

PIGMENT DARKENING

UVR-induced skin pigmentation occurs in three distinct phases; that is, immediate pigment darkening, persistent pigment darkening, and delayed tanning.

Immediate Pigment Darkening

Immediate pigment darkening (IPD) occurs as a response to low doses ($1–5$ J/cm^2) of UVA; it appears almost immediately after exposure and usually fades within 10 to 20 minutes (44). Clinically, it manifests as grey-brown color. It is thought to result from oxidation and redistribution of pre-existing melanin; no new melanin synthesis occurs.

Persistent Pigment Darkening

At higher UVA doses (>10 J/cm^2), pigment darkening can persist for two hours to 24 hours; this is termed persistent pigment darkening (PPD) (44). Clinically, it appears as brown color, similar to IPD. It is also due to oxidation and redistribution of pre-existing melanin. Protection against the development of PPD is the most commonly used surrogate worldwide for the assessment of UVA protectiveness of sunscreen.

Delayed Tanning of the Skin
Nature of the Tanning Response
Tanning is a delayed effect of UVR. In contrast to IPD and PPD, delayed tanning is associated with synthesis of new melanin. Both UVB and UVA are capable of inducing tanning, although UVB is more efficient. A study on the action spectrum for melanogenesis in human skin in vivo showed that peak melanogenesis occurs at about 290 nm, similar to the peak for erythema (6). Because UVB is more erythemogenic than UVA, UVB-induced delayed tanning is always preceded by erythema. In contrast, UVA can induce tanning without noticeable redness. While both UVB and UVA can induce melanogenesis, UVB, additionally, induces epidermal thickening. This is reflected by the observation that for visually identical tan, UVB-induced tan resulted in a protection factor of 3 against UVB-induced erythema, while UVA-induced tan only conferred a protection factor of 1.4 (45).

Tanning occurs as a response to UVR-induced damage of the skin and may serve to limit the amount of subsequent damage caused by continued UVR exposure. Sun reactive skin types 3 and 4 and higher display a high ability to tan, whereas sun reactive skin types 1 and 2 show a poor ability to tan. This clinical observation is supported by a study of solar-simulated, radiation-induced tanning. Whereas tanning was associated with some protection against DNA damage in skin types 3 and 4, no protection was seen in skin types one and two (2).

Time Course
Delayed tanning (melanogenesis) becomes visible at around 72 hours following UV exposure. Melanin is formed and distributed within the basal layer of the epidermis. As cells move upward through the layers of the epidermis, the melanin eventually reaches the outer layer of the skin, that is, the stratum corneum, resulting in the tan fading as the surface layer is shed.

Mechanism and Mediators of Melanogenesis
It has been hypothesized that melanogenesis may be initiated by DNA excision repair (Table 2). This is supported by in vitro studies showing an increase in melanin content in human melanocytes following their exposure to thymidine dinucleotides, which mimic DNA excision fragments (46). Delayed tanning is associated with increases in both the number of melanocytes and melanocytic activity (47). The latter is characterized by increased tyrosinase activity, elongation of dendrites, and increased transfer of melanosomes to keratinocytes.

TABLE 2   Mediators of Melanogenesis

DNA excision repair fragments	Nitric oxide
α-Melanocyte stimulating hormone	Histamine

Following UVR exposure, keratinocytes release a melanocortin, α-melanocyte stimulating hormone (α-MSH), which stimulates melanin production in melanocytes (48). UVR also regulates the α-MSH receptors on melanocytes. The melanin is distributed in melanosomes through the dendritic processes of the melanocytes where it absorbs and scatters UVR, thus protecting other epidermal cells from damage. In particular, melanin forms "nuclear caps" over the nuclei of basal keratinocytes. Hence, the epidermis is protected. However, the amount of protection varies between individuals.

Two types of melanin are formed, eumelanin and phaeomelanin. Whereas eumelanin provides additional protection by acting as a free-radical scavenger, phaeomelanin can increase oxidative stress. Furthermore, not all melanocytes are responsive to α-MSH (49). In skin phototypes 1 and 2, a lack of responsiveness to α-MSH is associated with melanocortin 1 receptor (MC1R) variants, resulting in the production of little of the photoprotective eumelanin and clinically showing a weak pigmentary response.

Mediators that have been implicated in melanogenesis include nitric oxide, which may act in both an autocrine and paracrine manner to regulate pigmentation (50). Topical application of the NOS inhibitor L-NAME (N-nitro-L-arginine methylester hydrochloride) to guinea pig skin reduces the melanin content of melanocytes (51). Additionally, nitric oxide has been reported to enhance the dendricity of melanocytes (52). In vivo studies in guinea pig skin also support a role for histamine in UVR-induced melanogenesis (53). In vitro experiments suggest that nitric oxide, along with histamine, may play a role in setting the eumelanin/phaeomelanin ratio in melanocytes (54). It is uncertain how nitric oxide exerts this effect, although it may play a major role through the activation of tyrosinase (52).

EPIDERMAL HYPERPLASIA

Hyperproliferation of epidermal cells begins soon after UVB exposure and leads to epidermal thickening, which is histologically evident within days and persists for some weeks, following exposure. There is a several-fold increase in thickness, particularly affecting the stratum corneum, and along with melanogenesis this conveys some protection against further UVR damage. Dermal thickening may also occur.

VITAMIN D SYNTHESIS

The major and best understood beneficial effect of acute UVR on skin is the synthesis of vitamin D_3. The action spectrum for this lies in the UVB waveband (55).

Sources of Vitamin D
There are two forms of vitamin D, vitamin D_3 and vitamin D_2. Vitamin D_3 is synthesized in the epidermis, and is available through naturally occurring food sources. However, it is found naturally in few foods, the main sources being oily fish (e.g., herring, salmon, sardines), liver, and egg yolk; therefore, the amount obtained from dietary sources is generally low, typically around 10% of the body's source. Vitamin D_3 is available as a vitamin supplement. Vitamin D_2 is present in plants. It is the most widely used form in vitamin supplements, and is in fortified milk, margarine, butter, and cereals.

Cutaneous Synthesis of Vitamin D
The initial step in vitamin D formation is the rapid conversion of 7-dehydrocholesterol to previtamin D (cholecalciferol), by UVB. Previtamin D undergoes thermal isomerization to vitamin D_3, the isomer mixture reaching a pseudoequilibrium in sunlight that limits the previtamin D that can be formed in a single UVB exposure, to 10% to 20% of the epidermal 7-dehydrocholesterol concentration. The vitamin D benefit of sunlight is reached long before any risk of sunburn, and further sun exposure is of no benefit, only serving to increase UVR hazards. Incidental sun exposure during normal daily activity along with balanced diet is probably sufficient for most individuals to achieve adequate vitamin D levels. For those at a high risk to develop vitamin D insufficiency, such as a elderly, home-bound individuals, those with dark skin, and indoor workers, vitamin D_3 supplement should be taken (56,57).

Metabolism of Vitamin D

Vitamin D derived from either cutaneous or dietary source is biologically inactive and undergoes two hydroxylation steps. Firstly, it is metabolized in the liver to 25-hydroxy vitamin D (25OHD), the main circulating storage form. Then it is converted under strict metabolic control in the kidney to 1,25-dihydroxy vitamin D (1,25D), which promotes intestinal absorption of calcium and facilitates bone mineralization.

Vitamin D and Bone Health

It is well established that severe vitamin D deficiency leads to rickets and osteomalacia. Circulating 25OHD levels above 5 ng/ml are sufficient to prevent these extreme health effects (58). However, it has relatively recently been recognized that 25OHD values between 5 and 20 ng/mL are associated with secondary hyperparathyroidism, with consequent bone loss and osteoporotic fractures (59–61). Counter-intuitively, a study of over 36,000 women followed for 7 years showed that daily supplements of vitamin D_3 (400 IU) and calcium (1000 mg) did not significantly reduce hip fractures (62). Elderly individuals and people with darker skin appear particularly at risk of low serum 25OHD levels, due to low amounts of vitamin D that may be achieved through both oral and cutaneous routes (63,64).

Vitamin D and Other Disorders

Circumstantial evidence is accumulating that inadequate vitamin D levels may have other adverse health consequences, including the risk of a range of malignancies, hypertension and diabetes mellitus (56,57,65,66). These are largely based on epidemiologic studies examining the relationship between the prevalence or mortality of a range of disorders and latitude (67–70). However, a 7-year study of over 36,000 women failed to show any protective effects of vitamin D_3 (400 IU/day) and calcium (1000 mg/day) supplements on the incidence of colorectal cancer (71).

Although the concept is unproven, data from a variety of experimental approaches provides support for the hypothesis that, via effects on vitamin D synthesis, UVR may convey chemoprotective properties (72,73). Many tissues including colon, skin, breast, and prostate are now known to synthesize 1,25D locally from precursor 25OHD. The antiproliferative effect of 1,25D in tumor cell lines provides a potential mechanism for its postulated anticarcinogenic properties (73).

Vitamin D Controversies

Strategies to protect against skin cancer include avoidance of the midday sun and the use of sunscreens and photoprotective clothings, both of which reduce the amount of UVB reaching the skin (74,75) and thus may reduce cutaneous vitamin D synthesis. However, it is debatable how completely the public follows these recommendations, including adequacy of sunscreen application and use. At northern latitudes, there is insufficient ambient UVB to initiate vitamin D synthesis in skin during the winter (55) and excess vitamin D formed in the summer months is stored in fat for use throughout the winter months. However, stores may be inadequate to maintain an optimal vitamin D status all year round, and strategies may be needed to combat this. Whereas there is good evidence for the relationship between low 25OHD levels and bone health, other potential benefits of vitamin D are speculative, and the subject of considerable international debate (57,56,76). Recent efforts have focused on defining an optimal circulating 25OHD level. Many suggest that this is around 80 nmol/L (or 32 μgm/L) (77,78), a level anticipated to be adequate for bone health plus giving a margin for other potential health benefits; this can be achieved with 800 to 1000 IU of daily vitamin D_3, or 50,000 IU of monthly vitamin D_3 (79).

PHOTOIMMUNOSUPPRESSION
The Nature of Photoimmunosuppression in Human Skin

The induction of immunosuppression in human skin by UVR is a "normal" phenomenon occurring in all individuals. This topic is discussed in greater detail in chapter 5. It is established from several studies, that UVR exposure of human skin results in downregulation of delayed hypersensitivity (DTH) responses, a measure of T cell function (80). It has been demonstrated that UVR suppresses the contact hypersensitivity (CHS) responses to nickel in nickel-sensitive individuals (81), and to DNCB (82). Further studies of CHS responses to DNCB designated 40% of volunteers as UVB-susceptible (83). Furthermore, the same investigators found that 92% of skin cancer patients fell into the UVB-susceptible category, thus implying that UVB-induced suppression of CHS may be a risk factor for skin cancer. Studies by Cooper et al. (84) illustrated, however, that a clear division into UVR-susceptible and UVR-resistant individuals might be too simplistic.

Action Spectrum

It has previously been assumed that UVB is the waveband of importance when considering immunosuppression. However, there has been increasing interest in the effects of UVA over the last 10 years, and it is now clear that this waveband also has important immunosuppressive properties. This is likely to be of clinical relevance when considering the high proportion of UVA compared to UVB in sunlight (UVA 95%, UVB 5%); the augmentation of this difference by the use of sunscreens, which are more effective at blocking UVB than UVA, and enable the individual to stay longer in the sunlight without sunburn; and the growing popularity of the use of commercial sunbeds.

Mechanisms of Photoimmunosuppression

UVR-induced immunosuppression appears as a complex phenomenon, including the interactive processes mediated by resident keratinocytes and endothelial cells and infiltrating lymphocytes. These cells play important signalling roles, mediated by cell surface molecules and soluble factors, which then influence the responses of skin immune cells. The following are components of this response.

Antigen Presenting Cells

UVR modulates the number and function of epidermal Langerhans cells, a key antigen-presenting cell. Following UVR exposure, Langerhans cells are observed to round up morphologically into their migratory form, and to disappear from the epidermis. This could result in diminished antigen presentation by these cells, that is, a reduction of their immunosurveillance role. The phenomenon may be mediated through UVR induction of cytokines, particularly TNF-α and IL-1β (85), and there is also evidence for the involvement of eicosanoids, particularly PGE$_2$ (86). Furthermore, UVR causes an influx of CD11+ macrophages with immunosuppressive properties, which may largely be conveyed through their secretion of the immunosuppressive cytokine, IL-10 (87).

Alteration of the Th1/Th2 Cytokine Profile

UVR alters the skin lymphocyte profile, such that there is a relative reduction in the secretion of Th1 cytokines such as IL-12 and Gamma Interferon (IFN-γ), which mediate the immune responses of CHS and DTH, and a relative increase in Th2 cytokines, including IL-4 and IL-10, which are immunosuppressive. IL-10 reduces T-lymphocyte responses by inhibiting antigen presentation by antigen presenting cells. IL-10 is secreted by a range of cells including T- and B-lymphocytes, monocytes, macrophages, and keratinocytes (88), and there is evidence for its induction by both UVB and UVA (89).

Other Mediators of Immunosuppression

Several mediators other than Th2 cytokines mediate immunosuppression, many of which are also active in conveying UVR-induced skin inflammation. This includes TNF-α, which plays a role in the sunburn response, but also causes Langerhans cell migration away from the skin (90). PGE$_2$, a major mediator of sunburn erythema, is also a potent mediator of immunosuppression; as with TNF-α, there is evidence that it stimulates the migration of Langerhans cells out of the epidermis. The neuropeptide, calcitonin gene related peptide (CGRP), and nitric oxide are also implicated in UVR-induced immunosuppression (91). In humans, topical application of a NOS inhibitor prevented both the suppression of recall immunity to nickel, and the loss of epidermal Langerhans cells from the skin (92).

Candidate Chromophores: Urocanic Acid and DNA

The chromophore(s) of photoimmunosuppression are unknown, although both urocanic acid and DNA have been speculated to play this role.

Urocanic Acid

Urocanic Acid (UCA) exists in two forms, the *cis* and the *trans* forms. It is normally found in its *trans* form in the stratum corneum, and UVR causes its isomerization from the *trans* to the *cis* form, which is associated with cutaneous immunosuppression. UCA has the capacity to reduce Langerhans cell numbers (93) and to suppress contact hypersensitivity (CHS) in mice (94). However, it remains uncertain what role UCA actually plays in skin in view of studies revealing an inconsistent effect on CHS (95) and the apparent lack of correlation between the action spectra for CHS suppression and UCA photoisomerization (96).

DNA

DNA dimer formation has been associated with UVR-induced immunosuppression. The application of the excision repair enzyme T4 endonuclease V (T4 N5), which increases dimer removal, is associated with reversal of UVR-induced suppression of CHS and delayed hypersensitivity (97).

Innate Immunity

UVR causes a dose-dependent inhibition of the activity of natural killer (NK) cells, which are part of the innate immune system (98). In vivo studies in humans have confirmed that NK cell function is reduced during a course of solarium tanning, (99) and in psoriasis patients during a course of UVB therapy (100). Circulating NK cell numbers also fall following solarium treatment but not during UVB therapy.

Oxidative Stress

It is likely that oxidative stress plays a larger role in UVA-induced immunosuppression than UVB-induced immunosuppression. However, more work needs to be done to clarify the pathways of action of UVA (101). Antioxidant supplementation studies have demonstrated that ROS are involved in UVR-induced immunosuppression in animals (102) and humans (103).

Sunscreens and Immune Protection

Sunscreens have been developed to protect against the sunburn response, rather than immunosuppression, but attempts are in progress to develop a system for assessing the immune protection factor of sunscreens, in addition to their erythema protection [sun protection factor (SPF)] (101,104,105). Sunscreens combining a high SPF with high-UVA protection appear most effective (106). Research continues with dietary and topical antioxidant agents, in an attempt to improve the immunoprotection conveyed by traditional sunscreens (14,80,101).

OTHER ACUTE EFFECTS OF ULTRAVIOLET RADIATION
Photosensitivity Disorders

Unlike the other UVR effects described in this chapter, the photosensitivity disorders do not represent a "normal" response of the skin to UVR. Rather, they involve abnormal responses of the skin to low doses of UVA, and/or UVB, and/or visible light. The underlying etiology shows wide diversity, including immune malfunction, biochemical disorders, and DNA repair deficiency. It has been speculated that some of the immune mediated photosensitivity disorders may result from a failure of "normal" photoimmunosuppression of skin, thus permitting photoprovocation to occur (107). Photosensitivity conditions, which manifest with a range of symptoms and/or signs following exposure to sunlight or artificial radiation sources, will be discussed further in Section III of this book.

Disturbance of Skin Barrier Function

High-dose UVR causes alterations in epidermal barrier function, which become evident at around 72 hours postexposure and manifest as increased transepidermal water loss. This delayed barrier disruption appears to occur when lamellar body-deficient keratinocytes arrive at the stratum granulosum/stratum corneum interface (108), suggesting that failure of secretion of lamellar body-derived lipids to the stratum corneum is at least partially responsible for the reduced barrier function. T cell dependent epidermal hyperproliferation (109) and reduced stratum corneum ceramide content (110) also correlate with the barrier disturbance. Rapid recovery is seen.

ACKNOWLEDGMENT

With gratitude to Mrs. Vivien Robinson for her dedication in the preparation of this text.

REFERENCES

1. Everett MA, Yeargers E, Sayre RM, et al. Penetration of epidermis by ultraviolet rays. Photochem Photobiol 1966; 5:533–542.
2. Young AR, Potten CS, Chadwick CA, et al. Photoprotection and 5-MOP photochemoprotection from UVR-induced DNA damage in humans: the role of skin type. J Invest Dermatol 1991; 97:942–948.
3. Barker JNWN, Mitra RS, Griffiths CEM, et al. Keratinocytes as initiators of inflammation. Lancet, 1991; 337:211–214.
4. Rhodes LE, Joyce M, West DC, et al. Comparison of changes in endothelial adhesion molecule expression following UVB irradiation of skin and a human dermal microvascular cell line (HMEC-1). Photodermatol Photoimmunol Photomed 1996; 12:114–121.
5. Storey A, McArdle F, Friedmann PS, et al. Eicosapentaenoic acid and docosahexaenoic acid reduce UVB- and TNF-α-induced IL-8 secretion in keratinocytes and UVB-induced IL-8 in fibroblasts. J Invest Dermatol 2005; 124:248–255.
6. Parrish JA, Jaenicke KF and Anderson RR. Erythema and melanogenesis action spectrum of normal human skin. Photochem Photobiol 1982; 36:187–191.
7. Diffey BL, Farr PM and Oakly AM. Quantitive studies on UVA-induced erythema in human skin. Br J Dermatol 1987; 117:57–66.
8. Rhodes LE, Belgi G, Parslew R, et al. Ultraviolet-B-induced erythema is mediated by nitric oxide and prostaglandin E_2 in combination. J Invest Dermatol 2001; 117:880–885.
9. Hawk JLM, Murphy GM, Holden CA. The presence of neutrophils in human cutaneous ultraviolet-B-induced inflammation. Br J Dermatol 1988; 118:27–30.
10. Rosario R, Mark GJ, Parrish JA, et al. Histological changes produced in skin by equally erythemogenic doses of UV-A, UV-B, UV-C and UVA with psoralens. Br J Dermatol 1979; 120:767–777.
11. Yarosh DB, Klein J, Kibetel J, et al. Enzyme therapy of xeroderma pigmentosum: safety and efficacy testing of T4N5 liposome lotion containing a prokaryotic DNA repair enzyme. Photodermatol Photoimmunol Photomed 1996; 12:122–130.
12. Young AR. Chromophores in human skin. Phys Med Biol 1997; 42:789–802.
13. Heck DE, Gerecke DR, Vetrano AM, et al. Solar ultraviolet radiation as a trigger of cell signal transduction. Toxicol Appl Pharmacol 2004; 195:288–297.
14. Swindells K, Rhodes LE. Influence of oral antioxidants on ultraviolet radiation-induced skin damage in humans. Photodermatol Photoimmunol Photomed 2004; 20 (6):297–304.
15. Terui T, Okuyama R, Tagami H. Molecular events occurring behind ultraviolet-induced skin inflammation. Curr Opin Allergy Clin Immunol 2001; 1:461–467.
16. Black AK, Greaves MW, Hensby CN, et al. The Effects of indomethacin on arachidonic acid and prostaglandins E_2 and F_2 alpha levels in human skin 24 h after UVB and UVC irradiation. Br J Clin Pharmacol 1978; 6:261–266.
17. Crunkhorn P, Willis AL. Cutaneous reactions to intradermal prostaglandins. Br J Pharmacol 1971; 41:49–56.
18. Greenberg RA, Eaglstein WH, Turnier H, et al. Orally given indomethacin and blood flow response to UVL. Arch Dermatol 1975; 111:328–330.
19. Snyder DS, Eaglstein WH. Topical indomethacin and sunburn. Br J Dermatol 1974; 90, 91–93.
20. Farr PM, Diffey BL. A quantitative study of the effect of topical indomethacin on cutaneous erythema induced by UVB and UVC radiation. Br J Dermatol 1986; 115, 453–466.
21. Kuhn A, Fehsel K, Lehmann P, et al. Aberrant timing in epidermal expression of inducible nitric oxide synthase after UV irradiation in cutaneous lupus erythamatosus. J Invest Dermatol 1998; 111, 149–153.

22. Kang-Rotondo CH, Major S, Chiang TM, et al. Upregulation of nitric oxide synthase in cultured human keratinocytes after ultraviolet B and bradykinin. Photodermatol Photoimmunol Photomed 1996; 12(2):57–65.

23. Sasaki M, Yamaoka J, Miyachi Y. The effect of ultraviolet B irradiation on nitric oxide synthase expression in murine keratinocytes. Exp Dermatol 2000; 9:417–422.

24. Hruza LL, Pentland AP. Mechanisms of UV-induced inflammation. J Invest Dermatol 1993; 100:355–415.

25. Farr PM, Diffey BL, Humphreys F. A quantitive study of the effect of terfenadine on cutaneous erythema induced by UVB and UVC irradiation. J Invest Dermatol 1986; 87:771–774.

26. Anderson PH, Abrams K, Maibach H. Ultraviolet B dose-dependant inflammation in humans: a reflectance spectroscopic and laser Doppler flowmetric study using topical pharmacologic antagonists on irradiated skin. Photodermatol Photoimmunol Photomed 1992; 9:17–23.

27. Hawk JL, Black AK, Jaenicke KF, et al. Increased concentrations of arachidonic acid, prostaglandins E_2, D_2, and 6-oxo-F1α, and histamine in human skin following UVA irradiation. J Invest Dermatol 1983; 80:496–499.

28. Oxholm A, Oxholm P, Staberg B, et al. Immunohistological detection of interleukin 1-like molecules and tumour necrosis factor in human epidermis before and after UVB-irradiation in vivo. Br J Dermatol 1988; 118:369–376.

29. Kock A, Schwartz T, Kirnbauer R, et al. Human keratinocytes are a source for tumour necrosis factor alpha: evidence for synthesis and release upon stimulation with endotoxin or ultraviolet light. J Exp Med 1990; 172:1609–1614.

30. Kupper TS, Chua AO, Flood P, et al. Interleukin 1 gene expression in cultured human keratinocytes is augmented by ultraviolet irradiation. J Clin Invest 1987; 80:430–436.

31. Oxholm A. Epidermal expression of interleukin-6 and tumour necrosis factor-alpha in normal and immunoinflammatory skin states in humans. APMIS Suppl 1992; 24:1–32.

32. Kondo S, Kono T, Sauder DN, et al. IL-8 gene expression and production in human keratinocytes and their modulation by UVB. J Invest Dermatol 1993; 101:690–694.

33. Strickland I, Rhodes LE, Flanagan BF, et al. TNF-α and IL-8 are upregulated in the epidermis of normal human skin after UVB-exposure, correlation with neutrophil accumulation and E-selectin expression. J Invest Dermatol 1997; 108:763–768.

34. Shen J, Bao S, Reeve VE. Modulation of IL-10, IL-12 and IFN-γ in the epidermis of hairless mice by UVA (320–400 nm) and UVB (280–320 nm) radiation. J Invest Dermatol 1999; 113:1059–1064.

35. Barr RM, Walker SL, Tsang W, et al. Suppressed alloantigen presentation, increased TNF-α, IL-1, IL-1Ra, IL-10 and modulation of TNF-R in UV-irradiated human skin. J Invest Dermatol 1999; 112:692–698.

36. Murphy GM, Dowd PM, Hudspith BN, et al. Local increase in interleukin-1-like activity following UVB irradiation of human skin in vivo. Photodermatol 1989; 6:268–274.

37. Granstein RD, Sauder DN. Whole body exposure to ultraviolet radiation results in increased serum interleukin-1 activity in humans. Lymphokine Res 1987; 6:193–197.

38. Urbanski A, Schwarz T, Neuner P, et al. Ultraviolet light induces circulating interleukin-6 in humans. J Invest Dermatol 1990; 94:808–811.

39. Norris DA, Lyons MB, Middleton MH, et al. Ultraviolet radiation can either suppress or induce expression of intercellular adhesion molecule 1 (ICAM-1) on the surface of cultured human keratinocytes. J Invest Dermatol 1990; 95:132–138.

40. Krutmann J, Kock A, Schauer E, et al. Tumor necrosis factor beta and ultraviolet radiation are potent regulators of human keratinocyte ICAM-1 expression. J Invest Dermatol 1990; 95:127–131.

41. Norris P, Poston RN, Sian TD, et al. The expression of endothelial adhesion molecules (ICAM-1) and vascular cell adhesion molecule-1 (VCAM-1) in experimental cutaneous inflammation: a comparison of ultraviolet B erythema and delayed hypersensitivity. J Invest Dermatol 1991; 96:763.

42. Heckmann M, Eberlein-Konig B, Wollenberg A, et al. Ultraviolet-A radiation induces adhesion molecule expression on human dermal microvascular endothelial cells. Br J Dermatol 1994; 131:311–318.

43. Olaizola-Horn S, Christoph H, Budnik A, et al. Ultraviolet A1 radiation induced immunomodulation is mediated via the generation of singlet oxygen. J Invest Dermatol 1994; 103:429.

44. Hönigsmann H. Erythema and pigmentation. Photodermatol Photoimmunol Photomed 2002; 18: 75–81.

45. Gange RW, Blackett AD, Matzinger EZ, et al. Comparative protection efficiency of UVA- and UVB-induced tans against erythema and formation of endonuclease-sensitive sites in DNA by UVB in human skin. J Invest Dermatol 1985; 85:362–364.

46. Gilchrest BA, Zhai S, Eller MS, et al. Treatment of human melanocytes and S91 melanoma cells with the DNA repair enzyme T4 endonuclease V enhances melanogenesis after ultraviolet irradiation. J Invest Dermatol 1993; 101:666–672.

47. Stierner U, Rosdahl I, Augustsson A, et al. UVB irradiation induces melanocyte increase in both exposed and shielded human skin. J Invest Dermatol 1989; 92:561–564.

48. Archambault M, Yaar M, Gilchrest BA. Keratinocytes and fibroblasts in a human skin equivalent model enhance melanocyte survival and melanin synthesis after ultraviolet irradiation. J Invest Dermatol 1995; 104:859–867.

49. Hunt G, Todd C, Thody AJ. Unresponsiveness of human epidermal melanocytes to melanocyte-stimulating hormone and its association with red hair. Mol Cell Endocrinol 1996; 116:131–136.

50. Cals-Grierson MM, Ormerod AD. Nitric oxide function in the skin. Nitric Oxide 2004; 10: 179–193.

51. Horikoshi T, Nakahara M, Kaminaga H, et al. Involvement of nitric oxide in UVB-induced pigmentation in guinea pig skin. Pigment Cell Res 2000; 13:358–363.

52. Romero-Graillet C, Aberdam E, Biagoli N, et al. Ultraviolet B radiation acts through the nitric oxide and cGMP signal transduction pathway to stimulate melanogenesis in human melanocytes. J Biol Chem 1996; 271:28052–28056.

53. Yoshida M, Hirotsu S, Nakahara M, et al. Histamine is involved in ultraviolet B-induced pigmentation of guinea pig skin. J Invest Dermatol 2002; 118:255–260.

54. Lassalle MW, Igarashi S, Sasaki M, et al. Effects of melanogenesis-inducing nitric oxide and histamine on the production of eumelanin and pheomelanin in cultured human melanocytes. Pigment Cell Res 2003; 16:81–84.

55. Webb AR, Kline L, Holick MF. Influence of season and latitude on the cutaneous synthesis of vitamin D3: exposure to winter sunlight in Boston and Edmonton will not promote vitamin D3 synthesis in human skin. J Clin Endocrinol Metab 1988; 67:373–378.

56. Wolpowitz D, Gilchrest BA. The vitamin D questions: How much do you need and how should you get it? J Am Acad Dermatol 2006; 54:301–317.

57. Lim, HW, Gilchrest BA, Cooper KD, et al. Sunlight, tanning booths, and vitamin D. J Am Acad Dermatol 2005; 52:868–876.

58. Berry JL, Davies M, Mee AP. Vitamin D metabolism, rickets, and osteomalacia. Semin Musculoskelet Radiol 2002; 6:173–182.

59. Gomez-Alonso C, Naves-Diaz ML, Fernandez-Martin JL, et al. Vitamin D status and secondary hyperparathyroidism: the importance of 25-hydroxyvitamin D cut off levels. Kidney Int 2003; 63:S44–S48.

60. LeBoff MS, Kohlmeier L, Hurwitz S, et al. Occult vitamin D deficiency in postmenopausal US women with acute hip fracture. JAMA 1999; 281:1505–1511.

61. Lukert BP, Higgins J, Stosopf M. Menopausal bone loss is partially regulated by dietary intake of vitamin D. Calcif Tissue Int 1992; 51:173–179.

62. Jackson RD, LaCroiz AZ, Gass M, et al. Calcium plus vitamin D supplementation and the risk of fractures. N Engl J Med 2006; 354(7):669–683.

63. Bischoff-Ferrari HA, Dietrich T, Orav EJ, et al. Positive association between 25-hydroxy vitamin D levels and bone mineral density: a population-based study of younger and older adults. Am J Med 2004; 116:634–639.

64. Young AR, Walker SL. UV radiation, vitamin D and human health: an unfolding controversy introduction. Photochem Photobiol 2005; 81(6):1243–1245.

65. Holick MF. Vitamin D: importance in the prevention of cancers, type 1 diabetes, heart disease, and osteoporosis. Am J Clin Nutr 2004; 79:362–371.

66. Giovannucci E, Liu Y, Rimm EB, et al. Prospective study of predictors of vitamin D status and cancer incidence and mortality in men. J Natl Cancer Inst 2006; 98:451–459.

67. Garland CF, Garland FC. Do sunlight and vitamin D reduce the likelihood of colon cancer? Int J Epidemiol 1980; 9:227–231.

68. Hanchette CL, Schwartz GG. Geographic patterns of prostate cancer mortality. Evidence for a protective effect of ultraviolet radiation. Cancer 1992; 70:2861–2869.

69. Leftkowitz ES, Garland CF. Sunlight, vitamin D and ovarian cancer mortality rates in US women. Int J Epidemiol 1994; 23:1133–1136.

70. Grant WB. An estimate of premature cancer mortality in the US due to inadequate doses of solar ultraviolet-B radiation. Cancer 2002; 94:1867–1875.

71. Wactawski-Wende J, Kotchen JM, Anderson GL, et al. Calcium plus vitamin D supplementation and the risk of colorectal cancer. N Engl J Med 2006; 354(7):684–696.

72. Moon SJ, Fryer AA, Strange RC. Ultraviolet radiation, vitamin D and risk of prostate cancer and other diseases. Photochem Photobiol 2005; 81:1252–1260.

73. Holick MF. A perspective on the beneficial effects of moderate exposure to sunlight: bone health, cancer prevention, mental health and well being. In: Giacomoni PU, ed. Comprehensive Series in Photosciences. Sun Protection in Man. Vol 3, Elsevier Science 2001:11–37.

74. IARC Handbooks of Cancer Prevention. Volume 5: Sunscreens. International Agency for Research on Cancer. Lyon, World Health Organization, 2001.

75. Matsuoka L, Wortsman J, Hanifan N, et al. Chronic sunscreen use decreases circulating concentrations of 25-hydroxyvitamin D. Arch Dermatol 1988; 124:1802–1804.

76. McKinlay A. Workshop round-up session. Rapporteur's report. Prog Biophys Mol Biol 2006; 92:179–184.
77. Heaney RP. Vitamin D: How much do we need, and how much is too much? Osteoporos Int 2000; 11:553–555.
78. Hollis BW. Circulating 25-hydroxyvitamin D levels indicative of vitamin D sufficiency: implications for establishing a new effective dietary intake recommendation for vitamin D. J Nutr 2005; 135: 317–322.
79. Lehmann B. The vitamin D3 pathway in human skin and its role for regulation of biological processes. Photochem Photobiol 2005; 81(6):1246–1251.
80. Duthie MS, Kimber I, Norval M. The effects of ultraviolet radiation on the human immune system. Br J Dermatol 1999; 140:995–1009.
81. Sjovall P, Christensen OB. Local and systemic effect of ultraviolet irradiation (UVB and UVA) on human allergic contact dermatitis. Acta Dermato-venereologica (Stockh) 1986; 66:290–294.
82. Friedmann PS, White SI, Parker S, et al. Antigenic stimulation during ultraviolet therapy in man does not result in immunological tolerance. Clin Exp Immunol 1989; 76:68–72.
83. Yoshikawa T, Rae V, Bruins-Slot W, et al. Susceptibility to effects of UVB radiation on induction of contact hypersensitivity as a risk factor for skin cancer in humans. J Invest Dermatol 1990; 95:530–536.
84. Cooper KD, Oberhelman L, Hamilton TA, et al. UV exposure reduces immunization rates and promotes tolerance to epicutaneous antigens in humans: relationship to dose, CD1a—DR + epidermal macrophage induction, and Langerhans cell depletion. Proc Natl Acad Sci USA. 1992; 89:8497–8504.
85. Cumberbatch M, Bushan M, Dearman RJ, et al. IL-1 beta-induced Langerhans cell migration and TNF-α production in human skin: regulation by lactoferrin. Clin Exp Immunol 2003; 132:352–359.
86. Gualde N, Harizi H. Prostanoids and their receptors that modulate dendritic cell-mediated immunity. Immon Cell Biol 2004; 82:353–360.
87. Kang K, Hammerberg C, Meunier L, et al. CD11b+ macrophages that infiltrate human epidermis after in vivo ultraviolet exposure potently produce IL-10 and represent the major secretory source of epidermal IL-10 protein. J Immunol 1994; 153:5256–5264.
88. DeVries JE. Immunosuppressive and anti-inflammatory properties of Interleukin 10. Ann Med 1995; 27:537–541.
89. Grewe M, Gyufko K, Krutmann J. Interleukin-10 production by cultured human keratinocytes: regulation by ultraviolet B and ultraviolet A1 radiation. J Invest Dermatol 1995; 104:3–6.
90. Cumberbatch M, Kimber I. Dermal tumour necrosis factor-alpha induces dendritic cell migration to draining lymph nodes, and possibly provides one stimulus for Langerhans' cell migration. Immunology 1992; 75:257–263.
91. Gillardon F, Moll I, Michel S, et al. Calcitonin gene-related peptide and nitric oxide are involved in ultraviolet radiation-induced immunosuppression. Eur J Pharmacol 1995; 293:395–400.
92. Kuchel JM, Barnetson RS, Halliday GM. Nitric oxide appears to be a mediator of solar-simulated ultraviolet radiation-induced immunosuppression in humans. J Invest Dermatol 2003; 121:587–593.
93. Moodycliffe AM, Kimber I, Norval M. The effect of ultraviolet B irradiation and urocanic acid isomers on dendritic cell migration. Immunology 1992; 77:394–399.
94. Ross JA, Howie SE, Norval M, et al. Systemic administration of urocanic acid generates suppression of the delayed type hypersensitivity response to herpes simplex virus in a murine model of infection. Photodermatol 1988; 5:9–14.
95. El-Ghorr AA, Norval M. A monoclonal antibody to cis-urocanic acid prevents the ultraviolet-induced changes in Langerhans cells and delayed hypersensitivity responses in mice, although not preventing dendritic cell accumulation in lymph nodes draining the site of irradiation and contact hypersensitivity responses. J Invest Dermatol 1995; 105:264–268.
96. Reeve VE, Boehm-Wilcox C, Bosnic M, et al. Lack of correlation between suppression of contact hypersensitivity by UV radiation and photoisomerization of epidermal urocanic acid in the hairless mouse. Photochem Photobiol 1994; 60:268–273.
97. Applegate LA, Ley RD, Alcalay J, et al. Identification of the molecular target for the suppression of contact hypersensitivity by ultraviolet radiation. J Exp Med 1989; 170:1117–1131.
98. Schater B, Lederman MM, LeVine MJ, et al. Ultraviolet radiation inhibits human natural killer activity and lymphocyte proliferation. J Immunol 1983; 130:2484–2487.
99. Hersey P, Magrath H, Wilkinson F. Development of an in vitro system for the analysis of ultraviolet radiation-induced suppression of natural killer cell activity. Photochem Photobiol 1993; 57:279–284.
100. Gilmour JW, Vestey JP, George S, et al. Effect of phototherapy and urocanic acid isomers on natural killer cell function. J Invest Dermatol 1993; 101:169–174.
101. Halliday GM. Inflammation, gene mutation and photoimmunosuppression in response to UVR-induced oxidative damage contribute to photocarcinogenesis. Mutation Res 2005; 571:107–120.
102. Yuen KS, Halliday GM. Alpha-Tocopherol, an inhibitor of epidermal lipid peroxidation, prevents ultraviolet radiation from suppressing the skin immune system. Photochem. Photobiol 1997; 65(3):587–592.

103. Fuchs J, Packer L. Antioxidant protection from solar-simulated radiation-induced suppression of contact hypersensitivity to the recall antigen nickel sulfate in human skin. Free Rad Biol Med 1999; 27:422–477.
104. Rhodes LE, Callaghan TM. Beyond sun protection factor testing. Int J Cosmet Sci 2004; 26:207–214.
105. Fourtanier A, Moyal D, Maccario J, et al. Measurement of sunscreen immune protection factors in humans: a consensus paper. J Invest Dermatol 2005; 125(3):403–409.
106. Poon TS, Barnetson RS, Halliday GM. Prevention of immunosuppression by sunscreens in humans is unrelated to protection from erythema and dependent on protection from ultraviolet A in the face of constant ultraviolet B protection. J Invest Dermatol 2003; 121:184–190.
107. Van de Pas CB, Kelly DA, Seed PT, et al. Ultraviolet-radiation-induced erythema and suppression of contact hypersensitivity responses in patients with polymorphic light eruption. J Invest Dermatol 2004; 122(2):295–299.
108. Holleran WM, Uchida Y, Halkier-Sorensen L, et al. Structural and biochemical basis for the UVB-induced alterations in epidermal barrier function. Photodermatol Photoimmunol Photomed 1997; 13:117–128.
109. Haratake A, Uchida Y, Schmuth M, et al. UVB-induced alterations in permeability barrier function: roles for epidermal hyperproliferation and thymocyte-mediated response. J Invest Dermatol 1997; 108:769–775.
110. Meguro S, Arai Y, Masukawa K, et al. Stratum corneum lipid abnormalities in UVB-irradiated skin. Photochem Photobiol 1999; 69:317–321.
111. Rhodes LE. Mechanisms of UVB-induced erythema. MD Thesis, University of Liverpool, Liverpool, UK, 1995.
112. Moyal D, Fourtanier A. Acute and chronic effects of UV on skin: what are they and how to study them? In: Rigel DS, Weiss RA, Lim HW, Dover JS, eds. Photoaging. New York: Marcel Dekker, Inc., 2004:15–32.

7 | The Chronic Effects of Ultraviolet Radiation on the Skin: Photoaging

Mina Yaar
Department of Dermatology, Boston University School of Medicine, Boston, Massachusetts, U.S.A.

- UVA, UVB, and infrared irradiation induce cutaneous photodamage.

- UV irradiation leads to DNA damage and also invokes membrane signaling resulting in decreased collagen production and increased degradation.

- Telomere signaling could be mediating DNA damage responses to UV irradiation.

- Different ethnic groups display diverse photodamage responses.

- Several tools are currently available to assess skin aging and photoaging.

INTRODUCTION

Skin aging has been viewed as two distinct phenomena: intrinsic aging, changes attributable to the passage of time alone; and photoaging, the superposition of changes attributable to chronic ultraviolet (UV) exposure on intrinsic aging. UV irradiation is harmful to the skin invoking damage to DNA, proteins, and lipids and adversely affecting the skin structure and function. Intrinsically aged skin appears finely wrinkled, lax, dry, and rough; it displays a variety of benign neoplasms (1). Photoaged skin by definition is present in areas that are habitually exposed to the sun. It prominently affects the face with its abundant vasculature and other unique anatomic features, as well as the dorsal hands and forearms, upper chest, and other areas more readily contrasted with less-exposed "control" areas. The rate and degree of photoaging are determined by poorly understood genetic factors such as tanning ability and DNA damage repair capacity. Generally, fair-skinned individuals are more severely affected; however, individuals with darker skin phototypes are affected as well. Eventually, photodamage may lead to the development of skin cancer.

MECHANISMS OF PHOTOAGING
General Aspects

UV irradiation (wavelengths 100–400 nm) comprises only 5% of the terrestrial solar irradiation. It is arbitrarily divided into UVA (320–400 nm), UVB (280–320 nm), and UVC (100–280 nm) [for review, see (2)]. The UVC portion of the spectrum is not present in terrestrial sunlight, except at high altitudes, as it is absorbed by the atmospheric ozone layer. The predominant component of solar UV irradiation is UVA, the intensity of which varies little with season or during the day, and unlike UVB irradiation is not blocked by glass (3). Although the energy per photon delivered by UVA irradiation is approximately 1000-fold weaker than that of UVB, because of its longer wavelengths, UVA penetrates into the skin to reach deeper dermal layers.

Most of UVA adverse effects in skin are assumed to be the result of oxidative damage mediated through UVA absorption by cellular chromophores such as urocanic acid, riboflavin, and melanin precursors that act as photosensitizers leading to the generation of reactive oxygen species (ROS) and free radicals (4). Interestingly, advanced glycation endproducts that accumulate with aging in long-lived proteins like those of the extracellular matrix also act as UVA chromophores to become photosensitizers and affect dermal fibroblasts. ROS also directly damage dermal matrix components inducing collagen oxidation and degradation [for review, see (5)]. However, although it is evident that UV irradiation plays a role in cutaneous photodamage, it is not clear what changes are the result of UVA irradiation and what changes are induced by UVB irradiation (see subsequently further discussion).

UVB irradiation primarily affects the epidermis. It is directly absorbed by cellular DNA, leading to the formation of DNA lesions, mainly cyclobutane dimers and pyrimidine (6-4) pyrimidone photoproducts (6). Despite comprehensive nuclear DNA damage repair systems, DNA damage is rarely completely repaired. When cells sustain abundant DNA damage, they undergo apoptosis [for review, see (1)], a process mediated largely by the tumor suppressor p53 protein. p53 also participates in DNA damage repair and in transient cell cycle arrest after DNA damage. However, those cells that have not undergone apoptosis and in which the damage is not completely repaired risk developing mutations, eventually become cancerous. This is particularly important in view of recent epidemiologic studies showing that more than 90% of epidermal squamous cell carcinomas and more than 50% of basal cell carcinomas display UV-induced mutations that inactivate p53 (7). Furthermore, p53 mutations are present in the premalignant actinic keratoses, suggesting that p53 mutations occur early, increasing the risk for malignant transformation of affected cells.

Apart from its direct effect on epidermal DNA, studies in the murine system show that UVB irradiation affects both the cutaneous and systemic immune responses leading to defective antigen presentation and formation of suppressor T cells, allowing the propagation of cancerous cells that would otherwise be rejected [for review, see (8)]. In this regard, it was suggested that UVA, by inducing lipid peroxidation, stimulates the outward migration of immune-responsive cells from the epidermis and thus further contributes to immunosuppression (8). Also, UVB irradiation induces the secretion of epidermal cytokines, and evidence suggests that, of these cytokines, tumor necrosis factor-α and interleukin-10 play a major role in UVB-induced immunosuppression.

In addition to UV irradiation, sunlight also transmits infrared (IR) irradiation (760 nm– 1 mm) [for review, see (9)]. Wavelengths of 760 to 1400 nm can penetrate the skin to reach the subcutaneous tissue without inducing a significant increase in skin temperature. In contrast, wavelengths 1400 nm to 1 mm are primarily absorbed in the epidermis and considerably increase the skin temperature (10). IR is particularly important in regions of high insulation, and studies suggest that in addition to UV, IR contributes to cutaneous photoaging (discussed subsequently).

UV-Induced Membrane Signaling

In addition to its well-known effects on DNA, UV irradiation directly activates cell surface receptors, in part possibly through ROS generation, to induce intracellular signaling by activating the nuclear transcription complex AP-1, composed of the proteins c-Jun and c-Fos [for review, see (11)] (Fig. 1). UV also activates NF-κB, a ubiquitous transcription factor composed of Rel family members, which controls the expression of a large array of genes involved in immune function and cell survival [for review, see (12)]. In intact human skin, even suberythemogenic doses of UVB [$\sim$0.1 minimal erythema dose (MED)] transcriptionally upregulate and activate AP-1 (13). Increased AP-1 activity interferes with synthesis of the major dermal collagens I and III by blocking the effect of transforming growth factor-β (TGF-β), a cytokine that enhances collagen gene transcription (11,13). AP-1 also decreases the level of TGF-β receptors, further inhibiting collagen transcription (14), and also antagonizes retinoid effects in skin, leading to a functional retinoid deficiency and reducing collagen synthesis normally promoted by retinoic acid bound to its nuclear receptors. Hence, in photodamaged skin, there is an overall reduction in collagen synthesis (15).

Increased AP-1 activity also increases the levels and activity of several enzymes that degrade extracellular matrix components, notably the matrix metalloproteinases (MMP)-1 (collagenase), MMP-3 (stromelysin-1), and MMP-9 (92-kd gelatinase) (11,16). Degradation of matrix proteins is aggravated by NF-κB that increases the levels of MMP-1 and MMP-9 (13). Finally, matrix degradation is further exacerbated by MMP-8 (collagenase) of neutrophil

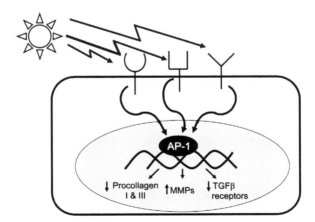

FIGURE 1 Ultraviolet (UV) irradiation induces membrane signaling. UV irradiation directly activates cell surface receptors, initiating intracellular signaling that eventually activates the nuclear transcription complex AP-1. AP-1 increases transcription of matrix metalloproteinases and decreases expression of the procollagen I and III genes and transforming growth factor-β receptors, with a final consequence of reduced dermal matrix. *Abbreviations*: MMPs, matrix metalloproteinases; TGFβ, transforming growth factor β. *Source*: Adapted from Refs. 11, 81.

origin, following neutrophil infiltration of UV-irradiated skin (17). Although there is also a concomitant upregulation of tissue inhibitors of metalloproteinases (TIMPs) that limit further
matrix degradation, TIMPs presumably are not completely effective in blocking cumulative
damage to dermal collagen (18).

UV-induced collagen degradation is generally incomplete, leading to accumulation of
partially degraded collagen fragments in the dermis, thus reducing the structural integrity
of the skin (11). In addition, the large collagen degradation products inhibit new collagen synthesis (19), and thus, collagen degradation itself negatively regulates new collagen synthesis.
Interestingly, increased MMP levels and reduced collagen production have been documented
also in intrinsically aged skin (20), suggesting that similar mechanisms may contribute to
chronologic aging, perhaps again through the generation of ROS, as discussed above.

Mitochondrial Damage

Mitochondria are cellular organelles that produce energy (ATP) by consuming oxygen.
Although equipped with antioxidant defense systems, studies suggest that continuous generation of ROS damages mitochondrial DNA (mtDNA). To date, machinery to remove bulky
DNA lesions has not been identified in mitochondria, although they display capacity for
base excision repair and repair of oxidative damage. Still, mtDNA mutation frequency is
approximately 50-fold higher than that of nuclear DNA, and photodamaged skin has higher
mtDNA mutation frequency when compared with sun-protected skin, displaying large-scale
DNA deletions (21–24) and resulting in decreased mitochondrial function, as a result of
faulty respiratory chain leading to further accumulation of ROS. Also, a correlation
was noted between decreased mitochondrial function and increased MMP-1 levels without
concomitant increases in MMP-1-specific TIMP (21), further exacerbating collagen degradation
(21–24) and aggravating skin photoaging.

Telomeres
Telomere Shortening
The terminal portions of eukaryotic chromosomes are termed telomeres. In all mammals, they
are composed of repeats of the short DNA sequence TTAGGG (25) and in man are several thousand bases in length. Telomeres appear to protect the chromosomes from degradation or fusion
(26). As well, because DNA polymerase, the enzyme that replicates chromosomes, cannot repli-
cate the final base pairs of each chromosome, chromosomes shorten after each round of DNA
replication (27), and the presence of telomeric repeats at the chromosome ends prevents loss of
critical-coding sequences (Fig. 2). Finally, by shortening with each round of cell division, telomeres serve as the biological clock, informing cells that they are young or old. Both epidermal
keratinocytes and dermal fibroblasts from older individuals have shorter telomeres than do
younger individuals (27,28), and telomeres of patients with disorders of premature aging,
such as Werner's syndrome and progeria, are shorter than those of age-matched controls
(27,29). Germline cells as well as immortalized cell lines and almost all malignant cells
express the enzyme telomerase that adds bases to telomeres and thus maintains their length,
despite repeated cell divisions (30). In contrast, somatic cells generally lack this enzyme and
have a finite proliferative ability.

Telomeres and DNA Damage
A recent model proposes that telomere function is determined by more than just length. Telomere ends appear to exist in a "capped" (hidden) or "uncapped" (exposed) form and, when
uncapped, cause DNA damage responses in the cell (Fig. 2) (25). It is known that telomeres
are normally present in a loop configuration (31) and that the loop is held in place by the
final 150 to 200 bases of the TTAGGG repeats on the 3′ strand that forms a single-stranded overhang and insert into the proximal telomeric double helix (31). Further, when the loop is disrupted experimentally, the overhang is digested and the cell mounts DNA damage responses,
including entry into senescence in some cell types (32,33). It was reported that oligonucleotides homologous to the telomere overhang sequence ("T-oligos") are taken up into the cell
nucleus and cause identical responses (34,35). These findings suggest that the physiological

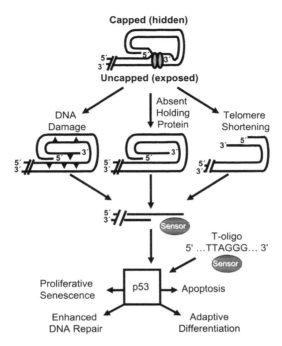

FIGURE 2 Cellular responses induced by exposure of the telomere repeat sequence. Telomeres normally exist in a loop configuration, held in place by the final 150 to 200 bases (TTAGGG repeats) on the 3′ strand that form a single-stranded overhang. When the loop is disrupted experimentally, for example, by interfering with the synthesis of the protein that holds the loop together, the cell mounts DNA damage responses that, depending on the cell type, include senescence or apoptosis. We speculate that the 3′ telomere overhang may also be exposed when telomeres become critically short, for example, after repeated cell divisions, or when telomeres are damaged as a result of UV irradiation or other DNA damage. A sensor protein that invokes the DNA damage responses recognizes the exposed overhang. We have shown that introducing oligonucleotides homologous to the telomere overhang sequence (T-oligo) into cells invokes the same responses in the absence of telomere disruption and propose that a common molecular pathway, involving the tumor suppressor protein p53, mediates the responses independent of the initiating event. *Source*: From Ref. 81.

signal for cells to enter senescence following acute DNA damage or critical telomere shortening may be exposure of the TTAGGG overhang sequence, an event mimicked by T-oligos in the absence of telomere disruption (Fig. 3). In all instances, the responses are mediated by the same molecular pathways, centrally involving the tumor suppressor protein p53 (34,35).

It is well documented that many DNA damaging agents also produce aging-like changes. Such agents include UV irradiation, ROS, cigarette smoke (presumably the carcinogen benzo(a)pyrene), and many chemotherapeutic drugs, notably cisplatin (36). UV irradiation causes pyrimidine dimers, most commonly between adjacent thymidines (37), ROS primarily cause 8-oxo-guanine, and the other agents form adducts that alter DNA at guanine nucleotides (38,39). In this context, it is interesting that one-third of the TTAGGG telomere overhang repeat sequence is dithymidines (TT) and half is guanine (G) residues (35). The resultant concentration of UV or chemical carcinogen damage in the telomere might therefore reasonably lead to disruption of the loop structure and exposure of the overhang, followed by DNA damage signaling. Certainly, signaling through the p53 pathway is well documented after exposure to UV (40) or other DNA-damaging agents (41), as well as during entry into senescence [for review, see (42)].

Repeated UV irradiation and/or prolonged exposure to ROS would thus be expected to accelerate cellular senescence, as documented to occur during experimental loop disruption (32) and/or as a consequence of compensatory cell divisions required to replace cells lost to apoptosis. This model is supported by the findings that abnormally short telomeres are found in cells after long exposure to oxidative stress or cisplatin (38,39).

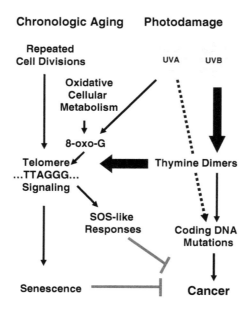

FIGURE 3 Hypothetical common mechanism for intrinsic aging and photoaging. Repeated cell divisions shorten telomeres. Exposure to ROS during aerobic cellular metabolism may also damage guanine residues in telomeres. During the repair of such damage, the telomere loop would be temporarily disrupted. Both critical telomere shortening and telomere loop disruption would invoke signaling leading to SOS-like responses, proliferative senescence, or apoptosis, all of which interfere with carcinogenesis. Photodamage leads to thymine dimers (UVB) and ROS (both UVA and UVB) that damage genomic DNA and give rise to mutations that may lead to cancer development. However, these lesions also damage telomeres, disrupting the telomere loop. Consequent signaling through the exposed TTAGGG sequence would lead to SOS-like responses, senescence, or apoptosis that would interfere with carcinogenesis. *Abbreviation*: ROS, reactive oxygen species. *Source*: From Ref. 81.

A concept thus emerges that nature may employ the same molecular defenses against DNA damage, with its inherent cancer risk, whether the damage is severe and acute or subtle but cumulative over many rounds of cell division. Specifically, both extensive damage to thymidine dinucleotides and to guanines within the TTAGGG tandem repeat sequence and age-associated telomere shortening may lead to disruption of the telomere loop that in turn activates p53 and other mediators of cell cycle arrest, apoptosis, and/or senescence. Within this concept, the "genetic" or intrinsic component of aging that relies on progressive telomere shortening during serial cell division and the "environmental" or "wear and tear" component that in the skin results primarily from UV irradiation and oxidative cellular metabolism similarly disrupt the telomere loop structure and activate a common final pathway (Fig. 3). This concept explains the stereotyped predictable character of photoaged skin and the substantial clinical overlap between intrinsically aged and photoaged skin. The unique features of photoaged skin, including its predisposition to skin cancer, are likely attributable to UV-induced mutations in key regulatory genes that accumulate during the telomere-driven aging process.

ACTION SPECTRUM FOR PHOTOAGING

The action spectrum for human photoaging has not clearly been determined, and hence the relative contribution of the various spectral bands within sunlight is unknown. There is no truly appropriate animal model. In rodent skin, an elastosis-like condition can be produced by prolonged intense irradiation with either a predominantly UVB or UVA source, but attempts to determine the action spectrum for murine elastosis have yielded conflicting results (43,44). Using UVA irradiation and the hairless mouse model, studies showed decreased activity of the enzyme prolyl-hydroxylase that participates in post-translational modification of collagen (45).

In contrast to UVB, which renders collagen more susceptible to enzymatic degradation, irradiation with UVA rendered dermal collagen more resistant to degradation, in part as a result of increased cross-linking of the fibers.

As mentioned above, UVB photons are on average 1000 times more energetic than UVA photons and are overwhelmingly responsible for sunburn, suntanning, and photocarcinogenesis following sun exposure (46), although UVA also contributes to these endpoints (47,48). UVA is suspected of playing a proportionately larger role in photoaging because of its minimally 10-fold greater abundance in terrestrial sunlight, far greater year-round and day-long average irradiance, and greater average depth of penetration into the dermis compared with UVB. Moreover, human skin exposed daily for only one month to suberythemogenic doses of UVA alone demonstrates epidermal hyperplasia, stratum corneum thickening, Langerhans cell depletion, and dermal inflammatory infiltrates with deposition of lysozyme on the elastic fibers (49). These latter changes have been interpreted to suggest that frequent casual exposure to sunlight containing principally UVA, for example, while wearing a UVB-absorbing sunscreen, eventually may result in damage to dermal collagen and elastin in ways expected to produce photoaging. Indeed, studies using reconstructed human skin in vitro containing live fibroblasts in a dermal equivalent and differentiated epidermis showed that UVB primarily affected epidermal cells, giving rise to cyclobutane–pyrimidine dimers and sunburn cells, whereas UVA induced apoptosis of fibroblasts located in the upper dermal compartment as well as secretion of MMPs (50,51).

Initially, histological changes in elderly sun-exposed skin were described by experienced investigators as differing only in degree from those in elderly sun-protected skin at both the light microscopic and electron microscopic levels. Many of the age-associated physiological decrements, such as slowed wound healing and loss of immunoresponsiveness, also appear to be accelerated in sun-exposed skin. Furthermore, cells cultured from chronically sun-exposed skin sites differ from cells cultured from sun-protected sites of the same donors in having shortened culture life spans, slower growth rates, lower saturation densities, and altered responsiveness to retinoic acid (52), all changes also observed as a function of advanced chronological donor age. Only in recent decades have qualitative differences in the dermal fibrous proteins and microvasculature of paired sun-exposed and sun-protected sites been documented. On a theoretical level, several of the mechanisms known to be involved in UV-mediated cellular damage are also postulated to underlie chronological aging (53,54). These include DNA injury and/or decreased DNA repair, oxidative damage, lysosomal disruption, and altered collagen structure.

In addition to UV irradiation, IR aggravates UVA-induced dermal changes producing severe elastosis in a guinea pig model. Even when delivered without UV, IR affects dermal elastic fibers and increases the amount of dermal ground substance (10). In the hairless mouse model, IR contributes to UV-induced thickening of the epidermis and dermis and alone induces the expression of MMP-3 and the mouse equivalent of MMP-1 (9). Furthermore, in human skin, the expression of tropoelastin, a major component of elastic fiber that associates with microfibrils, is increased as a result of IR, and IR induces the expression of fibrillin-1, a component of the microfibrils (55). In addition, the level of MMP-12, the enzyme that degrades elastin, is increased (55). Thus, IR appears to contribute to UV-induced photoaging.

CLINICAL CHANGES

The features of actinically damaged skin are listed in Table 1. Photodamaged skin is characteristically described as dry and sallow, displaying increases in both fine and deep wrinkling. In addition, facial skin may display a pattern of papular elastosis with open comedones (Favre–Racouchot disease) and telangiectasis [for review, see (56)]. Other changes include irregular pigmentation manifesting as freckling, lentigines, and guttate hypomelanosis and a variety of premalignant lesions, such as actinic keratoses (56). Functionally, photodamaged skin displays decreased resilience and elasticity, increased fragility, and decreased capacity for wound healing.

However, sun-induced cutaneous changes vary considerably among individuals, undoubtedly reflecting inherent differences in vulnerability and repair capacity for the solar

TABLE 1   Features of Actinically Damaged Skin[a]

Clinical Abnormality	Histologic Abnormality
Dryness (roughness)	Increased compaction of stratum corneum, increased thickness of granular cell layer, reduced epidermal thickness, reduced epidermal mucin content
Actinic keratoses	Nuclear atypia, loss of orderly, progressive keratinocyte maturation; irregular epidermal hyperplasia and/or hypoplasia; occasional dermal inflammation
Irregular pigmentation	
Freckling	Reduced or increased number of hypertrophic, strongly dopa-positive melanocytes
Lentigines	Elongation of epidermal rete ridges; increases in number and melanization of melanocytes
Guttate hypomelanosis	Reduced number of atypical melanocytes
Persistent hyperpigmentation	Increased number of dopa-positive melanocytes and increased melanin content per unit area and increased number of dermal melanophages
Wrinkling	
Fine surface lines	None detected
Deep furrows	Contraction of septae in the subcutaneous fat
Stellate pseudoscars	Absence of epidermal pigmentation, altered fragmented dermal collagen
Elastosis (fine nodularity and/or coarseness)	Nodular aggregations of fibrous to amorphous material in the papillary dermis
Inelasticity	Elastotic dermis
Telangiectasia	Ectatic vessels often with atrophic walls
Venous lakes	Ectatic vessels often with atrophic walls
Purpura (easy bruising)	Extravasated erythrocytes and increased perivascular inflammation
Comedones (maladie de Favre et Racouchot)	Ectatic superficial portion of the pilosebaceous follicle
Sebaceous hyperplasia	Concentric hyperplasia of sebaceous glands

[a]Basal cell carcinoma and squamous cell carcinoma also occur in actinically damaged skin but, unlike the table entries, affect only a small minority of individuals with photoaging.
Source: From Ref. 2.

insult but may also be the result of different culturally based behavior when outdoors. Even among whites, the gross appearance of photodamaged skin of individuals with skin types I and II differs from that of individuals with skin types III and IV, the former generally showing atrophic skin changes with less wrinkles and at times focal depigmentation (gutate hypomelanosis) and dysplastic changes such as actinic keratoses and epidermal malignancies (Fig. 4A). In contrast, hypertrophic responses such as deep wrinkling, coarseness, leathery appearance of the skin, and lentigines appear in individuals with skin types III and IV (Fig. 4B). With time, exposed skin may remain persistently hyperpigmented (permanently "tanned" or "bronzed") even in the absence of further UV exposure. One study has noted that white patients presenting with basal cell carcinomas are less wrinkled than peers of similar complexion and degree of photodamage (57), suggesting that different factors determine these two responses to chronic UV exposure.

    Photoaging occurs not only in Caucasians but also in Asians, Hispanics, and African Americans. The differences in clinical appearance of photoaged skin between Caucasians and other ethnic groups is primarily due to differences in their UV defense systems. In the latter three groups, melanin is the major form of protection, whereas in Caucasians, in addition to melanin, stratum corneum thickening plays an important role. Indeed, the sun protection factor (SPF) for black epidermis is 13.4 when compared with 3.4 for white epidermis (58). Accordingly, black epidermis allows for approximately 6% of UVB to be transmitted into the dermis when compared with almost 30% penetration into white dermis (58). Furthermore, only ~18% of UVA is transmitted into black dermis when compared with more than 55% into white dermis (58). Interestingly, in black skin, most of the UV irradiation is filtered in

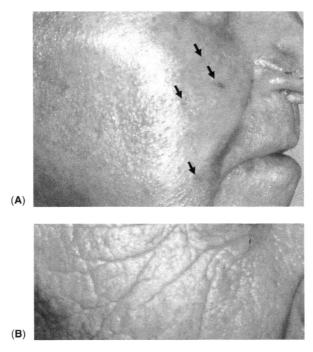

FIGURE 4 Photoaging. (**A**) An individual with skin type I displaying atrophic skin photodamage response with relatively few wrinkles but with several actinic keratoses (*arrows*) and a site of previous basal cell carcinoma over the lateral aspect of the nose. (**B**) An individual with skin type IV displaying hypertrophic skin photodamage response with deep wrinkles and leather-like coarse skin.

the malpighiam layer when compared with the stratum corneum as a major area of filtration in white skin [for review, see (59)].

The major clinical mark of photoaging in Asian people is pigmentary changes including solar lentigines, flat seborrheic keratoses, and mottled pigmentation [for review, see (60)]. Also, sun-induced melasma is common in Asians and is considered a clinical sign of photodamage in this ethnic group. Nevertheless, moderate to severe wrinkling is also documented in Asians but only in the sixth decade of life and only in individuals who spent more than five hours per day in the sun (61).

There are no specific studies addressing photoaging in Hispanics. It appears that fair-skinned Hispanics display clinical photoaging signs similar to darker skin Caucasians, whereas Hispanics with darker skin phototypes are more similar to Asians and display fine wrinkling and mottled pigmentation occurring late in the fourth through the sixth decade (60). Published studies on photoaging of black skin have been conducted only in African-Americans. Naturally, African-Americans with lighter complexions show signs of photoaging, but usually not until the fifth or sixth decades of life (62) and these include fine wrinkling and mottled pigmentation (60,62).

Wrinkling of photodamaged skin is exacerbated by cigarette smoking (63) and possibly other environmental factors. The apparent influence of sex on the prevalence of certain photoaging features undoubtedly reflects different hair styles, patterns of dress, and nature of sun exposure (occupational vs. recreational) between men and women over the past several generations. Other sex differences, such as epidermal thickness and sebaceous gland activity, and as yet unrecognized effects of circulating sex hormones also may influence their development. The characteristic distribution of different lesions is a complex function of relative sun exposure for different body sites, anatomic distribution of the participating cutaneous structures (e.g., melanocytes and sebaceous glands), and other poorly understood factors.

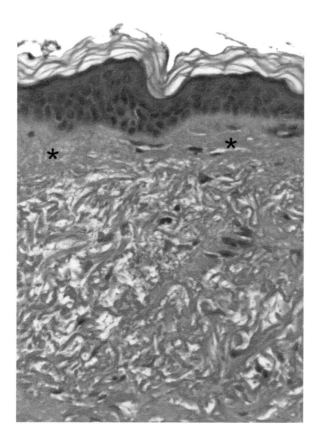

FIGURE 5 Histological appearance of photo-damaged skin. Hematoxylin and eosin (H&E) staining of photodamaged skin displaying bluish masses of deranged elastic fibers characteristic of solar elastosis. A thin subepidermal Grenz zone (*asterisk*) is present. *Source*: Courtesy of Jag Bhawan, M.D. From Ref. 8.

HISTOLOGICAL CHANGES

Photodamage affects both the epidermis and the dermis. In contrast to chronologically aged skin, photodamaged epidermis is frequently acanthotic, although as discussed above, severe atrophy also can be seen. The epidermis displays, in addition, loss of polarity and cellular atypia. Also, there is a decrease in the number and function of Langerhans cells.

The dermis displays loss of mature collagen and the remaining collagen shows basophilic degeneration [for review, see (5)]. Also, there is a reduction in the density of anchoring fibrils affecting epidermal adhesion to the dermis (5). A major component of photodamaged dermis is elastosis, a material characterized histologically by tangled masses of degraded elastic fibers that further deteriorate to form an amorphous mass composed of disorganized tropo-elastin and fibrillin (Fig. 5). Although fibrillin is abundant in the elastotic material deeper in the dermis, in the upper portions of the dermis at the dermo-epidermal junction, fibrillin is reduced (62). The amount of ground substance, largely composed of glycosaminoglycans and proteoglycans, increases in photodamaged dermis (5). In contrast to aged sun-protected skin that demonstrates hypocellularity, photodamaged skin frequently displays inflammatory cells, including mast cells, histiocytes, and other mononuclear cells, giving rise to the term heliodermatitis (literally, "cutaneous inflammation due to sun"). Fibroblasts are also more numerous in photodamaged skin than in aged sun-protected skin and display an irregular stellate shape. Ultrastructurally, these cells contain active endoplasmic reticulum, consistent with enhanced biosynthetic activity (2,5).

METHODS FOR MEASURING CUTANEOUS PHOTOAGING

In the clinical setting, it is important to develop a systematic approach of assessing and advising a patient regarding potential interventions that could improve the appearance of photoaged skin. The correlation between clinical signs of actinically damaged skin to their histological presentation is summarized in Table 1. The use of objective methods for assessing the different parameters that affect skin photoaging could be beneficial for determining treatment efficacy. The following paragraphs describe different methodologies currently available to assess skin aging and photoaging.

Photonumeric Scales

In 1992, Griffiths et al. (64) proposed assessing several cutaneous aging parameters using a photonumeric scale. They selected representative photographs of patients displaying different grades of photodamage and assigned a progressive scale of nine grades to assess the different parameters (0, none; 8, severe). Seven experienced dermatologists were asked to determine the degree of photodamage of 25 patients by matching it to the photonumeric scale. In addition, the dermatologists were asked to assess the degree of photodamage of 25 different patients as determined by reading a written description of the different photodamage parameters. The assessed parameters were fine wrinkling, coarse wrinkling, mottled pigmentation, and sallowness. Using the photonumeric scale for assessment, the examiners agreed on the severity (grade) of photodamage in 80% of the subjects. In contrast, when they used the descriptive scale, they agreed only on 36% of the subjects. Furthermore, when the examiners assessed the same patients a week later, they reached the same conclusions only when they used the graded images, demonstrating that photonumeric scales based on representative images are superior to written descriptions in assessing photodamage.

Photonumeric scales are easy to use and can be generated to assess different segments of the face like the peri-orbital region. Because of the reproducibility of the assessment, photonumeric scales are also useful in assessing treatment outcome and can easily be used in the outpatient office setting and when performing clinical studies.

Measuring Cutaneous Mechanical Properties

Different instruments were developed to assess the mechanical properties of the skin. To investigate cutaneous limpness, a simple instrument called DensiScore was devised (65). The device is attached to the patient's skin and pressure is applied by pushing the two arms of the instrument, compressing the skin horizontally, generating consistently the same level of compression. Studies have shown that in young skin, horizontal compression results in the generation of thin folds, whereas the number of folds and their width increase with patient age. This instrument provides a simple straightforward technique for measuring age-associated decrements of this mechanical property of the skin.

Different from the DensiScore, the Extensometer is an instrument composed of two plates. Instead of compressing the skin, the device stretches it (66). A sensor records the extent to which the skin can be pulled and its ability to stretch directly correlates with cutaneous elasticity and suppleness.

A more sophisticated device that measures rotational deformation and recovery is the Twistometer or Dermal Torque Meter (67). The instrument is equipped with a rotating head that gently twists the skin. By applying a constant torque for a specific time interval, the investigator measures the degree of deformation imparted on the skin and the time required for the deformation to return to its baseline condition. The measurements allow the investigator to calculate cutaneous extensibility, viscosity, and recovery. Elasticity can then be calculated as the ratio between recovery and extensibility.

Another instrument called Cutometer measures cutaneous elasticity by applying vacuum to the skin pulling the skin vertically into the Cutometer probe (68). The resistance to the deformation generated by the vacuum correlates with cutaneous elasticity.

Measuring Skin Surface Properties

One of the most noticeable changes that occur in photodamaged skin is loss of surface smoothness and increased coarseness, often interpreted as dry skin. As it is difficult to objectively measure skin smoothness, different methodologies were developed to assess this parameter.

Classically, to examine skin topography, investigators used silicone molds creating a "negative" replica of the skin surface. This replica could be scanned into a computer or it can be scanned by a laser beam that accurately measures 3D surfaces and converts them into an image—a technique called laser profilometry (69). Naturally, these procedures are expensive and time-consuming and cannot routinely be performed by the practicing dermatologist.

However, recently an instrument called Dermascore, a modified version of the dermatoscope, was developed to assess skin topography (70). In addition to providing information on surface morphology and pore size, by using polarized light and by rotating the instrument 90°, the dermatologist can assess cutaneous pigmentary and vascular homogeneity.

Measuring Skin Structure

Although it is convenient to evaluate photoage-associated changes in the structure of the skin using skin biopsies, this method is invasive. Ultrasound echography is an alternative method to skin biopsy for assessing cutaneous structure. Like all ultrasound-based techniques, the instrument is attached to the skin and utilizes a transducer that emits ultrasonic sound waves. The sound waves bounce off the skin like an echo; they are then picked up by the transducer and converted into an electronic image of the skin (71,72). Using this methodology, the investigator can measure skin thickness.

Magnetic resonance imagery (MRI), a technique widely used for various diagnostic procedures of other body parts, for a long time was not suitable for use on the skin because of failure to obtain high spatial resolution. However, the recent development of a device that can be attached to the standard MRI machine and that allows for a higher image resolution now permits the use of this technology to assess skin structure (73). In particular, the device is useful in obtaining a 3D structure of the hypodermis that can be used to evaluate changes that take place in this cutaneous compartment.

Confocal microscopy is a noninvasive imaging methodology that allows for analysis of different skin layers in vivo. By sensing light that is emitted from specific focal planes in the skin, the confocal microscope permits the visualization of the skin layer by layer (74). Confocal microscopic devices with spatial resolution of 1 μm enable the examiner to visualize separately each layer of the epidermis. Ultrasound echography and MRI are more suitable to visualize the dermis and hypodermis, respectively, whereas confocal micrsocopy is an excellent method to visualize the stratum corneum, the epidermis, and the papillary dermis. Indeed, using this technology on volar forearm skin of young (18–25 years) versus old (>65 years) individuals, a layer by layer analysis of the epidermis and papillary dermis showed no age-associated changes in the stratum corneum, an age-associated increase in the granular cell layer, an increased thickness of the basal cell layer, and a significant decrease in the number of dermal papillae (75).

Measuring Cutaneous Hydration

Barrier function of the skin is largely dependent on water and lipid content of the stratum corneum. Stratum corneum hydration can be evaluated using a device called Corneometer that measures the electrical properties of this cutaneous layer, specifically its capacitance (76). The device has a probe that acts as a capacitor, an apparatus that accumulates electrical charges. The ability of the probe to store the charges is proportional to the water content of the stratum corneum. Stratum corneum hydration can also be measured using skin surface hygrometer (77). The device has two electrodes and it measures conductance capacity by determining stratum corneum resistance to electrical current. Conductance is proportional to the water content of the stratum corneum. Thus, both the corneometer and the skin surface hygrometer provide straightforward, reliable, and easy methods for measuring water content of the stratum corneum.

Another method that measures skin barrier examines the rate of trans-epidermal water loss using a device called Evaporimeter, which is a hygrometer that measures the amount of water vapor that is lost at a given time (78,79).

Measuring Sebum Production

Skin surface lipids and sebaceous gland activity can be measured using a device called Lipometer or Sebumeter and Sebutape, a tape that absorbs sebum (80). The tape is an opaque film that becomes transparent upon contact with cutaneous lipids. To measure sebum production, the tape is applied to the skin surface for a specific length of time and then it is inserted into the lipometer that registers the size and the number of the transparent areas. From these measurements, sebum output can be calculated.

CONCLUSION

The rapid increase in older individuals in the population of developed countries has focused the attention of dermatologists on issues associated with photoaging impacting the individual's quality of life. Older individuals displaying photodamage, even when otherwise healthy, direct their attention to their appearance and seek dermatologic advice with the hope of reversing the damage. Dermatologists need to understand the mechanisms that contribute to photoaging as well as the functional and structural changes displayed in photoaged skin in order to better address prevention and treatment of photoaging.

REFERENCES

1. Gilchrest BA, Eller MS, Geller AC, Yaar M. The pathogenesis of melanoma induced by ultraviolet radiation. N Engl J Med, 1999; 340:1341–1348.
2. Yaar M, Gilchrest BA. Aging of the skin. In: Fitzpatrick TB, Eisen AZ, Wolff K, Freedberg IM, Austen KF. eds. Dermatology in General Medicine. New York: McGraw-Hill, 2003.
3. Johnson JA, Fusaro RM. Broad-spectrum photoprotection: the roles of tinted auto windows, sunscreens and browning agents in the diagnosis and treatment of photosensitivity. Dermatology 1992; 185:237–241.
4. Gasparro FP. Sunscreens, skin photobiology, and skin cancer: the need for UVA protection and evaluation of efficacy. Environ Health Perspect 2000; 108(suppl 1):71–78.
5. Wlaschek M, Tantcheva-Poor I, Naderi L, et al. Solar UV irradiation and dermal photoaging. J Photochem Photobiol B 2001; 63:41–51.
6. Eller MS. Repair of DNA photodamage in human skin. In: Gilchrest BA, ed. Photodamage. Cambridge: Blackwell, 1995: 26–50.
7. Brash DE, Ziegler A, Jonason AS, Simon JA, Kunala S, Leffell DJ. Sunlight and sunburn in human skin cancer: p53, apoptosis, and tumor promotion. J Investig Dermatol Symp Proc 1996; 1:136–142.
8. Granstein RD. Photoimmunology. In: Freedberg IM, Eisen AZ, Wolff K, Austen KF, Goldsmith LA, Katz SI, eds. Fitzpatrick's Dermatology in General Medicine. Vol. 1. New York: McGraw-Hill, 2003: 378–386.
9. Kim HH, Lee MJ, Lee SR, et al. Augmentation of UV-induced skin wrinkling by infrared irradiation in hairless mice. Mech Ageing Dev 2005; 126:1170–1177.
10. Schieke SM, Schroeder P, Krutmann J. Cutaneous effects of infrared radiation: from clinical observations to molecular response mechanisms. Photodermatol Photoimmunol Photomed 2003; 19:228–234.
11. Fisher GJ, Kang S, Varani J, et al. Mechanisms of photoaging and chronological skin aging. Arch Dermatol 2002; 138:1462–1470.
12. Ruland J, Mak TW. Transducing signals from antigen receptors to nuclear factor kappaB. Immunol Rev 2003; 193:93–100.
13. Fisher GJ, Datta SC, Talwar HS, et al. Molecular basis of sun-induced premature skin aging and retinoid antagonism. Nature 1996; 379:335–339.
14. Quan T, He T, Voorhees JJ, Fisher GJ. Ultraviolet irradiation blocks cellular responses to transforming growth factor-beta by down-regulating its type-II receptor and inducing Smad7. J Biol Chem 2001; 276:26349–26356.
15. Fisher GJ, Datta S, Wang Z, et al. c-Jun-dependent inhibition of cutaneous procollagen transcription following ultraviolet irradiation is reversed by all-*trans* retinoic acid. J Clin Invest 2000; 106:663–670.

16. Angel P, Szabowski A, Schorpp-Kistner M. Function and regulation of AP-1 subunits in skin physiology and pathology. Oncogene 2001; 20:2413–2423.

17. Fisher GJ, Choi HC, Bata-Csorgo Z, et al. Ultraviolet irradiation increases matrix metalloproteinase-8 protein in human skin in vivo. J Invest Dermatol 2001; 117:219–226.

18. Sudel KM, Venzke K, Knussmann-Hartig E, et al. Tight control of matrix metalloproteinase-1 activity in human skin. Photochem Photobiol 2003; 78:355–360.

19. Varani J, Spearman D, Perone P, et al. Inhibition of type I procollagen synthesis by damaged collagen in photoaged skin and by collagenase-degraded collagen in vitro. Am J Pathol 2001; 158:931–942.

20. Varani J, Warner RL, Gharaee-Kermani M, et al. Vitamin A antagonizes decreased cell growth and elevated collagen-degrading matrix metalloproteinases and stimulates collagen accumulation in naturally aged human skin. J Invest Dermatol 2000; 114:480–486.

21. Berneburg M, Plettenberg H, Krutmann, J. Photoaging of human skin. Photodermatol Photoimmunol Photomed 2000; 16:239–244.

22. Yang JH, Lee HC, Lin KJ, Wei YH. A specific 4977-bp deletion of mitochondrial DNA in human aging skin. Arch Dermatol Res 1994; 286:386–390.

23. Berneburg M, Gattermann N, Stege H, et al. Chronically ultraviolet-exposed human skin shows a higher mutation frequency of mitochondrial DNA as compared to unexposed skin and the hematopoietic system. Photochem Photobiol 1997; 66:271–275.

24. Birch-Machin MA, Tindall M, Turner R, Haldane F, Rees JL. Mitochondrial DNA deletions in human skin reflect photo- rather than chronologic aging. J Invest Dermatol 1998; 110:149–152.

25. Blackburn EH. Telomere states and cell fates. Nature 2000; 408:53–56.

26. Cervantes RB, Lundblad V. Mechanisms of chromosome-end protection. Curr Opin Cell Biol 2002; 14:351–356.

27. Allsopp RC, Vaziri H, Patterson C, et al. Telomere length predicts replicative capacity of human fibroblasts. Proc Natl Acad Sci USA 1992; 89:10114–10118.

28. Nakamura K, Izumiyama-Shimomura N, Sawabe M, et al. Comparative analysis of telomere lengths and erosion with age in human epidermis and lingual epithelium. J Invest Dermatol 2002; 119:1014–1019.

29. Schulz VP, Zakian VA, Ogburn CE, et al. Accelerated loss of telomeric repeats may not explain accelerated replicative decline of Werner syndrome cells. Hum Genet 1996; 97:750–754.

30. Ahmed A, Tollefsbol T. Telomeres and telomerase: basic science implications for aging. J Am Geriatr Soc 2001; 49:1105–1109.

31. Griffith JD, Comeau L, Rosenfield S, et al. Mammalian telomeres end in a large duplex loop. Cell 1999; 97:503–514.

32. Karlseder J, Smogorzewska A, de Lange T. Senescence induced by altered telomere state, not telomere loss. Science 2002; 295:2446–2449.

33. Kruk PA, Rampino NJ, Bohr VA. DNA damage and repair in telomeres: relation to aging. Proc Natl Acad Sci USA 1995; 92:258–262.

34. Li GZ, Eller MS, Firoozabadi R, Gilchrest BA. Evidence that exposure of the telomere 3′ overhang sequence induces senescence. Proc Natl Acad Sci USA 2003; 100:527–531.

35. Eller MS, Puri N, Hadshiew IM, Venna SS, Gilchrest BA. Induction of apoptosis by telomere 3′ overhang-specific DNA. Exp Cell Res 2002; 276:185–193.

36. Wang X, Wong SC, Pan J, et al. Evidence of cisplatin-induced senescent-like growth arrest in nasopharyngeal carcinoma cells. Cancer Res 1998; 58:5019–5022.

37. Patrick MH. Studies on thymine-derived UV photoproducts in DNA—I. Formation and biological role of pyrimidine adducts in DNA. Photochem Photobiol 1977; 25:357–372.

38. Oikawa S, Kawanishi S. Site-specific DNA damage at GGG sequence by oxidative stress may accelerate telomere shortening. FEBS Lett 1999; 453:365–368.

39. Ishibashi T, Lippard SJ. Telomere loss in cells treated with cisplatin. Proc Natl Acad Sci USA 1998; 95:4219–4223.

40. Zhan Q, Carrier F, Fornace AJ, Jr. Induction of cellular p53 activity by DNA-damaging agents and growth arrest. Mol Cell Biol 1993; 13:4242–4250.

41. Pei XH, Nakanishi Y, Takayama K, Bai F, Hara, N. Benzo[a]pyrene activates the human p53 gene through induction of nuclear factor kappaB activity. J Biol Chem 1999; 274:35240–35246.

42. Stein GH, Dulic V. Molecular mechanisms for the senescent cell cycle arrest. J Investig Dermatol Symp Proc 1998; 3:14–18.

43. Kligman LH, Sayre RM. An action spectrum for ultraviolet induced elastosis in hairless mice: quantification of elastosis by image analysis. Photochem Photobiol 1991; 53:237–242.

44. Wulf HC, Poulsen T, Davies RE, Urbach, F. Narrow-band UV radiation and induction of dermal elastosis and skin cancer. Photodermatol 1989; 6:44–51.

45. Johnston KJ, Oikarinen AI, Lowe NJ, Clark JG, Uitto, J. Ultraviolet radiation-induced connective tissue changes in the skin of hairless mice. J Invest Dermatol 1984; 82:587–590.

46. Kochevar IE. Molecular and cellular effects of UV radiation relevant to chronic photodamage. In: Gilchrest BA, ed. Photodamage. Cambridge, MA: Blackwell Science, 1995: 51.

47. Ying CY, Parrish JA, Pathak MA. Additive erythemogenic effects of middle-(280–320 nm) and long-(320–400 nm) wave ultraviolet light. J Invest Dermatol 1974; 63:273–278.
48. Kligman LH. UVA enhances low dose UVB tumorigenesis. Photochem Photobiol 1988; 47:8s.
49. Lavker RM, Gerberick GF, Veres D, Irwin CJ, Kaidbey KH. Cumulative effects from repeated exposures to suberythemal doses of UVB and UVA in human skin. J Am Acad Dermatol 1995; 32:53–62.
50. Bernerd F, Asselineau D. Successive alteration and recovery of epidermal differentiation and morphogenesis after specific UVB-damages in skin reconstructed in vitro. Dev Biol 1997; 183:123–138.
51. Bernerd F, Asselineau, D. UVA exposure of human skin reconstructed in vitro induces apoptosis of dermal fibroblasts: subsequent connective tissue repair and implications in photoaging. Cell Death Differ 1998; 5:792–802.
52. Gilchrest BA. In vitro studies of aging human epidermis. In: Rothstein M, ed. Review of Biological Research. Vol. 4. New York: Alan R. Liss, 1990: 281.
53. Lopez-Torres M, Shindo Y, Packer L. Effect of age on antioxidants and molecular markers of oxidative damage in murine epidermis and dermis. J Invest Dermatol 1994; 102:476–480.
54. Gilchrest BA, Bohr VA. Aging processes, DNA damage, and repair. FASEB J 1997; 11:322–330.
55. Chen Z, Seo JY, Kim YK, et al. Heat modulation of tropoelastin, fibrillin-1, and matrix metalloproteinase-12 in human skin in vivo. J Invest Dermatol 2005; 124:70–78.
56. Yaar M, Gilchrest, BA. Skin aging: postulated mechanisms and consequent changes in structure and function. In: Gilchrest BA, ed. Clinics in Geriatric Medicine. Vol. 17. Philadelphia: W.B. Saunders, 2001: 617–630.
57. Brooke RC, Newbold SA, Telfer NR, Griffiths CE. Discordance between facial wrinkling and the presence of basal cell carcinoma. Arch Dermatol 2001; 137:751–754.
58. Kaidbey KH, Agin PP, Sayre RM, Kligman AM. Photoprotection by melanin—a comparison of black and Caucasian skin. J Am Acad Dermatol 1979; 1:249–260.
59. Munavalli GS, Weiss RA, Halder RM. Photoaging and nonablative photorejuvenation in ethnic skin. Dermatol Surg 2005; 31:1250–1260; discussion 1261.
60. Halder RM, Richards GM. Photoaging in patients of skin of color. In: Rigel DS, Weiss RA, Lim HW, Dover JS, eds. Photoaging. New York: Marcell Dekker, Inc., 2004: 55–63.
61. Chung JH, Lee SH, Youn CS, et al. Cutaneous photodamage in Koreans: influence of sex, sun exposure, smoking, and skin color. Arch Dermatol 2001; 137:1043–1051.
62. Halder RM. The role of retinoids in the management of cutaneous conditions in blacks. J Am Acad Dermatol 1998; 39:S98–S103.
63. Smith JB, Fenske NA. Cutaneous manifestations and consequences of smoking. J Am Acad Dermatol 1996; 34:717–732.
64. Griffiths CE, Wang TS, Hamilton TA, Voorhees JJ, Ellis CN. A photonumeric scale for the assessment of cutaneous photodamage. Arch Dermatol 1992; 128:347–351.
65. L'Oreal observing the skin: firm and supple. http://www.loreal.com/_en/_ww/loreal-skin-science/vivre/ferme.aspx.
66. Quan MB, Edwards C, Marks R. Non-invasive in vivo techniques to differentiate photodamage and ageing in human skin. Acta Derm Venereol 1997; 77:416–419.
67. Boyce ST, Supp AP, Wickett RR, Hoath SB, Warden GD. Assessment with the dermal torque meter of skin pliability after treatment of burns with cultured skin substitutes. J Burn Care Rehabil 2000; 21:55–63.
68. Nishimori Y, Edwards C, Pearse A, Matsumoto K, Kawai M, Marks R. Degenerative alterations of dermal collagen fiber bundles in photodamaged human skin and UV-irradiated hairless mouse skin: possible effect on decreasing skin mechanical properties and appearance of wrinkles. J Invest Dermatol 2001; 117:1458–1463.
69. Leveque JL. Quantitative assessment of skin aging. In: Gilchrest BA, ed. Clinics in Geriatric Medicine. Philadelphia: W.B. Saunders, 2001: 673–689.
70. Musnier C, Piquemal P, Beau P, Pittet JC. Visual evaluation in vivo of 'complexion radiance' using the C.L.B.T. sensory methodology. Skin Res Technol 2004; 10:50–56.
71. Sandby-Moller J, Thieden E, Philipsen PA, Schmidt G, Wulf HC. Dermal echogenicity: a biological indicator of individual cumulative UVR exposure? Arch Dermatol Res 2004; 295:498–504.
72. Sandby-Moller J, Wulf HC. Ultrasonographic subepidermal low-echogenic band, dependence of age and body site. Skin Res Technol 2004; 10:57–63.
73. Liffers A, Vogt M, Ermert H. In vivo biomicroscopy of the skin with high resolution magnetic resonance imaging and high frequency ultrasound. Biomed Tech (Berl), 2003; 48:130–134.
74. Cullander C. Light microscopy of living tissue: the state and future of the art. J Investig Dermatol Symp Proc 1998; 3:166–171.
75. Sauermann K, Clemann S, Jaspers S, et al. Age related changes of human skin investigated with histometric measurements by confocal laser scanning microscopy in vivo. Skin Res Technol 2002; 8:52–56.

76. Alanen E, Nuutinen J, Nicklen K, Lahtinen T, Monkkonen J. Measurement of hydration in the stratum corneum with the MoistureMeter and comparison with the Corneometer. Skin Res Technol 2004; 10:32–37.

77. Mosely H, English JSC, Coghill GM, Mackie RM. Assessment and use of a new skin hygrometer. Bioeng Skin 1985; 1:177–192.

78. Wheldon AE, Monteith JL. Performance of a skin evaporimeter. Med Biol Eng Comput 1980; 18:201–205.

79. Shah JH, Zhai H, Maibach HI. Comparative evaporimetry in man. Skin Res Technol 2005; 11:205–208.

80. Pierard-Franchimont C, Pierard GE. Postmenopausal aging of the sebaceous follicle: a comparison between women receiving hormone replacement therapy or not. Dermatology 2002; 204:17–22.

81. Halachmi S, Yaar M, Gilchrest BA. Advances in skin aging/photoaging: theoretical and practical implications. Ann Dermatol Venereol 2005; 132:362.

8 | The Chronic Effects of Ultraviolet Radiation on the Skin: Photocarcinogenesis

Antony R. Young
Division of Genetics and Molecular Medicine, St. John's Institute of Dermatology, King's College London, London, England, U.K.

Norbert M. Wikonkál
Department of Dermatology, Semmelweis University, School of Medicine, Budapest, Hungary

- Skin cancers are among the most common types of cancer in humans, and their incidence has been steadily increasing for several decades. These cancers can be divided into three main types: malignant melanoma (MM), basal cell carcinoma (BCC), and squamous cell carcinoma (SCC). SCC and BCC are often collectively referred to as nonmelanoma skin cancer.

- The clinical behavior of these three tumor types differs greatly. MM is one of the most aggressive cancers seen in adults with early metastatic capacity, such that the vast majority of skin cancer deaths results from MM that normally account for less the 10% of all skin cancers. SCC can also metastasize, but mainly only at advanced stages, whereas BCC almost completely lacks the ability to metastasize.

- Epidemiology supports a relationship between solar radiation and skin cancer, and a definitive role for ultraviolet radiation (UVR) was first established in animals.

- In the "normal" population, the main risk factor for all types of skin cancer is skin phototype, based on the Fitzpatrick classification.

- A direct role for UVR in SCC and BCC has been established in recent years by the identification of UVR "signature mutations." However, as yet there is very little molecular evidence to confirm the relationship between UVR and MM.

- Missense mutations are mostly manifest by impairing the function of the translated protein. Tumor suppressor genes are particularly important and perturbations of these genes greatly increase the likelihood of loss of genetic surveillance with the consequent potential of favoring a clone of cells that can progress into cancer. Probably, the most extensively studied tumor suppressor gene is TP53, which translates into a protein that acts as a transcription factor for a number of genes, including those that regulate cell cycle, DNA synthesis, and programmed cell death (apoptosis).

- Skin cancer remains a major public health problem, and the best advice for persons with susceptible skin types is to minimize solar exposure. Many campaigns advocate the use of sunscreens that one might reasonably expect to reduce skin cancer risk. Admittedly, the human evidence for this is not very strong, except for actinic keratoses, and there is no evidence that sunscreen use has any effect on MM.

INTRODUCTION: SKIN CANCER

Skin cancers are among the most common types of cancer in countries where good registration data exist, and their incidence has been steadily increasing for several decades. These cancers, of epidermal origin, can be divided into three main types: malignant melanoma (MM), basal cell carcinoma (BCC), and squamous cell carcinoma (SCC). SCC and BCC are often collectively referred to as nonmelanoma skin cancer (NMSC). However, this historic classification has little relevance to the pathogenesis of these tumors whose similarity is mostly confined to their being derived from the keratinocyte. This also explains their lack of pigmentation, although this is occasionally seen in BCC. In contrast, MM originates from epidermal melanocytes that accounts for their usual dark pigmentation, although amelanotic MM do occur. The clinical behavior of these three tumor types differs greatly. MM is one of the most aggressive cancers seen in adults with early metastatic capacity, such that the vast majority of skin cancer deaths result from MM that normally account for less than 10% of all skin cancers. SCCs can also metastasize, but mainly at advanced stages only; whereas BCC almost completely lack the ability to metastasize, leading some to argue that BCC should not be termed a "cancer." BCCs are generally tumors of the elderly, but dermatologists are more likely to find BCC on a younger patient than SCC. A genodermatosis with autosomal dominant inheritance, the Gorlin-Goltz syndrome is known to predispose to BCC at a very early age as shown in Figure 1.

The Gorlin-Goltz syndrome has been shown to be the result of a mutation of the human homologue of the Drosophila "patched" gene, PTCH (1,2). Another member of the hedgehog signal transduction pathway, sonic hedgehog (Shh) (Fig. 2), has also been shown to have a pronounced effect on keratinocyte proliferation: overexpression of Shh in keratinocytes resulted in a BCC-like phenotype after grafting on immunodeficient mice (3) (see Athar et al. (4) for recent review).

PHENOTYPIC AND SOLAR EXPOSURE RISK FACTORS FOR SKIN CANCER

In the "normal" population the main risk factor for all types of skin cancer is skin phototype, based on the Fitzpatrick classification, as shown in Table 1. Thus, fair-skinned sun-sensitive skin types I and II, who tan poorly if at all, are more susceptible than sun-tolerant skin types III and IV who tan well. Skin types V (brown) and VI (black) with high levels of constitutive pigmentation have the lowest incidence of skin cancer.

The risk for skin cancer, especially BCC and MM, is closely related to the number of sunburn episodes in the person's life, which is influenced by the skin color. Very light skin

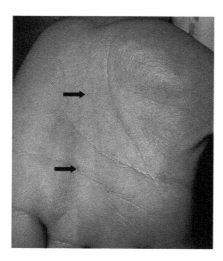 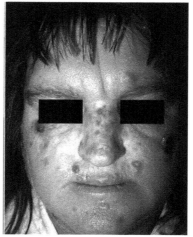

FIGURE 1   Gorlin-Goltz syndrome. *Left panel*: Arrowheads indicate the keratotic pitting of the palms. *Right panel:* A large number of basal cell cancers on the face of a female patient in her late 30s.

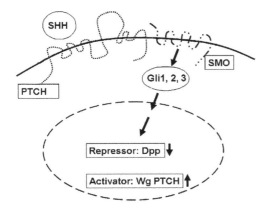

FIGURE 2 The sonic hedgehog (Shh) signal transduction pathway. The receptor for Shh is the product of PTCH; PTCH acts as a negative regulator of Shh, without which PTCH represses the activation smoothened (SMO). This inhibits the expression of various downstream target genes, which include members of the TGF-β family, gli, and PTCH itself. *Abbreviations*: PTCH; Drosophila "patched" gene; Shh, sonic hedgehog; SMO, smoothened.

color may increase skin cancer incidence up to 1100-fold compared to darkly pigmented individuals depending on the level of ultraviolet radiation (UVR) exposure (5). An important factor is the melanin content of keratinocytes, as complete lack of melanin in cases of albinism predisposes to a higher rate of NMSC in both human and mouse (6,7). Human skin and hair color is determined largely by one gene, the melanocortin 1 receptor (MC1R) gene (8). The human MC1R gene encodes a 317 amino acid protein, a seven-pass transmembrane G protein coupled receptor. This family has further members, such as MC2R, the receptor for ACTH and MC4R, which play a crucial role in body-weight regulation. The cleavage of the proopiomelanocortin (POMC) protein generates the melanocyte-stimulating hormone alpha (αMSH) that serves as a ligand for the MC1R gene product. Its activation results in an increase in cellular cAMP that leads to activation of protein kinase A, which then leads to increased transcription of microphthalmia transcription factor (MITF). MITF directly regulates melanogenesis by activating the transcription in several genes that also include tyrosinase and tyrosinase-related protein 1 and 2 (9). POMC is synthesized in the pituitary gland; but, in humans, keratinocytes are a more important source of this peptide as they produce acetylated αMSH, a more powerful agonist of the human MC1R. Thus, skin pigmentation is primarily regulated by locally produced αMSH that acts as paracrine and/or autocrine mediator of UVR-induced pigmentation (10). Melanin is an organic polymer originated from the amino acid tyrosine with an oxidation reaction by the tyrosinase enzyme. Two types of melanin are synthesized: (*i*) a cysteine-rich red–yellow form known as pheomelanin, and (*ii*) a less-soluble black–brown form known as eumelanin. MC1R activation results in primarily the synthesis of eumelanin (11).

TABLE 1 A Classification of Skin Phototypes Based on Susceptibility to Sunburn in Sunlight, Tanning Ability, and Skin Cancer Risk, Together with Indicative Minimal Erythema Doses that Might Be Expected Following UVR Exposure on Unacclimatized Skin

Skin phototype	Sunburn susceptibility	Tanning ability	Skin cancer risk	No. SED[a] for 1 MED
I	High	None	High	1–3
II	High	Poor	High	
III	Moderate	Good	Low	3–7
IV	Low	Very good	Low	
V	Very low	Excellent	Very low	7–>12
VI	Very low	Excellent	Very low	

[a]A standard erythema dose (SED) is equivalent to an erythemally effective radiant exposure of 100 Jm^{-2} (12). About 3 SEDs are required to produce just perceptible MEDs in the unacclimatized white skin of the most common northern European skin types (13). See Chapter 2.
Abbreviations: MED, minimal erythema dose; SED, standard erythema dose.

Despite the extremely large differences between individuals' skin color, light and dark skin have similar numbers of melanocytes; the major difference lies in the size, number, and pigment content of pigment-containing organelles, the melanosomes (14).

Melanin protects epidermal DNA by various mechanisms, and induced pigmentation offers protection factors in the region of 3 (15). Protective melanin caps are often seen over basal layer nuclei. Melanin also scavenges reactive oxygen species (ROS), although the two major forms, pheomelanin and eumelanin, are not equally effective in this role (16).

In contrast to the above mentioned protective effects of melanin, it is also capable of generating ROS upon UV irradiation (17–19). It is now presumed that sunlight sensitivity of individuals with pheomelanin, that is, the fair-skinned population, contributes to three-fold greater DNA damage after UVB than eumelanin along with less efficient protection (19).

Solar exposure has long been presumed to play a role in the development of skin cancer, and this has been supported by extensive clinical observation and epidemiological data. The most direct association is for SCCs, which rarely appear before the age of 60 and are usually seen in patients with habitual long-term solar exposure. Furthermore, these patients usually have other signs of chronic photodamage such as photoaging with loss of skin elasticity, deep wrinkles, and numerous solar lentigines. SCC is an occupational hazard for outdoor workers such as farmers, but is also prevalent in avid golfers and boaters. SCC has a precancerous lesion known as a solar or actinic keratosis (AK) that appears as a scaling reddish papule or plaque that consists of aberrantly differentiating and proliferating cells. These precancers may regress (20), but one in a thousand are thought to progress to carcinoma in situ and then SCC (21). AKs are also biomarkers for SCC risk. Intermittent high-dose solar exposure is thought to provoke BCC rather than regular moderate doses of UVR (22). Unlike SCCs, BCCs never appear on mucus membranes and have no precursor/biomarker lesions.

Solar exposure is the major environmental risk factor for MM. A recent meta-analysis has supported the conclusions of many individual case-control studies that intermittent sun exposure is the most predictive environmental risk factor for melanoma [relative risk (RR) = 1.6, 95% confidence interval (CI) 1.3–2.0] and that sunburn, especially in childhood, is a significant risk factor (23). This analysis also suggested a highly significant effect for sunburn at any age (RR = 2.0, 95% CI 1.7–2.4). There was no evidence for a causal effect of chronic sun exposure on MM risk (RR = 1.0, 95% CI 0.9–1.0). Further evidence for a role of sun exposure in MM comes from penetrance studies for the melanoma susceptibility gene CDKN2A, in which there was evidence for an interaction between susceptibility genes and latitude of residence, so that penetrance was highest in families with germline CDKN2A mutations living in Australia when compared with those in Europe (24).

Many case-control studies have established that phenotypic characteristics associated with sun sensitivity are risk factors for MM and this has been confirmed in a recent meta-analysis of 60 such studies (25). This showed that skin type I (vs. IV) was associated with a RR of 2.1 for melanoma (95% CI 1.7–2.6). A high density of freckles was associated with a RR of 2.1 (95% CI 1.8–2.5), eye color (Blue vs. Dark: RR = 1.5, 95% CI 1.3–1.7), and hair color (Red vs. Dark: RR = 3.6, 95% CI 2.6–5.4). Risk of melanoma is also greater in patients with larger numbers of melanocytic nevi, whether banal or clinically atypical. A meta-analysis of case-control studies by Gandini et al. (26) showed that the number of common nevi was confirmed as an important risk factor for MM with a substantially increased risk associated with the presence of 101 to 120 nevi compared with <15 (RR = 6.9; 95% CI: 4.6, 10.3), as was the number of atypical nevi (RR = 6.4 95%; CI: 3.8, 10.3; for 5 vs. 0).

EVIDENCE FOR A ROLE OF UVR IN SKIN CANCER

Epidemiology supports a relationship between solar radiation and skin cancer, but terrestrial sunlight contains visible and infrared as well as UVR. A definitive role for UVR was first established in animals.

Detailed wavelength dependency (action spectrum) studies for SCC in mice have shown that UVB (280–315 nm) is much more carcinogenic than UVA (315–400 nm). The animal data

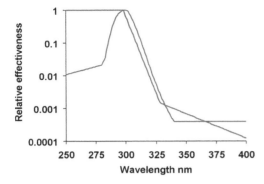

FIGURE 3   The CIE reference action spectrum for erythema in human skin (12) (red) and the estimated CIE action spectrum for human squamous cell carcinoma (27) (blue) based on mouse studies. See Chapter 2.

have been used to generate a human action spectrum for SCC that is very similar to that for human erythema as shown in Figure 3. This modeling implicates UVB as the main cause of human SCC, and the recent development of mouse model for MM also indicates that UVB is much more important than UVA (28). BCC animal models, such as Shh overexpressing (29) and Ptch heterozygous mice (30) only incompletely reproduce this skin cancer. However, no wavelength dependence studies have been done.

A direct role for UVR in SCC and BCC has been established in recent years by the identification of UVR "signature mutations" in these tumors as described subsequently. However, as yet there is very little molecular evidence to confirm the relationship between UVR and MM.

DNA PHOTODAMAGE AND UVR SIGNATURE MUTATIONS

DNA is a major epidermal chromophore with absorption spectrum maximum in the nonterrestrial UVC range, at 260 nm. However, there is also significant absorption in the UVB region and to a much lesser extent in the UVA region. This absorption of UVR photon energy can result in its dissipation by the rearrangement of electrons to form new bonds resulting in the structural alteration of adjacent DNA pyrimidine bases into two major classes of DNA photolesions as described further and shown in Figure 4. Thus, the target sites for UVR damage are determined by the DNA-base sequence as well as the chemical structure of individual bases.

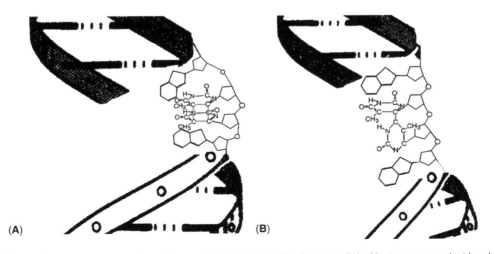

(A)   **(B)**

FIGURE 4   **(A)** Cyclobutane pyrimidine dimer. Two adjacent pyrimidine bases are linked by two new covalent bonds to form a 4-C atom ring. **(B)** Pyrimidine-pyrimidone (6-4) photoproduct. A single new covalent bond is formed that distorts the DNA helix.

Cyclobutane Pyrimidine Dimers

The most prevalent photoproduct is the cyclobutane pyrimidine dimer (CPD) that results from a UVR photon's energy splitting the C5=C6 double bonds of each of the pyrimidine bases [thymine (T) and cytosine (C)], after which their electrons form two new covalent bonds between the bases that results in a 4-carbon cyclobutane ring. Simulated solar UVR readily induces CPD in human epidermis in vivo with an action spectrum that is very close to that for human erythema. Peak efficacy in vivo is at 300 nm rather than shorter wavelengths (31), most probably because of screening by other skin chromophores such as stratum corneum-bound urocanic acid, as well as DNA itself (32).

6-4 Photoproducts

The second major photoproduct is the pyrimidine-pyrimidone (6-4) [(6-4)PP] photoproduct. In this case, the C5=C6 double bond breaks and the surplus energy results in the rotation of one of the pyrimidine rings, which offers its C4 to form a new bond with the C6 of the adjacent ring. In this case, only one new bond is formed. This structure causes a more significant distortion in the double helix than the cyclobutane ring.

Dipyrimidine lesions interfere with base pairing during DNA replication. The "A rule" results in the correct pairing for T but not for C (33). Thus, C can be replaced by T (C → T mutation) and sometimes two adjacent C are changed to T (CC → TT, known as a tandem mutation). These changes are known as "UVR signature mutations" because they are almost exclusively due to UVR (34–36). Repair mechanisms are capable of monitoring and restoring genetic integrity and may prevent mutation. In all systems studied, including human skin, the repair of (6-4)PP is much faster than CPD, which probably explains why the CPD has been demonstrated to be more important in skin cancer models. As discussed elsewhere, the extremely high incidence of skin cancer in xeroderma pigmentosum (XP) patients, who are deficient in DNA repair, demonstrates the crucial role of DNA repair mechanism in the prevention of skin cancer. The enhancement of DNA repair, in particular of CPD, has been shown to inhibit photocarcinogenesis in different animal models, and the application of a topical DNA repair enzyme has been shown to reduce the incidence of AK in XP patients (37). Recently, length mutations of mitochondrial DNA has also been proposed to play a role as deletions and tandem duplications were found in tissues of AK, BCC, SCC, and sun-exposed normal skin but not sun-protected skin (38).

UVR SIGNATURE MUTATIONS IN TUMOR SUPPRESSOR GENES

In general, the causes of cancer-inducing mutations are unknown. However, the specificity of UVR-induced mutations enables the detection of the early molecular events in skin carcinogenesis. Missense mutations are mostly manifest by impairing the function of the translated protein. The significance of a given mutation, in principle, is determined by the role of the protein for which the mutated gene is coding. In functional terms, tumor suppressor genes are particularly important, and perturbations of these genes greatly increase the likelihood of loss of genetic surveillance with the consequent potential of favoring a clone of cells that can progress into cancer. Probably, the most extensively studied tumor suppressor gene is TP53, which translates into a 53-kDa molecular-weight protein that acts as a transcription factor for a number of genes including those that regulate cell cycle, DNA synthesis, and programmed cell death (apoptosis) reviewed by Fisher (39). TP53 is mutated in about 50% of human cancers and is considered a tumor suppressor gene, because its mutations inactivate its ability to suppress tumor cell growth in culture (40). In addition, such mutations inactivate its transcriptional activator function.

TP53 and Programmed Cell Death

In skin, UVB irradiation leads to the formation of "sunburn cells" (SBCs) that are apoptotic keratinocytes (41). Apoptosis can also be induced by UVB in cultured human keratinocytes. Mouse studies have shown that the TP53 tumor suppressor gene plays a role in SBC, but apoptosis can also occur via a TP53 independent pathway, recently reviewed by Raj et al. (42). The TP53 protein is thought to participate in a surveillance pathway that monitors the integrity of the genome. In some cells, this appears to be a "guardian of the genome" route in which DNA damage induces TP53 protein, leading to transient cell cycle arrest at a G_1 checkpoint (43). In other cases, however, the endpoint is TP53-dependent apoptotic death of the damaged cell. This pathway has been termed "cellular proofreading" because it aborts the aberrant cell rather than restoring its genome [for reviews see Sheehan and Young (44), Harris and Levine (45)]. SBCs are evidently the end result of such a TP53-dependent DNA surveillance mechanism, in which keratinocytes with unrepaired UVR lesions are killed by apoptosis. SBC formation thus appears to be one way that nature prevents skin cancer. Apoptosis can also be induced by cell cycle abnormalities caused by a defective Rb gene or excessive E2F-1 (46). This apoptosis pathway has a complex relation to TP53-dependent apoptosis and the two act together as cellular proofreading of potentially precancerous cells.

TP53 in Squamous Cell Carcinoma

Induction of epidermal TP53 can be seen as early as 30 minutes after exposure to UVR (47). This is a translational, rather than a transcriptional, event because no increase in its mRNA is observed. The half-life of wild-type TP53 protein is short and its signal usually disappears within a few hours of induction (48). However, mutated TP53 is relatively resistant to degradation and this phenomenon can be used immunohistochemically to detect cells that are likely to harbor mutated TP53 (49). This technique uses a mono- or polyclonal antibody to detect epitopes of the TP53 protein, and the antigen-antibody binding is visualized as a nuclear staining. The skin has a low background expression level of TP53 protein, which means that a positive reaction is indicative of either: (*i*) expression in response to a very recent challenge, in which case TP53 is likely to be wild-type; or (*ii*) the protein was not degraded and is likely to be mutant. Some antibodies have been targeted against epitopes that are most frequently mutated, which allows some selective detection of mutated TP53, as shown in Figure 5. However, unlike sequencing, an immunohistochemical approach cannot confidently distinguish between mutated TP53 protein and overexpressed wild-type protein.

Sections from BCC and SCC usually contain many cells that are positive for TP53 antibody (50–52). Sequencing data from a large number of tumors show that TP53 is mutated in more than 90% of SCCs (50,51,53–55), the vast majority of which are UVR signature mutations. The most common is C → T at dipyrimidine sites in about 70% of the cases. Tandem CC → TT mutations were also found with the frequency of 10%. Hence, two important pieces of the cancer-formation puzzle became apparent: (*i*) UVR is the most prominent mutagen, and (*ii*) TP53 is the gene that undergoes mutations. The high frequency and nature

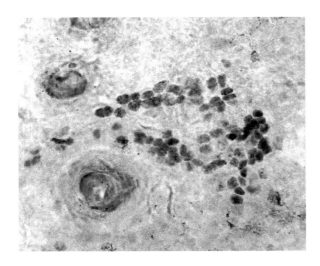

FIGURE 5 TP53-positive cells in murine epidermal sheet detected by CM-5 antibody. The darkly staining nuclei are the TP53 mutant cells.

of TP53 mutations in SCC strongly suggest that this modification is a significant contributor to skin tumors. The SCC (and BCC) of XP patients contains high frequencies of UVR signature mutations. One must note, however, that even though TP53 mutations are not exclusive to skin cancer and such mutations are present in half of all human cancers, TP53 mutations in internal cancers are more diverse with hardly any characteristic UVR signature mutations (56).

The assumption that UVR-induced TP53 mutations result in SCC leads one to assess TP53 status in AK that may progress to SCC, especially as the transition from severe sun damage to AK, and from AK to in situ SCC have clear and seemingly sequential histological features with increasing numbers of cell divisions, more apparent cellular atypia, and the appearance of the horn cysts characteristic of SCC. Work in several laboratories shows a molecular similarity between AK and to SCC with AK also containing anti-TP53 positive cells. Moreover, these cells contain mutations with patterns similar to those of SCC (57). These observations further support the view that TP53 mutations are an early event and play a critical role in the development of skin cancer (58). Indeed, using the same anti-TP53 antibody approach, clones of 60 to 1000 positive cells have been identified in healthy human sun-exposed epidermis prior to any micro- or macroscopic sign of skin cancer. These experiments also demonstrated that sun-shielded skin harbors very few TP53-positive cells that appear singly or in very small groups. Chronically sun-exposed skin, on the other hand, contains more patches of TP53-positive-staining cells than sun-protected skin and these patches are also greater in size. Sequencing TP53-positive cells from sun-exposed and sun-shielded sites revealed TP53 mutations in sun-exposed skin only. The presence of large numbers of TP53-positive clones on sun-exposed skin strongly suggests that only a small percentage of these cells gives rise to actual tumors. These clones are present in such a surprisingly large number that a comparison with the incidence of skin tumors leaves one to conclude that most of these clones disappear. In fact, the frequency of apoptosis in AK is high, which supports the clinical observations that these lesions often regress if further sun-exposure is prevented (20).

TP53-positive clones have also been shown in mouse skin exposed to UVB for 17 days, which supports the theory that these clones arise as daughter cells of a single TP53-mutated cell. However, these clones gradually disappear after the UVR exposure ceases (59). UVA, by itself, in high doses, is also capable of inducing skin tumors, although its carcinogenesis shows less of a dose-dependency than UVB (60). Psoralens in combination with UVA radiation also give rise to mutations in the TP53 gene (61). Similarly to the human experiments, groups of keratinocytes with mutated TP53 could be shown in murine epidermis (62). In a set of experiments, wild-type C57BL/6 mice were shaved on the back and regularly irradiated with a UVB source. At the end of the irradiation most of the dorsal skin was excised in whole and the epidermis was peeled off in one sheet to stain for immunoreactive cells with an anti-T53 antibody. At a time- and dose-dependent manner, the progression of clones of TP53-positive cells could be shown in which process-continued UVB irradiation was required for mutated cells to break in neighboring epidermal proliferation units, thus allowing the growth of preclinical tumors.

TP53 in Basal Cell Carcinoma

Clinical differences between BCC and SCC may result from differences at the gene level. Mutation analysis of TP53 in BCC showed that 60% of tumors contained TP53 gene mutations (51). Some studies, based on the analysis of very small foci from the tumor tissue, have also shown that all BCCs harbor TP53 mutations (63). It is important to consider the sample size for mutation analysis. Current technology allows the extraction of DNA from a very small cluster of cells (e.g., 50–100 cells) (64) and the demonstration of genetic alteration after several amplification steps in a thermocycler. However, this exquisite sensitivity can confound data interpretation, and it is, therefore, desirable that mutation reports indicate the sample size analyzed and the intensity of the mutated allele compared to its wild type, so that readers can draw their own conclusions. BCCs have also been found to contain UVR signature mutations in the human homologue of the PTCH gene (65), which suggests that this gene is important for this type of tumor. Its function is less clear than that of TP53, but it is part of the hedgehog signal transduction pathway that transmits extracellular growth and differentiation signals to the nucleus. Interestingly, PTCH does not seem to play a role in SCC, leaving TP53 as the only gene known to lead to SCC upon inactivation.

CONCLUSIONS

UVR has been established as a skin carcinogen by a combination of epidemiological, animal, and molecular studies. The molecular evidence is very strong in the case of SCC and BCC, whereas the vast majority of the evidence for MM is epidemiological. The phenotypic risk factors for all types of skin cancer are well understood but we lack understanding of the genetic basis of these factors. Skin cancer remains a major public health problem, and the best advice one can give at the moment is for persons with susceptible skin types to minimize solar exposure, as is done in many public health campaigns. Many such campaigns advocate the use of sunscreens that one might reasonably expect to reduce skin cancer risk. However, the human evidence for this is not very strong, except for AK (66), and there is no evidence that sunscreen use has any effect on MM (67).

ACKNOWLEDGMENTS

We thank Professor Brian Diffey for his contributions to Table 1 and Figure 3.

REFERENCES

1. Gailani MR, Bale SJ, Leffell DJ, et al. Developmental defects in Gorlin syndrome related to a putative tumor suppressor gene on chromosome 9. Cell 1992; 69:111–117.
2. Gailani MR, Stahle-Backdahl M, Leffell DJ, et al. The role of the human homologue of Drosophila patched in sporadic basal cell carcinomas. Nat Genet 1996; 14(1):78–81.
3. Fan H, Oro AE, Scott MP, et al. Induction of basal cell carcinoma features in transgenic human skin expressing Sonic Hedgehog. Nat Med 1997; 3(7):788–792.
4. Athar M, Tang X, Lee JL, et al. Hedgehog signalling in skin development and cancer. Exp Dermatol 2006; 15(9):667–677.
5. Urbach F. The cumulative effects of ultraviolet radiation on the skin: photocarcinogenesis. In: Hawk J, ed. Photodermatology. London: Arnold Publishers, 1999:89–111.
6. Perry PK, Silverberg NB. Cutaneous malignancy in albinism. Cutis 2001; 67(5):427–430.
7. Kripke ML. Latency, histology, and antigenicity of tumors induced by ultraviolet light in three inbred mouse strains. Cancer Res 1977; 37(5):1395–1400.
8. Rees JL. Genetics of hair and skin color. Annu Rev Genet 2003; 37:67–90.
9. Bertolotto C, Abbe P, Hemesath TJ, et al. Microphthalmia gene product as a signal transducer in cAMP-induced differentiation of melanocytes. J Cell Biol 1998; 142(3):827–835.
10. Tsatmali M, Ancans J, Yukitake J, et al. Skin POMC peptides: their actions at the human MC-1 receptor and roles in the tanning response. Pigment Cell Res 2000; 13(suppl 8):125–129.
11. Barsh GS. What controls variation in human skin color? PLoS Biol 2003; 1(1):E27.
12. CIE. Erythema reference action spectrum and standard erythema dose. Vienna: Commission Internationale de l'Éclairage; 1998. Report No.: CIE S ed 007/E.
13. Harrison GI, Young AR. Ultraviolet radiation-induced erythema in human skin. Methods 2002; 28(1):14–19.
14. Szabo G, Gerald AB, Pathak MA, et al. Racial differences in the fate of melanosomes in human epidermis. Nature 1969; 222(198):1081–1082.
15. Agar N, Young AR. Melanogenesis: a photoprotective response to DNA damage? Mutat Res 2005; 571(1–2):121–132.
16. Rees JL. The genetics of sun sensitivity in humans. Am J Hum Genet 2004; 75(5):739–751.
17. Ortonne JP. Photoprotective properties of skin melanin. Br J Dermatol 2002; 146(suppl 61):7–10.
18. Hill HZ, Li W, Xin P, Mitchell DL. Melanin: a two-edged sword? Pigment Cell Res 1997; 10(3):158–161.
19. Takeuchi S, Zhang W, Wakamatsu K, et al. Melanin acts as a potent UVB photosensitizer to cause an atypical mode of cell death in murine skin. Proc Natl Acad Sci USA 2004; 101(42):15076–15081.
20. Marks R, Foley P, Goodman G, et al. Spontaneous remission of solar keratoses: the case for conservative management. Br J Dermatol 1986; 115(6):649–655.
21. Callen JP, Bickers DR, Moy RL. Actinic keratoses. J Am Acad Dermatol 1997; 36(4):650–653.

22. Kricker A, Armstrong BK, English DR, et al. Does intermittent sun exposure cause basal cell carcinoma? A case-control study in Western Australia. Int J Cancer 1995; 60(4):489–494.
23. Gandini S, Sera F, Cattaruzza MS, et al. Meta-analysis of risk factors for cutaneous melanoma: II. Sun exposure. Eur J Cancer 2005; 41(1):45–60.
24. Bishop JA, Corrie PG, Evans J, et al. UK guidelines for the management of cutaneous melanoma. Br J Plast Surg 2002; 55(1):46–54.
25. Gandini S, Sera F, Cattaruzza MS, et al. Meta-analysis of risk factors for cutaneous melanoma: III. Family history, actinic damage and phenotypic factors. Eur J Cancer 2005; 41(14):2040–2059.
26. Gandini S, Sera F, Cattaruzza MS, et al. Meta-analysis of risk factors for cutaneous melanoma: I. Common and atypical naevi. Eur J Cancer 2005; 41(1):28–44.
27. CIE. Action spectrum for photocarcinogenesis (non-melanoma skin cancers). Vienna: Commission Internationale de l'Éclairage; 2000. Report No.: CIE 132/2; TC 6-32 ed.
28. De Fabo EC, Noonan FP, Fears T, et al. Ultraviolet B but not ultraviolet A radiation initiates melanoma. Cancer Res 2004; 64(18):6372–6376.
29. Xie J, Murone M, Luoh SM, et al. Activating smoothened mutations in sporadic basal-cell carcinoma. Nature 1998; 391(6662):90–92.
30. Aszterbaum M, Epstein J, Oro A, et al. Ultraviolet and ionizing radiation enhance the growth of BCCs and trichoblastomas in patched heterozygous knockout mice. Nature Medicine 1999; 5(11):1285–1291.
31. Young AR, Chadwick CA, Harrison GI, et al. The similarity of action spectra for thymine dimers in human epidermis and erythema suggests that DNA is the chromophore for erythema. J Invest Dermatol 1998; 111(6):982–988.
32. Young AR. Chromophores in human skin. Phys Med Biol 1997; 42(5):789–802.
33. Loeb LA, Preston BD. Mutagenesis by apurinic/apyrimidinic sites. Annu Rev Genet 1986; 20:201–230.
34. Miller JH. Mutagenic specificity of ultraviolet light. J Mol Biol 1985; 182:45–68.
35. Brash DE, Seetharam S, Kraemer KH, et al. Photoproduct frequency is not the major determinant of UV base substitution hot spots or cold spots in human cells. Proc Natl Acad Sci USA 1987; 84:3782–3786.
36. Drobetsky EA, Grosovsky AJ, Glickman BW. The specificity of UV-induced mutations at an endogenous locus in mammalian cells. Proc Natl Acad Sci USA 1987; 84:9103–9107.
37. Yarosh D, Klein J, O'Connor A, et al. Effect of topically applied T4 endonuclease V in liposomes on skin cancer in xeroderma pigmentosum: a randomised study. Xeroderma Pigmentosum Study Group. Lancet 2001; 357(9260):926–929.
38. Yang JH, Lee HC, Chung JG, et al. Mitochondrial DNA mutations in light-associated skin tumors. Anticancer Res 2004; 24(3a):1753–1758.
39. Fisher DE. Apoptosis in cancer therapy: crossing the threshold. Cell 1994; 78(4):539–542.
40. Kemp CJ, Donehower LA, Bradley A, et al. Reduction of p53 gene dosage does not increase initiation or promotion but enhances malignant progression of chemically induced skin tumors. Cell 1993; 74:813–822.
41. Danno K, Horio T. Sunburn cell: factors involved in its formation. Photochem Photobiol 1987; 45:683–690.
42. Raj D, Brash DE, Grossman D. Keratinocyte apoptosis in epidermal development and disease. J Invest Dermatol 2006; 126(2):243–257.
43. Lane DP. p53, guardian of the genome. Nature 1992; 358:15–16.
44. Sheehan JM, Young AR. The sunburn cell revisited: an update on mechanistic aspects. Photochem Photobiol Sci 2002; 1(6):365–377.
45. Harris SL, Levine AJ. The p53 pathway: positive and negative feedback loops. Oncogene 2005; 24(17):2899–2908.
46. DeGregori J, Leone G, Miron A, et al. Distinct roles for E2F proteins in cell growth control and apoptosis. Proc Natl Acad Sci USA 1997; 94(14):7245–7250.
47. Maltzman W, Czyzyk L. UV irradiation stimulates levels of p53 cellular tumor antigen in nontransformed mouse cells. Mol Cell Biol 1984; 4(9):1689–1694.
48. Ljungman M, Zhang F. Blockage of RNA polymerase as a possible trigger for u.v. light-induced apoptosis. Oncogene 1996; 13(4):823–831.
49. Hall PA, Lane DP. p53 in tumour pathology: can we trust immunohistochemistry?—Revisited: [editorial] [see comments]. J Pathol 1994; 172(1):1–4.
50. Brash DE, Rudolph JA, Simon JA, et al. A role for sunlight in skin cancer: UV-induced p53 mutations in squamous cell carcinoma. Proc Natl Acad Sci USA 1991; 88:10124–10128.
51. Ziegler A, Leffell DJ, Kunala S, et al. Mutation hotspots due to sunlight in the p53 gene of nonmelanoma skin cancers. Proc Natl Acad Sci USA 1993; 90:4216–4220.
52. Wikonkál NM, Berg RJ, van Haselen CW, et al. bcl-2 vs p53 protein expression and apoptotic rate in human nonmelanoma skin cancers. Arch Dermatol 1997; 133(5):599–602.

53. Campbell C, Quinn AG, Ro YS, et al. p53 mutations are common and early events that precede tumor invasion in squamous cell neoplasia of the skin. J Invest Dermatol 1993; 100(6):746–748.
54. Ren ZP, Hedrum A, Pontén F, et al. Human epidermal cancer and accompanying precursors have identical p53 mutations different from p53 mutations in adjacent areas of clonally expanded non-neoplastic keratinocytes. Oncogene 1996; 12(4):765–773.
55. Jonason AS, Kunala S, Price GJ, et al. Frequent clones of p53-mutated keratinocytes in normal human skin. Proc Natl Acad Sci USA 1996; 93(24):14025–14029.
56. Greenblatt MS, Bennett WP, Hollstein M, et al. Mutations in the p53 tumor suppressor gene: clues to cancer etiology and molecular pathogenesis. Cancer Res 1994; 54(18):4855–4878.
57. Ziegler A, Jonason AS, Leffell DJ, et al. Sunburn and p53 in onset of skin cancer. Nature 1994; 372(22):773–776.
58. Wikonkál NM, Brash DE. Ultraviolet radiation induced signature mutations in photocarcinogenesis. J Invest Dermatol Symp Proc 1999; 4(1):6–10.
59. Berg RJ, van Kranen HJ, Rebel HG, et al. Early p53 alterations in mouse skin carcinogenesis by UVB radiation: immunohistochemical detection of mutant p53 protein in clusters of preneoplastic epidermal cells. Proc Natl Acad Sci USA 1996; 93(1):274–278.
60. de Laat A, van der Leun JC, de Gruijl FR. Carcinogenesis induced by UVA (365-nm) radiation: the dose-time dependence of tumor formation in hairless mice. Carcinogenesis 1997; 18: 1013–1020.
61. Nataraj AJ, Black HS, Ananthaswamy HN. Signature p53 mutation at DNA cross-linking sites in 8-methoxypsoralen and ultraviolet A (PUVA)-induced murine skin cancers. Proc Natl Acad Sci USA 1996; 93(15):7961–7965.
62. Zhang W, Remenyik E, Zelterman D, et al. Escaping the stem cell compartment: sustained UVB exposure allows p53-mutant keratinocytes to colonize adjacent epidermal proliferating units without incurring additional mutations. Proc Natl Acad Sci USA 2001; 98(24):13948–13953.
63. Pontén F, Berg C, Ahmadian A, et al. Molecular pathology in basal cell cancer with p53 as a genetic marker. Oncogene 1997; 15(9):1059–1067.
64. Pontén F, Williams C, Ling G, et al. Genomic analysis of single cells from human basal cell cancer using laser-assisted capture microscopy. Mutat Res 1997; 382(1–2):45–55.
65. Hahn H, Wicking C, Zaphiropoulous PG, et al. Mutations of the human homolog of Drosophila patched in the nevoid basal cell carcinoma syndrome. Cell 1996; 85(6):841–851.
66. IARC. Suncreens. Lyon: International Agency for Cancer Prevention; 2001.
67. Huncharek M, Kupelnick B. Use of topical sunscreens and the risk of malignant melanoma: a meta-analysis of 9067 patients from 11 case-control studies. Am J Public Health 2002; 92(7):1173–1177.

9 The Epidemiology of Skin Cancer

Luigi Naldi
Centro Studi GISED, Ospedali Riuniti, Bergamo, Italy

Thomas Diepgen
*Department of Clinical Social Medicine, Occupational and Environmental Dermatology,
Heidelberg, Germany*

- Melanoma is the 19th most frequent tumor worldwide. Its incidence varies over 100-fold around the world.

- The increase in melanoma incidence in recent decades is accompanied by a much smaller increase in mortality and, after a steady increase, mortality is now levelling off in many countries.

- Basal cell carcinoma is the most common cancer in white populations. As compared to basal cell carcinoma, the incidence rates for squamous cell carcinoma are four times lower in males, and six times lower in females. The high incidence rates of these tumors are not paralleled by increased mortality rates.

- The incidence of nonmelanoma skin cancer is remarkably high in organ transplanted patients.

- Exposure to ultraviolet radiation appears as the major environmental risk factor for nonmelanoma skin cancer and melanoma, and is the most important avoidable cause.

WHAT IS "SKIN CANCER"?

The term "skin cancer" is nonspecific. Different clinico-pathological entities with different etiologic factors, presentation, clinical course, and prognosis come under such a heading. A distinction is usually made between "cutaneous melanoma" and "nonmelanoma skin cancer." The term "nonmelanoma skin cancer" includes a large number of different disorders. Nonetheless, it is common practice to use it with reference to only two entities, which, by far, are the most frequent ones, namely, basal cell carcinoma and squamous cell carcinoma, also collectively labeled as "keratinocyte carcinomas" or "epidermal skin cancer" (1). Besides the aforementioned disorders, a large number of clinicopathological entities may be listed as representing "skin cancer" (Table 1). Only a short mention will be made of the epidemiology of clinicopathological entities other than cutaneous melanoma, basal cell carcinoma, and squamous cell carcinoma.

EPIDEMIOLOGY: PURPOSES AND MEASURES

Epidemiology is mainly concerned with measuring disease frequency in a given population and with the evaluation of variations with disease frequency in different populations and/or according to the presence of specific factors, which may represent causal factors for the disease (risk factors). In addition, epidemiology describes how a given disease progresses once it has been developed and assesses those factors, which may affect the outcome of a disease (prognostic factors). The final aim is to provide clues to prevent disease onset and to

TABLE 1 Classification of Skin Cancer

	Example
Epidermal skin tumors	Basal cell carcinoma
	Squamous cell carcinoma
	Paget's disease
	Keratoacantoma
Tumors of skin appendages	
Hair-follicle tumors	Pilary complex carcinoma
Sebaceous glands	Sebaceous carcinoma
Apocrine gland tumors	Apocrine carcinoma
Eccrine gland tumors	Sweat-gland carcinoma
	Microcystic adnexal carcinoma
	Eccrine epithelioma
	Mucinous eccrine epithelioma
	Adenoid cystic carcinoma
	Lymphoepithelioma-like carcinoma
Melanocytic tumors	Melanoma
	Malignant blue naevus
Langerhans cell tumors	Histiocytosis X
Mast cell tumors	Lymphadenopatic mastocytosis and eosinophilia
Subcutaneous tissue tumors	Liposarcoma
Fibrohistiocytic tumors	Dermatofibrosarcoma protuberans
	Atypical fibroxanthoma
	Malignant fibrous histiocytoma
Neoplasms of the vessel wall	Angiosarcoma
	Kaposi's sarcoma
Smooth muscle tumors	Superficial leiomyosarcoma
Neural and neuroendocrine tumors	Granular cell tumor
	Neuroendocrine and Merkel cell carcinoma
Cutaneous lymphoproliferative disease	
T cell	Mycosis fungoides
	Sézary syndrome
	Adult T-cell leukaemia/lymphoma
	Primary cutaneous CD30+ lymphoproliferative disorders
B cell	Primary cutaneous marginal zone B-cell lymphoma
	Primary cutaneous diffuse large B-cell lymphoma, leg type
Precursor hematologic neoplasms	

reduce morbidity and mortality associated with disease in humans. A number of measures are usually adopted in epidemiological research. The most common are "incidence," "prevalence," and the "relative risk" (2). Incidence is defined as the number of new cases of a disease occurring in a population during a defined time interval. By population, it is meant not only natural populations, that is, all the inhabitants of a given country or area, but also groups of people identified by a common characteristic, for example, organ transplant patients. Person-time incidence rate (or incidence density) is calculated for dynamic populations, that is, populations that gain and lose members over time, such as all the natural populations. This is the number of new cases that occur in a defined period divided by the sum of the different times each individual was at risk of the disease (person-time). Alternatively, the average size of the population during the period may be used, which is calculated as the estimated population at the mid-period. In follow-up studies with no censoring, cumulative-incidence measures may be used, which are calculated by dividing the number of new cases in a specified period by the initial size of the cohort being followed. A special case of cumulative incidence is the "lifetime incidence rate or risk," which reflects the probability of a single individual of an exposed group to develop a given disease at any time during life. When studying diseases like cancer, which carry a relevant mortality, mortality rates can be used as a surrogate for incidence. Mortality rates are easy to calculate from routinely collected data and are particularly useful to assess the disease burden, and to compare it among different countries. The numerator is the number of persons dying during the examined period of the disease of interest (as resulting from death certificates) while the denominator is usually the mid-period population.

Prevalence is defined as the number of individuals with a certain disease in a population at a specified time divided by the number of individuals in the population at that time. The time interval considered may be short (point prevalence) or may extend over a longer period (period prevalence). The "lifetime prevalence" refers to the total number of persons known to have had the disease for at least part of their life. New cases enter the prevalence pool and remain there until recovery or death. Prevalence measures are affected not only by incidence but also by the duration of the disease, being roughly measured by the product of the incidence and the average duration of the disease. To illustrate, a disease that is easily transmitted but has a short duration may have a low prevalence and a high incidence.

Age and gender, among the others, may strongly influence the rate of a disease and should be taken into account when comparing disease frequencies among different countries or populations. Age- and sex-specific rates can be adopted. Alternatively, and more efficiently, a set of techniques can be used to standardize the measures. Direct standardization involves, using as weights the distribution of a specified standard population. Directly standardized rates represent what the rate would have been in the study population if that population had the same distribution in terms of age and sex (or other variables of interest) as the standard population. Indirect methods involve calculation of standardized morbidity or mortality ratio, that is, the ratio of the number of events observed in the study population to the number that would be expected, if the study population had the same specific rates as the standard population. In looking at trends of the incidence of a disease over time, at least three factors need to be considered. These are the age at which the subject is diagnosed with the disease (age effect), the calendar year of diagnosis (period effect), and the year of birth of the subject (cohort effect). Age is usually considered when describing the incidence of cancer, therefore, the problem remains in separating period and cohort effects. The effects of periods may reflect changes in community activities such as education and screening programs, while cohort effects may be the consequence of specific exposure early in life. Age-period-cohort models are used to allow an analysis of incidence or mortality data, according to these different effects. A number of methods can also be used to model the spatial distribution of disease incidence, analyzing spatial patterns such as clustering or dispersion as well as identifying the potential role of environmental exposure.

A more refined analysis of the effect of candidate etiologic factors on the disease occurrence is offered by analytical epidemiology methods, that is, cohort and case-control studies. A cohort study involves following-up over time subjects with different levels of exposure to a candidate etiologic factor comparing the incidence of diseases of interest in these subjects. A case-control study involves comparing previous exposure to etiologic factors in a group of people diagnosed with a disease of interest (cases) and in a group of people, otherwise comparable, without the disease (controls). The measure adopted to express the link between the exposure and the disease is the "relative risk." This is the ratio of the incidence of a disease among the exposed to the risk among the unexposed. Odds ratios, that is, the ratio of the odds in favor of getting disease, if exposed to the odds in favor of getting the disease, if otherwise, can be calculated from case-control studies as an estimate of the relative risk. The approximation works well for rare disorders. Multivariate models can be used to simultaneously control the effects of variables other than the one of interest, when calculating relative risks or odds ratios.

THE WORLD BURDEN OF SKIN CANCER

Skin cancer is by far the most common kind of cancer diagnosed in many western countries. The chance of developing a skin cancer in British Columbia, Canada is approximately one in seven, over a lifetime (3). This corresponds to, perhaps, one in three for a white population in California (4), and even higher for a white population in Queensland, Australia (5). The most common skin cancer is basal-cell carcinoma, followed by squamous carcinoma and melanoma. The chance of developing a malignant melanoma during a lifetime, in North America, is in the order of 1 in 100 (6). This is a startling increase over the figures of, for instance, 1935, when the risk was 1 in 1500. Predictions of future incidence of skin cancer in the Netherlands suggest that if the rates continue to increase and population growth and ageing remain unabated, a rise in annual demand for care of more than 5% could occur by the year 2015, a heavy burden on the health system (7).

DESCRIPTIVE EPIDEMIOLOGY OF MELANOMA

The incidence of malignant melanoma varies over 100-fold around the world (Figs. 1 and 2). According to data provided in Cancer Incidence in Five Continents, the lowest rates reported around 1993–1997 were 0.3 to 0.5 per 100,000 person-years, in parts of Asia, and in Asian and black people in the United States, while the highest were up to 50 per 100,000 in Queensland, Australia (8). Overall, melanoma is the 19th most frequent tumor worldwide (Fig. 3). Incidence

Melanoma of skin, Males
Age-Standardized incidence rate per 100,000

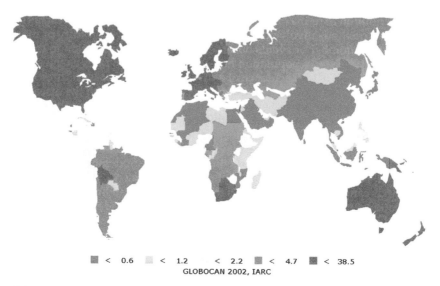

■ < 0.6 ░ < 1.2 ░ < 2.2 ■ < 4.7 ■ < 38.5
GLOBOCAN 2002, IARC

FIGURE 1   Melanoma of skin, males—ages-standardized incidence rate per 100,000. *Source*: From Ref. 126.

Melanoma of skin, Females
Age-Standardized incidence rate per 100,000

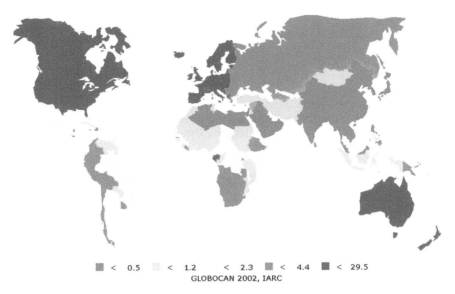

GLOBOCAN 2002, IARC

FIGURE 2   Melanoma of skin, females—ages-standardized incidence rate per 100,000. *Source*: From Ref. 126.

rates has risen significantly over the last 30 to 40 years, and continues to increase in the United States, Canada, Australia, and Europe, being perceived as a major public health concern. A number of campaigns to increase melanoma awareness have been developed in many areas of the world. A sharp increase in melanoma incidence above preceding long-term trends has

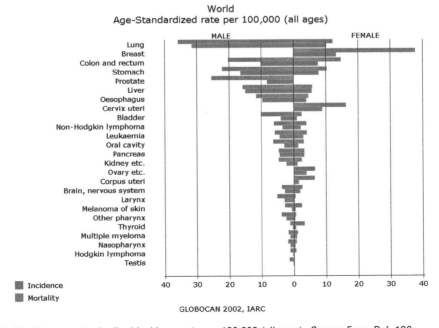

GLOBOCAN 2002, IARC

FIGURE 3   World—ages-standardized incidence rate per 100,000 (all ages). *Source*: From Ref. 126.

been observed in Australia, with doubling in as little as two years, mainly linked to thin melanoma (<1.5 mm thick), thicker melanoma not showing a levelling in incidence. Such an increase was paralleled by a rise in excision of pigmentary lesions. It has been suggested that the advancement of the time of diagnosis could not explain all of the increase and increased diagnosis of a pre-existing, nonmetastasizing form of thin melanoma could also contribute (9). In Switzerland, the increase in incidence of cutaneous melanoma over the period 1978–2002, was mainly due to lentigo maligna and superficial spreading melanoma, nodular melanoma remaining stable (10). In contrast to populations of mainly European origin, there has been no consistent upward trend over the full period from the early 1960s to the late 1980s in population of mainly non-European origin.

Geographic variations with incidence of cutaneous melanoma appears to reflect the combined effect of constitutional characteristics and latitude. Epidemiological data from the United States and Australia show that melanoma incidence in whites increases the closer to the equator people live.

Variations by body site have been documented. It is of interest to consider not only frequency but also density per unit of body surface area. While the greatest numbers of melanomas are found on the intermittently exposed areas of the back and legs, the greatest density is on the more continuously exposed areas of the head and neck. Recent increases in incidence in populations of European origin have been most pronounced on the trunk and other intermittently exposed areas, particularly in men, while the incidence of melanoma of the face has remained reasonably stable over time (11–15). The anatomical distribution in black people and people of Asian origin is quite different with most melanomas occurring on the soles of the feet (16,17).

Even if the increase in incidence in the last decades has been greater among women than men, the overall incidence of melanoma tends to be higher in men compared to women. Age-standardized incidence rates in more developed countries, according to Globocan data (2002), were 1.8 per 100,000 in men and 1.2 in women. Melanoma is rare before age 15. Thereafter incidence increases steadily and more or less linearly with age up to 45 to 49 years. From 50 to 55 years of age the curves for men and women diverge, climbing much more steeply in men than women. The incidence rate of melanoma in those who had already had one is much higher than in those who had never had one. At 20 years, the cumulative incidence of a second melanoma approaches 5%. Interestingly, at variance with most epithelial cancers whose incidence rises with a power of age, second melanoma presents a high constant incidence curve compatible with the occurrence of a single mutational event in a population of susceptible individuals (18).

It is remarkable that the strong increase in melanoma incidence in many populations is accompanied by a much smaller increase in mortality. Mortality from cutaneous malignant melanoma has been increasing until the late 1980s in young and middle-aged populations from most European countries, as well as from North America, Australia, and New Zealand (19,20). A recent update of trends in skin cancer (mostly represented by malignant melanoma) among young and middle-aged adults indicates that mortality from melanoma, after a steady increase, is now levelling off in the European Community, following a similar tendency observed in the United States (21,22), Australia (21,23), and New Zealand (15). In particular, a decline in mortality can be observed among young adults from several European countries (24). Trends in middle-aged adults are less favorable, with some countries still reporting an increase, even if they started to level off in the mid-1990s, as well. The favorable mortality trends in young people are of particular interest, since they suggest that a further decline in mortality from melanoma in Europe is likely to occur over the next few years (25). Less favorable trends in middle-aged adults could be a consequence of comparatively heavier sun exposure experienced at younger ages. Although some investigations reported less favorable mortality trends for melanoma in men (12,21,26), characterized also by a worse prognosis and survival in comparison with women (12,27), the analysis of mortality in different European countries did not show meaningful differences in trends between men and women. Particularly favorable trends have been observed in some northern European countries, characterized by a high melanoma cancer incidence and mortality (28). Conversely, in countries from southern Europe, such as France, Italy, and Spain, with lower skin cancer rates in the past, smaller

declines in mortality rates have been observed (21). This could be an effect of a higher awareness in high-incidence countries, as a consequence of earlier preventive campaigns and intervention programs launched (29,30). It is, however, possible that in the high-incidence countries
of northern Europe a peak has already been reached.

DESCRIPTIVE EPIDEMIOLOGY OF BASAL CELL CARCINOMA AND SQUAMOUS CELL CARCINOMA

As already discussed, basal cell and squamous cell carcinoma are usually considered together
under the heading "nonmelanoma skin cancer" but they present rather different distribution
and etiologic factors. The two tumors share the difficulties of obtaining reliable incidence
data, and the limited contribution of mortality to understand their distribution and burden.
Incidence estimates for "cancer of the skin, other than melanoma," based on registry data,
range from around 0.5 per 100,000 in Hispanics, Blacks, and Asian people to more than 100
per 100,000 in white people in Switzerland and Ireland (8). However, few cancer registries
provide reliable data on nonmelanoma skin cancer, and ad hoc studies need to be conducted
in a better way. To give an example, the cancer registry from Queensland, Australia, provides
estimates of 1.5 per 100,000, which are lower than the incidence for melanoma. A few ad hoc
studies have been performed providing specific incidence rates for basal cell and squamous
cell carcinoma. Based on these estimates, basal cell carcinoma appears as the most common
cancer in white people in the United States, Australia, and Europe.

A fundamental study to provide a reliable picture of the descriptive epidemiology of nonmelanoma skin cancer was the one conducted by Scotto et al. in several areas in the United
States, in two separate periods, that is, 1971–1972 and 1977–1978 (31). The locations varied
in latitude from 47.5 at Seattle to 30.0 at New Orleans. In the period 1977–1978, indices of
solar radiation were obtained from Robertson-Berger meters placed at National Weather
Service stations, located at airports in metropolitan areas. Annual UVB estimates were
derived from data provided by the National Oceanic and Atmospheric Administration. In
the period 1977–1978 the annual age-adjusted incidence rate for nonmelanoma skin cancer
among whites was 232.6 per 100,000 population, while the corresponding rate among blacks
being only 3.4. Hispanics also showed low incidence rates. On the average, the incidence
rates for basal cell carcinoma among whites were four times higher than squamous cell carcinoma in males, and six times higher in females. However, as the UVB index increased, the
ratio of basal cell to squamous cell carcinomas decreased. On the whole, 10% of the cases had
skin cancer of multiple sites, usually diagnosed simultaneously, with the proportion of multiple
tumors being higher in southern areas. In a small proportion of all patients (2.5%), both basal
cell and squamous cell carcinomas were reported. Over 80% of all patients had at least one
skin cancer on the face, head, or neck. The risk for males was greater than for females, with a
two-fold excess risk apparent in many locations. However, women were at higher risk of
tumors of the lower extremities, presumably because of clothing habits and differential ultra-
violet-light exposure. The incidence rates for squamous cell carcinoma began to rise rapidly
around age forty, and showed a sharper increase with age than did basal cell carcinoma. In
addition, the male excess of squamous cell carcinoma was present throughout life in all
areas, while the sex disparity for basal cell carcinoma appeared at older ages. A model of the
relation between UVB intensity and nonmelanoma skin cancer was developed, the log of the
age-adjusted rates for each sex and each cell type being a linear function of UVB intensities.
In general, a 1% relative increase in UVB may result in a 2% increase in skin cancer incidence.
The increases in UVB exposure appeared to have a greater relative impact on the risk of squamous cell than basal cell carcinoma. Although only four locations and six months were covered
in the survey period of 1971–1972, the results were consistent with the study conducted in the
period 1977–1978. After making adjustments for the month of diagnosis, there was a 15% to
20% increase in the age-adjusted rates for nonmelanoma skin cancer in the period 1977–1978
compared to the period 1971–1972. More recently, an overall increase in incidence among
people younger than 40 years was documented in Olmsted County, Minnesota, and notably,
a disproportionate increase in the incidence of basal cell carcinoma among young women (32).

Particular attention has been paid to the epidemiology of nonmelanoma skin cancer in Australia, where the highest ever incidence rates have been documented. In a study among 2095 inhabitants of Queensland, Australia, the incidence rate of nonmelanoma skin cancer in individuals aged 20 to 69 was 2389 per 100,000 person-years for males; 1908 per 100,000 person-years for females. The incidence of basal cell carcinoma was 4.5 times higher than that of squamous cell carcinoma (33). The population with skin type 1 in Queensland is considered a unique group for studying induction of skin cancer by sunlight. Another important study is the five-year longitudinal study (1982–1986) performed in 2669 people over 40 years of age, living in Maryborough, 180 kilometers north of Melbourne. The annual incidence rate for basal cell carcinoma was estimated as 672 per 100,000, and for squamous cell carcinoma was 201 per 100,000. The ratio of the incidence of basal cell carcinoma to that of squamous cell carcinoma was 33. Age, sex, skin reaction to sunlight, and occupation were all significant factors in the determination of the risk of developing nonmelanoma skin cancer (34). Recent data from Australia suggest that, after a steady increase of incidence rates in recent decades, a stabilization of incidence may have been reached in people younger than 60 years who were exposed to skin cancer prevention programs in their youth (5). Similarly, in south-eastern Arizona of the United States, where very high incidence rates compared to northern parts of the United States have been reported, this high incidence is not increasing further and especially the incidence of squamous cell carcinoma declined between 1985 and 1996 (35). Downward trends of squamous cell carcinoma over the past decades are also observed from Singapore, while the incidence of basal cell carcinoma increased on an average by 3% every year over the years 1968–1997 (36).

More sparse data are available from other countries and a number of studies are summarized in Table 2 (37–51). Common features include the epidemic increase of incidence during the last decades, the larger proportion of basal cell carcinoma as compared to squamous cell carcinoma, a male excess, which is greater for squamous cell carcinoma than for basal cell carcinoma, with a two-fold excess risk apparent in many locations, the preferential location (on the average, 80% of lesions) on sun exposed areas, the rarity among blacks, Asian people, and Hispanics. To give an example, in the period 1990–1992 the overall incidence rate of nonmelanoma skin cancer in the African population of Harare, Zimbabwe, was estimated as 4 per 100,000 (52). When phenotype is distributed uniformly, a UVB gradient is also clearly evident, with skin cancer incidence rates being highest in geographic areas of relatively higher UVB exposure.

One special population where the incidence of nonmelanoma skin cancer appears as remarkably high worldwide is represented by organ transplanted patients (53), where the increase is associated with immunosuppression and possibly human papilloma virus infection (54). According to data from cohort studies, the cumulative incidence of nonmelanoma skin cancer in transplanted patients increases from 10% after 10 years to 40% after 20 years of survival of the graft (53–58). Increased age at transplantation and male gender are established risk factors. No clear-cut variations in risk, according to the transplanted organ or the immunosuppressive regimen adopted, have been documented. Post-transplant immunosuppression appears to promote squamous cell carcinoma to a greater degree than basal cell carcinoma with a reversal of the ratio between the two tumors observed in the general population. Interestingly, such a reversal is seen much more dramatically in Northern European and Australian transplant patients (55,56) than in Mediterranean transplant populations (57,58). It has been repeatedly documented that once a person has developed a nonmelanoma skin cancer there is a significantly increased risk of developing subsequent skin cancers at other sites. The risk of a second basal cell carcinoma, after a first one is in the order of 40% after 20 years, and the risk is greater at younger age (59). A first basal cell carcinoma or a first squamous cell carcinoma both are also associated with increased risk of another nonmelanoma skin cancer, melanoma, non-Hodgkin lymphoma, and cancer of the salivary glands (60,61).

It is worth considering that the high incidence rates of basal cell and squamous cell carcinomas are not paralleled by increased mortality rates. On the contrary, mortality rates for "nonmelanoma skin cancer" are steadily decreasing in many geographic areas, for example, Germany, Finland, and the United States (62–64). In Germany, the age-standardized mortality rate for nonmelanoma skin cancer decreased from 0.56 per 100,000 in 1968 to 0.24 per 100,000 in

TABLE 2 Incidence Rates of Basal Cell Carcinoma and Squamous Cell Carcinoma in Selected Studies

Country	Period	Incidence rates × 100,000 person-years[a]	
		Basal cell carcinoma	**Squamous cell carcinoma**
U.S.A. and Canada			
U.S.A.	1971–1972	202.1 (M); 115.8 (F)	65.5 (M); 21.8 (F)
	1977–1978	246.6 (M); 150.1 (F)	65.4 (M); 23.6 (F)
Minnesota (U.S.A.)	1984–1992	180 (M); 105 (F)	48 (M); 16 (F)
Olmsted county, U.S.A. (≤40 yrs)	1976–2003	22.9–26.7 (M); 13.4–31.6 (F)	1.3–4.2 (M); 0.6–4.1 (F)
New Hampshire	1993–1994	309.9 (M); 165.5 (F)	97.2 (M); 32.4 (F)
New Mexico	1998–1999	930.3 (M); 485.5 (F)	356.2 (M); 150.4 (F)
Arizona	1996	935.9 (M); 497.1 (F)	270.6 (M); 112.1 (F)
Kauai, Hawaii	1983–1997		
Japanese		22 (M); 41 (F)	11 (M); 36 (F)
Filipinos		17 (M); 7 (F)	3 (M); 0 (F)
British Columbia (Canada)	1973–1987	70.7–120.4 (M); 61.5–92.2 (F)	16.6–31.2 (M); 9.4–16.9 (F)
Manitoba (Canada)	1960–2000	30.7–93.9 (M); 25.7–77.4 (F)	7.2–26.1 (M); 2.8–12.1 (F)
Australia			
Australia	1985	735 (M); 593 (F)	209 (M); 122 (F)
	1990	849 (M); 605 (F)	338 (M); 164 (F)
	1995	955 (M); 629 (F)	419 (M); 228 (F)
	2002	1541 (M); 1070 (F)	772 (M); 442 (F)
North Queensland	1997	2058 (M); 1195 (F)	1332 (M); 755 (F)
Europe			
The Netherlands	1975–1988	45.6 (M); 30.3 (F)	10.9 (M); 3.4 (F)
Norway	1982–1996	42.8 (M); 38.7 (F)	6.4 (M); 3.2 (F)
Denmark	1988	30.4 (M); 23.7 (F)	6.7 (M); 2.5 (F)
Finland	1985	43.7 (M); 31.7 (F)	5.6 (M); 3.9 (F)
South Wales (U.K.)	1988	112.2 (M); 54.1 (F)	31.7 (M); 6.2 (F)
South Wales (U.K.)	1998	128 (M); 105 (F)	25 (M); 9 (F)
Schleswing-Holstein (Germany)	1998–2001	80.8 (M); 63.3 (F)	18.2 (M); 8.5 (F)
Saarland (Germany)	1995–1999	43.7 (M); 31.7 (F)	11.2 (M); 4.4 (F)
Trento (Italy)	1992–1997	72.7 (M); 53.9 (F)	23.4 (M); 11.2 (F)
Vaud (Switzerland)	1976–1985	51.6 (M); 38 (F)	16.1 (M); 7.7 (F)
Vaud (Switzerland)	1995–1998	75.1 (M); 66.6 (F)	28.9 (M); 17.1 (F)
Slovakia	1993–1995	38.0 (M); 29.2 (F)	6.7 (M); 3.8 (F)
Asia			
Singapore, China	1993–1997	6.4 (M); 5.8 (F)	3.2 (M); 1.8 (F)

Note: M, male; F, female.
[a]Adjusted by age.
Source: Adapted from Refs. 3, 5, 7, 31, 32, 35–51.

1999 among men, and from 0.42 to 0.11 among women. Age-cohort-period regression models of the mortality data showed that the declining mortality was driven by both cohort and period effect, the latter probably resulting from increased awareness of skin cancer (62). In Rhode Island, U.S.A., in the period between 1988 and 2000, mortality rate from nonmelanoma skin cancer was 0.91 per 100,000 person-years of which almost half (0.45) was due to genital carcinoma. Skin cancers originating on the ear were responsible for more than a quarter of all deaths caused by nongenital lesions. Many individuals had co-morbid psychiatric disorders or evidence of unreasonable delay in seeking medical care for their lesions (64).

Some controversies exist about the recognition of actinic keratosis as precursor lesions versus in situ squamous cell carcinoma (65,66). From an epidemiological point of view, actinic keratosis should be better considered as separate from established and invasive squamous cell carcinoma. Actinic keratoses are highly prevalent in the general population and are usually manifested in multiple lesions. In the first Health and Nutrition Examination Survey (HANES I) conducted in the United States, the overall point prevalence increased from 15.9 per 1000 at age 45 to 54 to 65.1 per 1000 at age 65 to 74 (67). However, much higher estimates has been obtained in other studies. In Nambour (Queensland, Australia), 44% of men and 37% of women between the age of 20 and 69 years had at least one actinic keratosis of head, neck, hands, and arms (68). In a survey in South Wales, involving 1034 subjects aged 60 years or older, the prevalence was 23% (69) while in another study in the Mersey region in north-west England of people over 40 years of age the prevalence was 15.4% in men and 5.9% in women (70). In the community of Freixo de Espada à Cinta in northeast Portugal, actinic keratosis were identified in 9.6% of people (71). The fact that actinic keratoses are not established tumors is supported by the high-turnover rate for actinic keratosis, which has been documented in the Australian population, with a high rate of spontaneous regression and the appearance of new lesions over time (72), and by the acceleration of regression of actinic keratoses through regular use of sunscreens (73). In any case, the risk of progression of actinic keratoses to invasive squamous cell carcinoma is remarkably low, being much lower than 1 lesion in 1000 per year (74). These data, coupled with the lack of evidence, concerning the benefit of treating individual actinic keratoses to prevent invasive skin cancer, support a view of actinic keratosis as a risk marker prompting the adoption of sun protective habits, and regular examinations, rather than a view of these lesions as representing early squamous cell carcinoma that need individual lesion removal and consequent histologic documentation.

LIMITED DATA ON LESS COMMON SKIN CANCERS

Sparse data exist on the epidemiology of skin tumors other than melanoma, squamous cell, and basal cell carcinomas. Of interest, in this respect, were surveys conducted in Rochester, Minnesota, the United States, and Kauai, Hawaii (40). Table 3 presents some data on rare tumors (40,75).

ANALYTIC EPIDEMIOLOGY OF SKIN CANCER

Most of the discussion concerning environmental risk factors for skin cancer is centered around the exposure to sun and ultraviolet radiation and its interaction with constitutional characteristics. Light skin complexion (especially light skin and blond-red hair), freckling, and tendency to burn, not tan, after sun exposure, are constitutional variables, which affect the risk of skin cancer (76,77). People from Southern European ethnic origin are at a significantly lower risk than those from English, Celtic, and Scandinavian origin. Those who migrate early in their life from such regions to lower latitudes increase their exposure levels to sunlight and show a higher risk of developing skin cancer (78).

In spite of some variations among the different studies available, mainly explained by the latitude where the studies were conducted and the type of controls adopted, it can be stated that the timing and character of sun exposure may affect differently for the risk of different

TABLE 3   Incidence Rates for Some Unusual and Rare Skin Cancers

Cancer	Country (period)	Incidence rates × 100,000 person-years
Dermatofibrosarcoma protuberans	Minnesota (1973–1984)	0.45
Adenocarcinoma of sweat gland	Minnesota (1973–1984)	0.27
Merkel cell carcinoma	Minnesota (1973–1984)	0.16
	SEER U.S.A. (2000)	0.34 (M); 0.17 (F)
Extramammary Paget's disease	Minnesota (1973–1984)	0.19
Liposarcoma	Minnesota (1973–1984)	0.16
Cutaneous T cell lymphoma	Minnesota (1973–1984)	0.9
Keratoacantoma	Hawaii (1983–1987)	
White		104
Japanese		13
Filipinos		7
Hawaiians		6

Note: M, male; F, female.
Abbreviation: SEER, Surveillance Epidemiology and End Results Program.
Source: Adapted from Refs. 40, 75.

skin cancers. Both basal cell carcinoma and melanoma are most significantly linked to early exposure to ultraviolet light. Intermittent sun exposure and sunburn history are more important than cumulative dose in predicting adult risk for these tumors (79–81). Basal cell carcinoma and melanoma tumors appear to have a rapidly accelerating relative risk with relatively low exposures, followed by a broad plateau. Among sensitive individuals, sun avoidance behavior in adulthood may not markedly reduce risk for these tumors.

On the contrary, squamous carcinoma is associated with total lifetime sun exposure (80,82,83). Overall, high occupational exposure is inversely associated with melanoma and directly related to the risk of squamous cell carcinoma (79–83). Late stage solar exposure may play an important role in the development of squamous cell carcinoma, since sunlight exposure just prior to diagnosis is associated with an increased risk of the tumor. Actinic keratoses are well-established precursor lesions and recent sun exposure is connected to their development (84). Actinic keratoses may spontaneously disappear in people who limit solar exposure, and their progression to malignancy seems to require continued exposure to relatively high doses of ultraviolet light.

Variations in risk profiles have been proposed for both basal cell carcinoma and melanoma at different locations and with different clinicopathological variants. The frequency of superficial basal cell carcinoma appears to be higher in females and seen in younger patients as compared with nodular lesions. The latter occur mainly in the head/neck region while superficial lesions occur mainly on the trunk. Chronic sun exposure may be an etiologic factor for nodular lesions while intermittent sun exposure may play a role in superficial basal cell carcinoma (85,86). Similarly, heterogeneity of risk by anatomical site, suggesting multiple causal pathways, have been proposed for melanoma, with chronic sun exposure influencing the risk of melanoma of the head, and neck and intermittent sun exposure associated with a nevus-prone phenotype influencing the risk of melanoma elsewhere (87). However, limited data have been published on these issues.

The single greatest predictor of risk for developing melanoma is the total number of nevi (88). Studies over the last decades have revealed a great deal about the way nevi develop and the relationship between nevi and melanoma. Cross-sectional and cohort studies in schoolchildren are, particularly, informative since most nevi develop by the age of 20 (89–95). The following aspects of the epidemiology of melanocytic nevi are well established:

1. Boys develop more nevi than girls;
2. While the number of nevi increases with age up to 18 to 20 years, nevus density (i.e., number per square meter of body surface area) reaches a plateau earlier in life, between the age nine and 10 years, suggesting a genetic influence for such a variable;
3. Nevi are more common in children with lighter phenotype who burn and do not tan easily in the sun, and with freckling. However, red-haired subjects have fewer nevi than other children;
4. Higher counts are seen in children with a family history of skin cancer;
5. The number of nevi increases among children who live closer to the equator;
6. The number of nevi increases with increased history of sunburns.

It appears from these data that nevi are a complex exposure variable combining constitutional and environmental effects. Reducing nevi in children may substantially lower melanoma rates as they move into adulthood. Interestingly, red-haired children have a reduced count of nevi as compared to other skin phenotypes, but a higher melanoma risk, suggesting different pathways to melanoma development.

Other risk factors considered for the development of skin cancers are listed in Table 4. Smoking and other types of tobacco use are clearly associated with squamous cell carcinoma of the lip. Squamous cell carcinoma at other sites of the skin has been positively related to cigarette smoking in some studies (96,97), but negative results have also been reported (98). A two-fold increase in risk has been calculated (99).

The relationship between squamous cell carcinoma and diet or serum levels of nutrients has been investigated by a few studies. A high intake of *n*-3 fatty acids was associated with a lower risk of squamous cell carcinoma in a case-control study (100). The incidence of squamous cell carcinoma was not influenced by beta-carotene supplementation in a large-scale interventional study (101).

TABLE 4 Summary of Risk Factors for Skin Cancer

Risk factor	Melanoma	Nonmelanoma skin cancer
Age	Peak frequency in early adulthood, but age-related incidence rises with increasing age	More common with increasing age
Chemicals and exposures	PUVA therapy probably increases risk	Ionizing radiation increases risk. The use of coal–tar products and PUVA therapy increase risk. Tobacco increases risk for squamous cell carcinoma
Family history	Occurrence of melanoma in a first- or second-degree relative confers increased risk. Familial atypical mole melanoma syndrome confers even higher risk	Family history is associated with increased risk for basal cell carcinoma but not squamous cell carcinoma
Gender	Slight male predominance	Substantially more common in males
Geographic location	Higher incidence in whites living near the equator	Higher incidence in whites living near the equator
Medical conditions	Xeroderma pigmentosum, immuno-suppression, other malignancies, and previous nonmelanoma skin cancer all increase risk	Chronic osteomyelitis sinus tracts, burn scars, chronic skin ulcers, xeroderma pigmentosum, immuno-suppression, and possibly human papillomavirus infection all increase risk
Nevi	A large number of melanocytic nevi, and giant pigmented congenital nevi confer increased risk. Melanocytic nevi are markers for risk, not precursor lesions	Limited influence on risk
Occupation	Higher incidence in indoor workers, as well as those with higher education and income	Higher incidence in outdoor workers for squamous cell carcinoma
Previous history of skin cancer	Previous melanoma is associated with increased risk	36–52% chance of a new skin cancer of any kind within five years of index case
Race	More common in whites	More common in whites
Skin type/ethnicity	Increased incidence in those with fair complexions; those who burn easily, tan poorly and freckle; those who have red, blonde or light brown hair; and those of Celtic ancestry	Increased incidence in those with fair complexions; those who burn easily, tan poorly and freckle; those who have red, blonde or light brown hair; and those of Celtic ancestry
Sun exposure		
Cumulative	Probably does not influence risk	Single greatest risk factor for squamous cell carcinoma; 80% of lifetime sun exposure is obtained before 18 years of age
Episodic	Intense, intermittent exposure and blistering sunburns in childhood and adolescence are associated with increased risk	Intense, intermittent exposure and blistering sunburns in childhood and adolescence are associated with increased risk of basal cell carcinoma but not squamous cell carcinoma

Abbreviation: PUVA, psoralen plus ultraviolet A.

Ionizing radiation has been shown to cause nonmelamoma skin cancer (102). For low-level radiation, an increased risk has been documented in uranium miners and radiologists. Also among survivors of the nuclear bomb there is an increased risk of basal cell carcinoma (103). The risk of basal cell carcinoma is increased among persons exposed to occupational radiation, and among patients receiving therapeutic ionizing radiation before the age of 40 (102).

There is a synergistic acceleration of the risk of skin cancer through cumulative DNA damage by a combination of exposure to UVA radiation, environmental carcinogens, and benz[a]pyrene (104). Exposure to arsenic, not only occupational but also environmental via drinking water, has been associated with an increased risk of skin cancer, especially squamous cell carcinoma (105).

Outdoor workers such as farmers, welders, watermen, police officers, physical education teachers, pilots, and cabin attendants have an increased risk of skin cancer (106). There is scientific and epidemiological evidence to recognize squamous cell carcinoma induced by occupational UV-light exposure as an occupational disease, since a doubling of risk due to occupational UV-radiation can be demonstrated (107).

Of particular interest, is the association of skin cancer with Psoralen plus Ultraviolet A (PUVA) therapy and to a lesser extent ultraviolet B treatment. The best evidence on chronic toxicity of PUVA therapy comes from an ongoing study of more than 1300 people, who first received PUVA treatment in 1975 (108). The study found a dose-dependent increased risk of squamous cell carcinoma, basal cell carcinoma, and, possibly, malignant melanoma compared with the risk in the general population (109). A systematic review (search date 1998) of eight additional studies has confirmed the findings concerning nonmelanoma skin cancer (110). After less than 15 years, about a quarter of people exposed to 300 or more treatments of PUVA had at least one squamous cell carcinoma of the skin, with particularly high risk in people with skin type 1 and 2. A combined analysis of two cohort studies of 944 people treated with bath PUVA, excluded a three-fold excess risk of squamous cell carcinoma after a mean follow up of 14.7 years, suggesting that bath PUVA is possibly safer than conventional PUVA (111). One systematic review (search date 1996) estimated that the excess annual risk of nonmelanoma skin cancer associated with ultraviolet B radiation was likely to be less than 2% (112).

Limited data suggest that the use of tanning devices that emit ultraviolet radiation, such as tanning lamps and tanning beds, may be associated with a two-fold increased risk of squamous cell carcinoma, and a more limited increased risk of basal cell carcinoma, and, possibly, melanoma (113,114). Negative results have also been published (115). Most exposures to ultraviolet A tanning devices began after 1980; therefore, epidemiologic studies have difficulty in revealing any increase in risk of melanoma and/or basal cell carcinoma because of the latent period between exposure and occurrence of these tumors.

SKIN CANCER PREVENTION AND EDUCATION

Nonmelanoma skin cancer is seldom lethal, but if advanced can cause disfigurement and morbidity. Although malignant melanoma represents only 9% of all skin cancers, it occurs relatively early in life and causes more than 90% of overall skin cancer mortality.

In spite of the limitations in knowledge we have outlined earlier, exposure to ultraviolet radiation appears as the major environmental risk factor for nonmelanoma skin cancer and melanoma, and the most important avoidable cause. The aim of primary skin cancer prevention is therefore to limit ultraviolet light exposure. Campaigns to prevent skin cancer have incorporated numerous messages, including the need to avoid sunburn and, generally, to reduce exposure to ultraviolet radiation, especially midday sun (between 11 AM and 3 PM), wearing protective clothing, seeking shade, and applying sunscreen (116). Additional public health messages focus on prompt seeking medical attention when noticing suspicious or changing skin lesions. The detection of skin cancer at an early stage when it is most likely to be cured, by simple outpatient excision, is classified as secondary prevention.

Skin cancer educational programs have been increasingly common in recent years (117,118). However, there is no standardized procedure for these programs, which range from broad community campaigns to those targeted at particular population subgroups (e.g., school children, outdoor workers, teachers, pharmacists). Community-wide educational campaigns generally promote protection from sun exposure to reduce risk of skin cancer in later life. It is difficult to evaluate directly the overall effectiveness of such campaigns, and surveys on Australian population suggest that adequate, regular sun-protection measures are used by only a small proportion of high-risk population (119).

Different forms of educational programs have been proposed, from standardized print materials (e.g., pamphlets and posters) to more complex interventions (e.g., multimedia programs and written materials, combined with a supply of sunscreen samples). Even if some experiences have suggested that awareness and attitudes may be changed by educational efforts, there is little evidence that sun protection behavior has been significantly changed by these interventions, or that any behavioral changes have been maintained in the longer term. Changing human behavior is not easy, and the more complex the behavior, the more difficult it is to change. The most effective behavioral interventions have been based on sound theoretical models for decision-making and cognitive development. A United States study identified adolescents' readiness to change their sun protection practices on the basis of the transtheoretical model of behavior change (120). The conceptual framework on which this model is based has been applied to many health behaviors, including sun protection practices. The model postulates incremental stages from precontemplation of a behavior, to contemplation, preparation, action, and maintenance. For sun protection practices amongst adolescents, it has been reported that over half the surveyed adolescents were in precontemplative stage, 8% were in contemplative stage, none were in preparation stage, 4.4% were in action stage, and over a third identified themselves as being in the maintenance stage. These results have implications for choice of effective skin cancer educational programs and may partly explain the variable effectiveness of different educational programs. Halpern and Kopp found significant differences in skin cancer awareness and sun protection behaviors among Australia, United States, and Europe (121). In Australia, where the incidence of skin cancer is high, more than 80% of respondents expressed concern over skin cancer. In comparison, Germany (30%) and France (34%) demonstrated the lowest level of concerns about the risk of developing skin cancer. This survey also demonstrated that the main source of information, through which awareness was attained, was the media and not qualified healthcare representatives, and support the importance of increased patient education by medical professionals in the context of routine medical care.

The effectiveness of skin cancer educational programs depends on several factors, including the perceived, likely outcome of behavior change and the magnitude of the value attached to the outcome. Tangible immediate outcomes are more salient, and tend to have a greater influence on behavior than theoretical long-term outcomes. Even if people are well informed about skin cancer, they may not comply with prevention advice. Most health educators agree that the greatest long-term benefits are expected to occur when targeting children. Childhood is an excellent time to form life-long prevention habits, and early preventive behaviors may be less resistant to change than those acquired in adulthood. The best way to assess the effectiveness of an educational campaign is by a randomized controlled trial (sometimes with clusters), that compare either two or more alternative educational strategies, or one strategy with no strategy at all (i.e., no specific educational intervention). Relevant outcomes are influences on incidence/mortality of skin cancer. Behavior attitudes with reduction in sun exposure and number of sunburns are a surrogate outcome measure. A recent systematic review concluded that there was some evidence that approaches to increasing sun-protective behaviors were effective when implemented in primary schools and in recreational settings, but found insufficient evidence when implemented in other settings (117).

No sound data exist about the effectiveness of early diagnosis programs or screenings. A significant proportion of patients with one skin cancer will develop a second cancer. Subjects with atypical nevi and a family history of melanoma have a high chance of developing melanoma in their lifetime. Significantly, freckled individuals are at high risk for melanoma, as are those with nevi numbering more than 50. All of these must be taken into account when recommending appropriate follow-up examinations.

SUNSCREEN USE AND SKIN CANCER

The mainstay of sun protection is through avoidance of deliberate sun tanning, and use of adequate protection measures such as wearing wide-brimmed hats, sunglasses and protective clothing, and avoidance of peak hours for UV light. Sunscreens cannot be a substitute for other protective means.

Broad-spectrum sunscreens can prevent sunburns, some aspects of photoaging, and actinic keratoses (67). Some pre-existing actinic keratoses can regress as well. Squamous cell carcinoma may also be prevented, since actinic keratoses are precursors of this condition. Evidence does not suggest that sunscreens directly prevent basal cell carcinoma or melanoma (122–124). Concern has also been raised that they may directly or indirectly increase the risk of malignancy, primarily, because of poor application and increased exposure to the sun. The thickness of application has been shown to be less than half that is officially tested, and key exposed sites are often missed completely (125).

REFERENCES

1. Weinstock MA. Controversies in the public health approach to keratinocyte carcinomas. Br J Dermatol 2006; 154(suppl):3–4.
2. Last A, Robert A, Spasoff RA, Harris SS. A Dictionary of Epidemiology. 4th ed. Oxford University Press, New York, 2000.
3. Demers AA, Nugent Z, Mihalcioiu C, Wiseman MC, Kliewer EV. Trends of nonmelanoma skin cancer from 1960 through 2000 in a Canadian population. J Am Acad Dermatol 2005; 53:320–328.
4. Rigel DS, Friedman RJ, Kopf AW. Lifetime risk for development of skin cancer in the U.S. population: current estimate is now 1 in 5. J Am Acad Dermatol 1996; 35:1012–1013.
5. Staples MP, Elwood M, Burton RC, Williams JL, Marks R, Giles GG. Non-melanoma skin cancer in Australia: the 2002 national survey and trends since 1985. Med J Aust 2006; 184:6–10.
6. Merrill RM, Feuer EJ. Risk-adjusted cancer-incidence rates (United States). Cancer Cause Control 1996; 7:544–552.
7. de Vries E, van de Poll-Franse LV, Louwman WJ, de Gruijl FR, Coebergh JW. Predictions of skin cancer incidence in the Netherlands up to 2015. Br J Dermatol 2005; 152:481–488.
8. Parkin DM, Whelan SL, Ferlay J, Storm H. Cancer Incidence in Five Continents. Volumes I to VIII. IARC CancerBase No. 7, Lyon, 2005.
9. Burton RC, Armstrong BK. Recent incidence trends imply a nonmetastasizing form of invasive melanoma. Melanoma Res 1994; 4:107–113.
10. Levi F, Te VC, Randimbison L, La Vecchia C. Trends in incidence of various morphologies of malignant melanoma in Vaud and Neuchatel, Switzerland. Eur J Cancer 2004; 40:1630–1633.
11. Osterlind A, Engholm G, Jensen OM. Trends in cutaneous malignant melanoma in Denmark 1943–1982 by anatomic site. APMIS 1988; 96:953–963.
12. Thorn M, Bergstrom R, Adami HO, Ringborg U. Trends in the incidence of malignant melanoma in Sweden, by anatomic site, 1960–1984. Am J Epidemiol 1990; 132:1066–1077.
13. Dennis LK, White E, Lee JA. Recent cohort trends in malignant melanoma by anatomic site in the United States. Cancer Cause Control 1993; 4:93–100.
14. Chen YT, Zheng T, Holford TR, Berwick M, Dubrow R. Malignant melanoma incidence in Connecticut (United States): time trends and age-period-cohort modeling by anatomic site. Cancer Cause Control 1994; 5:341–350.
15. Bulliard JL, Cox B. Cutaneous malignant melanoma in New Zealand: trends by anatomical site, 1969–1993. Int J Epidemiol 2000; 29:416–423.
16. Cress RD, Holly EA. Incidence of cutaneous melanoma among non-Hispanic whites, Hispanics, Asians, and blacks: an analysis of California cancer registry data, 1988–1993. Cancer Cause Control 1997; 8:246–252.
17. Stevens NG, Liff JM, Weiss NS. Plantar melanoma: is the incidence of melanoma of the sole of the foot really higher in blacks than whites? Int J Cancer 1990; 45:691–693.
18. Levi F, Randimbison L, Te VC, La Vecchia C. High constant incidence rates of second cutaneous melanomas. Melanoma Res 2005; 15:73–75.
19. La Vecchia C, Lucchini F, Negri E, Boyle P, Levi F. Trends in cancer mortality in the Americas. Eur J Cancer 1993; 29:431–470.
20. Jemal A, Devesa SS, Fears TR, Hartge P. Cancer surveillance series: changing patterns of cutaneous malignant melanoma mortality rates among whites in the United States. J Natl Cancer Inst 2000; 92:811–818.
21. Severi G, Giles GG, Robertson C, Boyle P, Autier P. Mortality from cutaneous melanoma: evidence for contrasting trends between populations. Br J Cancer 2000; 82:1887–1891.

22. Scotto J, Pitcher H, Lee JAH. Indication of future decreasing trends in skin melanoma mortality among whites in the United States. Int J Cancer 1991; 49:490–497.
23. Giles GG, Armstrong BK, Burton RC, Staples MP, Thursfield VJ. Has mortality from melanoma stopped rising in Australia? Analysis of trends between 1931 and 1994. BMJ 1996; 312:1121–1125.
24. Bosetti C, La Vecchia C, Naldi L, Lucchini F, Negri E, Levi F. Mortality from cutaneous malignant melanoma in Europe. Has the epidemic levelled off? Melanoma Res 2004; 14:301–309.
25. La Vecchia C, Negri E, Levi F, Decarli A, Boyle P. Cancer mortality in Europe: effects of age, cohort of birth and period of death. Eur J Cancer 1998; 34:118–141.
26. Streetly A, Markowe H. Changing trends in the epidemiology of malignant melanoma: gender differences and their implications for public health. Int J Epidemiol 1995; 24:897–907.
27. MacKie R, Aitchison TC, Hunter JAA, et al., for The Scottish Melanoma Group. Cutaneous malignant melanoma, Scotland, 1979–1989. Lancet 1992; 339:971–975.
28. de Vries E, Bray FI, Coebergh JW, Parkin DM. Changing epidemiology of malignant cutaneous melanoma in Europe 1953–1997: rising trends in incidence and mortality but recent stabilizations in western Europe and decreases in Scandinavia. Int J Cancer 2003; 107:119–126.
29. MacKie RM, Hole D, Hunter JA, et al. Cutaneous malignant melanoma in Scotland: incidence, survival, and mortality. The Scottish Melanoma Group, 1979–1994. BMJ 1997; 315:1117–1121.
30. Melia J, Pendry L, Eiser JR, Harland C, Moss S. Evaluation of primary prevention initiatives for skin cancer: a review from a UK perspective. Br J Dermatol 2000; 143:701–708.
31. Scotto J, Fears TR, Fraumeni JF. Incidence of non-melanoma skin cancer in the United States. NIH Pub. no. 83-2433. Bethesda, MD: U.S. Dept. of Health and Human Services, National Institutes of Health, 1983.
32. Christenson LJ, Borrowman TA, Vachon CM, et al. Incidence of basal cell and squamous cell carcinomas in a population younger than 40 years. JAMA 2005; 294:681–90.
33. Green A, Battistutta D. Incidence and determinants of skin cancer in a high-risk Australian population. Int J Cancer 1990; 46:356–361.
34. Marks R, Jolley D, Dorevitch AP, Selwood TS. The incidence of non-melanocytic skin cancers in an Australian population: results of a five-year prospective study. Med J Aust 1989; 150:475–478.
35. Harris RB, Griffith K, Moon TE. Trends in the incidence of nonmelanoma skin cancers in southeastern Arizona, 1985–1996. J Am Acad Dermatol 2001; 45:528–536.
36. Koh D, Wang H, Lee J, Chia KS, Lee HP, Goh CL. Basal cell carcinoma, squamous cell carcinoma and melanoma of the skin: analysis of the Singapore Cancer Registry data 1968–1997. Br J Dermatol 2003; 148:1161–1166.
37. Gray DT, Suman VJ, Su WP, Clay RP, Harmsen WS, Roenigk RK. Trends in the population-based incidence of squamous cell carcinoma of the skin first diagnosed between 1984 and 1992. Arch Dermatol 1997; 133:735–740.
38. Karagas MR, Greenberg ER, Spencer SK, Stukel TA, Mott LA. Increase in incidence rates of basal cell and squamous cell skin cancer in New Hampshire, USA. New Hampshire Skin Cancer Study Group. Int J Cancer 1999; 81:555–559.
39. Athas WF, Hunt WC, Key CR. Changes in nonmelanoma skin cancer incidence between 1977–1978 and 1998–1999 in Northcentral New Mexico. Cancer Epidemiol Biomarkers Prev 2003; 12:1105–1108.
40. Chuang TY. Skin cancer II. Nonmelanoma skin cancer. In: Williams HC, Strachan DP, eds. The Challenge of Dermatoepidemiology. Boca Raton: CRC Press, 1997:209–222.
41. Gallagher RP, Ma B, McLean DI, et al. Trends in basal cell carcinoma, squamous cell carcinoma, and melanoma of the skin from 1973 through 1987. J Am Acad Dermatol 1990; 23:413–421.
42. Buettner PG, Raasch BA. Incidence rates of skin cancer in Townsville, Australia. Int J Cancer 1998; 78:587–593.
43. Magnus K. The Nordic profile of skin cancer incidence. A comparative epidemiological study of the three main types of skin cancer. Int J Cancer 1991; 47:12–19.
44. Roberts DL. Incidence of non-melanoma skin cancer in West Glamorgan, South Wales. Br J Dermatol 1990; 122:399–403.
45. Holme SA, Malinovszky K, Roberts DL. Changing trends in non-melanoma skin cancer in South Wales, 1988–98. Br J Dermatol 2000; 143:1224–1229.
46. Katalinic A, Kunze U, Schafer T. Epidemiology of cutaneous melanoma and non-melanoma skin cancer in Schleswig-Holstein, Germany: incidence, clinical subtypes, tumour stages and localization (epidemiology of skin cancer). Br J Dermatol 2003; 149:1200–1206.
47. Stang A, Stegmaier C, Jockel KH. Nonmelanoma skin cancer in the Federal State of Saarland, Germany, 1995–1999. Br J Cancer 2003; 89:1205–1208.
48. Boi S, Cristofolini M, Micciolo R, Polla E, Dalla Palma P. Epidemiology of skin tumors: data from the cutaneous cancer registry in Trentino, Italy. Ann Epidemiol 2003; 13:436–442.
49. Levi F, La Vecchia C, Te VC, Mezzanotte G. Descriptive epidemiology of skin cancer in the Swiss Canton of Vaud. Int J Cancer 1988; 42:811–816.

50. Levi F, Te VC, Randimbison L, Erler G, La Vecchia C. Trends in skin cancer incidence in Vaud: an update, 1976–1998. Eur J Cancer Prev 2001; 10:371–373.

51. Plesko I, Severi G, Obsitnikova A, Boyle P. Trends in the incidence of non-melanoma skin cancer in Slovakia, 1978–1995. Neoplasma 2000; 47:137–142.

52. Watts T, Siziya S, Chokunonga E. Cancer of the skin in Zimbabwe: an analysis based on the Cancer Registry 1986 to 1992. Cent Afr J Med 1997; 43:181–184.

53. Berg D, Otley CC. Skin cancer in organ transplant recipients: Epidemiology, pathogenesis, and management. 1. J Am Acad Dermatol 2002; 47:1–17.

54. Bouwes Bavinck JN, Feltkamp M, Struijk L, ter Schegget J. Human papillomavirus infection and skin cancer risk in organ transplant recipients. J Investig Dermatol Symp Proc 2001; 6:207–211.

55. Lindelof B, Sigurgeirsson B, Gabel H, Stern RS. Incidence of skin cancer in 5356 patients following organ transplantation. Br J Dermatol 2000; 143:513–519.

56. Ong CS, Keogh AM, Kossard S, Macdonald PS, Spratt PM. Skin cancer in Australian heart transplant recipients. J Am Acad Dermatol 1999; 40:27–34.

57. Naldi L, Fortina AB, Lovati S, et al. Risk of nonmelanoma skin cancer in Italian organ transplant recipients. A registry-based study. Transplantation 2000; 70:1479–1484.

58. Fuente MJ, Sabat M, Roca J, Lauzurica R, Fernandez-Figueras MT, Ferrandiz C. A prospective study of the incidence of skin cancer and its risk factors in a Spanish Mediterranean population of kidney transplant recipients. Br J Dermatol 2003; 149:1221–1226.

59. Levi F, Randimbison L, Maspoli M, Te VC, La Vecchia C. High incidence of second basal cell skin cancers. Eur J Cancer 2006; 42:656–659.

60. Levi F, La Vecchia C, Te VC, Randimbison L, Erler G. Incidence of invasive cancers following basal cell skin cancer. Am J Epidemiol 1997; 146:734–739.

61. Levi F, Randimbison L, La Vecchia C, Erler G, Te VC. Incidence of invasive cancers following squamous cell skin cancer. Int J Cancer 1997; 72:776–779.

62. Stang A, Jockel KH. Changing patterns of skin melanoma mortality in West Germany from 1968 through 1999. Eur J Cancer 2005; 41:45–60.

63. Hannuksela-Svahn A, Pukkala E, Karvonen J. Basal cell skin carcinoma and other nonmelanoma skin cancers in Finland from 1956 through 1995. Arch Dermatol 1999; 135:781–786.

64. Lewis KG, Weinstock MA. Nonmelanoma skin cancer mortality (1988–2000): the Rhode Island follow-back study. Arch Dermatol 2004; 140:837–842.

65. Lober BA, Lober CW, Accola J. Actinic keratosis is squamous cell carcinoma. J Am Acad Dermatol 2000; 43:881–882.

66. Flaxman AB. Actinic keratoses- Malignant or not? J Am Acad Dermatol 2001; 45:466–467.

67. Johnson M.-LT, Roberts J. Skin conditions and related need for medical care among person 1–74 years. US Department of Health Education and Welfare, Hyattsville, 1978.

68. Frost CA, Green AC, Williams GM. The prevalence and determinants of solar keratoses at a subtropical latitude (Queensland, Australia). Br J Dermatol 1998; 139:1033–1039.

69. Harvey I, Frankel S, Marks R, Shalom D, Nolan-Farrell M. Non-melanoma skin cancer and solar keratoses. I. Methods and descriptive results of the South Wales skin cancer study. Br J Cancer 1996; 74:1302–1307.

70. Memon AA, Tomenson JA, Bothwell J, Friedmann PS. Prevalence of solar damage and actinic keratosis in a Merseyside population. Br J Dermatol 2000; 142:1154–1159.

71. Massa A, Alves R, Amado J, et al. Prevalence of cutaneous lesions in Freixo de Espada a Cinta. Acta Med Port 2000; 13:247–254.

72. Frost C, Williams G, Green A. High incidence and regression rates of solar keratoses in a Queensland community. J Invest Dermatol 2000; 115:273–277.

73. Thompson SC, Jolley D, Marks R. Reduction of solar keratoses by regular sunscreen use. N Engl J Med 1993; 329:1193–1194.

74. Marks R, Rennie G, Selwood TS. Malignant transformation of solar keratoses to squamous cell carcinoma. Lancet 1988; 1:795–797.

75. Agelli M, Clegg LX. Epidemiology of primary Merkel cell carcinoma in the United States. J Am Acad Dermatol 2003; 49:832–841.

76. Gandini S, Sera F, Cattaruzza MS, et al. Meta-analysis of risk factors for cutaneous melanoma: III. Family history, actinic damage and phenotypic factors. Eur J Cancer 2005; 41:2040–2059.

77. Zanetti R, Rosso S, Martinez C, et al. The multicentre south European study "Helios." I: Skin characteristics and sunburns in basal cell and squamous cell carcinomas of the skin. Br J Cancer 1996; 73(11):1440–1446.

78. Whiteman DC, Green AC. Melanoma and sun exposure: where are we now? Int J Dermatol 1999; 38:481–489.

79. Gandini S, Sera F, Cattaruzza MS, et al. Meta-analysis of risk factors for cutaneous melanoma: II. Sun exposure. Eur J Cancer 2005; 41:28–44.

80. Rosso S, Zanetti R, Martinez C, et al. The multicentre south European study "Helios." II: Different sun exposure patterns in the etiology of basal cell and squamous cell carcinomas of the skin. Br J Cancer 1996; 73:1447–1454.

81. Gallagher RP, Hill GB, Bajdik CD, et al. Sunlight exposure, pigmentary factors, and risk of nonmelanocytic skin cancer. I. Basal cell carcinoma. Arch Dermatol 1995; 131:157–163.

82. Gallagher RP, Hill GB, Bajdik CD, et al. Sunlight exposure, pigmentation factors, and risk of nonmelanocytic skin cancer. II. Squamous cell carcinoma. Arch Dermatol 1995; 131:164–169.

83. Vitasa BC, Taylor HR, Strickland PT, et al. Association of nonmelanoma skin cancer and actinic keratosis with cumulative solar ultraviolet exposure in Maryland watermen. Cancer 1990; 65:2811–2817.

84. Harvey I, Frankel S, Marks R, Shalom D, Nolan-Farrell M. Non-melanoma skin cancer and solar keratoses. II analytical results of the South Wales skin cancer study. Br J Cancer 1996; 74:1308–1312.

85. Bastiaens MT, Hoefnagel JJ, Bruijn JA, Westendorp RG, Vermeer BJ, Bouwes Bavinck JN. Differences in age, site distribution, and sex between nodular and superficial basal cell carcinoma indicate different types of tumors. J Invest Dermatol 1998; 110:880–884.

86. Lovatt TJ, Lear JT, Bastrilles J, et al. Associations between ultraviolet radiation, basal cell carcinoma site and histology, host characteristics, and rate of development of further tumors. J Am Acad Dermatol 2005; 52:468–473.

87. Siskind V, Whiteman DC, Aitken JF, Martin NG, Green AC. An analysis of risk factors for cutaneous melanoma by anatomical site (Australia). Cancer Cause Control 2005; 16:193–199.

88. Gandini S, Sera F, Cattaruzza MS, et al. Meta-analysis of risk factors for cutaneous melanoma: I. Common and atypical naevi. Eur J Cancer 2005; 41:28–44.

89. English DR, Armstrong BK. Melanocytic nevi in children. I. Anatomic sites and demographic and host factors. Am J Epidemiol 1994; 139:390–401.

90. Kelly JW, Rivers JK, MacLennan R, Harrison S, Lewis AE, Tate BJ. Sunlight: a major factor associated with the development of melanocytic nevi in Australian schoolchildren. J Am Acad Dermatol 1994; 30:40–48.

91. Dennis LK, White E, Lee JA, Kristal A, McKnight B, Odland P. Constitutional factors and sun exposure in relation to nevi: a population-based cross-sectional study. Am J Epidemiol 1996; 143:248–256.

92. Dulon M, Weichenthal M, Blettner M, et al. Sun exposure and number of nevi in 5- to 6-year-old European children. J Clin Epidemiol 2002; 55:1075–1081.

93. Carli P, Naldi L, Lovati S, La Vecchia C; Oncology Cooperative Group of the Italian Group for Epidemiologic Research in Dermatology (GISED). The density of melanocytic nevi correlates with constitutional variables and history of sunburns: a prevalence study among Italian schoolchildren. Int J Cancer 2002; 101:375–379.

94. MacLennan R, Kelly JW, Rivers JK, Harrison SL. The Eastern Australian Childhood Nevus Study: site differences in density and size of melanocytic nevi in relation to latitude and phenotype. J Am Acad Dermatol 2003; 48:367–375.

95. Wiecker TS, Luther H, Buettner P, Bauer J, Garbe C. Moderate sun exposure and nevus counts in parents are associated with development of melanocytic nevi in childhood: a risk factor study in 1,812 kindergarten children. Cancer 2003; 97:628–638.

96. Doll R. Cancers weakly related to smoking. Br Med Bull 1996; 52:35–49.

97. Moore S, Johnson N, Pierce A, Wilson D. The epidemiology of lip cancer: a review of global incidence and aetiology. Oral Dis 1999; 5:185–195.

98. Green A, Battistutta D, Hart V, Leslie D, Weedon D. Skin cancer in a subtropical Australian population: incidence and lack of association with occupation. The Nambour Study Group. Am J Epidemiol 1996; 144:1034–1040.

99. De Hertog SA, Wensveen CA, Bastiaens MT, et al. Relation between smoking and skin cancer. J Clin Oncol 2001; 19:231–238.

100. Hakim IA, Harris RB, Ritenbaugh C. Fat intake and risk of squamous cell carcinoma of the skin. Nutr Cancer 2000; 36:155–162.

101. Green A, Williams G, Neale R, et al. Daily sunscreen application and betacarotene supplementation in prevention of basal-cell and squamous-cell carcinomas of the skin: a randomized controlled trial. Lancet 1999; 354:723–729.

102. Lichter MD, Karagas MR, Mott LA, Spencer SK, Stukel TA, Greenberg ER. Therapeutic ionizing radiation and the incidence of basal cell carcinoma and squamous cell carcinoma. The New Hampshire Skin Cancer Study Group. Arch Dermatol 2000; 136:1007–1011.

103. Ron E, Preston DL, Kishikawa M, et al. Skin tumor risk among atomic-bomb survivors in Japan. Cancer Cause Control 1998; 9:393–401.

104. Saladi R, Austin L, Gao D, et al. The combination of benzo[a]pyrene and ultraviolet A causes an in vivo time-related accumulation of DNA damage in mouse skin. Photochem Photobiol 2003; 77:413–419.

105. Yu RC, Hsu KH, Chen CJ, Froines JR. Arsenic methylation capacity and skin cancer. Cancer Epidemiol Biomarkers Prev 2000; 9:1259–1262.
106. Ramirez CC, Federman DG, Kirsner RS. Skin cancer as an occupational disease: the effect of ultraviolet and other forms of radiation. Int J Dermatol 2005; 44:95–100.
107. Diepgen TL, Drexler H. Skin cancer and occupational disease. Hautarzt 2004; 55:22–27.
108. Stern RS, Laird N. The carcinogenic risk of treatments for severe psoriasis. Photochemotherapy follow-up study. Cancer 1994; 73:2759–2764.
109. Stern RS, Nichols KT, Vakeva LH. Malignant melanoma in patients treated for psoriasis with methoxsalen (psoralen) and ultraviolet A radiation (PUVA). The PUVA Follow-Up Study. N Engl J Med 1997; 336:1041–1045.
110. Stern RS, Lunder EJ. Risk of squamous cell carcinoma and methoxsalen (psoralen) and UVA radiation (PUVA). A meta-analysis. Arch Dermatol 1998; 134:1582–1585.
111. Hannuksela-Svahn A, Sigurgeirsson B, Pukkala E, et al. Trioxsalen bath PUVA did not increase the risk of squamous cell skin carcinoma and cutaneous malignant melanoma in a joint analysis of 944 Swedish and Finnish patients with psoriasis. Br J Dermatol 1999; 141:497–501.
112. Pieternel CM, Pasker-de-Jong M, Wielink G, et al. Treatment with UVB for psoriasis and nonmelanoma skin cancer. A systematic review of the literature. Arch Dermatol 1999; 135:834–840.
113. Autier P, Dore JF, Lejeune F, et al. Cutaneous malignant melanoma and exposure to sunlamps or sunbeds: an EORTC multicenter case-control study in Belgium, France and Germany. EORTC Melanoma Cooperative Group. Int J Cancer 1994; 58:809–813.
114. Karagas MR, Stannard VA, Mott LA, Slattery MJ, Spencer SK, Weinstock MA. Use of tanning devices and risk of basal cell and squamous cell skin cancers. J Natl Cancer Inst 2002; 94:224–246.
115. Bajdik CD, Gallagher RP, Astrakianakis G, Hill GB, Fincham S, McLean DI. Non-solar ultraviolet radiation and the risk of basal and squamous cell skin cancer. Int J Cancer 1994; 58:809–813.
116. Fry A, Verne J. Preventing skin cancer. BMJ 2003; 326:114–115.
117. Saraiya M, Glanz K, Briss PA, et al. Interventions to prevent skin cancer by reducing exposure to untraviolet radiation: a systematic review. Am J Prev Med 2004; 27:422–466.
118. Stoebner-Dalbarre A, Dafez C, Borrel E, Sancho-Garnier H, Guillot B, Group Epi-CES. Prevention of skin cancer programs: analysis of the impact of randomised trials. Ann Dermatol Venereol 2005; 132:641–647.
119. Livingston PM, White V, Hayman J, Dobbinson S. Sun exposure and sun protection behaviours among Australian adolescents: trends over time. Prev Med 2003; 37:577–584.
120. Prochaska JO. Strong and weak principles for progressing from precontemplation to action on the basis of twelve problem behaviors. Health Psychol 1994; 13:47–51.
121. Halpern AC, Kopp LJ. Awareness, knowledge and attitudes to non-melanoma skin cancer and actinic keratosis among the general public. Int J Dermatol 2005; 44:107–111.
122. Vainio H, Miller AB, Bianchini F. An international evaluation of the cancer-preventive potential of sunscreens. Int J Cancer 2000; 88:838–842.
123. Bastuji-Garin S, Diepgen TL. Cutaneous malignant melanoma, sun exposure, and sunscreen use: epidemiological evidence. Br J Dermatol 2002; 146(suppl. 61):24–30.
124. Dennis LK, Beane Freeman LE, VanBeek MJ. Sunscreen use and the risk for melanoma: a quantitative review. Ann Intern Med 2003; 139:966–978.
125. Johnson K, Davy L, Boyett T, Weathers L, Roetzheim RG. Sun protection practices for children: knowledge, attitudes, and parent behaviors. Arch Pediatr Adolesc Med 2001; 155:891–896.
126. http://www-dep.iarc.fr. (GLOBOCAN 2002 database).

10 | Evaluation of the Photosensitive Patient

Henry W. Lim
Department of Dermatology, Henry Ford Hospital, Detroit, Michigan, U.S.A.

John L. M. Hawk
Photobiology Unit, St. John's Institute of Dermatology, St. Thomas' Hospital, King's College of London, London, England, U.K.

- Systematic evaluation of photosensitive patients includes a thorough history, physical examination, phototesting, and as needed, photopatch testing and laboratory evaluation.

- Polymorphous light eruption, chronic actinic dermatitis, solar urticaria, and photosensitivity secondary to systemic medications are the most frequently encountered photodermatoses in photodermatology centers around the world.

INTRODUCTION

Photodermatoses can be classified into four categories: (*i*) immunologically mediated photodermatoses, (*ii*) drug- and chemical-induced photosensitivity, (*iii*) photodermatoses associated with defective DNA nucleotide excision repair, and (*iv*) photoaggravated dermatoses (Table 1). Systematic evaluation of patients with photosensitivity is an important step in establishing the appropriate diagnosis. One of the earliest documented examples of such an approach was reported by Wilkinson in 1961. He evaluated several patients with photo-distributed eruptions. By history, he noted that these patients were all working in the same factory, and the eruption was exacerbated by exposure to sunlight. Patch testing with a germicidal agent that the workers were exposed to, tetrachlorosalicylanilide, was positive in many patients; the reaction was intensified by exposure to ultraviolet (UV) radiation. Biopsy specimens from these patients showed changes consistent with photoallergic contact dermatitis. Wilkinson (1) published these patients as examples of those with photosensitivity to tetrachlorosalicylanilide.

Wilkinson's approach exemplified the appropriate steps in evaluating the photosensitive patient. This evaluation should include a thorough history-taking, complete cutaneous examination and, when appropriate, phototesting for the determination of the minimal erythema dose (MED), photopatch testing and laboratory evaluation, such as skin biopsy, ANA panel, and/or plasma porphyrin profile (Table 2). These steps will be discussed in detail in this chapter.

HISTORY

Thorough history-taking with special attention to the relationship between sun exposure and the features of the skin eruption is an important step in the evaluation of photosensitivity. This is outlined in Table 3, and discussed subsequently.

Age of Onset

The age of onset of photosensitivity frequently assists in the diagnosis (Table 4) (2). It should be noted that the most common immunologically mediated photodermatosis, polymorphous light eruption, and related disorders (juvenile spring eruption, actinic prurigo) tend to have their onset in childhood and/or early adulthood. Photosensitivity associated with two of the cutaneous porphyrias, congenital erythropoietic porphyria and erythropoietic protoporphyria,

---

TABLE 1 Classification of Photodermatoses

Immunologically mediated
  Polymorphous light eruption
  Juvenile spring eruption
  Actinic prurigo
  Hydroa vacciniforme
  Chronic actinic dermatitis
  Solar urticaria
Drug- and chemical-induced
  Exogenous: phototoxicity and photoallergy
  Endogenous: cutaneous porphyrias
Defective DNA repair
  Xeroderma pigmentosum
  Cockayne syndrome
  UV-sensitive syndrome
  Trichothiodystrophy
  Bloom syndrome
  Rothmund–Thomson syndrome
  Kindler syndrome
Photoaggravated
  Lupus erythematosus
  Dermatomyositis
  Others

TABLE 2   Evaluation of the Photosensitive Patient

History
Physical examination
Phototesting for MED and abnormal morphological responses
Photopatch testing
Laboratory: skin biopsy, ANA panel, plasma porphyrin (and complete porphyrin profile if necessary)

Abbreviations: ANA, antinuclear antibodies; MED, minimal erythema dose.

have their onsets in infancy and early childhood, respectively. In contrast, chronic actinic dermatitis, another immunologically mediated photodermatosis, and drug-induced photosensitivity, most frequently manifest themselves in individuals older than 60 years; reflecting the increased exposure to precipitating agents of sunlight and exacerbating airborne allergens in this cohort of individuals.

Exposure to Photosensitizers

Possible exposure to known photosensitizers should be obtained in the history taking. Questions should be asked not only about the intake of oral prescription medications, but also over-the-counter oral agents, as well as topical agents. The more common photosensitizers are listed in Table 5 (3). Examples of over-the-counter oral and topical photosensitizers include nonsteroidal anti-inflammatory drugs, St. John's wort, tar and tar-containing products, sunscreen agents, and fragrances such as musk ambrette.

Seasonal Variation, Interval Before Onset, and Duration of the Eruption

An important part of the history is information about the relationship of sun exposure and cutaneous eruption. For patients living in temperate climates, all photodermatoses are almost always very severe in the sunny season, although actinic prurigo is very occasionally worse in winter, or during spring and fall. While most photodermatoses tend to persist during spring and summer, polymorphous light eruption (also known as polymorphic light eruption) often has a rather unusual time course. It tends to manifest itself in greatest severity in the early part of the sunny season and becomes less severe as the season progresses, a phenomenon of the development presumed immunological tolerance, commonly referred to as the "hardening" reaction.

   The interval between sun exposure and the development of cutaneous lesions is also characteristic for many of the photodermatoses. For example, in polymorphous light eruption, patients typically notice development of the eruption after a few hours of exposure to the sun, frequently by the evening of the day of the sun exposure, and rarely after a day or so of continuing sun exposure. In contrast, lesions in solar urticaria generally appear within five to ten minutes of sun exposure. In porphyria cutanea tarda (PCT), while the erosions and blisters are on sun-exposed areas, patients may not notice the direct correlation between sun exposure and the development of these lesions at all. Photo-provocation of lesions in patients with lupus erythematosus may not appear for a few days after the exposure to sunlight.

TABLE 3   Evaluation of Photodermatoses: History

Age of onset
Exposure to oral or topical photosensitizers
Seasonal variation
Interval between sun exposure and skin eruption
Duration of lesions
Effect of window glass
Family history of photosensitivity
Systemic symptoms
History of connective tissue disease

TABLE 4 Evaluation of Photodermatoses: Age of Onset

Infancy
  Congenital erythropoietic porphyria (Günther disease)
Childhood
  Juvenile spring eruption (a variant of polymorphous light eruption)
  Polymorphous light eruption
  Actinic prurigo
  Hydroa vacciniforme
  Erythropoietic protoporphyria
Adulthood
  Polymorphous light eruption
  Drug-induced photosensitivity
  Solar urticaria
  Lupus erythematosus
  Porphyria cutanea tarda
Old age
  Chronic actinic dermatitis
  Drug-induced photosensitivity
  Dermatomyositis

Source: Adapted from Ref. 2.

The duration of the persistence of the lesions also gives a clue to the diagnosis. In the absence of additional sun exposure, lesions in patients with polymorphous light eruption tend to last for a few days. In contrast, those in solar urticaria resolve within one to two hours, whereas those of chronica actinic dermatitis and PCT usually persist throughout the sunny season.

TABLE 5 Common Phototoxic and Photoallergic Agents

Common phototoxic agents	Common photoallergic agents
Antiarrhythmics	*Topical agents*
Amiodarone	Sunscreen agents
Quinidine	Fragrances
Diuretics	6-Methylcoumarin
Furosemide	Musk ambrette
Thiazides	Sandalwood oil
Nonsteroidal anti-inflammatory drugs	Antibacterial agents
Nabumetone	Bithionol
Naproxen	Chlorhexidine
Piroxicam	Hexachlorophene
Phenothiazines	Others
Chlorpromazine	Chlorpromazine
Prochlorperazine	Fenticlor
Psoralens	Promethazine
5-Methoxypsoralen	*Systemic agents*
8-Methoxypsoralen	Antiarrhythmics
4,5′,8-Trimethylpsoralen	Quinidine
Quinolones	Antifungal
Ciprofloxacin	Griseofulvin
Lomefloxacin	Antimalarial
Nalidixic acid	Quinine
Sparfloxacin	Antimicrobials
St. John's wort	Quinolone
Hypericin	Sulfonamides
Tar	Nonsteroidal anti-inflammatory drugs
Tetracyclines	Ketoprofen
Demeclocycline	Piroxicam
Doxycycline	

Source: Adapted from Ref. 3.

Window Glass

Whether or not an eruption can be induced by window glass-filtered sunlight gives some information on the action spectrum of the photodermatosis. However, it should be noted that while window glass is known to filter out UVB, the long-standing belief that UVA regularly penetrates window glass well is no longer accurate. New developments in the glass industry in the past ten years have resulted in a significant improvement of the UV-filtering property of window glass. Currently, there are many types of glass used in buildings and in the automobile industry that have excellent UVB and UVA2 (320–340 nm) filtering properties. Some would even filter efficiently a good proportion of UVA1 (340–400 nm), allowing only UV wavelength greater than 380 nm to penetrate the glass; this results in glass that would allow only <1% of wavelength below 380 nm to be transmitted (4). Obviously, unless the glass is opaque, visible light always penetrates through the glass.

For safety reasons, windshields of cars are made of laminated glass, so that if the glass is broken, fragments will adhere to a polyvinyl butyral interlayer rather than falling free, hence reducing the likelihood of injury. Side and back windows of cars are made of nonlaminated glass. Laminated glass is more efficient at filtering UVA than nonlaminated glass. Since the occupants in cars are seated more closely to side windows than the windshield, there is a significant risk that the side window-filtered sunlight will precipitate lesions in patients with photodermatoses. These factors should be taken into account in obtaining the history in relation to window glass-filtered sunlight.

Family History

Family history is another aspect that needs to be obtained during the history taking. This is most relevant in evaluating patients who may have one of the cutaneous porphyrias (chap. 15). The mode of inheritance of these porphyrias is shown in Table 6. In addition, a study from the United Kingdom indicated that polymorphous light eruption and actinic prurigo also appeared to have an important familial tendency (5).

Systemic Abnormalities

A history of acute abdominal pain, and peripheral neuropathy and paresis in a patient with photosensitivity should lead one to consider the possibility of variegate porphyria or hereditary coproporphyria. It should be noted that acute intermittent porphyria, which is also associated with abdominal and neurologic symptoms, is not associated with any cutaneous eruption. A history of Raynaud's phenomenon, cutaneous ulcerations, thrombosis, livedo reticularis, and muscle weakness should raise the possibility of lupus erythematosus or dermatomyositis.

Photodermatoses associated with defective DNA nucleotide excision repair are rare. These patients have multiple organ involvement; these disorders are covered in chapter 16.

PHYSICAL EXAMINATION

The second part of the evaluation is a complete physical examination of the skin, paying special attention to sun-exposed and sun-protected areas. The eruption may not always be present in intermittent conditions, such as polymorphous light eruption and solar urticaria; however, in which case, a very careful history of the eruption as described earlier is of particular importance in formulating the likely diagnosis. Virtually all photodermatoses when

TABLE 6 Mode of Inheritance of the Cutaneous Porphyrias

Porphyria	Inheritance
Congenital erythropoietic porphyria (Günther disease)	Autosomal recessive
Porphyria cutanea tarda (familial type)	Autosomal dominant
Hereditary coproporphyria	Autosomal dominant
Variegate porphyria	Autosomal dominant
Erythropoietic protoporphyria	3 allele model[a]

[a]N, normal; M, mutant; n, low output normal.

present demonstrate the most severe eruptions on the sun-exposed areas of the skin, which include the forehead, cheeks, V-region of neck, nape of neck, dorsum of the hands, and extensor aspects of forearms. In addition, examination of exposed but relatively sun-protected areas of the skin will also give important indication of the photosensitivity. These areas include nasolabial folds, postauricular area, upper eyelids, peri-orbital area in patients who wear glasses, superior aspects of the pinna, which may be covered by hair, especially in women, and area underneath the chin. These areas tend to be spared in patients with photodermatosis. In contrast, they will frequently be involved in patients with airborne allergic contact dermatitis.

While skin surfaces covered by clothing, such as the chest, back, and buttocks are generally spared; it should be noted that in markedly photosensitive patients, the eruption might also occur to a lesser extent in these covered areas; especially if an area is covered by clothing, which allows some penetration of UV radiation. The UV photoprotectivity of a garment is indicated by its ultraviolet protection factor (UPF), which is an in vitro determination on the degree of UV transmission through the fabric. However, many do not carry this label. A practical rule of thumb is that while holding a fabric up to visible light, the more transparent the fabric, the more UV is likely to penetrate.

The morphology of the skin eruption is also very important in determining the diagnosis (Table 7). Urticaria is seen in association with pruritus in patients with solar urticaria. The erythropoietic protoporphyria (EPP) is most commonly associated with no eruption, but just severe pain within about half an hour of sun exposure. In some patients, an even, skin-colored or pink edematous swelling with a sharp cut-off at clothing lines may be observed within a couple of hours after sun exposure; very rarely vesicles or urticarial lesions may occur. A papular eruption is commonly seen in patients with polymorphous light eruption, and sometimes in the acute exacerbations of chronic actinic dermatitis. In polymorphous light eruption, urticarial papules are the most common morphology for fair-skinned individuals, whereas in dark-skinned individuals, pinpoint papules are the most frequently observed lesions (6). Patients with polymorphous light eruption can also present with vesicular or very rarely bullous eruption, especially in those who are acutely exposed to intense UV radiation as most commonly seen during short vacations to resorts in tropical or subtropical climates (7). Juvenile spring eruption, a variant of polymorphous light eruption occurring mostly in young boys, usually presents with vesicles on the superior aspect of the pinna, and sometimes also on the back of the hands.

Eczematous vesicular eruptions are possible in photoallergy, while phototoxicity presents with acute inflammatory vesicles and bullae. Such vesicles and bullae are commonly seen

TABLE 7 Morphology of Lesions

Morphology	Possible diagnoses[a]
Urticaria or urticarial	Solar urticaria Erythropoietic protoporphyria (rare)
Papule	Polymorphous light eruption Actinic prurigo Chronic actinic dermatitis (acute eruption)
Vesicle	Polymorphous light eruption Juvenile spring eruption (ears) Porphyria cutanea tarda Phototoxicity Photoallergy Hydroa vacciniforme
Erosion, crust	Porphyria cutanea tarda Actinic prurigo (lips) Hydroa vacciniforme Variegate porphyria Congenital erythropoietic porphyria Hereditary coproporphyria
Eczema and/or lichenification	Chronic actinic dermatitis

[a]Listed in an approximate order of probability.

on dorsa of the hands of patients with PCT. It should be noted that these lesions reflect the skin fragility that occurs in these patients; therefore, the patients may not directly relate the development of lesions to sun exposure. Trauma frequently induces the development of this photo-distributed eruption in PCT, resulting in erosions and crusting. Crusting of the lips, along with conjunctivitis, is a common presentation in patients with actinic prurigo seen in Central and South America. Marked lichenification of the sun-exposed skin from scratching is commonly seen in patients with chronic actinic dermatitis, reflecting the chronic and pruritic nature of the condition.

Patients with cutaneous porphyrias frequently have other characteristic lesions (chap. 15). Patients with PCT have peri-orbital hypertrichosis and mottled dyspigmentation, and sclero-dermoid changes in sun-exposed as well as in sun-protected areas. Patients with EPP may develop acute ecchymoses of sun-exposed areas, usually the dorsa of the hands or extensor forearms, along with chronic lesions of "cobble-stoning" of the knuckles of the hands, superficial waxy linear or punctuate scars of the cheeks and nose, and radial scarring around the lips. The exposed skin in these patients is often characteristically dry.

Heliotrope is frequently seen in patients with dermatomyositis, whereas periungal telangiectasia is often observed in patients with lupus erythematosus or dermatomyositis.

PHOTOTESTING

Phototesting is an integral part of the evaluation of the photosensitive patient (see Appendix A "Phototesting" for further information). Briefly, using a template, uninvolved skin of the patient's back or abdomen is exposed to different doses of UVB, UVA, and/or visible monochromatic or broad-spectrum radiation. Evaluation immediately after the exposure is performed to detect the development of solar urticaria. The patient is re-evaluated 24 hours later for the development of erythema. The minimal erythema dose (MED) is defined as the lowest dose of UVB, or UVA, that would produce just perceptible erythema, covering the entire irradiated area. It should be noted that, while erythema can be produced by UVB and UVA, positive response to visible light is most frequently the urticarial response of solar urticaria, although it may also rarely be the eczema of severe chronic actinic dermatitis. Appropriately preformed, phototesting often but not always confirms the presence of photosensitivity, though not necessarily the precise diagnosis, and helps to determine the action spectrum. The induction of lesions by phototesting, which may require three to four consecutive days of exposure to the same site, is known as photo-provocation testing. This latter test is often helpful in confirming the diagnosis of polymorphous light eruption, or photosensitive form of lupus erythematosus. In the former, lesions usually develop at third or fourth day of exposure. In lupus erythematous, lesions may develop within one to two weeks after the completion of either phototesting or provocative phototesting.

Expected phototest results for some of the more common photodermatoses are shown in Table 8.

PHOTOPATCH TESTING

Photopatch testing is performed in the evaluation of the photosensitive patient in whom photoallergic contact dermatitis is suspected. Such testing involves the application of duplicate sets of photoallergens on uninvolved sites of the skin, usually on the upper back. Twenty-four

TABLE 8 Expected Results in Phototest and Photopatch Test

Disorder	MED-A	MED-B	Visible light	Photopatch test
Polymorphous light eruption	Normal/ ↓	Normal/ ↓	Normal	Negative
Chronic actinic dermatitis	↓	↓	Normal/ ↓	±
Solar urticaria	Urticaria[a]	Urticaria[a]	Urticaria[a]	Negative
Phototoxicity	↓	Normal	Normal	Negative
Photoallergy	↓	Normal	Normal	+

[a]Minutes after exposure; negative at 24 hours.

TABLE 9 Interpretations of Results of Photopatch Test

Irradiated site	Nonirradiated site	Interpretation
+	—	Photoallergic contact dermatitis
++	+	Photoallergic contact dermatitis and allergic contact dermatitis
+	+	Allergic contact dermatitis
—	—	Normal

hours later, one set would be exposed to either 10 J/cm^2 of UVA, or in patients with a markedly decreased MED-A, to 50% of MED-A. Forty-eight hours after the initial application of the photoallergens, the reactions on the irradiated and unirradiated sides are evaluated. Table 9 summarizes the interpretation of photopatch results (see Appendix B "Photopatch Testing" for further information).

A summary of the photopatch test studies involving more than 100 patients is shown in Table 10. At the completion of the evaluation, the percentage of patients with a diagnosis of photoallergic contact dermatitis to a clinically relevant photoallergen ranged from 1.4% to 12%, with most series being in the 10% range (8–15).

LABORATORY EVALUATION

The diagnosis of a photodermatosis relies on the history, physical examination, phototest results, and if necessary, photopatch test results. Skin biopsy may be performed to help to confirm diagnosis. This is helpful in the diagnosis of polymorphous light eruption and chronic actinic dermatitis. Lymphoid follicles seen in biopsy specimens of the lip and conjunctiva of patients with actinic prurigo seen in Central and South America are considered to be diagnostic of that condition (16).

Descriptions of the skin biopsy results are discussed in Chapters 11–17 on the various photodermatoses. Immunophenotypic markers studies and gene rearrangement analyses are helpful in differentiating chronic actinic dermatitis from cutaneous T-cell lymphoma, which may share similarities in their clinical manifestations.

In patients with polymorphous light eruption and photoaggravated dermatoses, assessment of antinuclear antibody titers (ANA and ENA) is essential to exclude connective tissue diseases. An excellent screening test for all types of cutaneous porphyrias is the determination of plasma porphyrin level. Should the results be elevated, evaluation of the complete porphyrin profile, which should include determination of erythrocyte porphyrin, 24-hour urinary porphyrin, and stool porphyrin levels, is indicated.

STEPS IN THE EVALUATION OF THE PHOTOSENSITIVE PATIENT

These are summarized in Table 11. After obtaining the history and performing the physical examination, the next step is to schedule phototesting, and if photocontact allergic dermatitis

TABLE 10 Summary of Studies on Photopatch Testing

Reference	Location	Number of patients	% Diagnosed with photoallergic contact dermatitis
Thune et al. (8)	Scandinavia	1993	11
Hölzle et al. (9)	Germany, Austria, Switzerland	1129	7
DeLeo et al. (10)	New York, U.S.A.	187	11
Fotiades et al. (11)	New York, U.S.A.	138	12
Neumann et al. (12)	Germany, Austria, Switzerland	1129	4
Neumann et al. (12)	Germany, Austria, Switzerland	1261	8
Bell and Rhodes (13)	Liverpool, U.K.	167	10
Darvay et al. (14)	London, U.K.	2715	2.3
Crouch et al. (15)	Melbourne, Australia	172	1.4

TABLE 11 Schedule of Phototesting and Photopatch Testing

Day	Procedure
1	Phototesting: exposure to UVA, UVB, and visible light; immediate reading done (to detect solar urticaria) Duplicate set of photoallergens applied
2	MED reading One set of photoallergen sites exposure to UVA (the lower of 5–10 J/cm^2 or 50% MED-A)
3	Reading of the irradiated and unirradiated photopatch test sites
4–5	Reading of the irradiated and unirradiated photopatch test sites

Abbreviation: MED, minimal erythema dose.

TABLE 12 Frequency of Photodermatoses Diagnosed at Photodermatology Centers

					Detroit	
Diagnosis	New York City ($n = 203$) (%)	Melbourne ($n = 513$) (%)	Athens ($n = 310$) (%)	Singapore ($n = 141$) (%)	Blacks ($n = 135$) (%)	Caucasians ($n = 110$) (%)
Polymorphous light eruption	26	23	65	28	67	46
Photoaggravated dermatoses	—	23	—	26	—	—
Chronic actinic dermatitis	17	7	10	15	11	7
Systemic drug photosensitivity	7	5	—	15	13	11
Solar urticaria	4	8	18	7	2	8

Source: Adapted from Refs. 11, 15, 17, 18, 19.

is suspected, photopatch testing. The exposure of skin to the appropriate radiation sources is done on the first day, and the first reading should be done upon completion of the irradiation to observe for solar urticaria. The patient then comes back on the second day, when the MED reading is undertaken, and any reduction below expected range and any abnormal morphology of the responses are noted.

If the patient is to receive photopatch testing, a duplicate set of photoallergens is placed on symmetrical sites of the uninvolved skin on the patient's back on the first day of phototesting. On the second day, after the determination of MED-A, one set is exposed to UVA. If the MED-A is normal (i.e., greater than 18 or 20 J/cm^2), an exposure dose of 10 J/cm^2 is most commonly used, although some centers use the lower dose of 5 J/cm^2. If the patient has a low MED-A, 50% of the MED-A is used as the exposure dose. On the third day (i.e., 24 hours later), assessment of the responses at the irradiated and nonirradiated sites is done. Readings at 48 and 72 hours are also performed in some centers.

CONCLUSION

A systematic approach to the evaluation of the photosensitive patient should lead to the appropriate diagnosis (Table 8). With the approach outlined in this chapter, a summary of the frequency of photodermatoses reported from photodermatology centers in New York, Melbourne, Athens, Singapore, and Detroit is given in Table 12 (11,15,17–19). Polymorphous light eruption, chronic actinic dermatitis, solar urticaria, and photosensitivity secondary to systemic medications are the most frequently encountered photodermatoses in these centers. Photoaggravated dermatoses are also seen relatively frequently in Melbourne and Singapore, reflecting their geographic locations.

REFERENCES

1. Wilkinson DS. Photodermatitis due to tetrachlorosalicylanilide. Br J Dermatol 1961; 73:213–219.
2. Roelandts R. The diagnosis of photosensitivity. Arch Dermatol 2000; 136:1152–1157.
3. Lim HW, Hawk J. Photodermatoses. In: Bolognia JL, Jorizzo JL, Rapini RP, eds. Dermatology. 2nd ed. London: Mosby, 2007.

4. Tuchinda C, Srivannaboon S, Lim HW. Photoprotection by window glass, automobile glass and sunglasses. J Am Acad Dermatol 2006; 54:845–854.
5. McGregor JM, Grabczynska S, Vaughan R, Hawk JL, Lewis CM. Genetic modeling of abnormal photosensitivity in families with polymorphic light eruption and actinic prurigo. J Invest Dermatol 2000; 115:471–476.
6. Kontos A, Cusack C, Chaffins M, Lim HW. Polymorphous light eruption in African-Americans: pinpoint popular variant. Photodermatol Photoimmunol Photomed 2002; 18:303–306.
7. Elpern DJ, Morison WL, Hood AF. Papulovesicular light eruption. A defined subset of polymorphous light eruption. Arch Dermatol 1985; 121:1286–1288.
8. Thune P, Jansen C, Wennersten G, Rystedt I, Brodthagen H, McFadden N. The Scandinavian multi-center photopatch study 1980–1985: final report. Photodermatol 1988; 5:261–269.
9. Hölzle E, Neumann N, Hausen B, et al. Photopatch testing: the 5-year experience of the German, Austrian, and Swiss Photopatch Test Group. J Am Acad Dermatol 1991; 25:59–68.
10. DeLeo VA, Suarez SM, Maso MJ. Photoallergic contact dermatitis. Results of photopatch testing in New York, 1985 to 1990. Arch Dermatol 1992; 128:1513–1518.
11. Fotiades J, Soter NA, Lim HW. Results of evaluation of 203 patients for photosensitivity in a 7.3-year period. J Am Acad Dermatol 1995; 33:597–602.
12. Neumann NJ, Holzle E, Plewig G, et al. Photopatch testing: the 12-year experiences of the German, Austrian, and Swiss photopatch test group. J Am Acad Dermatol 2000; 42(2 Pt 1):183–192.
13. Bell HK, Rhodes LE. Photopatch testing in photosensitive patients. Br J Dermatol 2000; 142:589–590.
14. Darvay A, White IR, Rycroft RJ, Jones AB, Hawk JL, McFadden JP. Photoallergic contact dermatitis is uncommon. Br J Dermatol 2001; 145:597–601.
15. Crouch RB, Foley PA, Baker CS. Analysis of patients with suspected photosensitivity referred for investigation to an Australian photodermatology clinic. J Am Acad Dermatol 2003; 48:714–720.
16. Hojyo-Tomoka T, Vega-Memije E, Granados J. Actinic prurigo: an update. Int J Dermatol 1995; 34:380–384.
17. Stratigos AJ, Antoniou C, Papathanakou E, et al. Spectrum of idiopathic photodermatosis in a Mediterranean country. Int J Dermatol 2003; 42:449–454.
18. Wong SN, Khoo LSW. Analysis of photodermatoses seen in a predominantly Asian population at a photodermatology clinic in Singapore. Photodermatol Photoimmunol Photomed 2005; 21:40–44.
19. Kerr HA, Lim HW. A comparison of photosensitivity disorders in African Americans and Caucasians. Presented at the Skin of Color Society meeting, New Orleans, USA. 2005.

11 | Polymorphous Light Eruption, Hydroa Vacciniforme, and Actinic Prurigo

Herbert Hönigsmann
Department of Dermatology, Medical University of Vienna, Vienna, Austria

Maria Teresa Hojyo-Tomoka
Departamento de Dermatologia del Hospital General Dr. Manuel Gea González, Tlalpan, Mexico City, Mexico

- Photodermatoses, though not life-threatening, can severely impair the quality of life, particularly in outdoor workers and during leisure activities.

- Polymorphous light eruption, hydroa vacciniforme, and actinic prurigo belong to the group of so-called idiopathic photodermatoses. The term denotes skin diseases that occur in otherwise healthy individuals from exposure to natural or artificial light without the intervention of an exogenous photosensitizer. The diseases included in this group have two factors in common: first, they are precipitated by electromagnetic radiation in the ultraviolet or visible range; secondly, their exact pathomechanism remains to be elucidated, but is presumably immunologic in nature.

- Polymorphous light eruption is the most common photodermatosis, with a prevalence of as high as 10% to 20% in Western Europe and in the U.S.A. It starts during the second and third decades of life.

- Hydroa vacciniforme is a very rare photodermatosis that starts in childhood. Its name derives from pock-like scarring as the final state after healing of sunlight-induced vesicles.

- Actinic prurigo is a common chronic photodermatosis mainly affecting Mestizo populations of American countries, native American Indians, and Inuit people. Some sporadic cases do occur in Europe and Asia. There is a clear genetic predisposition with an association of specific alleles of the major histocompatibility complex.

POLYMORPHOUS (OR POLYMORPHIC) LIGHT ERUPTION

Polymorphous (or polymorphic) light eruption (PLE) is a common, recurrent, acquired sunlight-induced disorder of delayed onset. It is often incorrectly referred as to "sun allergy" by the lay press. The PLE is characterized clinically by the occurrence within hours to days of ultraviolet radiation (UVR) exposure of nonscarring, pruritic, erythematous papules, papulovesicles, vesicles or plaques on sun-exposed skin areas, generally symmetrically, which then resolve completely over several days to a week. It is commonly most severe in the spring or early summer, often diminishing in severity as summer progresses, before disappearing completely during the winter. Clinical manifestations may be manifold with a number of different yet overlapping clinical subtypes. Within each patient the single morphologic feature of the lesions mostly remains the same. The term "polymorphous" designates the inter-individual variation in the clinical appearance of the disease. The minimal erythema dose (MED) is usually normal.

Epidemiology

The PLE is the most common photosensitivity disease, and according to a survey of apparently healthy individuals (1), it may be even more common than one would assume when considering only the number of patients who seek medical advice. The prevalence is however inversely related to latitude: around 21% of Scandinavians appear to suffer from the condition (2) and 10% to 15% of those living in the Northern U.S. (1) and the U.K. (3), although only 5% of Australians (3) and 1% Singaporeans (4) have the disease.

The disorder (1,2,5,6) usually starts during the second and third decades of life and affects females twice to three times more often than males. It may also occur in all skin types and racial groups, but appears more commonly to affect relatively fair-skinned individuals. A positive family history is present in about one-sixth of patients (1).

Etiology and Pathogenesis

The condition has been considered for many years as a possible delayed-type hypersensitivity (DTH) response to endogenous, cutaneous photo-induced antigen (7), because of the hours or days delay between sun exposure and manifestation of PLE and the lesional histologic appearance, but firm evidence has been lacking.

The UV irradiation may convert some precursors in the skin to those antigens that cause the DTH reaction, resulting in the clinical appearance of the disease. The nature of the precursors or antigens, however, remains obscure. More recently, timed biopsies following irradiation with artificial light sources with doses below the MED have shown perivascular infiltrates of mainly CD4+ T lymphocytes within a few hours and CD8+ cells within days; an increased number of dermal and epidermal Langerhans cells (LC) and dermal macrophages has also been noted, a pattern suggestive overall of DTH as seen in the allergic contact dermatitis and tuberculin reactions (8). In addition, E-selectin, vascular cell adhesion molecule-1 (VCAM-1), and intercellular adhesion molecule-1 (ICAM-1), particularly a marked and characteristic staining of the latter on keratinocytes above areas of dermal leukocyte infiltration, are also expressed as in other DTH responses (9).

The UV-induced immunosuppression is a consistent finding in normal skin and it was speculated that this process might protect the skin from UV-induced photoallergens. Thus, susceptibility of individuals to PLE could arise from a failure of normal UV-induced immunosuppression.

Kölgen et al. (10) reported that the skin of PLE patients was less susceptible to UVB-induced migration of CD1+ LC. Following a six MED dose of UVB, there was a significant failure of LC to migrate from the epidermis of PLE compared with normal subjects. They also found a significant reduction in UVB-induced infiltration by CD11b+ macrophage-like cells in PLE compared with healthy skin, which was considered to represent an important finding in view of the prominent role of these cells in secretion of the immunosuppressive cytokine interleukin (IL)-10. It was therefore postulated that the pathologic defect underlying PLE might be a failure of normal photoimmunosuppression. Thus the balance of UV-induced suppression and UV-induced provocation would be altered, allowing sunlight exposure to provoke the PLE eruption (10). In a more recent study, Kölgen et al. assessed whether there are abnormalities of UV-induced secretion of tumor necrosis factor (TNF) α and IL-1β, cytokines known to be important in effecting LC migration. Secondly, they examined the effects of UV on secretion of T helper cell type 2 (T_H2) cytokines IL-4 and IL-10, which mediate immunosuppression. They concluded that the reduced expression of TNF-α, IL-4, and IL-10 in the UVB−irradiated skin of patients with PLE appears largely attributable to a lack of neutrophils, and is indicative of reduced Langerhans cell migration and reduced T_H2 skewing. An impairment of these mechanisms underlying UV-B−induced immunosuppression may be important in the pathogenesis of PLE (11).

Palmer and Friedmann (12) reported on functional studies examining DTH responses in PLE and concluded that the induction of sensitization by 2,4-dinitrochlorobenzene (DNCB) is suppressed less by UVR in patients with PLE than in healthy controls (12). Beyond this, van de Pas et al. (13) recently showed a reduction in UV-induced suppression of the DTH response to DNCB in PLE such that these patients are less easily sensitized to DNCB compared with healthy subjects (13). Schornagel et al. (14) also suggested a role for neutrophils in the pathogenesis of PLE by showing a relative reduction in UVB-induced neutrophilic infiltration. It is conceivable that abnormalities in both neutrophil and mononuclear cell activity could be involved in the pathogenesis of PLE.

However, the most recent findings on the effect of solar-simulated radiation on the elicitation phase of contact hypersensitivity revealed no significant difference between controls and patients with PLE. These results contrasted with previous findings of the same group that had indicated a resistance to UVR-induced suppression of sensitization to DNCB in PLE. This difference may reflect the greater importance of Langerhans cells in the sensitization phase, and is consistent with the hypothesis that PLE arises from impaired suppression of Langerhans cell activation or migration (15).

The reason for the occurrence of PLE appears likely to be genetic with a substantial environmental component, with 70% of the population perhaps having a tendency to the condition, but not all expressing it because of poor penetrance (16,17). Examination of 119 monozygotic twin pairs and 301 dizygotic twin pairs revealed an incidence of 21% among the monozygotic twins and 18% in dizygotic twins (16). However, the culprit gene has not been identified yet. This genetically-determined factor, which leads to the putative immune recognition of an autologous cutaneous antigen, is generated by UVR in PLE but not normal subjects, although the antigen is presumably expressed in all individuals. Inducing UV absorbers and antigens in PLE have not been characterized; however, one suggestion for the latter has been a form of heat-shock protein (18). A variety of such antigens within and between patients, however, seems more likely. In addition, the induction of lesions by a UVA sunbed in the non-tanning sacral pressure area (19) further suggests that the UV−chromophore interaction in at least some patients may be oxygen-independent.

Induction of Polymorphous Light Eruption

Difficulty in the reliable laboratory induction of clinical lesions has long frustrated investigations into the pathogenesis of PLE. Determination of the action spectrum of PLE by experimental reproduction of skin lesions using artificial radiation sources has led to conflicting results. A lack of response, often to adequate doses of artificially produced UV radiation, by patients who react readily to just suberythemogenic doses of natural sunlight may be attributed to a number of variables. These include the size of the UV irradiation site and its location, the irradiation of small, normally unaffected areas perhaps not eliciting sufficient immunologic stimulus to activate the response, but also to the UV spectrum, irradiation dose, dose rate, and degree of cutaneous immunologic tolerance, which may be increased by any recent prior exposure (20). There is also a lack of universally accepted, standardized phototest protocols.

The complex interrelationships between factors such as these have clearly contributed significantly to the conflicting nature of reports concerning the most effective wavelengths for PLE induction. In most series, UVA (320−400 nm) has been more reliably effective than

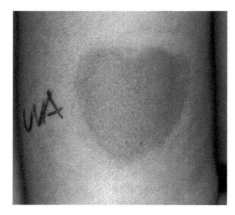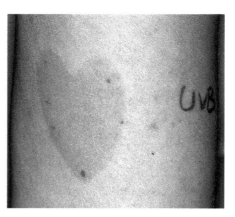

FIGURE 1 Polymorphous light eruption. Photoprovocation: small papulovesicles developing in the UVA-irradiated area (*left*) after three exposures with one minimal erythema dose on consecutive days. The UVB-irradiated site shows just erythema (*right*).

UVB (280–320 nm) (Fig. 1) (20–22). Thus, in one of these studies (21), following exposures of buttock skin to UVA or UVB daily for four to eight days, the action spectrum was in the UVA range in 56%, UVB in 17%, and both UVA and UVB in 27%. In another study (22), the ratio was: 68% triggered by UVA, 8% by UVB, and 10% by both wavelengths (Fig. 2). This apparent diversity in action spectrum for the induction of PLE is possibly the result of different UV-evoked inducing antigens, and perhaps also of different cutaneous levels for these antigens. Contradictory results regarding the action spectrum for PLE induction could also conceivably be accounted for by the presence of inhibitory wavelengths in some patients.

Variation in the proportions of UVA and UVB present in terrestrial sunlight may also explain certain clinical characteristics of PLE (23). Thus, the greater proportion of UVA to UVB in temperate climates and during the spring and fall months might be expected to contribute to a higher incidence of PLE in temperate rather than tropical regions (3), with greater susceptibility to the condition in spring and occasionally fall, rather than summer in most patients.

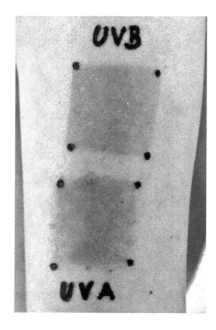

FIGURE 2 Polymorphous light eruption (PLE). Photoprovocation: PLE lesion induced after three exposures with one minimal erythema dose on consecutive days on both the UVA- and UVB-irradiated area. More pronounced with UVA.

Moreover, the higher proportion of UVB to UVA in summer sunlight also very probably inhibits PLE development through a predominantly UVB-induced cutaneous immunosuppressive mechanism (13,24). Older generation sunscreens that are protective primarily against UVB encouraged people to stay much longer in the sun, thereby receiving a much higher UVA dose than without UVB protection, did not provide adequate protection against provocation of PLE (23).

Clinical Features

Lesions generally develop symmetrically and affect only some sun-exposed areas of the skin, often those normally covered in winter, such as the V-area of the chest (Fig. 3), the external aspects of the arms and forearms, and lower anterior aspect of the neck. Occasionally, the face can be involved.

The PLE occurs more often in temperate areas. The eruption typically begins each spring or early summer, on sunny vacations, or after recreational sunbed use (25), often moderating with continuing exposure. An attack may also be induced by outdoor activities in winter or by exposure through window glass (26,27). The eruption develops after minutes to hours (on vacation, sometimes days) of sun exposure and lasts for one to several days or occasionally weeks, particularly with continuing exposure. The tendency to develop the condition, however, often fades or ceases as summer or the vacation proceeds. A polymorphic light eruption severity index (PLESI) has been proposed to produce a simple, valid and reproducible method to assess the severity of the disease (28).

In the absence of further exposure, all the lesions gradually subside completely without scarring over one to seven days, occasionally a week or two, or very rarely longer in severe cases. In a given patient, the eruption tends always to affect the same skin sites, although its distribution may gradually spread or recede overall.

Associated systemic symptoms are rare, but shivesing, headache, fever, nausea, and a variety of other sensations are possible. The condition may be lifelong, but gradually improves over years in many patients: Over seven years, 64 of 114 patients (57%) reported steadily diminishing sun sensitivity, including 12 (11%) who totally cleared (29).

The PLE has many morphologic variants. Lesions vary widely between patients, but are generally pruritic, grouped, erythematous or skin-colored papules of varying size not infrequently coalescing into large, smooth or rough-surfaced plaques (Fig. 4). Vesicles, bullae, and papulovesicles as well as confluent edematous swelling (particularly of the face) are also possible, while rarely erythema or pruritus alone (PLE sine eruptione) may occur (30). Insect bite-like and erythema multiform-like variants have also been described. In addition, the helices of the ears, particularly in boys because they are relatively more exposed, may be principally affected, often with vesicles, a form of PLE previously known as juvenile spring eruption (Fig. 5) (31). Such subdivisions do not apparently relate to differences in disease pathogenesis. The papular form, of either large or small separate or confluent lesions, and generally tending to be in clusters, is the most common, followed by the papulovesicular and

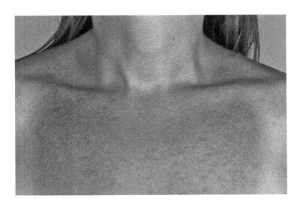

FIGURE 3 Polymorphous light eruption. Photoprovocation: classical papulovesicular rash at the V-area.

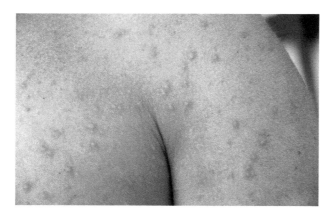

FIGURE 4   Polymorphous light ruption: close-up of papular rash.

plaque variants; the others are rare. The eczematous form probably does not exist, representing instead chronic actinic dermatitis, although PLE may on occasion become secondarily licheni-fied or eczematized during resolution. Differing morphologies may also occur at different skin sites in the same patient: diffuse facial erythema and swelling, for example, may accompany typical papular lesions at other sites. A final morphologic variant, a small papular form gener-ally sparing the face and occurring after several days' exposure on vacations, has been desig-nated as benign summer light eruption in Europe (32). Rarely, covered sites may be mildly affected, due to radiation penetration through clothes.

Histopathology

The histologic features of PLE are quite characteristic but not diagnostic and vary with the different clinical presentations (33,34). The epidermis shows edema, focal spongiosis, and occasionally small vesicles. Acanthosis, spongiosis focal parakeratosis, and basal vacuolization can be present. Sunburn cells are not a typical feature. There is a moderate-to-intense, super-ficial and deep dermal perivascular infiltrate in all clinical types, the infiltrate consisting

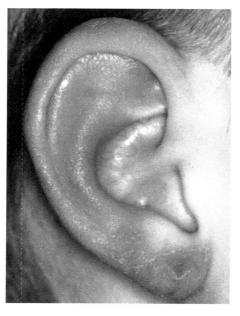

FIGURE 5   Juvenile spring eruption in a 10-year-old boy.

predominantly of T cells; while neutrophils and eosinophils are infrequent. Other common features are upper dermal and perivascular edema and endothelial cell swelling. Direct immunofluorescence is normal.

Diagnosis

The diagnosis of PLE is not difficult and is made largely on clinical grounds based on the typical morphology of the eruption. Although the diagnosis is mainly clinical, provocative phototesting may be valuable in winter, if no lesions are present, to confirm the diagnosis. The best way to do this is by using repetitive irradiations on the V area of the neck or forearms for one to four consecutive days. This can be done with high-intensity monochromatic UVA and UVB sources or with a solar simulator (UVA plus UVB). The doses needed are not necessarily erythemal. Readings are made immediately and up to 72 hours after the last irradiation. Abnormal cutaneous reactions can be provoked in more than 60% of patients. In most studies more patients reacted to UVA than to UVB (20,21,35).

There are no diagnostic laboratory tests available for PLE. Laboratory examinations are usually performed to exclude other dermatoses, such as erythropoietic protoporphyria and photosensitive lupus erythematosus. Subacute cutaneous lupus erythematosus, which is generally not itchy as PLE, must be excluded in some patients by determining antinuclear, Ro (SSA) and La (SSB) antibody titers. Persistent plaque-type PLE must also be differentiated from Jessner-Kanof's lymphocytic infiltration of the skin, while the photo-exacerbation of dermatoses, such as atopic and seborrheic eczema, may occur in susceptible subjects with the same time course as for PLE, but with differing and characteristic morphologies.

Treatment

The treatment of PLE has to be subdivided into therapy for the acute exacerbation and the prophylactic therapy before expected sun exposure (Table 1) (36).

TABLE 1 Treatment Measures

Disease	Treatment	Reference
Polymorphous light eruption		
First-line therapy (acute flare)	Topical/systemic corticosteroids	(38)
First-line therapy (prevention)	Moderation of sun exposure, high-factor broad-spectrum sunscreens, and avoidance of behavioral sunlight exposure and/or artificial tanning devices in more severe cases	(36)
Second-line therapy (prevention)	Narrowband UVB phototherapy or PUVA	(21,41–44)
Therapies of no or insufficiently documented efficacy	Antimalarials, β-carotene, nicotinamide, ω-3 polyunsaturated fatty acids, *Escherichia coli*-filtrate (Colibiogen) systemic antioxidants, and systemic immunosuppressive therapy	(45–51)
Hydroa vacciniforme		
First-line therapy (prevention)	High-factor broad-spectrum sunscreens and avoidance of behavioral sunlight exposure and/or artificial tanning devices	(58,59)
Second-line therapy (prevention)	Narrowband UVB phototherapy or PUVA	(58,60–62)
Therapies of no or insufficiently documented efficacy	Antimicrobials, antimalarials, and systemic immunosuppressive therapy, including corticosteroids, beta-carotene, and dietary fish oil	
Actinic prurigo		
First-line therapy (acute flare)	Thalidomide	(97,98)
First-line therapy (prevention)	High-factor broad-spectrum sunscreens and avoidance of behavioral sunlight exposure, protective hats and clothing, and sunglasses	
Second-line therapy (prevention)	PUVA (reportedly not always successful)	
Therapies of no or insufficient efficacy	Antimalarials, β-carotene, and antihistamines	

Abbreviation: PUVA, psoralen plus ultraviolet A.

The mild disease of many patients is satisfactorily controlled by the moderation of sun exposure at times of high UV intensity, use of protective clothing, and the regular application of broad-spectrum sunscreens with high protection factors, particularly against UVA. Combining a potent antioxidant with a broad-spectrum, highly UVA-protective sunscreen was reported to be more effective in preventing PLE than sunscreen alone. However, this will need further confirmation (37).

Patients with fully developed disease require topical corticosteroids, in some cases in the form of wet dressings, for several days. More severe attacks may be treated effectively with a short course of systemic (oral) corticosteroids (38). Since PLE will subside spontaneously and is not a life-threatening condition, all possible risks of therapy should be carefully considered.

Many patients will agree to undergo some sort of preventive measures. Prophylactic treatment consists of several approaches: avoidance of sunlight during the summer, the use of sunscreens with broadband filters, systemic treatment, and preventive phototherapy.

Severely affected subjects suffering frequent attacks of their disease throughout the summer may require courses of prophylactic photo(chemo)therapy before the expected sun exposure in the early spring. At first glance it appears somewhat bizarre to use light treatment to prevent a condition that is caused by light, and the mechanisms by which UVB and psoralen-photochemotherapy (PUVA) induce tolerance to sunlight are not completely understood. Pigmentation and thickening of the stratum corneum may be important factors for the protective effect, and UVB, high-dose UVA, and PUVA are efficient triggers of both. Although these local effects may provide some barrier against photosensitivity, they probably do not suffice to explain the degree of protection induced in many patients. Thus other mechanisms may be involved, since photodermatoses do occur in dark-skinned subjects (39). The ability of UV radiation to affect the skin immune system was first recognized in the early 1970s in numerous studies. It is therefore now generally accepted that UVA, UVB, and PUVA therapy exert a variety of immunomodulatory effects on human skin and that this is of critical importance for the therapeutic efficacy of phototherapy. Janssens et al. (40) showed that UVB hardening significantly normalizes UV-induced cell migratory responses of Langerhans cells and neutrophils in patients with PLE.

The PUVA is a very effective preventive (hardening) treatment. In approximately 70% of patients with this condition, a three- to four-week course of PUVA suffices to suppress the disease upon subsequent exposure to sunlight. The initial exposure and dose increments should be performed according to the guidelines outlined for psoriasis. The PUVA induces pigmentation rapidly and intensively at relatively low (suberythemogenic) UVA doses that usually remain well below the threshold doses for eliciting the PLE. About 10% of the patients develop typical lesions during the initial phase of PUVA. Interruption of treatment or reduction in the UVA dose is rarely required in such cases. Usually, brief symptomatic treatment with topical corticosteroids suffices (21,41,42). Treatment is given three times weekly over a period of four weeks in the early spring. The PUVA therapy protects only temporarily, and regularly repeated sun exposures are subsequently required to maintain protection. However, a considerable number of patients remain protected for two to three months, even after pigmentation has faded.

The use of narrowband 312 nm UVB phototherapy (TL-01 bulb) has become increasingly popular, being simpler to administer, possibly safer than, and apparently of comparable efficacy to PUVA (43,44). Also, exposure of prophylactic UVB may sometimes trigger the eruption, particularly in severely affected subjects, necessitating concurrent systemic corticosteroid therapy on occasion, which is usually effective.

Patients who only develop their disorder during infrequent vacations also generally respond well to oral corticosteroids prescribed for them in advance (38).

Other therapies are of uncertain efficacy. Such remedies include antimalarials, which have long been advocated (45), β-carotene (46), and nicotinamide (47). Likewise, probably only moderately effective are ω-3 polyunsaturated fatty acids (36). The efficacy of an *Escherichia coli*-filtrate (Colibiogen) awaits further confirmation (48). Also, systemic antioxidants did not reduce the severity of the disease (49). The use of immunosuppressants is certainly restricted to some rare, severe disabling cases (50,51).

HYDROA VACCINIFORME

Hydroa vacciniforme (HV) is a very rare photodermatosis of unknown etiology that principally starts in childhood, frequently resolving by adolescence or young adulthood. It is characterized by recurrent crops of papulovesicles or vesicles most commonly on the face and the dorsa of the hands, but other sun-exposed areas of the skin may also be involved. The vesicles resolve with pocklike scarring. The disease was first described by Bazin (52) in 1862, and it is possible that before the clear definition of erythropoietic protoporphyria by Magnus et al. (53), some cases may have been protoporphyria rather than hydroa because of the similarity of symptoms. Some recent reports of an association with Epstein–Barr virus (EBV) infection are interesting (54–56), but not all of the described cases are typical, associated with lymphoma (57) and may well be a different entity; but this is up to further investigations.

Epidemiology

Although it occurs in early childhood and may resolve spontaneously at puberty, some patients may suffer from life-long photosensitivity. There appears to be a male predominance for the severe manifestations, whereas milder forms (hydroa aestivale) are more common in females (58,59). Familial incidence is exceptional. In a recent study the estimated prevalence of HV was at least 0.34 cases per 100,000 with an approximately equal sex ratio. Males had a later onset and longer duration of disease than females (58).

Etiology and Pathogenesis

The pathogenesis of HV is unknown. No chromophores have been identified as yet. The UVB MED reaction is normal in the majority of the patient reported, but reduced UVA MED values have been found in some patients (58). Blood, urine, and stool porphyrins are negative and all other laboratory parameters including immunological tests are within normal limits. The course, distribution of lesions and histopathology with a perivascular lymphocytic infiltrate are somewhat reminiscent of PLE. However, the clinical features are quite different. Although the cause of the condition is unknown, its dermal, perivascular lymphocytic infiltrate suggests it may possibly be a scarring variant of PLE and thus conceivably also a delayed type hypersensitivity reaction. The action spectrum lies in the UVA region, and repetitive irradiation with broad spectrum UVA has been shown to elicit typical skin lesions that are clinically and histologically identical to those produced by natural sunlight and that heal with scarring (58–61).

Clinical Features

The HV usually presents in childhood with sometimes spontaneous improvement during adolescence. Erythema with a burning or itching sensation and sometimes associated swelling begins within hours of sufficient sun exposure in light-exposed skin areas, particularly on the face and the hands, followed by the appearance of symmetrically scattered tender papules within up to 24 hours; these generally later becoming vesicular, umbilicated, and occasionally confluent and hemorrhagic. Within a few weeks, crusting followed by detachment of the lesions leaves permanent, depressed, hypopigmented scars. Vesicles and bullae as well as the scars resemble the lesions of vaccinia (Fig. 6). Occasional systemic features include headache, malaise, and fever (59). The HV usually occurs only during the summer months, and sometimes but not always improves or resolves in adolescence (58,59). Parents generally seek specialist advice as their children are unable to tolerate sunshine (play outdoors or travel abroad) and because the eruption can result in considerable scarring, both causing significant morbidity.

Histopathology

Distinctive histologic changes include initial intraepidermal vesicle formation with later focal epidermal keratinocyte necrosis and spongiosis in association with dermal perivascular

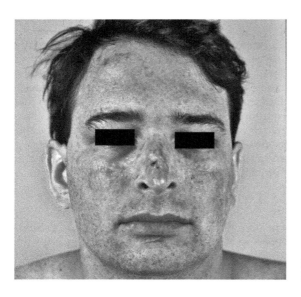

FIGURE 6 Hydroa vacciniforme: acute hemorrhagic lesions, crusting, and pock-like scarring on the face.

neutrophil leukocyte and lymphocyte infiltration. Vasculitic features have also been reported (59). Immunofluorescence findings are nonspecific.

Diagnosis

The differential diagnosis includes several photosensitivity states. However, the typical history and the clinical features are relatively characteristic. Of particular importance is the exclusion of erythropoietic protoporphyria, which may have similar morphology. An evaluation of erythrocyte protoporphyrin levels, red cell photohemolysis, and stool analysis will exclude protoporphyria.

Photoprovocation testing induces typical blisters (Fig. 7). There is now strong evidence that UVA radiation is the causal factor (58–62). In addition to reduced MED values to UVA, repetitive broad-spectrum UVA has been shown to reproduce lesions that are clinically and histologically identical to those produced by natural sunlight and that heal with scarring.

Serology for antinuclear antibody and extractable nuclear antigens (anti-Ro, La, and Sm), will exclude bullous lupus erythematosus, which quite commonly can be ruled out by its clinical symptoms. Screening for EBV is only indicated if lymphoma is suspected. However, atypical HV in patients with latent EBV infection could be reproduced by repeated UVA irradiations (63). Rare cases have been associated with metabolic disorders, such as Hartnup disease, so aminoaciduria should be ruled out (64).

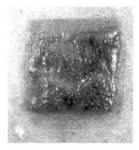 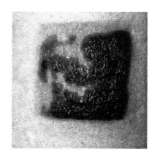 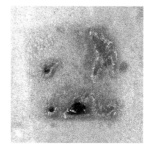

FIGURE 7 Hydroa vacciniforme. Photoprovocation: UVA irradiation (three times 30 J/cm² on three consecutive days). (*Left*) blistering after 24 hours; (*middle*) confluent hemorrhagic blisters after 48 hours; and (*right*) crusting and scar formation after two weeks.

Treatment

The HV is almost always refractory to any treatment, but restriction of sun exposure, appropriate clothing, and regular use of broad-spectrum sunscreens with an effective UVA filter can help in mild-to-moderate disease (Table 1). Windows in the car and home could be covered with certain films, which filter UV wavelengths less than 380 nm.

In patients with more severe disease, however, courses of narrow-band UVB phototherapy or PUVA administered as for PLE may occasionally help. Both phototherapy regimens usually consist of thrice weekly treatments for an average of three to four weeks. It is important to administer these therapies carefully in order not to provoke disease exacerbations (58,60–62). Antimicrobial therapy has also been tried, as have antimalarials (59,62) and systemic immunosuppressive therapy, including intermittent oral corticosteroids; although occasionally helpful, none of these appear to be reliably effective. β-carotene used in several studies, however, was mostly shown to be ineffective (60,62).

Anecdotally, dietary fish oil induced mild to good improvement in some patients (65). For severe and refractory HV unresponsive to other therapies, immunosuppressive agents, including azathioprine and cyclosporin (66), may be effective, but thalidomide does not seem to be (66). However, the use of immunosuppressive drugs for an admittedly unpleasant but otherwise benign disease should be considered carefully.

The rare nature of this condition means that there are no large or randomized trials. Evidence for treatment is based on case series or single reports.

ACTINIC PRURIGO

Actinic prurigo (AP) is a chronic photodermatosis of unknown etiology, frequent in Latin American mestizos (Caucasians and indigenous offspring) and in Amerindians living at high altitudes. A possible pathogenetic mechanism could consist of a delayed hypersensitivity reaction to UV-induced autoantigens in subjects with genetic susceptibility. The AP has been originally classified as a variant of PLE (67,68); however, there is now sufficient clinical, histologic, epidemiological, and immunogenetic data that confirm that AP and PLE are two different diseases (69).

The AP has been described under various names: solar dermatitis in 1954 (70), Guatemalan cutaneous syndrome in 1960 (71), solar prurigo in 1961 (72), light sensitive eruption in American Indians in 1961 (73), familial AP in 1968 (74), PLE (prurigo type) in 1975 (68,75), and hereditary PLE of American Indians in 1975 (76). The term that is used nowadays by most authors is "actinic prurigo," originally coined by Londoño in 1968 (74).

Epidemiology

The AP is a common chronic photodermatosis mainly affecting Mestizo populations of American countries (referring to people with mixed Indian and European ancestry), such as in Mexico, Central America, and most of South America. In the United States (77,78) and Canada (79,80), AP has been described in native American Indians and Inuit people, and some sporadic cases in Europe (81) and Asia (82).

The AP begins in the first decade of life usually around the age of four to five, affecting females more than males (ratio 2:1), and people living in regions located at altitudes higher than 1000 meters above sea level; although cases have been reported at lower altitudes. It runs a chronic course with partial or no remissions in patients living in tropical countries with intense sunlight the whole year round. In Canada, the United States, and England, the patient's condition flares during spring and summer and improves during the winter.

Etiology and Pathogenesis

In 1984, Moncada et al. (83) suggested an abnormal immune response in AP patients showing an increase of T lymphocytes in peripheral blood as well as a predominance of dermal T helper cells and Ia antigen-marked cells in the dermal infiltrate. Arrese et al. (84) re-examined the histologic characteristics of AP lesions and determined the possible role of various cell populations and mediators that participate in the pathogenesis. Immunohistochemical analysis of the dense inflammatory infiltrate showed a predominance of T helper cells clustered in the center of the lymphoid follicles and scattered in the diffuse inflammatory infiltrate. Keratinocytes showed abundant immunoreactivity for both calprotectin and TNF-α. Focal IgG and IgM deposits in the papillary dermis as well as IgM+ cells in the dense lymphocytic infiltrate and follicular center have also been demonstrated. The IL-2 was expressed in most inflammatory cells in the dermal infiltrate. It was concluded that in subjects genetically predisposed to AP, UV light might trigger excessive TNF-α production by keratinocytes whose sustained release in turn exerts its proinflammatory activity and deleterious epidermal effects.

Estrada et al. (85) described the effect of thalidomide on TNF-α serum levels, on IL-4, and on IFNγ-producing lymphocytes of AP patients. They showed that AP has indeed an immunologic component, as the clinical efficacy of thalidomide is exerted not only by inhibition of TNF-α synthesis but also by modulating of IFNγ-producing CD3+ cells, and these cells could be used as clinical markers for recovery.

Gomez et al. (86) compared cellular and humoral immunity by in vitro proliferation studies, ELISA, and immunofluorescence in AP patients and healthy controls. They found autoimmune reactivity in AP patients and postulated that AP patients may have one or more skin antigens that stimulate an autoimmune response.

For the prevalence of AP in Mestizo populations in American countries, it has been long suspected that AP patients may have a genetic predisposition that determines a particular inflammatory response to UV light. In several studies, a possible association of the expression of AP and specific alleles of the major histocompatibility complex (MHC) genes were investigated. In Saskatchewan, Canada, AP patients from the Cree Indian group had a high association with HLA-A24 and HLA-Cw4 (87), whereas in Colombia in the Chimila Indians, a high frequency of HLA-Cw4 was reported (88). In British and Irish patients, HLA-DR4 (DRB1*0407) was found to be significantly increasing in patients with AP as compared with patients with PLE (89,90). A recent study in the indigenous Chibcha family group from Colombia also revealed a high frequency of DRB1*0407 (91).

Mexican AP patients have shown a significantly increased frequency of HLA-A28 and HLA-B39 and HLA-DR4 (DRB1*0407) (92). In the Inuit people of Canada, an association with HLA-DR4 (DRB1*14) was found (93). Menagè et al. (81) suggested that the HLA type may have a causal role in patients with AP by determining the response to a particular peptide antigen, probably induced by UV radiation, to initiate the cutaneous response.

Induction of Actinic Prurigo

The AP lesions can be experimentally induced by repeated exposures to MEDs of UVA, with daily radiations of 2.5 J/cm^2 for ten days in 90% of the patients, and with UVB doses of 3 to 5 mJ cm/day for 15 days in 100% of the cases. It was shown that these patients react to broad-spectrum radiation (UVA and UVB), but their UVB and UVA MED is usually normal (94).

Clinical Features

The AP is characterized by symmetric involvement of sun-exposed areas of the skin, such as the face (eyebrows, malar regions, nose, and lips) (Fig. 8), neck, V-area of the chest, the external regions of the arms and forearms, as well as the dorsum of the hands. Lips and the conjunctiva are commonly affected (95).

The primary lesions are erythematous papules and excoriations, and crusts and lichenified plaques due to chronic scratching. Pruritus is always present and usually very intense. One important clinical feature that differentiates AP from PLE is the absence of vesicles as primary lesions in AP, although they can be seen as secondary lesions if eczema, impetigo, or contact dermatitis develops.

The lips are affected in 84% of the patients and show cheilitis with edema, crusts, fissures, ulcerations, and hyperpigmentation, whereas in mild cases only dry lips and scaling may be seen (Fig. 9).

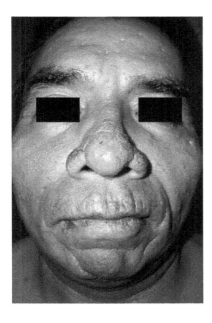

FIGURE 8   Actinic prurigo: involvement of the sun-exposed area of the face with lips affected.

Conjunctivae are affected in 45% of the patients in whom it manifests at the beginning with conjunctivitis, photophobia, watery eyes, and pruritus; after some years patients develop pigmentation and finally pseudopterygium, which in severe cases may even impair vision (Fig. 10) (96).

Histopathology

Histopathologic changes in AP have been considered nonspecific; however, it does have distinct microscopic findings. On the basis of data obtained from a large number of biopsies, an accurate diagnosis can be made and also allows to separate AP from other photodermatosis (97). Skin biopsies show hyperkeratosis, regular acanthosis, thickening of basal lamina, and a dense mainly lymphocytic perivascular infiltrate in the superficial dermis. The presence of lymphoid follicles can be observed in areas of ulceration, which supports the protective role of the stratum corneum and can explain why lymphoid follicles are more frequently found in mucosal lesions.

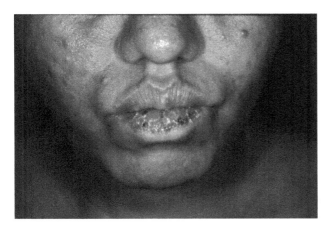

FIGURE 9   Actinic prurigo: severe lip involvement.

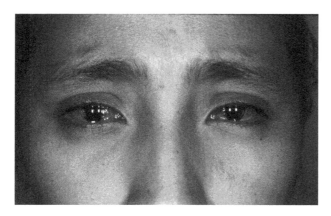

FIGURE 10 Actinic prurigo: chronic lesions of conjunctiva with pseudopteryrium.

Lip biopsies show hyperkeratosis with parakeratosis, regular acanthosis, spongiosis, and vacuolization of the basal cell layer, with areas of ulcerations in 50% of the biopsies. In the lamina propria, stromal edema, dilated capillaries are present and a dense lymphocytic infiltrate forming follicles with a prominent germinal center is found in up to 80% of the biopsies. Abundant eosinophils and mast cells are present, and in some cases the infiltrate tends to have a band-like distribution (Fig. 11).

Conjunctival biopsies exhibit areas of epithelial hyperplasia alternating with areas of atrophy. In 60% of the biopsies, marked vacuolization of basal cells and melanophages in the lamina propria are present, which are responsible for the brown discoloration observed clinically. The most constant findings are a dense lymphocytic infiltrate with follicular pattern in 88% of the biopsies.

Guevara et al. (98) in an immunohistochemical study reported an inflammatory infiltrate present in the skin, lips, and conjunctiva of AP patients, and they showed that T- and

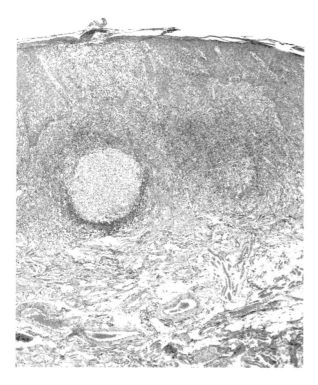

FIGURE 11 Actinic prurigo: histopathology of a lip lesion showing a dense lymphocytic infiltrate with follicular centers (10×).

B-lymphocytes are present in all of the biopsies. The B cells are in the center, and T cells are in the periphery of the lymphoid follicles.

Diagnosis

The diagnosis of AP is based on clinical and histopathological grounds. Lesions on the lips and conjunctiva are specific, and the skin offers an adequate histopathologic correlation. The experimental reproduction of AP lesions is possible with UVB and UVA.

The differential diagnoses of AP frequently include the following.

- Atopic dermatitis with photosensitivity, where the key findings are a familial incidence, an early infancy onset, the presence of xerosis, the sparing of the tip of the nose, and good response to topical corticosteroids and emollients.
- Chronic actinic dermatitis, which is quite rare, starts much later in life, and affects predominantly elderly men, with the UVB and UVA MED dramatically reduced. Histology reveals a dense lymphocytic infiltrate, which may sometimes resemble lymphoma.
- PLE is seen more frequently in Caucasian patients with no association to any particular HLA antigen. Vesicles and papulovesicles are the major part of the clinical picture and it does not affect lips or conjunctivas. Histologically it does not show follicle formation.

Treatment

Out of numerous treatment modalities that have been tried, only thalidomide has proved to be effective in most patients (Table 1). The excellent response is so constant that it can be used as a diagnostic marker of the disease (99,100). The initial daily dose is usually 100 mg, which is tapered as the patient shows clinical improvement. After several months of treatment, most patients can stop the drug and are maintained with sun-protective measures only. A few patients require maintenance doses of thalidomide as low as 25 mg weekly. Skin and lip lesions respond rapidly (within 1–2 months) but the conjunctival lesions tend to persist, although the symptoms disappear. Women of childbearing age must use adequate contraceptive measures with a very close follow-up because of the known teratogenicity. Thalidomide is usually very well tolerated, with somnolence as the most common side effect; peripheral neuropathy has not been a problem in most patient series.

Treatment modalities that are either ineffective or less effective than thalidomide are antimalarials, β-carotene, antihistamines, PUVA, and topical or systemic corticosteroids (which may be useful to treat lesions with secondary eczematization). Obviously, an essential part of AP treatment is adequate sun protection. Sunscreens, protective hats and clothing, sunglasses, and sun avoidance measures are usually enough for patients once they are clear of lesions and thalidomide is stopped. The problem is that AP affects more frequently people of lower economic status who work outdoors most of the time and in whom sun protection is almost always sub-optimal.

REFERENCES

1. Morison WL, Stern RS. Polymorphous light eruption: a common reaction uncommonly recognized. Acta Derm Venereol (Stockh) 1982; 62(3):237–240.
2. Ros AM, Wennersten G. Current aspects of polymorphous light eruption in Sweden. Photodermatology 1986; 3(5):298–302.
3. Pao C, Norris PG, Corbett M, Hawk JL. Polymorphic light eruption: prevalence in Australia and England. Br J Dermatol 1994; 130(1):62–64.
4. Khoo SW, Tay YK, Tham SN. Photodermatoses in a Singapore skin referral center. Clin Exp Dermatol 1996; 21(4):263–268.
5. Norris PG, Hawk JLM. The idiopathic photodermatoses: polymorphic light eruption, actinic prurigo and hydroa vacciniforme. In: Hawk JLM, ed. Photodermatology. London: Arnold, 1999:178–190.
6. Jansen CT. The natural history of polymorphous light eruptions. Arch Dermatol 1979; 115(2): 165–169.

7. Epstein S. Studies in abnormal human sensitivity to light. IV. Photoallergic concept of prurigo aestivalis. J Invest Dermatol 1942; 5:289–298.
8. Norris PG, Morris J, McGibbon DM, et al. Polymorphic light eruption: an immunopathological study of evolving lesions. Br J Dermatol 1989; 120(2):173–183.
9. Norris PG, Barker JNWN, Allen M, et al. Adhesion molecule expression in polymorphic light eruption. J Invest Dermatol 1992; 99(4):504–508.
10. Kölgen W, Van Weelden H, Den Hengst S, et al. CD11b+ cells and ultraviolet-B-resistant CD1a+ cells in skin of patients with polymorphous light eruption. J Invest Dermatol 1999; 113(1):4–10.
11. Kölgen W, van Meurs M, Jongsma M, et al. Differential expression of cytokines in UV-B-exposed skin of patients with polymorphous light eruption: correlation with Langerhans cell migration and immunosuppression. Arch Dermatol 2004; 140(3):295–302.
12. Palmer RA, Friedmann PS. Ultraviolet radiation causes less immunosuppression in patients with polymorphic light eruption than in controls. J Invest Dermatol 2004; 122(2):291–294.
13. van de Pas CB, Kelly DA, Seed PT, et al. Ultraviolet-radiation-induced erythema and suppression of contact hypersensitivity responses in patients with polymorphic light eruption. J Invest Dermatol 2004; 122(2):295–299.
14. Schornagel IJ, Sigurdsson V, Nijhuis EHJ, et al. Decreased neutrophil skin infiltration after UVB exposure in patients with polymorphous light eruption. Invest Dermatol 2004; 123(1):202–206.
15. Palmer RA, Hawk JL, Young AR, et al. The effect of solar-simulated radiation on the elicitation phase of contact hypersensitivity does not differ between controls and patients with polymorphic light eruption. J Invest Dermatol 2005; 124(6):1308–1312.
16. Millard TP, Bataille V, Snieder H, et al. The heritability of polymorphic light eruption. J Invest Dermatol 2000; 115(3):467–470.
17. McGregor JM, Grabczynska S, Vaughan RW, et al. Genetic modeling of abnormal photosensitivity in families with polymorphic light eruption and actinic prurigo. J Invest Dermatol 2000; 115(3):471–476.
18. McFadden JP, Norris PG, Cerio R, et al. Heat shock protein 65 immunoreactivity in experimentally induced polymorphic light eruption. Acta Derm Venereol 1994; 74(4):283–285.
19. Tegner E, Bradin AM. Polymorphous light eruption in hypopigmented pressure areas with a UVA sunbed. Acta Derm Venereol 1986; 66(5):446–448.
20. Hölzle E, Plewig G, Hofmann C, et al. Polymorphous light eruption: experimental reproduction of skin lesions. J Am Acad Dermatol 1982; 7(1):111–125.
21. Ortel B, Tanew A, Wolff K, et al. Polymorphous light eruption: action spectrum and photoprotection. J Am Acad Dermatol 1986; 14(5 Pt 1):748–753.
22. Van Praag MC, Boom BW, Vermeer BJ. Diagnosis and treatment of polymorphous light eruption. Int J Dermatol 1994; 33(4):233–239.
23. Farr PM, Diffey BL. Adverse effects of sunscreens in photosensitive patients. Lancet 1989; 1(8635):429–431.
24. Baadsgaard O, Cooper KD, Lisby S, et al. Dose response and time course for induction of T6-DR+; human epidermal antigen-presenting cells by in vivo ultraviolet A, B, and C irradiation. J Am Acad Dermatol 1987; 17(5 Pt 1):792–800.
25. Rivers JK, Norris PG, Murphy GM, et al. UVA sunbeds: tanning, photoprotection, acute adverse effects and immunological changes. Br J Dermatol 1989; 120(6):767–777.
26. Piletta PA, Salomon D, Beani JC, et al. A pilot with an itchy rash. Lancet 1996; 348(9035):1142.
27. Hampton PJ, Farr PM, Diffey BL, et al. Implication for photosensitive patients of ultraviolet A exposure in vehicles. Br J Dermatol 2004; 151(4):873–876.
28. Palmer RA, van de Pas CB, Campalani E, et al. A simple method to assess severity of polymorphic light eruption. Br J Dermatol 2004; 151(3):645–652.
29. Jansen CT, Karvonen J. Polymorphous light eruption. A seven-year follow-up evaluation of 114 patients. Arch Dermatol 1984; 120(7):862–865.
30. Dover JS, Hawk JLM. Polymorphic light eruption sine eruptione. Br J Dermatol 1988; 118(1):73–76.
31. Hawk J. Juvenile spring eruption is a variant of polymorphic light eruption. NZ Med J 1996; 109(1031):389.
32. Thomas P, Amblard P. Lucite estivale benigne. In: Thomas P, Amblard P, eds. Photodermatologie et Photothérapie, Paris: Masson, 1988:49–51.
33. Hawk JLM, Smith NP, Black MM. The photosensitivity disorders. In: Elder DE, Elenitsas R, Jaworsky C, Johnson B Jr, eds. Lever's Histopathology of the Skin. Philadelphia: Lippincott-Raven, 1997:305–310.
34. Hölzle E, Plewig G, von Kries R, et al. Polymorphous light eruption. J Invest Dermatol 1987; 88(suppl. 3):32s–38s.
35. van de Pas CB, Hawk JL, Young AR, et al. An optimal method for experimental provocation of polymorphic light eruption. Arch Dermatol 2004; 140(3):286–292.
36. Ling TC, Gibbs NK, Rhodes LE. Treatment of polymorphic light eruption. Photodermatol Photoimmunol Photomed 2003; 19(5):217–227.

37. Hadshiew I, Stab F, Untiedt S, et al. Effects of topically applied antioxidants in experimentally provoked polymorphous light eruption. Dermatology 1997; 195(4):362–368.
38. Patel DC, Bellaney GJ, Seed PT, et al. Efficacy of short-course oral prednisolone in polymorphic light eruption: a randomized controlled trial. Br J Dermatol 2000; 143(4):828–831.
39. Kontos AP, Cusack CA, Chaffins M, et al. Polymorphous light eruption in African Americans: pinpoint papular variant. Photodermatol Photoimmunol Photomed 2002; 18(6):303–306.
40. Janssens AS, Pavel S, Out-Luiting JJ, et al. Normalized ultraviolet (UV) induction of Langerhans cell depletion and neutrophil infiltrates after artificial UVB hardening of patients with polymorphic light eruption. Br J Dermatol 2005; 152(6):1268–1274.
41. Hönigsmann H. Polymorphous light eruption. In: Lim HW, Soter NA, eds. Clinical Photomedicine. New York: Marcel Dekker, 1993:167–179.
42. Murphy GM, Logan RA, Lovell CR, et al. Prophylactic PUVA and UVB therapy in polymorphic light eruption—a controlled trial. Br J Dermatol 1987; 116(4):531–538.
43. Bilsland D, George SA, Gibbs NK, et al. A comparison of narrow band phototherapy (TL-01) and photochemotherapy (PUVA) in the management of polymorphic light eruption. Br J Dermatol 1993; 129(6):708–712.
44. Man I, Dawe S, Ferguson J. Artificial hardening for polymorphic light eruption: practical points from ten years' experience. Photodermatol Photoimmunol Photomed 1999; 15(3–4):96–99.
45. Murphy GM, Hawk JLM, Magnus IA. Hydroxychloroquine in polymorphic light eruption: a controlled trial with drug and visual sensitivity monitoring. Br J Dermatol 1987; 116(3):379–386.
46. Corbett MF, Hawk JL, Herxheimer A, et al. Controlled therapeutic trials in polymorphic light eruption. Br J Dermatol 1982; 107(5):571–581.
47. Ortel B, Wechdorn D, Tanew A, et al. Effect of nicotinamide on the phototest reaction in polymorphous light eruption. Br J Dermatol 1988; 118(5):669–673.
48. Przybilla B, Heppeler M, Ruzicka T. Preventive effect of an E. coli-filtrate (Colibiogen) in polymorphous light eruption. Br J Dermatol 1989; 121(2):229–233.
49. Eberlein-Konig B, Fesq H, Abeck D, et al. Systemic vitamin C and vitamin E do not prevent photoprovocation test reactions in polymorphous light eruption. Photodermatol Photoimmunol Photomed 2000; 16(2):50–52.
50. Norris PG, Hawk JLM. Successful treatment of severe polymorphic light eruption with azathioprine. Arch Dermatol 1989; 125(10):1377.
51. Shipley DR, Hewitt JB. Polymorphic light eruption treated with cyclosporin. Br J Dermatol 2001; 144(2):446–447.
52. Bazin E: Leçons théorétiques et cliniques sur les affections génériques de la peau. Vol. 1. Paris: Delebrage, 1862:132.
53. Magnus IA, Jarret A, Prankerd TAJ, et al. Erythropoietic protoporphyria: a new porphyria syndrome with solar urticaria due to protoporphyrinaemia. Lancet 1961; 26(2):448–451.
54. Cho KH, Kim CW, Heo DS, et al. Epstein-Barr virus-associated peripheral T-cell lymphoma in adults with hydroa vacciniforme-like lesions. Clin Exp Dermatol 2001; 26(3):242–247.
55. Ohtsuka T, Okita H, Otuska S, et al. Hydroa vacciniforme with latent Epstein-Barr virus infection. Br J Dermatol 2001; 145(3):509–510.
56. Cho KH, Lee SH, Kim CW, et al. Epstein-Barr virus-associated lymphoproliferative lesions presenting as a hydroa vacciniforme-like eruption: an analysis of six cases. Br J Dermatol 2004; 151(2):372–380.
57. Steger GG, Dittrich C, Hönigsmann H, et al. Permanent cure of hydroa vacciniforme after treatment of Hodgkin's disease with C-MOPP/AS VD regimen. Br J Dermatol 1988; 119(5):684–685.
58. Gupta G, Man I, Kemmett D. Hydroa vacciniforme: a clinical and follow-up study of 17 cases. J Am Acad Dermatol 2000; 42(2 Pt 1):208–213.
59. Sonnex TS, Hawk JLM. Hydroa vacciniforme: a review of ten cases. Br J Dermatol 1988; 118(1):101–108.
60. Jaschke E, Hönigsmann H. Hydroa vacciniforme-Aktionsspektrum, UV-Toleranz nach Photochemotherapie. Hautarzt 1981; 32(7):350–353.
61. Halasz CL, Leach EE, Walther RR, et al. Hydroa vacciniforme: induction of lesions with ultraviolet A. J Am Acad Dermatol 1983; 8(2):171–176.
62. Goldgeier MH, Nordlund JJ, Lucky AW, et al. Hydroa vacciniforme: diagnosis and therapy. Arch Dermatol 1982; 118(8):588–591.
63. Heo EP, Park SH, Kim TH. Artificial reproduction of atypical hydroa vacciniforme caused by latent Epstein-Barr virus infection. Int J Dermatol 2003; 42(6):476–479.
64. Ashurst PJ. Hydroa vacciniforme occurring in association with Hartnup disease. Br J Dermatol 1969; 81(7):486–492.
65. Rhodes LE, White SI. Dietary fish oil as a photoprotective agent in hydroa vacciniforme. Br J Dermatol 1998; 138(1):173–178.
66. Blackwell V, McGregor JM, Hawk JLM. Hydroa vacciniforme presenting in an adult successfully treated with cyclosporin A. Clin Exp Dermatol 1998; 23(2):73–76.

67. Epstein JH. Polymorphous light eruption; phototest technique studies. Arch Dermatol 1962; 85(4):502–504.

68. Epstein JH. Polymorphous light eruption. J Am Acad Dermatol 1980; 3(4):329–343.

69. Addo HA, Frain-Bell W. Actinic prurigo—a specific photodermatosis? Photodermatol 1984; 1(3):119–128.

70. Escalona E. Dermatología. Lo esencial para el estudiante. México: Impresiones Modernas, S.A. 1964:194.

71. Cordero CFA. Síndrome cutáneo guatemalense en la dermatitis actínica. Med Cut ILA 1976; 4:393–400.

72. López González G. Prúrigo solar. Arch Argent Dermatol 1961; 11(9):301–318.

73. Everett MA, Crockett W, Lamb JH, et al. Light sensitive eruption in American Indians. Arch Dermatol 1961; 83(2):243–246.

74. Londoño F, Mundi F, Giraldo F, et al. Familial actinic prurigo. Arch Argent Dermatol 1966; 16(4):290–307.

75. Hojyo-Tomoka MT, Dominguez-Soto L. Clinical and epidemiological characteristics of polymorphous light eruption. Castellania 1975; 3:21–23.

76. Birt AR, Davis RA. Hereditary polymorphic light eruption of American Indians. Int J Dermatol 1975; 14(2):105–111.

77. Brandt R. Dermatological observations on the Navajo reservation. Arch Dermatol 1958; 71:681–685.

78. Fusaro RM, Johnson JA. Hereditary polymorphic light eruption in American Indians. Photoprotection and prevention of streptococcal pyoderma and glomerulonephritis. J Am Med Assoc 1980; 244(13):1456–1459.

79. Birt AR, Davis RA. Photodermatitis in North American Indians: familial actinic prurigo. Int J Dermatol 1971; 10(2):107–114.

80. Lane PR, Hogan DJ, Martel MJ, et al. Actinic prurigo: clinical features and prognosis. J Am Acad Dermatol 1992; 26(5 Pt 1):683–692.

81. Menagè HP, Vaughan RW, Baker CS, et al. HLA-DR4 may determine expression of actinic prurigo in British patients. J Invest Dermatol 1996; 106(2):362–364.

82. Wong NS, Khoo LS. Analysis of photodermatoses seen in a predominantly Asian population at a photodermatology clinic in Singapore. Photodermatol Photoimmunol Photomed 2005; 21(1):40–44.

83. Moncada B, Gonzalez-Amaro R, Baranda L, et al. Immunopathology of polymorphous light eruption. T lymphocytes in blood and skin. J Am Acad Dermatol 1984; 10(6):970–973.

84. Arrese JE, Dominguez-Soto L, Hojyo-Tomoka MT, et al. Effectors of inflammation in actinic prurigo. J Am Acad Dermatol 2001; 44(6):957–961.

85. Estrada I, Garibay-Escobar A, Núñez-Vazquez A, et al. Evidence that thalidomide modifies the immune response of patients suffering from actinic prurigo. Int J Dermatol 2004; 43(12):893–897.

86. Gomez A, Umaña A, Trespalacios AA. Immune responses to isolated human skin antigens in actinic prurigo. Med Sci Monit 2006; 12(3):BR106–BR113.

87. Sheridan DP, Lane PR, Irvine J, et al. HLA typing in actinic prurigo. J Am Acad Dermatol 1990; 22(6 Pt 1):1019–1023.

88. Bernal JE, Duran MM, Ordoñez CO, et al. Actinic prurigo among the Chimila Indians: HLA studies. J Am Acad Dermatol 1990; 22(6 Pt 1):1049–1051.

89. Grabczynska SA, McGregor JM, Kondeatis E, et al. Actinic prurigo and polymorphic light eruption: common pathogenesis and the importance of HLA-DR4/DRB1*0407. Br J Dermatol 1999; 140(2):232–236.

90. O'Reilly FM, Spencer S, Darke C, et al. HLA–DR4B1*0407 strong association with actinic prurigo in Ireland. Br J Dermatol 1996; 135(suppl. 47):65.

91. Suarez A, Valbuena MC, Rey M, et al. Association of HLA subtype DRB1*0407 in Colombian patients with actinic prurigo. Photodermatol Photoimmunol Photomed 2006; 22(2):55–58.

92. Hojyo-Tomoka T, Grados J, Vargas-Alarcon G, et al. Further evidence of the role of HLA-DR4 in the genetic susceptibility to actinic prurigo. J Am Acad Dermatol 1997; 36(6 Pt 1):935–937.

93. Wiseman MC, Orr PH, McDonald SM, et al. Actinic prurigo: clinical features and HLA associations in a Canadian Inuit population. J Am Acad Dermatol 2001; 44(6):952–956.

94. Hojyo-Tomoka MT. Pruebas fotobiológicas en prurigo actínico. Dermatol Hojyo-Tomoka MT 1993; 37(suppl. 1):328.

95. Hojyo-Tomoka MT, Vega-Memije ME, Cortes-Franco R, et al. Diagnosis and treatment of actinic prurigo. Dermatol Ther 2003; 16(1):40–44.

96. Hojyo-Tomoka T, Vega-Memije E, Granados J, et al. Actinic prurigo: an update. Int J Dermatol 1995; 44(6):380–384.

97. Vega ME. Características histopatológicas del prurigo actínico. Dermatol Rev Mex 1993; 37(suppl. 1):295–297.

98. Guevara E, Hojyo-Tomoka MT, Vega-Memije ME. Cortes-Franco R, Domínguez-Soto L. Estudio immunohistoquímico para demostrar la presencia de linfocitos T y B en el infiltrado inflamatorio de las biopsias de piel, labio y conjuntiva de pacientes con prurigo actínico. Dermatol Rev Mex 1997; 41:223–226.
99. Londoño F. Thalidomide in the treatment of actinic prúrigo. Int J Dermatol 1973; 12(5):326–328.
100. Vega E, Hojyo-Tomoka MT, Dominguez-Soto L. Tratamiento del prurigo actínico con talidomida: estudio de 30 pacientes. Dermatol Rev Mex 1993; 37(suppl 1):342–343.

12 | Chronic Actinic Dermatitis

John L. M. Hawk
Photobiology Unit, St. John's Institute of Dermatology, St. Thomas' Hospital, King's College of London, London, England, U.K.

Henry W. Lim
Department of Dermatology, Henry Ford Hospital, Detroit, Michigan, U.S.A.

- CAD is a form of eczema induced by ultraviolet and rarely also visible radiation.

- The inducing action spectrum frequently resembles that for sunburn in shape, although acting at lower doses and leading to eczema, but suggesting a similar or associated absorbing molecule may be responsible through a different mechanism.

- CAD has exactly the features of allergic contact dermatitis but seems to be a response instead to a photo-altered absorbing molecule as mentioned above rather than to an exogenous substance.

- Older people with outdoor interests, particularly gardening, are most affected, often following prior eczema, particularly atopic in younger people, later more frequently airborne contact or probably seborrheic, whereas HIV disease may also rarely be a predisposing factor.

- CAD affects exposed areas, initially patchily, later confluently, sometimes with marked lichenification or a pseudolymphomatous appearance previously known as actinic reticuloid, with rare late progression to erythroderma.

- The condition is harmless of itself but extremely persistent and distressing before not infrequent gradual resolution over decades, although in exceptionally rare instances it may perhaps represent a form of cutaneous lymphoma.

- The treatment of CAD requires restriction of exposure to the inducing ultraviolet and rarely visible wavelengths and to any contact allergens, wearing of ultraviolet-protective clothing, regular application of high protection factor, broad-spectrum sunscreens, topical eczema therapy with emollients, steroids, and if necessary calcineurin inhibitors, or in severe cases with immunosuppressive oral agents or rarely phototherapy.

INTRODUCTION

hronic actinic dermatitis (CAD), as originally proposed by Hawk and Magnus in 1979 (1), is a clinical entity embracing different presentations of the same condition, previously known separately and somewhat confusingly as actinic reticuloid (AR) (2), photosensitive eczema (3), and photosensitivity dermatitis (PD) (4), but now all shown to be variants of CAD. It was also noted as essentially synonymous with the PD/AR syndrome as used in a slightly less embracing way by Frain-Bell et al. (4), and the originally described form, persistent light reaction (reactivity) (PLR) (5), not understood at that stage. All the previous terms, although briefly mentioned for interest and historical reasons below, and except perhaps for the occasional use of AR to refer to the severest variant of CAD, should now be discarded for clarity.

PLR as first described by Wilkinson in 1962 (5) was a persisting eczema of light-exposed sites following an apparently completed episode of topical photoallergic contact dermatitis, thereafter remaining despite avoidance of the original allergen and irrespective of whether the currently affected sites had been previously exposed to allergen. The wavelengths responsible for the eruption were reported to be not only in the UVA (315–400 nm) waveband, generally responsible for photoallergenic responses, but also in the UVB (280–315 nm), thereby fulfilling the requirements later defined for CAD. PLR was first noted to occur following photoallergic contact sensitization to halogenated phenols (tetrachlorsalicylanilide and tribromosalicylanilide) (5), then antibacterial agents present in soaps, to antiseptics and toiletries such as bithionol (6), and later to the fragrance musk ambrette (7), a synthetic agent once used widely in aftershave preparations. Other occasionally implicated products have been quinoxaline-N-dioxide in animal foodstuffs (8), zinc pyrithione (9), and certain bleaching agents (10), but such substances have largely been withdrawn and PLR as originally described, although apparently an original precursor of CAD, now appears vanishingly rare.

AR was first reported in 1969 by Ive et al. (2), its major clinical characteristic being infiltrated erythematous, or reticuloid, plaques of the exposed skin of elderly men, arising on a background of eczematous, erythematous, or normal skin. A clinical resemblance to the features of severe photoallergic contact dermatitis was noted, but photopatch tests were generally negative and the eruption was inducible by UVB, UVA, and sometimes also visible irradiation, as later described for CAD. The histical features were often noted closely to resemble those of cutaneous T-cell lymphoma (CTCL). AR is still occasionally observed as the most severe variant of CAD but with a much reduced frequency, almost certainly because of earlier recognition, diagnosis, and treatment.

Photosensitive eczema, described by Ramsay and Kobza-Black in 1973 (3), was a much milder, purely eczematous photo-eruption, also of exposed sites, without detectable photoallergy. A resemblance to AR was noted but the disease action spectrum was essentially just in the UVB region.

PD, reported shortly after by Frain-Bell et al. in 1974 (4), was also an exposed site eczema but now with an action spectrum often extending beyond the UVB into the UVA.

Hawk and Magnus in 1979 (1) then demonstrated a significant overlap between the features of photosensitive eczema, AR, and by implication PD, describing patients with the clinical and histological changes of eczema and the photobiological abnormalities of AR, and vice versa. They had also noted transitions between these disease states (11) and, therefore, unified all the variants of what appeared to be the same condition within the term CAD. Transition from PLR to AR was also later observed, as well as overlaps between PLR and CAD (12). In 1990, it was therefore proposed that PLR should also be included within the term CAD (13,14), thus at once simplifying the disease terminology and relegating PLR, AR, photosensitive eczema, and PD to terms of predominantly historical interest. Finally, the introduction of unifying diagnostic criteria has led to a better understanding of CAD and facilitated its recognition (13,15,16). Thus CAD is an eczema of exposed skin generally induced by UVB, sometimes also UVA, and rarely visible light as well, although sensitivity to other combinations of the above spectra have occasionally been noted.

PATHOGENESIS

The pathogenesis of CAD remains incompletely understood, although many aspects of it have been elucidated, and the clinical and histological appearances of the disease and its immuno-histochemical abnormalities are all similar in nature to those of delayed type hypersensitivity (DTH) responses and, in particular, allergic contact dermatitis. This is further supported by the known responsiveness of the condition to immunosuppressive agents such as cyclosporine and azathioprine. It is therefore likely that CAD is of similar nature, but by inference a reaction against cutaneous photo-induced endogenous antigen rather than an external contact agent.

Thus, the often pseudolymphomatous clinical and histological appearances of severe forms of CAD, and the dermal infiltrate containing a predominance of CD8+ T cells (17), are exactly the same as those previously reported in persistent allergic contact dermatitis against phosphorus sesquisulphide (18).

Also, a variety of other studies characterizing the CAD dermal infiltrate have also shown it to contain predominantly T cells, which are always present in DTH reactions, both in fully evolved (19–22) and new lesions (23,24), together also characteristically with Langerhans cells, interdigitating reticulum cells, and monocyte-macrophages, particularly CD36+ (OKM5+), factor XIIIa+, CD11b+, CD11c+, and CD14+ cells (23,24). Leukocyte epidermotropism is also observed, whereas keratinocytes express major histocompatibility class II antigens in induced lesions (23,24).

Further, a predominance of CD4+ cells has been noted in some studies (20,23), equal ratios in others (20,21), and a predominance of CD8+ in others again (22,24), the last particularly in lesions with more florid histological changes (17), and most workers agree that CD4+ cells similarly predominate over CD8+ in the early stages of known DTH reactions (25,26), with CD8+ cells becoming more numerous later (24). In addition, the pattern and time course of the infiltrating cells in evoked lesions of the disease in one study (23), particularly of epidermal and dermal activated T cells, epidermal Langerhans cells, and monocyte-macrophages, all peaking around 24 to 48 hours, again resembled the changes of DTH (25), and clearly differed from those induced by UVB irradiation of normal skin in which T- and Langerhans cell epidermotropism is not observed (27).

Analysis of circulating blood lymphocyte CD4+ to CD8+ ratios in CAD is normal in some patients (17,28) and reduced in others (17,21,24), particularly in florid CAD (29), correlating with simultaneous changes in the cutaneous infiltrate (17).

Specific changes in the kinetics and pattern of cell surface adhesion molecule expression have also been reported in DTH, and in five patients with CAD, timed biopsies after several minimal lesion-inducing doses of solar-simulated radiation (less than a minimal sunburning dose in normal subjects) demonstrated the upregulated expression of perivascular ICAM-1, VCAM-1, and E-selectin, dermal interstitial ICAM-1 and VCAM-1, and basal and focal epidermal keratinocyte ICAM-1, from within a few hours up to several days (30). These changes again resemble those occurring in DTH reactions (31,32), further suggesting CAD is a similar process, and differ from normal reactions to UVB irradiation, in which E-selectin expression is less prolonged and keratinocyte ICAM-1 and VCAM-1 are not expressed, and to combined UVB and UVA irradiation, in which keratinocyte ICAM-1 expression in vitro is delayed by 48 hours (31,33).

Cytokine production by keratinocytes also plays an important role in the initiation and maintenance of the allergic contact dermatitis reaction. Studies on this in the pathogenesis of CAD lesions are limited, but one immunohistochemical time course study of induced lesions supports a pro-inflammatory role for interleukin-1α, regulated by its receptor and receptor antagonist (34), as also seen in delayed immunological reactions.

These presumed DTH changes might therefore be a response against putative antigen created either through direct ultraviolet skin molecular absorption and distortion, or through endogenously photosensitized secondary oxidative damage within the skin, suggestions supported by the fact that albumin for example may become antigenic in vitro through photo-oxidation of its component histidine (35). In addition, CAD often occurs in association with pre-existing widespread, often airborne, contact dermatitis to an exogenous sensitizer or photosensitizer (36), especially that reported from England and Scotland, or perhaps occasionally drug-induced photosensitivity (13,37), such reactions arguably enhancing cutaneous immune function during light exposure to a sufficient degree to enable presumed endogenous photo-antigen recognition. Instead or as well, chronic photo-damage may conceivably impair ultraviolet-induced cutaneous immunosuppression such that normal endogenous ultraviolet-induced skin photo-antigen is more easily recognized, as seemingly occurs genetically in polymorphic light eruption (38), particularly in that elderly outdoor workers or enthusiasts are most often affected in CAD (36). Further, their photo-aged skin may conceivably lead to slower presumed antigen removal, as well as easier associated contact allergen penetration, such that immune antigen recognition is further facilitated. Finally, CAD may also occasionally develop in patients with long-standing endogenous eczema, very possibly a reaction of equally predisposing nature to allergic contact dermatitis, although CAD may also apparently arise in previously normal skin. As the disorder then gradually progresses (39), so too do the characteristic irradiation abnormalities of CAD develop.

There is no evidence for a genetic susceptibility to CAD, no positive family history or significant HLA association (personal communication, H. du P. Menagé) having been noted in patients with the disease, suggesting that it is therefore acquired. This may perhaps occur through continuing solar and ambient allergen exposure as suggested above, particularly as the condition develops readily in those with outdoor occupations or hobbies, whereas a report of onset after accidental UVC exposure again suggests that excessive ultraviolet exposure may be contributory (40). Thus, environmental rather than genetic factors appear to explain why patients develop CAD, and perhaps also the male and elderly predominance of the disorder.

Determination of the action spectrum for the induction of CAD might also help establish the nature of the presumptive antigen. In fact, this action spectrum is often of the same shape as that for sunburn (41), but in the case of CAD, the eruption is eczematous, and much lower irradiation doses are generally needed to induce the response. Therefore, the ultraviolet-absorbing molecule in at least some CAD is likely to be a similar or associated molecule to that leading to sunburn, but now acting as an antigen, namely DNA (42), RNA, or the like. It seems likely to be a different molecule altogether in rarer instances, some patients seeming sensitive to just UVA (43), and possibly even more rarely to just 600 nm visible light (44). On the other hand, preliminary studies with the autologous mixed epidermal cell leukocyte culture reaction failed to detect antigen in lesional CAD dermal and epidermal skin (45), although this may have been the result of experimental difficulties in ensuring adequate antigen preservation within patient skin. Definitive evidence of an antigen-driven process as the basis for CAD is therefore still awaited.

Thus in summary, CAD is very likely an allergic contact dermatitis-like response against ultraviolet radiation-damaged DNA or a similar or associated molecule, at least in some instances, perhaps because of airborne contact dermatitis-enhanced immune reactivity, or else photo-damaged immunosuppressive activity, in often long-standing sunlight- and airborne allergen-exposed subjects.

CLINICAL ASPECTS (TABLE 1)

CAD is relatively uncommon, its incidence in Scotland for example being only around one in 6000 (46). Males are much more often affected, but women probably increasingly so, now

TABLE 1 Predisposing or Associated Features in Chronic Actinic Dermatitis

Male sex
Older age
Outdoor life style
Human immunodeficiency virus infection (probable, rare)
Chronic endogenous eczema, particularly atopic (early-onset disease), seborrheic, rarely palmar or plantar
Allergic contact dermatitis, often airborne
Topical photoallergic contact dermatitis (previously, then known as persistent light reactivity; probably no longer occurs)
Systemic drug photosensitivity (uncertain, rare)

representing between 10% (46) and 22% (47) of those with the disease. Older subjects are most at risk, the mean CAD patient age being 65 years (47), although younger people, particularly with atopic eczema (48), may occasionally be affected. White Caucasians are predominant, although Japanese (12,47), other Asians (49), Afro-Caribbeans (47), and African Americans (50) are not exempt. In fact, in the United States, CAD is commonly seen among individuals with dark skin (13). The disease appears to be more common in temperate climates, although it does represent 15% of patients with photodermatoses in a referral center in Singapore (49). Familial incidence is not reported. Outdoor workers and leisure enthusiasts, particularly gardeners, most commonly develop CAD, although it has also been reported in patients treated over long periods with potentially photosensitizing medications such as thiazide diuretics (37); nevertheless, since such medicines are most commonly used in the elderly, it is not absolutely certain that they may induce the disorder. CAD has finally been noted to occur on occasion in subjects with human immunodeficiency virus (HIV) infection (51,52).

Allergic contact dermatitis to ubiquitous, frequently airborne, allergens often accompanies CAD (46) and may precede its onset (39,53). Positive responses to at least one of these allergens are found in about 75% of patients and to two or more in 65% (47). Compositae plant extracts, and to a lesser extent fragrance compounds and colophony are most often incriminated, with metals, rubber, epoxy resins, phosphorus sesquisulphide, medicaments, preservatives, and vehicle bases being occasional offenders (36,47,53–57). Rarely, contact dermatitis to sunscreens also supervenes during the course of the disease (13,56). Photoallergic contact dermatitis is also possible but rare, although the disorder as originally reported regularly evolved from photocontact dermatitis, then being known as PLR; this progression has now essentially ceased presumably with the gradual removal of potential photocontact allergens from the environment.

Finally, a moderate number of CAD patients progress to the disorder following suffering other eczemas, particularly atopic, and probably also seborrheic, palmar, or plantar (2,3,44). Thus, only around 10% of those with CAD have had no previous contact, photocontact, or endogenous eczema (47).

CAD is generally more severe in spring and summer (Fig. 1), although its dependence on ultraviolet exposure is not always obvious to patient or physician. Thus, the eruption may not deteriorate for hours to days after irradiation, and it may also continue into winter, albeit usually in milder form. It may also become disguised further by progression toward erythroderma or the simultaneous presence of contact dermatitis. Nevertheless, many patients do recognize an exacerbation of their condition by sun exposure, especially early in the disease, increased itching, and worsening of the eruption occurring within minutes to hours of exposure.

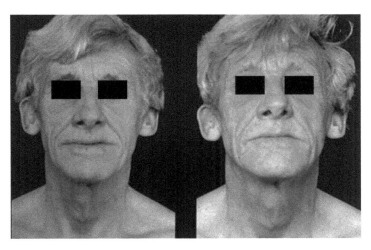

FIGURE 1 Chronic actinic dermatitis showing eczema of exposed facial skin worse in summer (*right*) than in winter (*left*). *Source*: Courtesy of H. du P. Menagé.

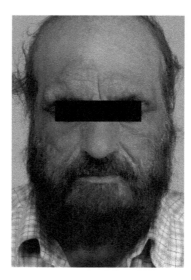

FIGURE 2 Chronic actinic dermatitis of exposed areas of face with clear cut-off on forehead where turban normally worn.

There is normally subacute or chronic, extremely pruritic eczema of predominantly sun-exposed sites, particularly face, back and sides of neck, upper chest, scalp, and backs of hands, characteristically with clear cut-off at lines of clothing (Figs. 2–4). In addition, the upper eyelids, submental area, areas behind the earlobes, skin creases and folds, and finger webs are often spared, more obviously when the eruption is confluent elsewhere (Fig. 5). In severely affected patients, generalization of the eruption to covered sites is possible (Fig. 6) and erythroderma may rarely develop. Lichenification is common in chronic disease, whereas in the most severely affected patients, probably following persistent failures of diagnosis or adequate treatment, shiny, infiltrated papules, and plaques mimicking those of cutaneous lymphoma may develop (2) (Fig. 7); palmar and occasionally plantar eczema may also supervene. Areas of hyper- or hypopigmentation too may occur in severe CAD, the latter tending to mimic vitiligo and probably occurring through melanocytic destruction by the disease process (58). Eyebrow and scalp hair may also be stubbly or lost from constant rubbing or scratching.

CAD patients in the past have on occasion committed suicide, probably because of the previously intractable nature of the condition (2), but this no longer seems to occur, almost

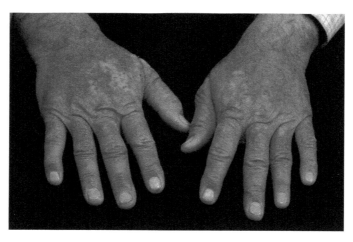

FIGURE 3 Chronic actinic dermatitis of backs of hands with cut-off at shirt cuffs at wrists.

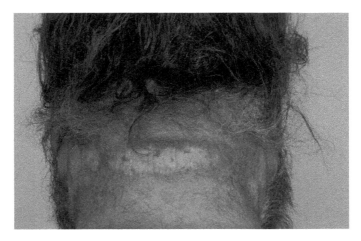

FIGURE 4 Chronic actinic dermatitis of back of neck with cut-off at shirt collar.

certainly because of better diagnosis and treatment. However, some patients may still be severely despondent.

Once established, CAD tends to persist over many years before not infrequent gradual resolution. It has been estimated that the probability of resolution by 10 years from diagnosis is 1 in 5; poorer prognosis is associated with severe abnormal UVB photosensitivity, and the identification of contact allergens in two or more patch test series (59). Malignant lymphomatous transformation has also been claimed on a number of occasions (60–63), arguably following chronic antigenic stimulation in long-standing, untreated disease (64), but it seems just as likely that these rarities are coincidental occurrences or diagnostic confusions rather than causal associations. Thus, a comparison of the incidence of lymphoma in CAD patients with that obtained from sex-matched national morbidity data did not indicate any increased risk (65), nor a study of the natural history of CAD over decades (59,66), nor again a flow cytometric study showing no evidence of DNA aneuploidy in the cutaneous infiltrate of CAD patients (67), nor finally T-cell receptor and immunoglobulin gene rearrangement studies demonstrating a lack of lymphoid clonality in the disorder (29). Thus, if present at all, the risk of lymphomatous transformation in CAD must be at most exceptionally rare. On the other hand,

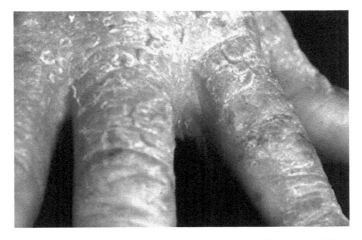

FIGURE 5 Chronic actinic dermatitis with sparing of finger-web skin.

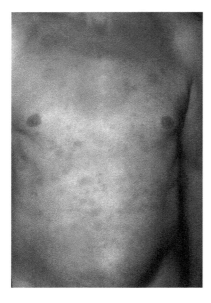

FIGURE 6 Chronic actinic dermatitis with sub-erythrodermic spread on to trunk.

importantly, very occasional malignant lymphomas may just perhaps be markedly light-sensitive of themselves (68).

HISTOPATHOLOGY

The histopathology of CAD (69) demonstrates epidermal spongiosis and acanthosis, on occasion with hyperplasia, along usually with a deep dermal, predominantly perivascular, often dense, mononuclear cell infiltrate, and not infrequently large, hyperchromatic, convoluted nuclei and mitotic figures. Macrophages, eosinophils, and plasma cells may also occur, whereas in extreme situations, the disorder may be impossible to differentiate from CTCL.

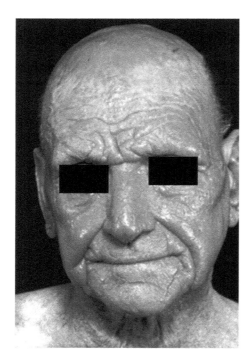

FIGURE 7 Chronic actinic dermatitis showing shiny pseudolymphomatous plaques of face in severe actinic reticuloid variant.

Immunophenotypic marker studies are then helpful, which usually show the predominance of CD8+ cells in CAD, and CD4+ cells in CTCL (17,70).

PHOTOTESTING

This is always abnormal in moderate to severe CAD, confirming the disorder, but in early, mild disease as is now fairly often seen because of better recognition, abnormal phototest results are not always observed. When the responses are abnormal, reduced ultraviolet doses are generally required to produce erythema at 24 hours, though sometimes earlier or later, and such reactions are morphologically different from those of sunburn, representing instead papular or eczematous lesions characteristic of the disease itself (4). They may also be pruritic and are usually to the UVB wavelengths, often also the UVA, and rarely visible light as well, but occasional abnormalities have been reported to just the UVA (4,43,50,71), and also very rarely to just 600 nm visible light (44,50,71). These latter cases, although not fulfilling the originally proposed diagnostic criteria (1), appear to be rare examples of otherwise typical CAD, presumably resulting from initial radiation absorption by other than usual chromophores.

    With the solar simulator or other broad spectrum sources, reduced minimal erythema doses are also often seen, except again perhaps in early, mild disease, whereas an appearance approximating eczema or else just a confluent raised erythematous plaque may regularly occur over the whole irradiation site. These areas may again be pruritic.

    If oral or topical steroids are needed to clear any eruption at the test site before exposure, testing should not take place until several days after their cessation, or the oral steroid dose has been minimal for at least a few days; otherwise, false negative results will very likely occur (72).

DIAGNOSIS (TABLE 2)

CAD is initially suggested by the patient's history and clinical appearance, assisted where necessary by the histological features of eczema, sometimes pseudolymphomatous in severe cases (Fig. 7). Abnormal phototest results following broad-band or monochromatic irradiation of unaffected skin are in all cases the preferred final method of disease confirmation. Such results were previously considered essential (1), but in early, very mild disease they may not always be present, and diagnosis based on compelling clinical and if necessary histological features seems acceptable in these occasional instances.

    Patch and photopatch testing should be undertaken in all patients and frequently reveals positive results to ubiquitous airborne, topical or rarely other allergens. These may have predisposed to onset of the CAD, but in any case, they contribute to the clinical picture and their avoidance is essential to optimal treatment of the patient.

    In relatively rare instances where CAD is suspected but the skin sites for phototesting or patch and photopatch testing are significantly eczematised, clearance of the eruption in a darkened room over days to a week or two is necessary prior to testing to avoid false negative

TABLE 2 Diagnosis of Chronic Actinic Dermatitis

Clinical features	Eczematous eruption of exposed areas, sometimes with pseudolymphomatous features in severe cases
Histology of lesional skin	Chronic eczema, sometimes with pseudolymphomatous features in severe cases, rarely indistinguishable from cutaneous T-cell lymphoma
Phototest responses	Irradiation monochromator: reduced 24-hr MED, papular responses to UVB representing disease itself, usually also to UVA, rarely visible light as well; occasionally to UVA alone; very rarely to long wavelength visible light alone; may not be any clear abnormality in very early disease
	Broad-band sources, preferably solar simulator: reduced 24-hr MED; induction of eczema possible, sometimes smooth confluent plaque
Patch and photopatch tests	Abnormalities frequently detected, often to widespread airborne allergens, less frequently topical medications
Blood, urine, and faecal porphyrins	Normal concentrations
Circulating lupus titres	Normal

Abbreviations: MED, minimal erythema dose; UVA, ultraviolet A; UVB, ultraviolet B.

results. If the disorder fails to settle, this makes the diagnosis of CAD unlikely. Also, as stated above, to avoid false negative results if oral or topical steroids are used, testing should not take place until several days after they have been stopped, or the oral steroid dose has been minimal for at least a few days (72).

Circulating lupus titres, and if there is doubt, blood, urine, and stool porphyrins should also be estimated but are always normal in CAD.

DIFFERENTIAL DIAGNOSIS (TABLE 3)

Contact dermatitis, especially to airborne allergens, and photocontact dermatitis may closely resemble CAD, but can usually be largely distinguished by the clinical history and examination, or more definitively in the presence of positive patch or photopatch tests, by their normal monochromatic irradiation tests, except at any sites of contact with the causative agent. Clinically, contact dermatitis is not confined to the sun-exposed areas, whereas airborne contact dermatitis usually affects exposed but also relatively photo-protected areas such as the postauricular areas, upper eyelids, and nasolabial folds. It should be remembered, however, that both contact, especially airborne, and photocontact dermatitis may occur in association with CAD as additional diagnoses.

Photoaggravated atopic or seborrheic eczema may also resemble CAD but can generally be distinguished clinically, whereas in more difficult cases, the cutaneous irradiation tests are generally essentially normal in the light-exacerbated conditions. Again, both eczemas may occur in association with CAD.

Erythrodermic CAD may be distinguished from other erythrodermas by its abnormal irradiation tests, after prior clearance of the eruption in darkened conditions over days to a week or two, essential to avoid false negative responses.

Systemic drug-induced photosensitivity may rarely suggest CAD in demonstrating an erythema but generally not eczema of the light-exposed areas, and is usually associated with either normal cutaneous irradiation tests or abnormalities only in the UVA range. In addition, withdrawal of the drug normally results in steady resolution of the clinical and any phototest abnormalities, generally rapidly but at most within a few months (73).

CTCL, including its Sézary form, may occasionally on examination and histologically be indistinguishable from severe widespread CAD, whereas CAD patients with erythroderma may demonstrate up to about 20% circulating Sézary cells (74). Analysis of phenotypic markers, T-cell receptor gene rearrangement studies, and lymphocyte morphometry are all helpful in distinguishing it from CAD (67,75). Further, clinical photosensitivity in CTCL is

TABLE 3 Differential Diagnosis of Chronic Actinic Dermatitis

Disease	Distinguishing features
Allergic or photoallergic contact dermatitis	Normal cutaneous irradiation tests in absence of antigen, and abnormalities generally in UVA alone; eruption generally localized only to sites of (photo)allergen contact
Systemic drug-induced photosensitivity	Normal cutaneous irradiation tests, or abnormalities usually just in UVA alone. Resolution of clinical and phototest abnormalities within months of drug withdrawal; eruption usually sunburn-like, urticarial, just painful without rash or fragile skin with bullae, not eczematous
Photoaggravated atopic eczema	Usually normal cutaneous irradiation tests; other features of atopic eczema
Photoaggravated seborrheic eczema	Usually normal cutaneous irradiation tests; other features of seborrheic eczema
Erythroderma of non-CAD etiology	Normal cutaneous irradiation tests undertaken after erythroderma is settled
Cutaneous T-cell lymphoma	Normal cutaneous irradiation tests or usually only minor abnormalities, predominantly in UVA
	Predominance of CD4+ circulating lymphocytes (CD8+ in severe CAD)
	Predominance of CD4+ lymphocytes in dermis (CD8+ in CAD)
	T-cell receptor gene rearrangement studies positive

Abbreviations: CAD, chronic actinic dermatitis; UVA, ultraviolet A.
Source: From Ref. 89.

normally at most minimal, as are any phototest abnormalities, principally to the UVA wavelengths (76), and thus out of keeping with the clinical disease severity. On the other hand, a recent report suggests that CTCL may very rarely be severely clinically photosensitive with markedly positive phototests, and thus essentially indistinguishable from CAD, except through T-cell receptor gene rearrangement studies (67), and these are always needed for definitive differentiation of the disorders in any case of diagnostic doubt. Finally, there is generally a CD8+ circulating lymphocyte predominance in CAD, particularly when severe (29), and a CD4+ preponderance in CTCL (77).

MANAGEMENT (TABLE 4)

CAD may often but not always be disabling and difficult to treat, imposing marked restrictions on a patient's lifestyle. Reduced exposure to solar ultraviolet radiation is the first line of management, time outdoors needing to be kept to a minimum whenever solar ultraviolet irradiance is high, namely in the middle of the day in summer or all year round at low latitudes. The UVA wavelengths, however, almost always at least partly responsible for inducing CAD, are more difficult to avoid, being present moderately throughout the whole day and year, and severely affected patients may need to stay indoors all day. Clothing offering high ultraviolet protection should also be worn, generally close-weave loose-fitting clothing opaque when held up to the light, although this may not always be so (78,79); clothing offering measured ultraviolet protection factors (UPFs) should probably be preferred when available, with high UPFs of 30 to 50 being most suitable. A broad-spectrum sunscreen offering high protection of around 50 or so with similar maximal UVA protection should also be liberally applied to exposed skin every hour or so during the day. Organic (i.e., chemical) and micronized inorganic (i.e., physical) filters now often provide such protection and are preferable to the older reflectant preparations for efficacy and cosmetic acceptability. Ultraviolet screening film applied to the windows of home or car may also be helpful, whereas fluorescent lamps for room lighting may affect sensitive patients, although tungsten bulbs, computer screens, and televisions are safe (80). Exposure to contact allergens, particularly airborne, should also be carefully avoided, whereas any apparent disease worsening may possibly be attributable to new contact or photocontact sensitization, particularly to a sunscreen (56).

All CAD needs regular treatment as for other eczemas, with emollients and usually potent topical steroids to all affected sites; for occasional severe flares, intermittent oral steroid courses may be necessary and helpful.

Difficult CAD, if moderate, or even occasionally severe, may sometimes settle with the topical calcineurin inhibitors, tacrolimus (81–83), or pimecrolimus (84), although responsiveness is unpredictable and they may cause annoying irritation. However, they should be tried if the prior measures are ineffective before the use of more aggressive treatment.

TABLE 4 Management of Chronic Actinic Dermatitis

In all patients	Avoidance of exposure to inducing UV wavelengths through avoidance of solar exposure when UV intensity high, use of UV-protective clothing, regular application of non-irritant, broad-spectrum sunscreening agents, avoidance of associated contact or photocontact allergens, regular use of emollients, intermittent use of topical corticosteroids.
For acute flares	Nursing in light-protected hospital cubicles or indoors with drawn blinds. Short-term oral corticosteroid therapy.
In resistant cases	Topical calcineurin inhibitors may occasionally be helpful. Oral cyclosporine 3.5–5 mg/kg/day, oral azathioprine 1–2.5 mg/kg/day, oral thioguanine 0.5–2 mg/kg/day, oral mycophenolate mofetil 15–40 mg/kg/day, in decreasing order of likely efficacy; careful supervision for varying possible side effects essential with each. Therapy should be discontinued if possible in winter. Very low-dose oral PUVA (with usually high-dose initial oral corticosteroid cover), gradually reducing in frequency as resolution sets in over months; low-dose three to four-weekly maintenance therapy likely to be necessary.

Abbreviation: PUVA, psoralen and UVA photochemotherapy.

For intractable disease, either psoralen photochemotherapy (PUVA) or oral immuno-suppressive agents may be required and are often helpful. Very low-dose PUVA is generally gradually effective over months although often poorly tolerated in the early stages, even under high-dose systemic steroid cover, whereas long-term maintenance therapy, possibly just of light-exposed sites, is generally required (85,86), often only every three to four weeks. The mode of action of PUVA is very likely through gradual cutaneous immunosuppression.

The oral immunosuppressive agent, cyclosporine, in doses of 3.5 to 5.0 mg/kg is usually helpful within weeks if tolerated (87), as to a lesser degree is azathioprine 1.0 to 2.5 mg/kg over several months (88). Mycophenolate mofetil 15 to 40 mg/kg may also be of benefit, but perhaps less reliably again. Finally, thioguanine 0.5 to 2.0 mg/kg in the experience of one of the authors (Hawk) may also help if the other drugs are not tolerated or ineffective, although care is needed to avoid the early sudden or later gradual onset of lymphopenia. If adverse effects occur with any of the drugs, often the case in elderly patients, two or more used in low doses may some-times be helpful while minimizing the individual drug drawbacks.

REFERENCES

1. Hawk JLM, Magnus IA. Chronic actinic dermatitis—an idiopathic photosensitivity syndrome includ-ing actinic reticuloid and photosensitive eczema. Br J Dermatol 1979; 101(suppl 17):24.
2. Ive FA, Magnus IA, Warin RP, et al. 'Actinic reticuloid': a chronic dermatosis associated with severe photosensitivity and the histological resemblance to lymphoma. Br J Dermatol 1969; 81:469–485.
3. Ramsay CA, Kobza-Black A. Photosensitive eczema. Trans St John's Hosp Dermatol Soc 1973; 59:152–158.
4. Frain-Bell W, Lakshmipathi T, Rogers J, et al. The syndrome of chronic photosensitivity dermatitis and actinic reticuloid. Br J Dermatol 1974; 91:617–634.
5. Wilkinson DS. Patch test reactions to certain halogenated salicylanilides. Br J Dermatol 1962; 74:302–306.
6. Jillson OF, Baughman RD. Contact photodermatitis from bithionol. Arch Dermatol 1963; 88:409–418.
7. Wojnarowska FT, Calnan CD, Hawk JLM. A study of patients with photocontact allergy to musk ambrette. Br J Dermatol 1982; 107(suppl 22):22.
8. Zaynoun S, Johnson BE, Frain-Bell W. The investigation of quindoxin photosensitivity. Contact Der-matitis 1976; 2:343–352.
9. Yates VM, Finn OA. Contact allergic sensitivity to zinc pyrithione followed by the photosensitivity dermatitis and actinic reticuloid syndrome. Contact Dermatitis 1980; 6:349–350.
10. Burckhardt W. Photoallergic eczema due to blankophores (optic brightening agents). Hautarzt 1957; 8:486.
11. Hawk JLM, Magnus IA. Resolution of actinic reticuloid with transition to photosensitive eczema. J Roy Soc Med 1978; 71:608.
12. Horio T. Actinic reticuloid via persistent light reactivity from photoallergic contact dermatitis. Arch Dermatol 1982; 118:339–342.
13. Lim HW, Buchness MR, Ashinoff R, et al. Chronic actinic dermatitis: study of the spectrum of chronic photosensitivity in 12 patients. Arch Dermatol 1990; 126:317–323.
14. Norris PG, Hawk JL. Chronic actinic dermatitis: a unifying concept. Arch Dermatol 1990; 126:376–378.
15. Milde P, Hölzle E, Neumann N, et al. Chronic actinic dermatitis. Concept and case examples. Hautarzt 1991; 2:617–622.
16. Roelandts R. Chronic actinic dermatitis. J Am Acad Dermatol 1993; 28:240–249.
17. Norris PG, Morris J, Smith NP, et al. Chronic actinic dermatitis: an immunohistologic and photobio-logic study. J Am Acad Dermatol 1989; 21:966–971.
18. Orbaneja JG, Diez LI, Lozano JLS, Salazar LC. Lymphomatoid contact dermatitis. A syndrome produced by epicutaneous hypersensitivity with clinical features and a histopathologic picture similar to that of mycosis fungoides. Contact Dermatitis 1976; 2:139–143.
19. Braathen LR, Førre Ø, Natvig JB. An anti-human T-lymphocyte antiserum: in situ identification of T-cells in the skin of delayed type hypersensitivity reactions, chronic photosensitivity dermatitis, and mycosis fungoides. Clin Immunol Immunopathol 1979; 13:211–219.
20. Ralfkiaer E, Lange Wantzin G, Stein H, et al. Photosensitive dermatitis with actinic reticuloid syndrome: an immunohistological study of the cutaneous infiltrate. Brit J Dermatol 1986; 114:47–56.
21. Takigawa M, Tokura Y, Shirahama S, et al. Actinic reticuloid: an immunohistochemical study. Arch Dermatol 1987; 123:296–297.
22. Toonstra H, van der Putte SCJ, Van Wichen DF, et al. Actinic reticuloid: immunohistochemical analysis of the cutaneous infiltrate in 13 patients. Br J Dermatol 1989; 120:779.

23. Menagé H du P, Sattar N, Hawk JLM, et al. Immunophenotyping of the inflammatory cell infiltrate during the evolution of induced lesions of chronic actinic dermatitis. J Invest Dermatol 1993; 100:482.
24. Fujita M, Miyachi Y, Horio T, et al. Immunohistochemical comparison of actinic reticuloid with contact dermatitis. J Dermatol Sci 1990; 1:289–296.
25. Poulter LW, Seymour GJ, Duke O, et al. Immunohistological analysis of delayed type hypersensitivity in man. Cellular Immunol 1982; 74:358–369.
26. Gawkrodger DJ, McVittie E, Carr MM, et al. Phenotypic characterisation of the early cellular responses in allergic and irritant contact dermatitis. Clin Exp Immunol. 1986; 66:590–598.
27. Vandervleuten CJM, Kroot EJA, Dejong EMJ, et al. The immunohistochemical effects of a single challenge with an intermediate dose of ultraviolet B on normal human skin. Arch Dermatol Res 1996; 288:510–516.
28. Kofoed ML, Munch-Petersen B, Larsen JK, et al. Non-replicative DNA synthesis detected in peripheral lymphocytes from a patient with actinic reticuloid. Photodermatol 1986; 3:158–163.
29. Menagé H du P, Whittaker SJ, Ng YI, et al. Analysis of T-cell receptor genes in chronic actinic dermatitis: no evidence of clonality. J Invest Dermatol 1992; 98:456.
30. Menagé H du P, Sattar N, Haskard DO, et al. A study of the kinetics and pattern of adhesion molecule expression in induced lesions of chronic actinic dermatitis. Br J Dermatol 1996; 134:262–268.
31. Norris DA, Bradley-Lyons, M, Middleton M, et al. Ultraviolet radiation can either suppress or induce expression of intercellular adhesion molecule-1 on the surface of cultured human keratinocytes. J Invest Dermatol 1990; 95:132–138.
32. Griffiths CEM, Barker JNWN, Kunkel S, et al. Modulation of leucocyte adhesion molecules, a T-cell chemotactin (IL-8), and a regulatory cytokine (TNF-a) in allergic contact dermatitis (rhus dermatitis). Br J Dermatol 1991; 124:519.
33. Norris PG, Poston RN, Thomas DS, et al. The expression of endothelial leukocyte adhesion molecule-1 (ELAM-1), intercellular adhesion molecule-1 (VCAM-1) in experimental cutaneous inflammation: a comparison of ultraviolet B erythema and delayed type hypersensitivity. J Invest Dermatol 1991; 96:763–770.
34. Menagé H du P, Kristensen M, Chu CQ, et al. Upregulation of interleukin 1, its receptor and interleukin 1 receptor antagonist levels in induced lesions of chronic actinic dermatitis. Br J Dermatol 1992; 127:429.
35. Kochevar IE, Harber LC. Photo-reactions of 3,3′,4′,5′-tetrachlorsalicylanilide with proteins. J Invest Dermatol 1977; 68:151–156.
36. Addo HA, Ferguson J, Johnson BE, Frain-Bell W. The relationship between exposure to fragrance materials and persistent light reaction in the photosensitivity dermatitis with actinic reticuloid syndrome. Br J Dermatol 1982; 107:261–274.
37. Robinson HN, Morison WL, Hood AF. Thiazide diuretic therapy and chronic photosensitivity. Arch Dermatol 1985; 121:522–524.
38. van de Pas CB, Kelly DA, Seed PT, et al. Ultraviolet-radiation-induced erythema and suppression of contact hypersensitivity responses in patients with polymorphic light eruption. J Invest Dermatol 2004; 122:295–299.
39. Murphy GM, White IR, Hawk JLM. Allergic airborne contact dermatitis to Compositae with photosensitivity: chronic actinic dermatitis in evolution. Photodermatol Photoimmunol Photomed 1990; 7:38–39.
40. Roelandts R, Huys I. Broad-band and persistent photosensitivity following accidental ultraviolet C overexposure. Photodermatol Photoimmunol Photomed 1993; 9:144–146.
41. Menagé H du P, Harrison GI, Potten CS, et al. The action spectrum for induction of chronic actinic dermatitis is similar to that for sunburn inflammation. Photochem Photobiol 1995; 62:976–979.
42. Freeman SE, Hacham H, Gange RW, et al. Wavelength dependence of pyrimidine dimer formation in DNA of human skin irradiated in situ with ultraviolet light. Proc Natl Acad Sci USA 1989; 86:5605–5609.
43. Patel DC, McGregor JM, Ross JS, Hawk JLM. UVA associated eczematous photosensitivity and multiple contact allergies: a further form of chronic actinic dermatitis? Br J Dermatol 1998; 139(suppl 51):27.
44. Yones SS, Palmer RA, Hextall JM, Hawk JL. Exacerbation of presumed chronic actinic dermatitis by cockpit visible light in an airline pilot with atopic eczema. Photodermatol Photoimmunol Photomed 2005; 21:152–153.
45. Sepulveda-Merrill C, Menagé H du P, Hawk JLM, et al. Functional studies of antigen presentation in induced lesions of chronic actinic dermatitis. J Invest Dermatol 1994; 102:603.
46. Ferguson J. Photosensitivity dermatitis and actinic reticuloid syndrome (chronic actinic dermatitis). Semin Dermatol 1990; 9:47–54.
47. Menagé H du P, Ross J, Hawk JLM, et al. Contact and photocontact sensitisation in chronic actinic dermatitis: sesquiterpene lactone mix is an important allergen. Br J Dermatol 1995; 132:543–547.

48. Kurumaji Y, Kondo S, Fukuro S, et al. Chronic actinic dermatitis in a young patient with atopic dermatitis. J Am Acad Dermatol 1994; 31:667–669.

49. Wong SN, Khoo LSW. Analysis of photodermatoses seen in a predominantly Asian population at a photodermatology clinic in Singapore. Photodermatol Photoimmunol Photomed 2005; 21:40–44.

50. Lim HW, Morison WL, Kamide R, et al. Chronic actinic dermatitis: an analysis of 51 patients evaluated in the United States and Japan. Arch Dermatol 1994; 130:1284–1289.

51. Pappert A, Grossman M, DeLeo V. Photosensitivity as the presenting illness in four patients with human immunodeficiency viral infection. Arch Dermatol Res 1994; 130:618–623.

52. Meola T, Sanchez M, Lim HW, Buchness MR, Soter NA. Chronic actinic dermatitis associated with human immunodeficiency virus infection. Br J Dermatol 1997; 137:431–436.

53. Sharma VK, Sethuraman G, Bhat R. Evolution of clinical pattern of parthenium dermatitis: a study of 74 cases. Contact Dermatitis 2005; 53:84–88.

54. Addo HA, Sharma SC, Ferguson J, et al. A study of Compositae plant extract reactions in photosensitivity dermatitis. Photodermatol 1985; 2:68–79.

55. Frain-Bell W, Hetherington A, Johnson BE. Contact allergic sensitivity to chrysanthemum and the photosensitivity dermatitis and actinic reticuloid syndrome. Br J Dermatol 1979; 101:491–501.

56. Green C, Catterall M, Hawk JLM. Chronic actinic dermatitis and sunscreen allergy. Clin Exp Dermatol 1991; 16:70–71.

57. Thune P. Allergy to lichens with photosensitivity. Contact Dermatitis. 1977; 3:213–214.

58. von den Driesch P, Fartasch M, Hornstein OP. Chronic actinic dermatitis with vitiligo-like depigmentation. Clin Exp Dermatol 1992; 17:38–43.

59. Dawe RS, Crombie IK, Ferguson J. The natural history of chronic actinic dermatitis. Arch Dermatol 2000; 136:1215–1220.

60. Ashinoff R, Buchness MR, Lim HW. Lymphoma in a black patient with actinic reticuloid treated with PUVA: possible etiologic considerations. J Am Acad Dermatol 1989; 21:1134–1137.

61. Jensen NE, Sneddon IB. Actinic reticuloid with lymphoma. Br J Dermatol 1970; 82:287–291.

62. Meynadier J, Peyron Jl, Barneon G, et al. Hodgkin's disease complicating actinic reticulosis. Ann Dermatol Venereol 1984; 111:999.

63. Thomsen K. The development of Hodgkin's disease in a patient with actinic reticuloid. Clin Exp Dermatol 1977; 2:109–113.

64. Tan RS, Butterworth CM, McLaughlin H, et al. Mycosis fungoides—a disease of antigen persistence. Brit J Dermatol 1974; 91:607–616.

65. Bilsland D, Crombie IK, Ferguson J. Is the photosensitivity dermatitis/actinic reticuloid syndrome associated with cutaneous lymphoma? Br J Dermatol 1993; 129(suppl 42):42.

66. Sigurdsson V, Toonstra J, Hezemans-Boer M, et al. Erythroderma. A clinical and follow-up study of 102 patients, with a special emphasis on survival. J Am Acad Dermatol 1996; 35:53–57.

67. Norris PG, Newton JA, Camplejohn RS, et al. A flow cytometric study of actinic reticuloid. Clin Exp Dermatol 1989; 14:128–131.

68. Morris SD, Hawk JLM, Russell-Jones R, Whittaker SJ. Severe photosensitivity in four patients with erythrodermic cutaneous T-cell lymphoma. Br J Dermatol 2002; 147(suppl 62):36–37.

69. Hawk JLM, Calonje E. The photosensitivity disorders. In: Elder DE, Elenitsas R, Johnson Jr BL, Murphy GF, eds. Lever's Histopathology of the Skin. 9th ed. Philadelphia, Pennsylvania: Lippincott Williams and Wilkins, 2005:345–353.

70. Heller P, Wieczorek R, Waldo E, et al. Chronic actinic dermatitis: An immunohistochemical study of its T cell antigenic profile with comparison to cutaneous T cell lymphoma. Am J Dermatopath 1994; 16:510–516.

71. Healy F, Rogers S. Photosensitivity dermatitis/actinic reticuloid syndrome in an Irish population: a review and some unusual features. Acta Dermatovenereol (Stockh). 1995; 75:72–74.

72. Lowe JG, Ferguson J. A double blind control study to assess the effect of pre-treatment with a potent topical steroid on the phototest response of photosensitivity dermatitis and actinic reticuloid syndrome (PD/AR). Scot Med J 1989; 34:509.

73. Bilsland D, Ferguson J. Management of chronic photosensitive eczema. Arch Dermatol 1991; 127:1065–1066.

74. Neild VS, Hawk JLM, Eady RAJ, et al. Actinic reticuloid with Sézary cells. Clin Exp Dermatol 1982; 7:143–148.

75. Preesman AH, Schrooyen SJ, Toonstra J, et al. The diagnostic value of morphometry in blood lymphocytes in erythrodermic actinic reticuloid. Arch Dermatol 1995; 131:1298–1303.

76. Volden G, Thune PO. Light sensitivity in mycosis fungoides. Br J Dermatol 1977; 97:279–284.

77. Chu AC, Robinson D, Hawk JLM, et al. Immunologic differentiation of the Sézary syndrome due to cutaneous T-cell lymphoma and chronic actinic dermatitis. J Invest Dermatol 1986; 98:134–137.

78. Davis S, Capjack L, Kerr N, et al. Clothing as protection from ultraviolet radiation: which fabric is most effective? Int J Dermatol 1997; 36:374–379.

79. Gambichler T, Rotterdam S, Altmeyer P, Hoffmann K. Protection against ultraviolet radiation by commercial summer clothing: need for standardised testing and labelling. BMC Dermatol 2001; 1:6.

80. Moseley H, Johnston S, Susskind W. Is viewing television harmful to actinic reticuloid patients? Photodermatol 1989; 6:191–193.
81. Uetsu N, Okamoto H, Fujii K, et al. Treatment of chronic actinic dermatitis with tacrolimus ointment. J Am Acad Dermatol 2002; 47:881–884.
82. Evans AV, Palmer RA, Hawk JLM. Erythrodermic chronic actinic dermatitis responding only topical tacrolimus. Photodermatol Photoimmunol Photomed 2004; 20:59–61.
83. Grone D, Kunz M, Zimmermann R, Gross G. Successful treatment of nodular actinic reticuloid with tacrolimus ointment. Dermatology 2006; 212:377–380.
84. Larangeira de Almeida H Jr. Successful treatment of chronic actinic dermatitis with topical pimecrolimus. Int J Dermatol 2005; 44:343–344.
85. Hindson C, Spiro J, Downey A. PUVA therapy of chronic actinic dermatitis. Br J Dermatol 1984; 113:157–160.
86. Hindson C, Downey A, Sinclair S, et al. PUVA therapy of chronic actinic dermatitis: a 5 year follow-up. Br J Dermatol 1990; 123:273.
87. Norris PG, Camp RDR, Hawk JLM. Actinic reticuloid: response to cyclosporin. J Am Acad Dermatol 1989; 21:307–309.
88. Murphy GM, Maurice PM, Norris PG, et al. Azathioprine in the treatment of chronic actinic dermatitis: a double-blind controlled trial with monitoring of exposure to ultraviolet radiation. Br J Dermatol 1989; 121:639–646.

13 | Solar Urticaria

Takeshi Horio
Department of Dermatology, Kansai Medical University, Osaka, Japan

Erhard Hölzle
Department of Dermatology and Allergology, Klinikum Oldenburg, Oldenburg, Germany

- Solar urticaria is an uncommon type of physical urticaria; the action spectrum ranges from UVB to visible light. It is most probably a type I allergic reaction to an as yet to be defined photoallergen.

- Spectrum of electromagnetic radiation that could inhibit, or augment, the development of solar urticaria is present in many patients.

- Exogenous agents such as tar and pitch, benoxaprofen, repirinast, and chlorpromazine have been reported to cause solar urticaria in rare instances.

- Association with PMLE, chronic actinic dermatitis, atopy, and elevated IgE has been reported in some studies.

- The course is chronic; 15% to 50% of patients are clear of disease within five years of the onset.

- Management includes photoprotection, oral antihistamines, desensitization with UVA or psoralen and UVA, cyclosporine, plasmapheresis, and photopheresis.

U rticaria is an extremely common disease that appears in 15% to 20% of the general population at some time in their lives (1). Among them, however, solar urticaria is a relatively rare type of physical urticaria. As Magnus (2) stated, the practicing clinician might expect to have an opportunity to see three or four patients in a professional lifetime. The present authors have seen about 100 patients with solar urticaria so far during the past 30 years. Careful and detailed examinations may reveal more cases than expected. The diagnosis of solar urticaria can be easily made from its characteristic features, although the causative factors, similar to other types of urticaria, are rarely found. Patients themselves usually recognize sunlight as a provocative agent. Wheal reaction can be easily reproduced in most patients with physical urticaria including solar urticaria. In this chapter, solar urticaria will be discussed focussing mainly on the pathomechanism of the disease.

DEMOGRAPHY

Patients with solar urticaria have been reported throughout the world without specific racial and geographic limitations. Forty-two Japanese and 31 German patients were extensively evaluated from 1973 to 2002 in our photodermatology sections. Table 1 shows the sex and age distribution at the onset of the disease. Thirty-nine (63%) of the subjects were female and 23 (37%) were male. Consistent with our findings, a slight preponderance in women has also been described in the literature. The onset is most common (43%) during the third decade in this series. All but two patients were less than 60 years old at the onset of solar urticaria. The earliest and the latest ages of onset were 13 and 73 years, respectively. In contrast, in 4 of 27 (15%) patients of Frain-Bell's cohort, the disease developed before the age of 10 years (3). To the best of our knowledge, there have been no familial or hereditary cases reported.

CLINICAL MANIFESTATIONS

Solar urticaria develops at the site of exposure to sunlight usually within a few minutes. Very rarely, it may appear a few hours after irradiation. Solar urticaria begins as an itching or burning sensation along with erythema and wheal. When the exposure time is short, the wheal may be minimal or absent, and only erythema of short duration develops. Within a few hours, the urticaria disappears completely without any residual skin changes, similar to other types of urticaria. When large areas of the body are exposed to sunlight for a long period of time, systemic symptoms can occur, such as dizziness, sleepiness, wheezing, dyspnea, and syncope. Seven of 61 patients in our series had experienced dyspnea and syncope following exposure of larger areas of the skin.

Regularly sun-exposed skin, such as the face, dorsal aspects of the hands, and extensor aspects of the forearms, are often less sensitive than are covered body areas due to a hardening phenomenon. In summer, solar urticaria may develop on covered parts of the body as a result of small amounts of UV radiation or visble light penetrating thin clothing. In visible light sensitive patients, artificial room light can produce urticaria.

TABLE 1   Disease Onset of 61 Japanese and German Patients with Solar Urticaria

Age of onset	Number of cases	Male	Female
0–9	0	0	0
10–19	9	2	7
20–29	23	11	12
30–39	11	6	5
40–49	6	2	4
50–59	10	2	8
60–69	1	0	1
70–79	1	0	1
80 and above	0	0	0
Total	61	23	38

In Europe, an uncommon variant of solar urticaria was described in which whealing occurred in a patchy pattern strictly localized to the same circumscribed skin areas (4,5). In these patients, wheals were reproducible in their pattern and location by eliciting radiation; the action spectra ranged 320 to 700 nm, 320 to 585 nm, and 400 to 560 nm, respectively. Intradermal injections of the patient's plasma following in vitro irradiation induced wheals only in the affected skin sites. For this subset of solar urticaria, the term "fixed solar urticaria" has been proposed. It is hypothesized that differences in the mast cell population of afflicted and nonafflicted skin sites account for the peculiar distribution pattern of lesions, since even the in vitro photo-activated serum or plasma of the patients containing the putative photoallergen failed to induce whealing in nonafflicted skin. Mast cells in affected skin sites contained numerous lipid bodies within the cytoplasm and were conspicuously devoid of association to fibrocytes as revealed by electron microscopical studies.

The fixed variant of solar urticaria seems to be associated with only a moderate degree of photosensitivity. The patients are usually able to manage their disease by themselves. Graduated exposures to natural sunlight induce hardening. Systemic symptoms are absent, probably due to the relatively small skin areas involved and the consequently small amount of mediators released. Thus, the patients are not dependent on medical assistance and this variant may be largely under-reported.

PHOTO-PROVOCATION AND ACTION SPECTRUM TESTS

When the patients visit dermatologists, skin changes of solar urticaria are not always observed. Therefore, to make an accurate diagnosis, urticaria reaction should be provoked by exposure to UV and visible light; however, whole body exposures must be avoided, since sycope may be an unwanted consequence. It is also important to determine the action spectrum for protection and treatment of solar urticaria. For experimental induction and action spectrum studies, we usually use a conventional slide projector for visible light source, fluorescent black light for UVA, and sunlamp as UVB source (Fig. 1). However, it should be kept in mind that the black light and sunlamp also emit a small amount of UVB and UVA, respectively.

Although the clinical features of solar urticaria are almost identical in all patients, the eliciting wavelengths (action spectra) are different among cases, ranging from UVB to visible light. This suggests that chromophores or photosensitizers responsible for solar urticaria are not uniform in all patients. We determined the action spectrum in 42 Japanese and in 31 German patients (Table 2). Among the Japanese group, 24 patients (57%) were sensitive only to visible light, which was the most common action spectrum in our series. Further studies using cut-off glass filters showed that the activating waveband occurs most often in a 400 to 500 nm region.

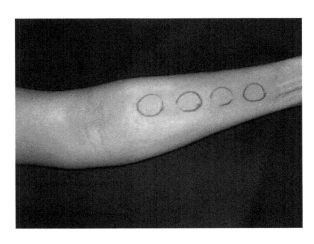

FIGURE 1 Urticaria following exposure to visible light. Note lesion also developed in area covered with one layer of clothing during the phototesting (e.g., antecubital fossa). *Source*: Courtesy of Henry W. Lim, MD.

TABLE 2   Action Spectrum of Solar Urticaria

Action spectrum	Number of cases	Male	Female
In 42 Japanese patients			
Visible light	24	12	12
UVA–visible	3	1	2
UVA	4	1	3
UVB	4	0	4
UVB–UVA	3	1	2
UVB–UVA–visible	4	2	2
Total	42	17	25
In 31 German patients			
Visible light	6	—	6
UVA–visible	7	4	3
UVA	6	3	3
UVB	—	—	—
UVB–UVA	8	2	6
UVB–UVA–visible	4	3	1
Total	31	12	19

In contrast, patients in Germany and other European countries have been reported to be activated most frequently by UV radiation. Table 2 shows the German data also. Six patients (19%) react to visible light only, all others to various parts of the UV spectrum with a preponderance for the UVA part. The majority (77%) of patients in Scotland reported by Frain-Bell reacted to a wide spectrum from UVB to visible light, and only 5 of 26 (19%) patients responded to visible light alone (3). In contrast, only 4 of the 42 patients seen in Japan, and 4 of the 31 patients seen in Germany, reacted across the spectrum from UVB to visible light. (Table 2) In a series of 25 cases reported from Belgium, five patients (20%) responded only to visible light (6). Although no specific explanation is available, there may be some geographical or ethnical differences in action spectrum of solar urticaria.

A wheal usually develops within 5 to 10 minutes after termination of the irradiation. However, in rare instances, urticaria may only appear hours after irradiation (7). The delayed onset of solar urticaria after light exposure may be due to the influence of an inhibition spectrum, which will be discussed later.

The activating wavelengths have been reported to vary from time to time with repeated phototesting in a few patients (8–10). The threshold dose to induce urticaria often varies depending on the time of the photo-provocation test and the test site. This most likely is due to the state of tolerance induced by repetitive irradiations.

INHIBITION SPECTRUM

An inhibition spectrum was first demonstrated in solar urticaria over 20 years ago (11). In this case, wheal formation induced by visible light was inhibited by immediate post-irradiation with longer wavelengths (>530 nm) than the action spectrum (400–500 nm). This phenomenon is not uncommon, and thereafter, similar cases have been further reported by other investigators. We have found the inhibition spectrum in 13 of 42 patients so far (Table 3). Wavelengths of inhibition spectrum were longer than those of action spectrum in all but one case (Patient 10). Inhibition spectra shorter than the activating one have been also reported by other authors (12). In 8 of 13 patients in our series, wheal formation was inhibited only when the skin was exposed to action spectrum and then to inhibition spectrum (postexposure). In four patients, exposures before and after exposure (pre- and postexposure) to the action spectrum showed inhibitory effect. In one patient, only pre-exposure was effective.

In some patients, only monochromatic radiation but not broadband spectrum can induce urticaria. In such instances, the broadband spectrum may include an inhibition spectrum. This could also be the explanation for urticaria reaction that appears with a long latent time after irradiation.

TABLE 3 Inhibition Spectrum in Solar Urticaria

Patient	Action spectrum (nm)	Inhibition spectrum (nm)	Pre or post[a]
1	400–500	>550	Post
2	400–500	>550	Post
3	380–500	>500	Post
4	320–420	>550–600	Pre- and post
5	400–500	500–600	Post
6	400–500	>550	Post
7	400–490	>550	Pre- and post
8	400–490	500–520	Post
9	300–400	>400	Pre and post
10	400–430	320–400	Pre-
11	300–320	>320	Pre- and post
12	300–380	400–500	Post
13	320–480	>500	Post

[a]Pre- or post-inhibition spectrum exerted its effect when irradiation was performed before or after exposure to the action spectrum, respectively.

The mechanism of inhibition has not been elucidated. In our examinations, the inhibition spectrum did not suppress the wheal formation induced by an intradermal injection of compound 48/80 or polymyxin B sulfate, mast cell degranulators (13). Therefore, it is unlikely that the inhibition spectrum suppresses mast cell degranulation or inactivation of released chemical mediators. An effect on vascular responses to chemical mediators is not likely also, since a wheal formation by histamine injection was not affected by exposure to the inhibition spectrum. In one patient, we observed that the photoallergen, which will be discussed later, produced by action spectrum was apparently inactivated by a subsequent exposure to the inhibition spectrum (13). Leenutaphong et al. (12) also described the similar reaction. However, it is difficult to evaluate the test, because the results were not always reproducible even in the same patient or were negative in other patients.

AUGMENTATION SPECTRUM

During the examination for an inhibition spectrum, we found that wavelengths apart from the action spectrum could enhance the wheal development, but by itself were ineffective (14). The action spectrum in this patient was defined in the 320 to 420 nm range using a monochromator. An exposure to longer wavelengths at 450 or 500 nm increased the reaction to 320 to 420 nm before but not after the irradiation with the action spectrum. Therefore, irradiation at 450 to 500 nm showed an augmentative rather than an additive effect with 320 to 420 nm light. If additive, the post-irradiation exposure should have the same effect as the pre-irradiation exposure. This theory was further supported by the observation that a monochromatic light of 450 nm showed a stronger enhancing effect than that of 360 nm, the peak of the action spectrum at the same irradiation dose. An augmentation spectrum was recognized only in 4 of 14 cases examined (29%). Interestingly, in one of these, longer wavelengths than the action spectrum showed both augmentative and inhibitory effects when exposed before and after the irradiation with the activating waveband (15). Danno and Mori (16) also reported two cases with augmentation spectrum. In their patients, however, only postirradiation but not preirradiation with the augmentation spectrum enhanced urticaria reactions.

In some patients with solar urticaria, a large amount of light dose is needed to induce an urticaria reaction from artificial light sources, whereas the urticaria can be easily produced by the natural sunlight. In such cases, the augmentation spectrum may play an important role in the development of clinical manifestations. The mechanism of the augmentation phenomenon has not been clarified. Various wavelengths simultaneously may exert complicated activating, inhibiting, and augmentating effects on wheal formation in solar urticaria.

PASSIVE TRANSFER

At the present time, the transfer of patients' sera to normal subjects is not ethical, because this test may transfer not only allergic reactions but also viral diseases. Until the 1970s, however, many important information for understanding immunological reactions had been obtained from passive transfer tests.

In 1942, Rajka (17) first demonstrated that solar urticaria could be passively transferred to normal subjects by means of an intradermal injection of serum from a patient and subsequent light exposure of injected skin (17). The passive transfer test in solar urticaria is a modification of the Prausnitz–Küstner technique classically used in immediate hypersensitivity reactions. Therefore, a positive result suggests that a specific IgE antibody to the urticaria development may exist in the patient's serum. In the passive transfer of this type, an incubation period of at least a few hours is needed between the injection of the patient's serum and antigen challenge. During this period, IgE antibody seems to adhere to the surface of mast cells. The original work by Rajka (17) showed that the incubation time was also necessary for the positive passive transfer reaction in solar urticaria. Kojima et al. (18) found that positive results were obtainable from the passive transfer test at two to six hours after the injection of serum, whereas the results were negative when the injection sites were irradiated at 30 minutes. These observations indicate that the positive reaction could not be due to a phototoxic substance in the patient's serum. An intradermal injection of a phototoxic substance can produce a wheal even if light exposure is administered immediately after the injection (19,20).

Rajka tried reverse passive transfer, by first exposing the skin of normal subjects and subsequently injecting the patient's serum to the irradiated skin; he obtained a negative result. In contrast, Epstein (21) reported reverse passive transfer with a positive result as well as passive transfer test. He assumed that the antigen of the urticaria reaction might be a normal photoproduct made in human skin by UVB radiation. However, the mechanism of a positive reverse passive transfer cannot be explained by IgE-mediated hypersensitivity, in which the antibody must be injected in the recipients at least a few hours before the antigen challenge. An explanation of this phenomenon could be the hypothesis of a type II solar urticaria in which the presumable precursor of the photoallergen as well as the photoallergen generated by irradiation occurs in both patients and normal subjects (22). In contrast, in type I solar urticaria, the precursor is apparently an abnormal endogenous substance present only in the patient.

PHOTOALLERGEN

The responsible photosensitizer has not been clearly identified in solar urticaria. Most patients develop an urticaria reaction at the site of injection of autologous serum, which has been previously irradiated in vitro with the action spectrum (Fig. 2) (23–26). This indicates that the wheal-forming factor is a substance that is produced by electromagnetic radiation energy in the patient's serum. The irradiated patient's serum does not produce the urticaria reaction in normal subjects. Therefore, the photoresponse is specific to the patients with solar urticaria; in other words, it may not be a phototoxic reaction. This is supported by positive passive transfer test, as described above. The results of serum examination are summarized in Table 4. In the Japanese study population, such a photoallergen was detected in 26 of 33 patients (79%) with any type of action spectrum (Table 5); similar data with 16 positive results in 26 patients (62%) were obtained from the German patients (Table 5).

After sunlight exposure, some patients developed easily or strongly a wheal at the skin which had received a bruise or puncture by injection needle. This might be due to the extravasation of serum into the skin by the physical trauma. This localized whealing is similar to but not identical with that in fixed solar urticaria reported by Reinauer et al. (4). Using ultrafiltration technique, we indicated that a serum factor with molecular weight more than 100 kDa might be transformed to the photoallergen after irradiation, in a patient sensitive to 400 to 500 nm radiation (24). In another patient, whose action spectrum ranged from UVA to 480 nm, the molecular weight was more than 300 kDa (15). However, Kojima et al. (18) reported that the molecular weight of the wheal-forming serum factor produced by light exposure was

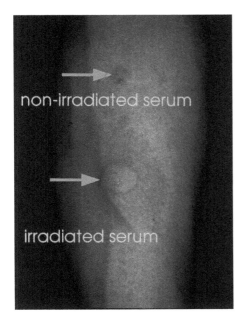

non-irradiated serum

irradiated serum

FIGURE 2 In vitro-irradiated autologous serum produced a wheal on a patient's skin.

25 to 45 kDa in three patients and 300 to 1000 kDa in one patient after gel filtration. Substances investigated in the serum differ between these two studies, in that chromophores were analyzed by us but photoproducts by Kojima et al. These examinations of molecular weight suggest that the photoallergens are not simple chemical substances with low molecular weight, although they vary among patients possibly depending upon the action spectra. The photoallergen can keep its wheal-forming ability after freezing and thawing.

Taking these results together, solar urticaria may be an immediate type of photoallergic reaction mediated by an IgE antibody to photoproducts of endogenous serum factors.

DRUG-INDUCED SOLAR URTICARIA

Solar urticaria may be an autoimmune disease, which is induced by endogenous factors. Very rarely, however, a solar urticaria-like phototoxic reaction can be induced by exogenous chemical substances, including tar and pitch (27), benoxaprofen (28), and repirinast (29). Chlorpromazine (CPZ) is also a phototoxic drug, but has been proved to be able to induce solar urticaria by immediate type of photoallergic reaction (30). In this case, the usual passive transfer study with the patient's serum and UVA was negative, but a modified technique produced a positive result. A wheal appeared immediately after UVA exposure at the site that had been injected with the patient's serum and subsequently with CPZ 24 hours later (Table 6). This is not a phototoxic reaction, because the injection of CPZ and subsequent exposure to UVA at

TABLE 4 Serum Examination in Solar Urticaria

Recipient	Injected serum	Response
Patient	Nonirradiated patient's serum	(−)
	In vitro-irradiated patient's serum	(+)
	Nonirradiated normal serum	(+) or (−)→(−)
	In vitro-irradiated normal serum	(−)→(+) or (−)
Normal control	Nonirradiated normal serum	(−)
	In vitro-irradiated normal serum	(−)
	Non irradiated patient's serum	(−)
	In vitro-irradiated patient's serum	(−)
	In vivo-irradiated patient's serum (passive transfer test)	(+)

TABLE 5 Serum Photoallergen in Patients with Solar Urticaria

Action spectrum	Number tested	(+)	(−)
Japanese			
Visible light	18	15	3
UVA–visible	3	3	0
UVA	2	1	1
UVB	4	3	1
UVB–UVA	3	3	0
UVB–UVA–visible	3	1	2
Total	33	26	7
German			
Visible light	5	3	2
UVA–visible	6	5	1
UVA	6	5	1
UVB	—	—	—
UVB–UVA	6	2	4
UVB–UVA–visible	3	1	2
Total	26	16	10

the same dose did not produce any reaction, but the presence of the patient's serum (antibody) was essential for the positive result.

CHEMICAL MEDIATORS

Some investigators have found elevated histamine levels in venous blood draining the skin in which urticaria had been induced (31,32), whereas others were unable to detect histamine and kinins in dermal perfusates (33). We measured plasma histamine levels by radioimmunoassay in a severe case of solar urticaria (15). The histamine level greatly increased after an exposure to visible light on a limited area of the forearm and reached more than 100 times the preexposure level in five minutes.

HISTOPATHOLOGY

Histopathological findings of solar urticaria are essentially identical to those of nonphotosensitive urticaria. There is edema in the upper and mid-dermis resulting in separation of the connective tissue. A minimal to moderate perivascular infiltrate, consisting of neutrophils, mononuclear cells, and sometimes a few eosinophils, is found. Norris et al. (34) observed histological alterations in urticaria lesions at five minutes to 24 hours after provocation by action spectrum radiation at various doses, ranging from 2 to 32 minimal whealing doses (MWDs). They found a significant increase in neutrophil and eosinophil numbers in the upper dermis at five minutes and two hours, but not at 24 hours, in a dose-dependent manner. The number of mononuclear cells did not change after an exposure to two MWDs at any time interval; however, after exposure to 32 MWDs, the number of mononuclear cells increased noticeably at 24 hours. Eosinophil degranulation associated with deposition of eosinophil major basic protein has been reported in solar urticaria (35). Armstrong et al. (36) observed histological findings of leukocytoclastic vasculitis, including dense infiltration of neutrophils,

TABLE 6 Passive Transfer of Immediate Drug Photoallergy

Serum	Drug	UVA	Wheal
Patient	(+)	(+)	(+)
Patient	(+)	(−)	(−)
Patient	(−)	(+)	(−)
—	(+)	(+)	(−)
Normal	(+)	(+)	(−)

nuclear dusts, and endothelial cell swelling, in a patient with unusual solar urticaria that appeared a few hours after exposure and persisted for days.

Sequential ultrastructural analysis demonstrated margination and activation of platelets, formation of interendothelial clefts, and alteration of nerve fibers as primary events in solar urticaria, preceding mast cell degranulation. Mediators other than histamine are most probably involved in the early stage of solar urticaria. Once the wheal is formed, mast cell degranulation is evident by dissolution of granular matrix, fusion of perigranular membranes including labyrinth formation and opening to the extracellular space. This is followed by extravasation of eosinophils, erythrocytes, and neutrophils. Nerve fibers, which initially demonstrate partial swelling, then show edema of endoneurium (37).

COEXISTING DISEASES

Solar urticaria usually occurs in otherwise healthy persons, but rarely is associated with other photosensitivity diseases. In a study of 87 patients with solar urticaria from Scotland, 23% had polymorphous light eruption (PMLE) and 3% had chronic actinic dermatitis (38). Two patients in our series had coexisting PMLE. Magnus et al. (39) reported a patient with erythropoietic proto-porphyria associated with features of solar urticaria. The patient developed a wheal immediately after the sunlight exposure, whereas edematous erythema with burning sensation, blisters, and scars, which are the typical manifestations of erythropoietic protoporphyria, were delayed. No additional case has been reported, and the authors have not seen such a patient. It is our opinion that this patient had erythropoietic protoporphyria with urticarial symptoms rather than solar urti-caria sensu strictu. More recently, a patient with coexisting porphyria cutanea tarda and solar urti-caria was reported (40). Although porphyrin is a phototoxic substance that is activated by visible light, solar urticaria is not observed in the vast majority of patients with porphyrias. Frain-Bell recorded two patients with solar urticaria that occurred in association with lymphocytoma (3). There are sporadic case reports of solar urticaria associated with other physical urticarias including cold urticaria (41), dermographism (14,41), heat urticaria (42), and pressure urticaria (43).

In our series, patients with solar urticaria lacked atopic dermatitis, and their total IgE levels were normal. Frain-Bell also found both personal and family history of atopy only in a minority of patients and stated that solar urticaria was not associated with an atopic back-ground (3). In contrast, 12 of 25 (48%) Belgian patients in Ryckaert and Roelandts' (6) survey had a personal history of atopy such as asthma, hay fever, or atopic dermatitis. A study of 57 patients from Italy reported the occurance of atopic dermatitis in 21% of the patients, asthma or rhinitis in 26%, and elevated serum immunoglobulin in 33% (42).

CLINICAL COURSE

The clinical course of solar urticaria is usually chronic and rather unpredictable. In the Japanese patients followed by one of the authors, the disease had lasted for 5 to 10 years before consul-tation in 7 of 42 patients and more than 10 years in five patients. Similarly, many of the patients studied by Ryckaert and Roelandts (6) had the disease for 4 to 11 years before consultation.

Follow-up study has not been done in our series. In the Frain-Bell's cohort, only 2 of 30 patients cleared completely (5). Five of 13 patients followed by Harber et al. (44) in the USA under-went spontaneous remission after an average of 4.5 years following the onset of the disease. Nearly half of the 57 patients reported from Italy were free of disease within five years of the onset of disease (42). On the basis of a study of 87 patients, the group in Scotland estimated that the prob-ability of disease resolution is 15%, 24%, and 46% in 5, 10, and 15 years, respectively (38).

TREATMENT

Multiple modalities need to be used since specific therapy is not available for solar urticaria (Table 7). For the treatment of urticaria, the prevention of its development is required, since the wheal, once appeared, spontaneously subsides in a short time.

Broadband sunscreening agents that contain both UVA and UVB filters are somewhat helpful for UV-sensitive patients, but have little effect for patients who react to visible light.

TABLE 7 Therapeutic Ladder in Solar Urticaria

Photoprotection
   Broad-spectrum sunscreen
   Clothing
   Wide-brimmed hat
Oral antihistamines
Desensitization/hardening
   UVA
   PUVA
Cyclosporine (3–5 mg/kg/day)
Plasmapheresis
Extracorporeal photochemotherapy (photopheresis)

In these cases, self-tanning agents containing dihydroxyacetone may be of some help. Photoprotection by the use of clothing, wide-brimmed hat, and gloves is an important measure to prevent wheal development.

Oral histamine H1 receptor antagonists have a beneficial effect to some degree in reducing the whealing and itching in patients with solar urticaria. Terfenadine, at doses higher than the conventional dose (up to 360 mg per day), has been reported to be effective (45,46). We observed that oral administration of terfenadine, 60 mg three times per day for three days, partially suppressed the histamine release in plasma after light exposure of a patient's skin (15). However, high-dose terfenadine must be used with caution because of the risk of life-threatening cardiac arrhythmias.

Other forms of antihistamines have also been widely used and reported to be at least partially effective (38,42). The new generation of histamine H1 receptor blocking agents, such as desloratadine and levocetiricine, are well tolerated and can be given in higher doses. Even if they are not sufficient to control solar urticaria by themselves, they are very helpful agents for combination therapy, For example, with broad-spectrum sunscreens, if the patient's action spectrum is in the UV region.

It is well known that the so-called "desensitization" or "hardening" can often occur in patients with solar urticaria. Skin constantly exposed to the sunlight and an area in which urticaria has recently been produced are tolerant to subsequent irradiation. Broadband UVA is the most commonly used radiation source in inducing hardening in patients with solar urticaria in patients whose action spectra include UVA (46,47). After determination of the MWD to UVA, 50% to 70% of MWD is delivered to localized area of the body, such as the sun-exposed areas only, or 25% of the body surface at each exposure. Single or multiple exposures with gradually increasing UVA doses (25–30% increase per exposure) can be done daily. However, caution must be taken in not exposing too large an area and not to increase the dose too rapidly to avoid systemic side effects that may include sycope.

The mechanism by which tolerance is induced is not clear, but may be partially due to the exhaustion of chemical mediators by repeated exposures (24). In a series of experiments, Leenutaphong et al. (48) showed that elevation of the mast cell degranulation threshold as proposed by Keahey et al. (49) due to direct exposure of mast cells to UV irradiaton is probably not the main underlying mechanism of tolerance. It is likely that the binding sites of IgE on mast cells remain occupied by the photoallergen during the state of tolerance and IgE-mediated histamine release from mast cells is blocked until new IgE is generated.

Photochemotherapy with psoralen and UVA (PUVA) has also been used with beneficial effect (50,51). The tolerance induced by PUVA therapy lasts longer than that obtained by phototherapy. PUVA therapy is effective not only in UVA-sensitive patients, but also in those in whom the action spectrum does not include UVA range. Therefore, the mode of action of PUVA appears to be different from that of the tolerance induced by action spectrum radiation.

The mechanism of PUVA-induced hardening has not been clarified. Photoprotection by PUVA-induced pigmentation and thickening of the stratum corneum may play a role. PUVA therapy has been used for the treatment of nonphotosensitive mast cell-mediated conditions, such as urticaria pigmentosa (52) and chronic urticaria (53), although the therapeutic effect on the latter is debatable (54). Therefore, it is possible that PUVA has direct effect on mast cells in patients with solar urticaria. This is supported by our observation that PUVA-inhibited mast cell degranulation and histamine release in animal models (55,56).

Cylosporine, at 4.5 mg/kg/day, has been successfully used to control solar urticaria in a patient; however, the effect is transient as the condition recurred one to two weeks after the discontinuation of the treatment (57).

Elimination of causative agent is very difficult in solar urticaria, because the photosensitizer is of endogenous origin in the majority of cases. Plasmapheresis has been used with a beneficial effect for the treatment of patients with solar urticaria in whom a photoallergen can be detected in the serum or plasma (58,59). Also, plasmapheresis followed by PUVA therapy has been proposed in order to prevent the formation of a new photoallergen after plasmapheresis (60). More recently, extracorporeal photochemotherapy (photopheresis) has been reported to be successful in one patient (61).

It should be emphasized that the use of a single treatment modality is not usually sufficient to obtain a complete prevention. Combination therapy is necessary depending upon the clinical response of the patients.

CONCLUSION

In the past, solar urticaria was often considered an idiopathic photodermatosis. However, more information about pathomechanisms are now available in solar urticaria; it is most probably a type I allergic reaction to an as yet to be defined photoallergen. Identification of this photoallergen is the most important issue remaining to be resolved in the future.

REFERENCES

1. Humphreys F, Hunter JAA. The characteristics of urticaria in 390 patients. Br J Dermatol 1998; 138:635–638.
2. Magnus IA. Solar urticaria. In: Magnus IA, ed. Dermatological Photobiology. Oxford: Blackwell Scientific Publications, 1976:202–210.
3. Frain-Bell W. Solar urticaria. In: Frain-Bell W, ed. Cutaneous Photobiology. Oxford: Oxford University Press, 1985:51–55.
4. Reinauer S, Leenutaphong V, Hölzle E. Fixed solar urticaria. J Am Acad Dermatol 1993; 29:161–165.
5. Schwarze HP, Marguery MC, Journe F, Loche E, Bazex J. Fixed solar urticaria to visible light successfully treated with fexofenadine. Photodermatol Photoimmunol Photomed 2001; 17:39–41.
6. Ryckaert S, Roelandts R. Solar urticaria—a report of 25 cases and difficulties in phototesting. Arch Dermatol 1998; 134:71–74.
7. Monfrecola G, Nappa P, Pini D. Solar urticaria with delayed onset; a case report. Photodermatol Photoimmunol Photomed 1988; 5:103–104.
8. Ravits M, Armstrong RB, Harber LC. Solar urticaria; clinical features and wavelength dependence. Arch Dermatol 1982; 118:228–231.
9. Murphy GM, Hawk JLM. Broadening of action spectrum in a patient with solar urticaria. Clin Exp Dermatol 1987; 12:455–456.
10. Ng JCH, Foley PA, Crouch RH, Baker CS. Changes of photosensitivity and action spectrum with time in solar urticaria. Photodermatol Photoimmunol Photomed 2002; 18:191–195.
11. Hasei K, Ichihashi M. Solar urticaria; detection of action and inhibition spectra. Arch Dermatol 1982; 118:346–350.
12. Leenutaphong V, von Kries R, Hölzle E, Plewig G. Solar urticaria induced by visible light and inhibited by UVA. Photodermatol 1988; 5:170–174.
13. Horio T, Yoshioka A, Okamoto H. Production and inhibition of solar urticaria by visible light exposure. J Am Acad Dermatol 1984; 11:1094–1099.
14. Horio T, Fujigaki K. Augmentation spectrum in solar urticaria. J Am Acad Dermatol 1988; 18:1189–1193.
15. Miyauchi H, Horio T. Detection of action, inhibition and augmentation spectra in solar urticaria. Dermatology 1995; 191:286–291.
16. Danno K, Mori N. Solar urticaria: report of two cases with augmentation spectrum. Photodermatol Photoimmunol Photomed 2000; 16:30–33.
17. Rajka E. Passive transfer in light urticaria. Clin Immunol 1942; 13:327–345.
18. Kojima M, Horiko T, Nakamura Y, Aoki T. Solar urticaria; the relationship of photoallergen and action spectrum. Arch Dermatol 1986; 122:550–555.

19. Kligman AM, Breit R. The identification of phototoxic drugs by human assay. J Invest Dermatol 1968; 51:90–99.

20. Kaidbey KH, Kligman AM. Identification of systemic phototoxic drugs by human intradermal assay. J Invest Dermatol 1978; 70:272–274.

21. Epstein S. Urticaria photogenica. Ann Allergy 1949; 7:443–457.

22. Leenutaphong, V., Hölzle, E., Plewig, G. Pathomechanism and classification of solar urticaria: a new concept. J Am Acad Dermatol 1989; 21:237–240.

23. Horio T, Minami K. Solar urticaria: photoallergen in a patient's serum. Arch Dermatol 1977; 113:157–160.

24. Horio T. Photoallergic urticaria induced by visible light: additional cases and further studies. Arch Dermatol 1978; 114:1761–1764.

25. Horio T. Solar urticaria—sun, skin and serum. Photodermatol 1987; 4:115–117.

26. Uetsu N, Miyauchi-Hashimoto H, Okamoto H, Horio T. The clinical and photobiological characteristics of solar urticaria in 40 patients. Br J Dermatol 2000; 142:32–38.

27. Crow KD, Alexander E, Buck WHL, Johnson BE, Magnus IA, Porter AD. Photosensitivity due to pitch. Br J Dermatol 1961; 73:220–232.

28. DeLeo VA, Hanson S, Scheide S. Benoxaprofen photosensitization of phospholipase activation in mammalian cells in culture. Toxicol Lett 1986; 32:215–220.

29. Kurumaji Y, Shono M. Drug-induced solar urticaria due to repirinast. Dermatology 1994; 188:117–121.

30. Horio T. Chlorpromazine photoallergy: coexistence of immediate and delayed type. Arch Dermatol 1975; 111:1469–1471.

31. Hawk JLM, Eady RAJ, Challoner AVJ, Kobza-Black A, Keahey TM, Greaves MW. Elevated blood histamine levels and mast cell degranulation in solar urticaria. Br J Clin Pharmacol 1980; 9:183–186.

32. Soter NA, Wasserman SI, Pathak MA, Parish JA, Austen KF. Solar urticaria: release of mast cell mediators in to the circulation after experimental challenge. J Invest Dermatol 1979; 72:282.

33. Sams WM Jr, Epstein JH, Winkelmann RK. Solar urticaria: investigation of pathogenetic mechanisms. Arch Dermatol 1969; 99:390–397.

34. Norris PG, Murphy GM, Hawk JLM, Winkelmann RK. A histological study of the evolution of solar urticaria. Arch Dermatol 1988; 124:80–83.

35. Leiferman KM, Norris PG, Murphy GM, Hawk JLM, Winkelmann RK. Evidence for eosinophil degranulation with deposition of granule major basic protein in solar urticaria. J Am Acad Dermatol 1989; 21:75–80.

36. Armstrong RB, Horan DB, Silver DN. Leukocytoclastic vasculitis in urticaria induced by ultraviolet irradiation. Arch Dermatol 1985; 121:1145–1148.

37. Behrendt, H., Lehmann, P., Leenutaphong, V., Hölzle, E., Plewig, G. Sequential ultrastructural analysis of solar urticaria: inflammatory cells, blood vessels, and nerve fibers. J Invest Dermatol 1989; 92:400a.

38. Beattie, PE, Dawe RS, Ibbotson SH, Ferguson J. Characteristics and prognosis of idiopathic solar urticaria: a cohort of 87 cases. Arch Dermatol 2003; 139(9):1149–1154.

39. Magnus IA, Jarrett A, Prankerd TAJ, Rimington C. Erythropoietic protoporphyria: a new porphyria syndrome with solar urticaria due to protoporphyrinaemia. Lancet 1961; 2:448–451.

40. Dawe RS, Clark C, Ferguson J. Porphyria cutanea tarda presenting as solar urticaria. Br J Dermatol 1999; 141:590–591.

41. Rantanen T, Suhonen R. Solar urticaria. A case with increased skin mast cells and good therapeutic response to an antihistamine. Acta Derm Venereol (Stockh) 1980; 60:363–365.

42. Monfrecola G, Masturzo E, Riccardo AM, Balato F, Ayala F, Di Costanzo MP. Solar urticaria: a report on 57 cases. Am J Contact Dermat 2000; 11(2):89–94.

43. Hölzle E. The idiopathic photodermatoses: solar urticaria. In: Hawk JLM, ed. Photodermatology. London: Arnold, 1999:113–125.

44. Harber LC, Bickers DR. Solar urticaria. In: Harber LC, Bickers DR, eds. Photosensitivity Diseases. 2nd ed. Toronto: B. C. Decker, 1989:209–218.

45. Diffey BL, Farr PM. Treatment of solar urticaria with terfenadine. Photodermatol 1988; 5:25–29.

46. Dawe RS, Ferguson J. Prolonged benefit following ultraviolet A phototherapy for solar urticaria. Br J Dermatol 1997; 137(1):144–148.

47. Beissert S, Stander H, Schwarz T. UVA rush hardening for the treatment of solar urticaria. J Am Acad Dermatol 2000; 42(6):1030–1032.

48. Leenutaphong V, Hölzle E, Plewig G. Solar urticaria: study on mechanisms of tolerance Br J Dermatol 1990; 122:601–606.

49. Keahey TM, Lavker RM, Kaidbey KH, Atkins PC, Zweiman B. Studies on the mechanism of clinical tolerance in solar urticaria.Br J Dermatol 1984; 110:327–338.

50. Hölzle E, Hofmann C, Plewig G. PUVA-treatment for solar urticaria and persistent light reaction. Arch Dermatol Res 1980; 269:87–91.

51. Parrish JA, Jaenicke KF, Morison WL, Momtaz K, Shea C. Solar urticaria: treatment with PUVA and mediator inhibitors. Br J Dermatol 1982; 106:575–580.
52. Christophers E, Hönigsmann H, Wolff K, Lagner A. PUVA treatment of urticaria pigmentosa. Br J Dermatol 1978; 98:701–702. Dermatology 1997; 195(1):35–39.
53. Midelfart K, Moseng D, Kavli G, Stenvold SE, Volden G. A case of chronic urticaria and vitiligo, associated with thyroiditis, treated with PUVA. Dermatologica 1983; 167:39–41.
54. Olafsson JH, Larkö O, Roupe G, Granerus G, Bengtsson U. Treatment of chronic urticaria with PUVA or UVA plus placebo: a double-blind study. Arch Dermatol Res 1986; 278:228–231.
55. Danno K, Toda K, Horio T. The effect of 8-methoxypsoralen plus long-wave ultraviolet (PUVA) radiation on mast cells: PUVA suppresses degranulation of mouse skin mast cells induced by compound 48/80 or concanavalin A. J Invest Dermatol 1985; 85:110–114.
56. Toda K, Danno K, Tachibana T, Horio T. Effect of 8-methoxypsoralen plus long-wave ultraviolet (PUVA) radiation on mast cells. II. *In vitro* PUVA inhibits degranulation of rat peritoneal mast cells induced by compound 48/80. J Invest Dermatol 1986; 87:113–116.
57. Edstrom DW, Ros AM. Cyclosporin A therapy for severe solar urticaria. Photodermatol Photoimmunol Photomed 1997; 13(1–2):61–63.
58. Duschet P, Leyen P, Schwarz T, Hocker P, Greiter J, Gschnait F. Solar urticaria: treatment by plasmapheresis. J Am Acad Dermatol 1986; 15:712–713.
59. Leenutaphong V, Hölzle E, Plewig G, Grabensee B, Kutkuhn B. Plasmapheresis in solar urticaria. Photodermatol 1987; 4:308–309.
60. Hudson-Peacock MJ, Farr PM, Diffey BL, Goodship TH. Combined treatment of solar urticaria with plasmapheresis and PUVA. Br J Dermatol 1993; 128:440–442.
61. Mang R, Stege H, Budde MA, Ruzicka T, Krutmann J. Successful treatment of solar urticaria by extracorporeal photochemotherapy (photopheresis)—a case report. Photodermatol Photoimmunol Photomed 2002; 18(4):196–198.

14 | Drug and Chemical Photosensitivity: Exogenous

James Ferguson
Photobiology Unit, Ninewells Hospital, Dundee, Scotland, U.K.

Vincent A. DeLeo
Columbia University, St Luke's—Roosevelt Hospital Center, New York, New York, U.S.A.

- The diagnosis of drug or chemical-induced photosensitization offers the opportunity of cure through removal of the chromophore.

- Topical agents produce photosensitization by a range of toxic and allergic mechanisms.

- The commonest recent photoallergens are sunscreens and topical non-steroidal anti-inflammatory agents.

- Systemic photoactive drugs most commonly produce phototoxicity; five distinguishable clinical patterns are seen.

- Drug phototoxicity can mimic chronic actinic dermatitis.

- Susceptibility to photosensitivity can persist for several months after cessation of a photoactive drug.

INTRODUCTION

W hen presented with an abnormally photosensitive patient, an important diagnostic group to be considered is that due to photosensitizing drugs and chemicals. The correct diagnosis offers the possibility of prevention by simply avoiding the agent. To miss that opportunity may result in a patient being considered as undiagnosed or worse, mis-diagnosed, perhaps leaving the clinic with an incorrect label of an endogenous photodermato-sis such as chronic actinic dermatitis (CAD). Systemic agents, either ingested or parenterally administered, are usually therapeutic chemicals with photosensitivity as an adverse effect (1).

The photosensitization reaction is a process in which normally ineffective ultraviolet (UV) and visible radiation interacts with a chromophore (a radiation-absorbing substance) producing an abnormal reaction, usually in the skin. The radiation element, which is frequently but not exclusively UVA (315–400 nm) dependent can extend to shorter or longer wavelengths. The clinical impact for the patient relates not only to the degree of sensitization, but also to the wavelength involved. A mild sensitivity to UVA is quite different in its consequences on the quality of life of a patient when compared with profound sensitivity to visible wavelengths, where severe reactions may occur in extreme latitudes, even in the winter season.

A range of mechanisms exist to explain how a therapeutic drug enhances the photosen-sitivity of cellular skin components. It does appear that phototoxicity, a nonimmunological event due to combination of a drug or metabolite, with light of appropriate wavelength, is the most commonly encountered mechanism. Other significant, less common, routes exist, which includes drug-induced photosensitive lichen planus and lupus erythematous, pellagra, photoallergy, and erythema multiforme. Although the latter mechanisms are uncommon, they should be remembered. Photosensitization, whether immune-based or not, can be reduced to the simple concept of absorption of radiant energy by a chromophore within the skin. Excitation of the electronic state from ground level with transfer of the radiant energy into a biologically active free radical species will induce cellular damage resulting in either direct toxicity, that is, phototoxicity, or via the immune system or other mechanisms.

Topical photosensitizers, that is, those in contact with the skin, are often nontherapeutic agents. A wide variety of plant materials and other chemicals, including sunscreens, and topical drugs are recognized to be responsible (2). This chapter will consider topical and systemic agents separately.

PHOTOSENSITIVITY INDUCED BY TOPICAL AGENTS

Many chemicals from the environment gain access to the skin from the topical route either intentionally or inadvertently. Some of these have the ability to absorb radiation from the sun or artificial sources. Usually, this radiation is in the UV and visible ranges and such agents can act as chromophores and become potential photosensitizers. In all such reactions, both chemicals and radiation are necessary for the photochemistry necessary to produce biological changes and disease.

The mechanism of the response can be either irritant (toxic) or allergic. The topical chemi-cal photosensitivities are therefore classified into two clinical entities: photoirritant (phototoxic) contact dermatitis (PICD) or photoallergic contact dermatitis (PACD).

The mechanism of action (allergic vs. toxic) is fairly easy to discern on the basis of clinical history and morphology in the case of topically applied chemicals (Table 1). The reaction occurs on first exposure to the chemical agent and light in PICD, whereas a sensitization delay is necessary for PACD.

Photopatch testing will confirm the diagnosis of the chemical-inducing PACD only in sensitized individuals and negative responses in the population in general. In contrast, photopatch testing of phototoxic agents in PICD is nondiscriminating since all or at least the vast majority of the population will develop positive reactions to photopatch testing of such chemicals.

The timing of the response in the clinical history of the eruption and in testing is delayed in PACD, as it is in allergic contact dermatitis. In PICD, the timing of the response varies depending on the chemical involved. Tars routinely induce an immediate response referred to as "tar smarts," which usually occurs while the patient is being exposed to radiation,

TABLE 1 Differences between Photoallergic and Phototoxic Contact Dermatitis

Feature	Photoallergic	Phototoxic
Incidence	Low	High
Occurrence on first exposure	No	Yes
Onset after ultraviolet exposure	24–48 hr	Minutes to days
Dose dependence		
Chemical	Not crucial	Important
Radiation	Not crucial	Important
Clinical morphological appearance	Eczematous	Erythematous and bullous, hyperpigmentation
Histology	Spongiotic dermatitis	Necrotic keratinocytes

whereas the reaction to psoralens, whether from natural or synthetic material, is delayed producing a response in skin 48 to 72 hours after exposure to light.

On clinical and histological examination, PACD presents as an eczematous response, whereas PICD appears clinically as erythema, edema, and bullous lesions and histologically as a toxic response with necrosis of keratinocytes.

The dose of both chemicals and radiation necessary to induce the response is more critical to the production of PICD when compared with PACD, but such factors may also play a role in PACD (3–6).

PICD is a clinical diagnosis made by a history of skin exposure to the photoirritant and a photodistributed eruption of the type described above. Photopatch testing in such patients is contraindicated, since a positive response might be severe and since, as stated above, such a positive response would be expected to occur in the general population and would not aid in the diagnosis.

The mechanism of action of PICD is dependent on the structure of the photosensitizing chemical. Certain agents like tar absorb radiation and transfer that energy to membranes of skin cells inducing cell damage. Furocoumarins like psoralens absorb radiation after intercalating into DNA and induce nuclear damage.

Although the mechanism of production has been extensively studied for a number of photoallergens, the process is still poorly defined. The pathophysiological mechanisms involved in production of the skin lesions, however, routinely reveal that the immunological process involved in this reaction is analogous to the process occurring in plain allergic contact dermatitis to a nonphotosensitized antigen.

The "action spectrum," that is, the wavelengths of the radiation inducing photocontact dermatitis, either toxic or allergic, falls almost always in the UVA-longwave (320–400 nm) and the visible ranges (400–800 nm) (5). This is of importance for a number of reasons. UVA and visible radiation penetrates most window glass so that patients have been reported to develop reactions to light coming through the windows of their cars and while sitting next to windows at home or at work. Rarely, particularly sensitive patients may react to artificial light from indoor lighting sources. Sunscreens that do not offer longwave protection offer little benefit in preventing photochemical sensitivity, and most importantly, a UVA light source is necessary for the performance of photopatch testing.

Photoirritant Contact Dermatitis

The incidence of PICD in the general population is unknown. Review of large studies of patients being evaluated for photosensitivity reveals a fairly low incidence of this diagnosis (7). This may be because the diagnosis is made clinically, since phototesting and photopatch testing are not done in these patients. For this reason, patients with PICD would not undergo testing and not appear in statistics. It is probably at least as common as PACD in the general population.

The agents that induce the response are listed in Table 2. The two general patterns in the history of individuals with PICD relate to either recreational or occupational exposure. As one might expect from the agents listed in Table 2, most individuals who experience occupationally related PICD are workers in outdoor occupations, but this is not always the case.

TABLE 2   Agents Commonly Inducing Photoirritant Contact Dermatitis

Tar-related products	
Therapeutic agents–tars	
Pitch	
Acridine	
Coal tar	
Anthracene	
Creosote	
Dyes	
Methylene blue	
Eosin	
Disperse blue 35	
Amino-benzoic acid derivative	
Amyl-*ortho*-dimethylaminobenzoic acid	
Furocoumarins	
Therapeutic	8-methoxypsoralen (Oxsoralen)
	4,5,8-trimethylpsoralen (Trisoralen)
	5-methoxypsoralen (Bergapten)
Fragrance materials[a]	
Plants[b]	
Rutaceace	Lime, lemon, bergamot, burning bush, bitter orange, gas plant, common rue
Umbelliferae	Carrots, cow parsley, wild chervil, fennel, dill, parsnip, cow parsnip, celery
Moraceae	Fig
Cruciferae	Mustard
Ranunculaceae	Buttercup

[a]Berloque dermatitis.
[b]Phytophotodermatitis (not all-inclusive).

All individuals with a photodistributed eruption should be suspected of having PICD. This necessitates a careful history for exposure to photosensitizers at home, in the work place, and in the recreational setting.

The diagnosis is suggested by the classic morphology, erythema and edema, with bullae in severe cases. Frequently, the lesions of PICD heal with pigmentation, especially when due to furocoumarin sensitizers. In fact, patients may present with only hyperpigmentation without a history of preceding inflammation. However, other clinical morphologies including psoriasiform dermatitis and even hypopigmentation after inflammation can occur.

Tar Products

Tar and related products produce a very distinctive photosensitive reaction known as "tar or pitch smarts" (8,9). The patients experience burning and stinging almost immediately on exposure to the sun. This can occur with very short exposure times. Roofers with exposure to pitch and coal tar are most susceptible and direct skin contact is not necessary, since aerosolized contact is sufficient to produce the reaction. Associated ophthalmological involvement may occur (10). The sensitizers in coal tar include acridine, anthracene, benzopyrene, and fluoranthene (11).

Reactions to creosote in roof paper and creosote-soaked wood products including saw dust and boxes have also been reported in a large number of workers (12,13).

Although not routinely reported, the other situation where "tar smarts" can occur is in the therapeutic setting. Since tar-based products such as creams, soaks, and shampoos are routinely used to treat skin disease, patients treated with these agents should be reminded that sun exposure can cause skin lesions.

Furocoumarins

Furocoumarins are photosynthesizing chemicals that occur in nature in wild and cultivated plants. Such agents have been synthesized for many uses including fragrances and as therapeutic agents. The most common agents used therapeutically, 8-methoxypsoralen and

5-methoxypsoralen, are also the ones most commonly present in plants that are potent photosensitizers.

Classically, these reactions have been divided into those produced by synthesized agents usually used as fragrances and called "berloque," the French word for pendant, dermatitis and those in which the photosensitizer is contacted inadvertently from plants, called "phytophotodermatitis."

When an individual develops PICD to a fragrance product, it usually appears as a hyperpigmented macule at the site of application—usually on the neck—and so the term berloque or pendant dermatitis (4). These reactions are relatively rare since most fragrance agents containing photosensitizers have been removed from products used in the United States and Western Europe. Many consumers, however, do continue to use containers of perfumes and colognes for many years or even decades.

Phytophotodermatitis is much more common. Although there have been reports of plants other than those containing furocoumarins causing phytophotodermatitis, they are exceedingly rare. For example, *Cneoridium dumosum*, a native bush, has been reported to cause photosensitivity in field worker-students in the chaparral vegetation zone in California and Mexico (14).

Unlike the reaction to tar-related products, the reaction to furocoumarins is delayed, occurring one to many days after the plant and light exposure. Healing is frequently accompanied with hyperpigmentation but in severe reactions hypopigmentation can occur.

The lime is the plant most often reported to induce phytophotodermatitis in our experience. Exposure to limes usually occurs in the recreational setting in sunny climates. Individuals usually report making and drinking cocktails which entail squeezing lime juice into their drinks. This process allows the furocoumarins from the exocarp, the outer green part of the lime skin, to be absorbed into the skin of the fingers. From the fingers, it can be transferred to other skin sites. Only short exposure to UVA radiation, just minutes of sun exposure, are needed to elicit a response. Since the response is delayed, individuals rarely recognize the association of exposure and skin lesions (Fig. 1).

The most common plant causing phytophotodermatitis in the workplace is celery. Initially, it was believed that a fungal parasite, pink-rot, infecting the celery was responsible for the reaction. It is now accepted that the infection induces increased productions of

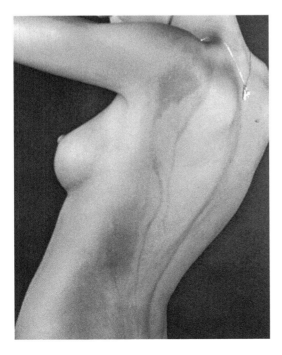

FIGURE 1 Hyperpigmented photo-irritant dermatitis ("berloque dermatitis"). This woman used a Brazilian oil bath that contained plant-derived furocoumarins.

furocoumarins in the celery and therefore leads to the reaction (15,16). Reactions have been reported in cannery workers, grocery store cashiers, baggers, produce clerks, and chefs (17). In addition to limes, other citrus also contain furocoumarins but not as high a concentration as the lime. However, handling of various citrus in great quantities may lead to phytophotodermatitis in bartenders. The lime still appears to be the most common cause of phytophotodermatitis in the nonoccupational setting (5).

Farmers and other outdoor workers as well as professional and recreational gardeners and others with outdoor recreational exposure to plants are at risk for developing phytophotodermatitis from exposure to the other plants listed in Table 3. Many such reactions will present with linear lesions as for poison ivy contact dermatitis.

Other Agents

Amyl *ortho*-dimethylaminobenzoic acid induced an immediate photosensitivity response followed by a second delayed erythema in workers formulating UV-cured inks (18) and similarly Disperse Blue Dye 35 produced a transient erythema and burning in workers on sun exposure (19).

Photoallergic Contact Dermatitis

The incidence of PACD in the general population is unknown but such reactions have become rarer in the last 25 years. The available incidence data are based on positive photopatch test results in groups of patients with presumed photosensitivity who were referred to tertiary care facilities for diagnostic photopatch testing. The rates of positive reactions and the diagnosis of PACD in groups ranged from 6% in a Canadian study to 25% in England in studies published in the 1970s (3). The Scandinavian Multicenter Photopatch Study (1988) reported 274 positive photopatch test results and 369 positive plain patch test responses in 1993 patients with a diagnosis of PACD in 11% of patients tested in the early 1980s (7,20). In the United States, in two studies done more recently, 11% and 20% of patients tested were reported to have PACD (21,22). Similarly, the North American Contact Dermatitis Group found approximately 20% of 250 patients tested in the 1990s to be diagnosed as having PACD after photopatch testing (DeLeo, personal communication). Unlike PICD, the only way to confirm a diagnosis of PACD is with photopatch testing. The technique is outlined in other sections and briefly reviewed here.

CAD is discussed in more detail in other sections. It should be remembered in the context of PACD that some patients with PACD may progress to persistent light reactions now classified as a type of CAD and continue to react to sun exposure even after removable of the antigen. These patients can be defined by phototesting with lowered minimal erythema doses (MEDs) in the UVB and/or UVA ranges and sometimes with sensibility in the visible light area. In the past, this reaction was more common than today. The most common agents were antibacterials, which are only rarely used today and primarily in the occupational setting and fragrances, especially musk ambrette, which is no longer used in colognes. It should be remembered that some patients with PACD, for example, to sunscreens, may react to light alone for a short period of time after removal of the antigen, probably because of antigen persistence in the skin. These patients, once called transient light reactors, will have normal MEDs on phototesting and as such will be distinguishable from those with CAD.

Photopatch Testing Techniques

Photopatch testing is patch testing with the addition of radiation to induce formation of the photoantigen. Application of antigens and scoring criteria are the same as those described for plain patch testing (5). The only additional equipment that is necessary is an appropriate light source and light opaque shielding for the period after removal of the Finn chambers before readings.

With very few exceptions, the radiation responsible for formation of the photoantigen and clinical PACD falls within the UVA spectrum (320–400 nm). The light source utilized should produce UVA radiation in a continuous spectrum (fairly uniform radiation from 320

TABLE 3

North American contact dermatitis group	European taskforce for photopatch testing	Henry Ford Health System
Sunscreens		
1—Octinoxate	Octyl methoxycinnamate (2-ethylhexyl-*p*-methoxycinnamate, Parsol MCX, Eusolex 2292)	Homosalate
2—Sulisobenzone (BZP-4)	Benzophenone-3 (2-hydroxy-4-methoxy benzophenone, oxybenzone, Eusolex 4360)	3-(4-methylbenzyliden) camphor (Eusolex 6300)
10—Oxybenzone (BZP-3)	Octyl dimethyl PABA (2-ethylhexyl-*p*-dimethyl-aminobenzoate, Escalol 507, Eusolex 6007)	Menthyl anthranilate
12—*Para*-aminobenzoic acid	PABA (4-aminobenzoic acid)	Octyl dimethyl *p*-aminobenzoic acid (PABA)
13—Octisalate	Butyl methoxydibenzoylmethane (Parsol 1789, Eusolex 9020)	Octyl methoxycinnamate
15—Menthylanthranilate	4-Methylbenzylidene camphor (Eusolex 6300, Mexoryl SD)	Benzophenone 3 (BZP-3)
19—2-Hydroxy-methoxy methyl benzophenone	Benzophenone-4 (2-hydroxy-4-methoxy-benzophenone-5-sulfonic acid, Uvenyl MS-40)	PABA
21—Octyl dimethyl PABA	Isoamyl *p*-methoxycinnamate (Neoheliopan, E1000)	Parsol 1789
23—Homosalate	Phenylbenzimidazole sulphonic acid (2-phenyl-5-benzimidazolsulphonic acid, Eusolex 232)	Benzophenone 4 (BZP-4)
24—Butyl methoxydibenzoylmethane		
22—Phenylbenzimidazole		
Antimicrobials		
4—Dichlorophene		Bithionol (thiobisdichlorophenol)
5—Triclosan		Chlorhexidine diacetate
6—Hexachlorophene		Dichlorophen
7—Chlorhexidine diacetate		Fenticlor (thiobisdichlorophenol)
11—Fenticlor (thiobis-chlorophenol)		Hexachlorophene
14—Tribromosalicylanilide		Tribromosalicylanilide (triclocarban)
20—Bithionol (thiobis-dichlorophenol)		
		Triclosan
Fragrances		
8—Sandalwood oil		Musk ambrette
9—Musk ambrette		6-methylcoumarin
		Sandalwood oil
Medicaments		
18—Ketoprofen	Naproxen	
	Ibuprofen	
	Diclofenac	
	Ketoprofen	
Plants		
16—Sesquiterpene lactone mix		Achillea millefolium (Yarrow)
17—Lichen acid mix		Alantolactone
		Alpha-methylene-gammabutyrolactone
		Arnica montana (mountain tobacco)
		Chamomilla Romana
		Chrysanthemum cinerariaefolium
		Diallyldisulfide
		Lichen acid mix
		Sesquiterpene lactone mix
		Tanacetum vulgare (tansy)
		Taraxacum officinale (dandelion)

Abbreviations: BZP-4, benzophenone-4; PABA, P-aminobenzoic acid.

to 400 nm) of sufficient irradiance and field size to allow irradiation of 20 to 25 antigen sites with a dose of 5 to 10 J/cm^2 within a reasonable time (about 30 minutes).

The dose of radiation used in photopatch testing has varied between 1 and 10 J/cm^2 in most studies. Theoretically, the largest dose not only induces erythema in skin but would be most likely to yield production of the photoallergy and a positive test response. Since the MED in the UVA range is between 20 and 60 J/cm^2, any dose that can be conveniently delivered below this level can be used, and 10 J/cm^2 has been selected more or less arbitrarily to fulfill these two criteria.

The photoallergens chosen for testing are determined by the usage patterns of photoallergens in a given population. Table 3 lists the photoallergen series of the North American Contact Dermatitis Group (DeLeo, personal communication), the Henry Ford Hospital System (23), and the Photopatch Testing Taskforce of European Academy of Dermatology and Venereology (24). The protocol for photopatch testing usually includes phototesting with UVA and UVB radiation alone to determine a baseline photopatch dose in the UVA range and to rule out other sensitivities in both the UVA and UVB ranges. Patches are applied in two sets, one to be irradiated and one left "dark" so as to differentiate between photocontact dermatitis and regular allergic contact dermatitis.

A positive response in the irradiated site and a negative in the covered site are diagnostic of photoallergy (Fig. 2). Equal positive responses in both irradiated and covered sites are diagnostic of plain contact allergy. When both sites are positive, but when the result in the irradiated patch is significantly more positive than in the covered site, this is considered by researchers either as simple allergic contact dermatitis or as allergic contact dermatitis with photocontact dermatitis.

Occasionally, irradiation appears to inhibit a positive patch test reaction—the nonirradiated site will be reactive, whereas the irradiated site will be negative. The pathophysiology of such an occurrence is not understood: neither are its clinical ramifications. Such a response, if clinically relevant, may be significant.

As with plain patch testing, false-positive and false-negative results can occur in photopatch testing. The former is particularly common with drugs such as ketoprofen, promethazine, and chlorpromazine (CPZ).

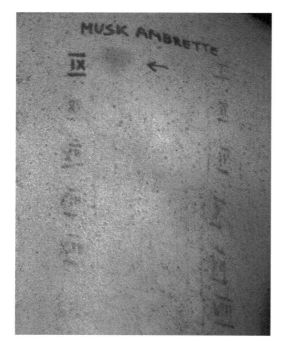

FIGURE 2   Positive photopatch test to musk ambrette and UVA.

Some antigens produce an immediate photoirritant response. Erythema is noted at the completion of the irradiation period. Rarely this is clinically relevant and may usually be disregarded unless the clinical history suggests an immediate reactivity.

In addition to the photoallergens in the tray, patients can be tested to their own products, particularly to sunscreens and fragrance-containing cosmetics. Industrial cleansers and the like, as well as personal-care cleansers, which may be the source for antibacterial agents, must be diluted appropriately.

Photosensitizing Agents

Sunscreens

Since the 1970s, people in the United States, Europe, and Australia have begun to increase their usage of sunscreens, as they were educated to the dangers of sun exposure. This is particularly true of outdoor workers and those seeking outdoor recreational activities. This has led to an increased exposure to active ingredients in these products. Therefore, it is not surprising that such agents induce contact allergy, and since such ingredients by definition absorb UV radiation, it is not surprising that they also induce PACD (Fig. 3). The incidence of these reactions in the sunscreen-using population is unknown, but it is probably very low. Sunscreen components were the most common group of agents producing relevant photopatch test reactions in many areas of the world (22) photopatch test series, but were less frequent than antimicrobials and fragrances in the Mayo Clinic and Scandinavian studies (7,20,21). The most common agents to induce this response are the benzophenones (oxybenzone and sulisobenzone), octyl-dimethyl P-aminobenzoic acid (PABA), and the dibenzoylmethanes.

Antibacterial agents

Tetrachlorosalicylanilide and *tetrabromosalicylanilide* the most potent of the photosensitizers caused an epidemic of PACD in many areas of the world. The former caused an outbreak in factory workers in Great Britain in 1960 (25,26). These agents were responsible for producing a large number of cases of debilitating CAD. Although these agents are no longer used in consumer cleaners, that is, bar soaps and shampoos, in the United States, they may still be used in industrial cleansers.

Triclosan (Irgasan DP 300) is a widely used antibacterial agent in bar soaps and deodorants. Most deodorant-type bar soaps marketed in the United States today contain this agent. It appears to be a very low level photosensitizer, and few cases have been reported despite its widespread usage patterns.

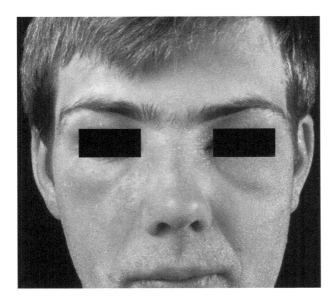

FIGURE 3 Eczematous photoallergic contact dermatitis to sunscreens in a patient photoallergic to oxybenzone.

Dichlorophene (G-4) is widely used in this country and in Europe in shampoos, dentifrices, antiperspirants, and "athlete's foot" powder. Dichlorophene is also used in the treatment of fabrics. It is a rarely reported photosensitizer.

Bithionol is a chlorinated phenol used in the 1960s in the United States and more extensively in Japan. It caused an epidemic of PACD in Japan, where it was present in bar soaps. It is banned in that country and is no longer used in bar soaps in the United States. It may still be used in industrial cleaners and agricultural and veterinary products marketed in the United States.

Fenticlor is a chlorinated phenol used as an antibacterial and antiseborrheic agent in hair-care products made primarily in Canada, the British Isles, and Australia. It was never used extensively in the United States. It appears to be a moderately potent photoallergen. It may produce false-positive responses in photopatch testing. Such responses have features of true photoallergy—they appear eczematous and occur in a delayed fashion with an increase in severity of response at second reading.

Hexachlorophene was a widely used antibacterial in over-the-counter skin cleansers in the United States. Reports of neurotoxicity resulted in a change of status to prescription only by the Food and Drug Administration (FDA). *pHisohex* is still used in the United States, but with much lower frequency. It is rarely reported photoallergen.

Chlorhexidine is used as an antibacterial in hospital cleansers for both skin and mucosa. It is also used as a dental rinse. It is a rare photoallergen.

Fragrances

A number of fragrance ingredients have been associated with PACD. The three most common include musk ambrette, 6-methylcoumarin, and sandalwood oil.

Musk ambrette is a synthetic fragrance fixative used primarily in men's cosmetics because of its potent floral odor. Related chemicals extracted from the scent glands of animals and some plants have been used for years as fixatives and enhancers in perfumes. In the 1970s and 1980s, huge quantities were used in the United States in various cosmetics, primarily men's after-shave lotions and colognes. Concentrations of musk ambrette as high as 15% were used in such products. In the late 1970s, reports of photoallergy began to appear in the literature. By the 1980s, this agent was the most frequently reported cause of PACD. Many of the men sensitized to musk ambrette developed persistent reactions now called CAD.

The International Fragrance Association has recommended that musk ambrette not be utilized in products that will have contact with skin. In other products, a concentration of ≤4% is recommended.

6-Methycoumarin is a synthetic fragrance that caused an epidemic of PACD when it was used in a sun-tanning lotion in the late 1970s. The reactions were particularly severe, requiring hospitalization in many cases. The morphology of many of the reactions suggested phototoxicity, but photoallergy was probably the underlying mechanism. The agent was removed from sun-related lotions and it is no longer recommended for use as a fragrance component. An early problem with the identification of this agent as etiologic occurred because of its apparent instability as a photoallergen once applied to skin. In routine photopatch testing, antigens are applied to skin 24 to 28 hours before UVA exposure. Such testing yielded negative results. When the antigen was applied shortly (30–60 minutes) before exposure, positive reactions were found in sensitized individuals. Testing with this agent is therefore done differently from the other routinely tested photoallergen.

Sandalwood oil is a "woodsy" smelling fragrance ingredient. It is a rarely reported photosensitizer.

Therapeutic agents

A number of systemic drugs that produce photosensitivity have been reported to cause PACD when contacted topically. Theoretically, this might occur with many such agents. The two most frequently reported are the phenothiazines, chlorpromazine hydrochloride (Thorazine) and promethazine (Phenergan). The PACD reported for the former has been found in health-care workers who have frequent skin contact with the agents.

The newest groups of photoallergens are topical nonsteroidal anti-inflammatory agents (NSAIDs). Since their entry into the marketplace in Europe, they have been widely used and are now the most common cause of PACD in some areas of Europe. Ketoprofen is the most common of these, and allergy to this agent is reported to cause cross-reactivity to benzophenones. These agents are not available for use in the United States (27,28).

Other agents

Quindoxin is a growth-promoting agent used in animal foodstuffs. It has been reported to cause PACD in farm workers handling the feed (29,30). It is no longer used.

Olaquindox similarly utilized in animal feed caused an outbreak of PACD in pig farmers (31).

Folpet and captan used by farmers and groundskeepers have been recently reported to induce PACD (32).

Air-Borne Contact Dermatitis

Photosensitivity can be mimicked by contact dermatitis in skin exposed to allergens, which can be aerosolized. In addition, some individuals with air-borne contact dermatitis have gone on to develop an idiopathic photosensitivity, CAD (discussed earlier). The major allergens in this group include occupationally acquired agents like chromates (33,34) and plants of the Compositae (35,36) and Lichen (37) families. An extensive review of this area as relates to the Compositae experience has revealed that this is not truly a PACD, but conversion to photosensitivity from contact dermatitis by an unknown mechanism. For this reason, as seen in Table 3, plant allergens are routinely tested in the photoallergen tray.

SYSTEMIC DRUG-INDUCED PHOTOSENSITIVITY

The incidence of phototoxicity due to systemic medication varies greatly from drug to drug and even within subjects taking a particular agent. It usually relates to drug dosage, the local intensity of the relevant wavelengths, and individual factors such as skin type and drug handling. This latter factor is as yet poorly understood, although it is to be anticipated that the current interest in pharmacogenomics will explain why some individuals experience idiosyncratic phototoxicity, whereas the majority taking that drug escape without problems.

Within a tertiary referral photobiology unit, the number of drug-induced photosensitive patients seen makes up a small proportion of the total workload (38). Although it might be inferred that systemic drug photosensitivity is a minor problem, it is highly likely that many are misinterpreted as sunburn and go unnoticed, whereas others are diagnosed by the family doctor or by patients themselves through reading the drug information leaflets. In countries with postmarketing surveillance, drug-induced photosensitivity is commonly reported, at least when a drug is new. Later, as the novelty reduces, further reports are often thought unnecessary. Publications using such data exist (2) and include lengthy lists of suspected drugs; there is no substitute for pre-registration data of knowledge regarding the photosensitizing potential of a molecule prior to the licensing and marketing of a particular drug.

Photosensitivity Testing of New Therapeutic Molecules Prior to Marketing

The pharmaceutical industry provides ever-increasing numbers of new molecules. While thankfully the days of discovering severe phototoxicity after regulatory authority approval and marketing are now rare, we cannot yet predict idiosyncratic phototoxicity and rarer mechanisms such as photoallergy, drug-induced lupus erythematosus (LE) or pellagra. Such cases only usually emerge with post-marketing surveillance. The move towards standardized pre-launch testing by the major regulatory authorities in North America, Europe, and Asia follows a simple pathway. A new molecule is required to have an absorption spectrum conducted. If it absorbs in the UVB/A or visible region and is known to be distributed to skin or the eye, standard in vitro testing with a fibroblast 3T3 model follows. If phototoxicity is detected, human volunteer testing may be recommended (40).

TABLE 4   Fluoroquinolone Phototoxicity Index Table

	Phototoxicity index
Absent phototoxicity	<1.4
Mild	1.3–3.0
Moderate	>3.0–6.0
Severe	>6.0

One early test system which involved "volunteers" being given a drug or placebo followed by a sunshine-soaked boat trip with erythema scoring thereafter did reveal some important information. Today, the system has evolved into a randomized controlled trial of healthy volunteers who have predrug phototesting using a relative monochromatic and solar simulated sources. Phototesting is repeated on drug/placebo/positive control with Good Laboratory and Good Clinical Practice standards of investigation. A within-individual phototoxic index (PI) or sensitization factor is produced. On code breakage, this index provides a clear indication of the degree of phototoxicity over a range of wave-lengths. The morphology of the reaction and importantly the duration of susceptibility postdrug cessation enable an overall picture of the molecule's phototoxic potential and its impact on later clinical usage. The PI can be graded into mild, moderate, or severe (Table 4). A high PI may for some drugs end their development, particularly when nonphotoac-tive alternatives exist, a situation particularly seen within the fluoroquinolone (FQ) family. Many phototoxic drugs that have been marketed for years have never been studied in such detail. Usually, they have postmarketing adverse reporting data, but limited other information, which historically were appropriate but now are out-of-date with standards that have improved considerably.

Drug Photosensitivity: Clinical Presentation

The wide spectrum of systemic therapies known to have a photosensitizing potential will be considered individually (Table 5).

In general, a particular family of photosensitizers produces a similar clinical type of presentation with a pattern of evolution that can be quite different from one family structure to another, for example, psoralens and FQs. When faced with a patient suspected of drug-induced photosensitivity, history taking and examination are equally important. Knowledge as to whether the eruption has been induced by light through thin clothing or window glass and how much light has been required often gives an indication of the responsible wavelength and severity. Examination for photosensitive site involvement such as forehead, cheeks, chin, rim of ears, back of hands, with a clothing cut-off, and the sparing of shadow sites such as beneath chin, behind ears, and within the hair, as well as under spectacle frames and watch strap, are often helpful in pinning down a photosensitive element. Having made a diagnosis of photosensitivity, a careful drug history and an idea of the mechanism involved will allow the correct diagnosis to emerge.

Phototoxicity, which will theoretically arise in any subject with sufficient exposure to light and chemical, has a number of presentations (Table 6). Although often thought of as an exaggerated sunburn, in fact an array of clinical features specific to each drug family is evident. Within each phototoxic drug family, although differences in wavelength dependency and morphology can be detected, these are the exceptions rather than the rule. In general, the susceptibility does vary with photo skin type (41) and drug dosage. However, idiosyncratic phototoxic skin reactions do occur with some photoactive drugs such as thiazides and quinine where only a minority of those prescribed will eventually develop photosensitivity. Often these patients describe it occurring after a number of years of drug taking rather than in weeks. In a similar fashion, many phototoxic drugs when administered do show a surprising variation and degree of photosensitivity independent of skin type. As pharmaco-logical drug handling does vary between subjects, it is not surprising that there are patients with more or less sensitivity with any group taking a particular phototoxic drug at a specific dosage.

TABLE 5 Photosensitizing Drugs

Antibiotics
    Fluoroquinolones
    Nalidixic acid
    Tetracyclines
    Sulphonamides
Antifungals
    Griseofulvin
Diuretics and cardiovascular agents
    Thiazides
    Furosemide
    Amiodarone
    Quinidine
Non-steroidal anti-inflammatory drugs
    Naproxen
    Tiaprofenic acid
    Piroxicam
    Azapropazone
Calcium channel antagonists
    Nifedipine
Psoralens
    8-methoxypsoralen
    5-methoxypsoralen
Psychoactive drugs
    Phenothiazines (chlorpromazine, thioridazine)
    Protriptyline
Retinoids
    Isotretinoin
    Etretinate
Photodynamic therapy agents
    Foscan
    Photofrin

Persistent Light Reactor

If an initial photoallergic episode is followed by a state of continuing photosensitivity, despite avoidance of the original photoallergen, the term "persistent light reactor" has been used. In fact, the evidence for this type of event is slight. Until more data emerges to support the concept, it seems sensible to use the term with caution, particularly as such a diagnosis may have considerable consequences if exposure was occupational. It does seem likely that some of those labeled as persistent light reactors do have CAD, a condition associated with multiple contact allergies and eczematous phototest reactions.

Wavelength dependency and duration of susceptibility after drug cessation
Phototoxic drugs do vary in the wavelength responsible for the clinical problem. Almost all involve the UVA spectrum (315–400 nm) with extension occasionally into the UVB or visible

TABLE 6 Major Patterns of Cutaneous Phototoxicity

Skin reactions	Photosensitizers
Prickling or burning during exposure; immediate erythema; edema or urticaria with higher doses; sometimes delayed erythema or hyperpigmentation	Photofrin, amiodarone, chlorpromazine
Exaggerated sunburn	Fluoroquinolone antibiotics, chlorpromazine, amiodarone, thiazide diuretics, quinine, demethylchlortetracycline, and other tetracyclines
Late-onset erythema, blisters with slightly higher doses, hyperpigmentation only with low doses	Psoralens
Increased skin fragility with blisters from trauma (pseudoporphyria)	Nalidixic acid, frusemide, tetracycline, naproxen, amiodarone, fluoro-quinolone antibiotics
Photoexposed site telangiectasia	Calcium channel antagonists

range. The degree of sensitization and the wavelength dependency are both key to predicting the environmental conditions causing the problems. Some agents, particularly the porphyrin-related systemic drugs used for photodynamic therapy for internal malignancy do have maximal activity in the visible region (400–700 nm). As would be expected, these latter patients would have a quite different susceptibility pattern in relation to light transmitted through cloud or clothing, or even artificial lighting conditions.

Drug-Induced Pseudoporphyria

This phenomenon, which is well recognized yet is uncommon, appears to have a porphyria cutanea tarda/variegate-like porphyric features in the presence of normal or near-normal values. Skin fragility/blistering of sunlight-exposed skin sites of face and hands are associated with the ingestion of a number of known phototoxic drugs including NSAID (42,43), tetracyclines, amiodarone, nalidixic acid, and voriconazole (44).

Duration of Susceptibility Following Drug Cessation

Although it would be expected that the duration of susceptibility to phototoxicity will relate to the elimination half-life of a drug, and this is often the case, considerable variation exists with some drugs, such as quinine and thiazide-induced photosensitivity lasting for up to nine months, yet the drugs themselves are usually eliminated rapidly, that is, within hours. Some pharmacological explanation will emerge, possibly related to an abnormal metabolite with a much longer half-life or perhaps tissue binding which only slowly resolves. In others where the duration of susceptibility is lengthy, such as is seen with amiodarone or photofrin, it does directly relate to the persistence of the photoactive molecule within the skin and circulation. Two of the most commonly encountered photoactive agents, psoralens and FQs, are rapidly eliminated from the vasculature and tissues. Within 24 to 48 hours of stopping these drugs, any increased susceptibility to photosensitive reactions has been lost.

Commonly Encountered Phototoxic Drugs

To a large extent, the responsible systemic agents encountered in the clinical setting relates to prescribing practice which varies from country to country and even between clinicians. In those latitudes furthest away from the equator, winter sunlight has little UVA and for many months of the year none of the UVB wavelengths. This results in increased susceptibility in spring when the UV environment does change significantly often occurring at a time when photo adaptation has been lost. In contrast, patients prescribed photoactive drugs who live near the equator, often have a greater UV-induced photoprotection due to high levels of the shorter pigmentogenic and epidermal thickening wavelengths. These can reduce the severity of reactions due to a natural "hardening" process. The phototoxic patients seen by clinicians do vary greatly. Secondary care specialists tend only to see the diagnostic problems. Drug photosensitivity as a diagnosis is well recognized by family doctors who are likely to see and recognize the majority of such problems without the need to refer on to photodermatology units.

Individual Drug Groups
Diuretics

Two subgroups are reported, the sulphonamide-based thiazide molecules and the loop diuretic furosemide. Members of the thiazide group appear capable of an idiosyncratic problem with phototoxicity, a lichen planus-like reaction (45) and a drug-induced lupus erythematosus reaction (Fig. 4) (46) being evident. The commonest of these by far appears to be the phototoxic dermatitis type of response (Fig. 5), which only occurs in a few patients taking a thiazide, often appearing sometimes years after starting to take the drug. This can have a presentation similar to CAD. The solution is to stop the agent and use a nonphotoactive substitute. Bumetanide, a loop diuretic, appears to have a lower phototoxic potential than thiazide and can be considered as an alternative (47).

When one considers how commonly frusemide is used, it is surprisingly rare to see a pseudoporphyric reaction with bullae and skin fragility (48).

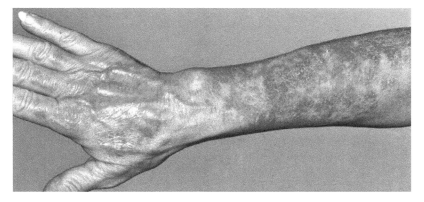

FIGURE 4 Drug-induced lupus erythematosus. Note the distribution over the dorsum of hand and proximal phalanges.

The Fluoroquinolones

This large group of antibiotics shows an interesting range of phototoxicity (49). Photoallergy, if it does occur, must be extremely rare. The chemical progenitor of the group nalidixic acid is itself a recognized photosensitive molecule. Introduction of fluorine at position 6 of the quinolone ring structure produced the first generation of FQs. Early molecules that were developed and marketed did show a phototoxic potential of a fairly marked type with erythema and blistering of the photoexposed sites only occurring in subjects who had taken a high-dose drug and been exposed to a significant amount of what seemed to be particular UVA wavelengths.

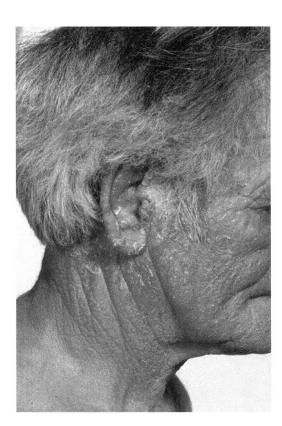

FIGURE 5 Thiazide-induced phototoxicity. Note the cut-off at the side of neck and similarity in penetration to chronic actinic dermatitis.

Lomefloxacin was first approved in 1992 in the United States. Following postmarketing surveillance, a large number of photosensitivity reports followed. Phototoxicity studies later showed it to have a PI of 3 to 6. Since then, the FQ group has been the most thoroughly studied family of molecules prior to licensing. A wide range of degree of phototoxicity has been observed from the nonphototoxic, even photoprotective moxifloxacin, to the extremely phototoxic molecule, clinafloxacin, which has PI values in some individuals as high as 90. The creation of extensive in vitro and human in vivo phototoxic data has allowed a comparison of the two methods. This has revealed FQ in vitro fibroblast study work to correlate with the in vivo monochromator phototest findings, the only family of drugs to date that has shown this correlation. The in vivo studies have revealed a predominantly UVA phenomenon with some molecules demonstrating an extension into the visible range. This latter finding raised the concern of ocular phototoxicity. Some FQs with encouraging broad-spectrum bactericidal activity have had their development terminated due to adverse effects including marked phototoxicity. Some FQs capable of severe phototoxicity have shown a marked pigmentary response of skin photoexposed sites that can last for two years.

Amiodarone

This drug, which is often used to control cardiac arrhythmias resistant to more conventional drug therapy, has a known phototoxic potential. The photosensitivity reaction is dose-related and is caused by UVA and visible wavelengths. It has two erythemal components, an immediate prickling burning erythema coupled to a 24-hour delayed erythema response. The problem is common, affecting 40% to 60% of those taking the drug (50,51). Elimination half-life is long (>200 days) so that those affected, if they come off the drug, will continue to have problems for many months. A complication seen in a number of patients is a golden or slate-gray pigmentation due to a lipofuscin-like pigment that contains the amiodarone metabolite, desethylamiodarone. In many patients, drug cessation is not a possibility, so broad-spectrum photoprotection/behavioural avoidance of the wavelengths and wearing dark clothing are advised. Occasionally, narrowband UVB phototherapy can help probably through a epidermal thickening and pigmentation effect (artificial hardening) (52). The persistence of pigmentation and photosensitivity can be protracted for years (53), although most generally clear over a two-year period.

Phenothiazine

CPZ which continues to be used, although less commonly than in the past, was first described in the 1950s as a photosensitizer. It is similar to amiodarone in that it produces a UV-induced abnormal burning immediate erythema of exposed sites (Fig. 6), which has a second erythema peak at approximately 24 hours. As a classical phototoxic drug, it is often used as an in vitro positive control. It has a dose-related effect that does cause severe pigmentation of both golden and slate-gray types. Both of these are reversible on drug cessation, although can

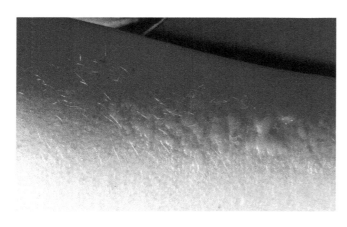

FIGURE 6 Chlorpromazine phototoxic blistering of photoexposed forearm.

take many months. Unlike amiodarone, CPZ phototoxicity quickly resolves following drug cessation.

It is interesting that CPZ is extensively metabolized with metabolites that are phototoxic. Variability in the breakdown/accumulation of these metabolites may explain the different degree of susceptibility to phototoxicity. CPZ has been reported capable of photoallergy. This may occur following exposure to crushed CPZ tablet dust, a problem no longer seen since the advent of CPZ syrup.

Quinine

Most commonly prescribed for night cramps, this agent occasionally produces an idiosyncratic photodistributed leukomelanoderma. Phototesting of these patients reveals sensitivity within the UVB/A region (54) with resolution of susceptibility lasting many months after taking the drug. A similar problem has been described with hydroxychloroquine (55); again it appears idiosyncratic. Laboratory studies suggest that the phototoxic mechanism is complex, raising the possibility of interindividual pharmacokinetic factors. Treatment alternatives for painful night cramps do exist. In those for whom that does not provide relief, drug dosage reduction is worth considering.

Tetracyclines

This family of anti-inflammatory antibiotics has a number of members that are photoactive. Originally, dimethylchlortetracycline (DMCT) was well recognized for phototoxicity, which follows a sunburn pattern. DMCT is now rarely used. Minocycline seems only rarely associated with sunburn-like phototoxicity, much more commonly reported is doxycycline, particularly when taken at the higher dose of 200 mg/day or above (56,57). Occasionally, photo-onycholysis is seen (58), although the majority shows the sunburn-like picture, rarely is pseudoporphyria reported.

Calcium channel antagonists

An unusual form of photosensitivity has been reported with nifedipine (59). Telangiectasia of photoexposed sites with sparing at clothing and watchstrap cut-off is seen when looked for. Some patients do describe an erythematous phototoxicity. Both appear reversible.

Photodynamic therapy reactions

Two intravenous photosensitizers used therapeutically to induce phototoxic damage of systemic tumors, include Photofrin® (porfimer sodium) and Foscan® (temoporfin). Both are associated with persistent phototoxicity, which is visible wavelength–dependent and potentially severe. Following intravenous injection, patients who have been administered Photofrin are encouraged to avoid bright sunlight and even incandescent light for four to six weeks. Some patients may develop severe phototoxicity within the infusion arm beyond this period suggesting that the drug persists at a higher concentration at that site much longer than elsewhere in the body. Work is underway to produce agents more rapidly eliminated, although such an agent, Verteporfin, has been associated with severe skin photosensitization (60).

A wide range of therapeutic agents is associated with photosensitive skin reactions. Fortunately, the majority of these therapies can be substituted by nonphotoactive alternatives. Predictable phototoxicity seen with the common drugs is rarely a diagnostic problem for clinicians. Much more of an issue are the idiosyncratic reactions as seen in the rarer forms of phototoxicity and other mechanisms.

REFERENCES

1. Ferguson J. Drug and chemical photosensitivity. In: Hawk JLM, ed. Photodermatology. New York: Oxford University Press, 1999:155–169.
2. Selvaag E. Clinical drug photosensitivity. A retrospective analysis of reports to the Norwegian Adverse Drug Reactions Committee from the years 1970–1994. Photodermatol Photoimmunol Photomed 1997; 13(1–2):21–23.
3. Cronin E. Contact Dermatitis. London: Churchill Livingstone, 1980.

4. DeLeo VA, Harber LC. Contact photodermatitis. In: Fisher AA, ed. Contact Dermatitis, 3rd ed. Philadelphia: Lea & Febiger, 1986.
5. Marks JG Jr, DeLeo VA. Contact and Occupational Dermatology. 2nd ed. St. Louis: Mosby-Yearbook, 1992.
6. Emmett EA. Phototoxicity and photosensitivity reactions. In: Adams RM, ed. Occupational Skin Disease. 2nd ed. Philadelphia: WB Saunders, 1990.
7. Thune P, Jansen C, Wennersten G, et al. The Scandinavian multicenter photopatch study: 1980 to 1985-final report. Photodermatology 1988; 5:261–269.
8. Crow KD, Alexander E. Buck WHL, Johnson BE, Magnus IA, Porter AD. Photosensitivity due to pitch. Br J Dermatol 1961; 73:220–232.
9. Emmett EA. Cutaneous and ocular hazards of roofers. Occup Med 1986; 1:307–322.
10. Emmett EA, Stetzer W, Taphorn B. Phototoxic keratoconjunctivitis from coal-tar pitch volatiles. Science 1977; 198:841–842.
11. Kochevar IE, Armstrong RB, Einbinder J, Walther RR, Harber LC. Coal tar phototoxicity: active compounds and action spectra. Photochem Photobiol 1982; 38(1):65–69.
12. Jonas AD. Creosote burns. J Ind Hyg Toxicol 1943; 25:418–420.
13. Heyl T, Mellett WA. Creosote dermatitis in an ammunition depot. S Afr Med J 1982; 62:66–67.
14. Tunget CL, Turchen SG, Manoguerra AS, et al. Sunlight and the plant: a toxic combination: severe phytophotodermatitis from Cneoridium dumosum. Cutis 1994; 54(6):400–402.
15. Klaber R. Phytophotodermatitis. Br J Dermatol 1942; 54:193–211.
16. Birmingham DJ, Key MM, Tubich GE, Perone VB. Phototoxic bullae among celery harvesters. Arch Dermatol 1961; 83:73–87.
17. Morbidity and Mortality Weekly Report. Phytophotodermatitis among grocery workers. JAMA 1985; 253:753.
18. Emmett EA, Taphorn BR, Kominsky JR. Phototoxicity occurring during the manufacture of ultraviolet cured ink. Arch Dermatol 1977; 113:770–775.
19. Gardiner JS, Dickson A, Macleod TM, Frain-Bell W. The investigation of photocontact dermatitis in a dye manufacturing process. Br J Dermatol 1972; 86:264.
20. Thune P. Contact and photocontact allergy to sunscreens. Photodermatology 1984; 1:5–9.
21. Menz MB, Sigfrid AM, Connolly SM. Photopatch testing: a six-year experience. J Am Acad Dermatol 1988; 18:1044–1047.
22. DeLeo VA, Suarez SM, Maso MJ. Photoallergic contact dermatitis: results of photopatch testing in New York—1985 to 1990. Arch Dermatol. 1992; 128:1513–1518.
23. Yashar SS, Lim HW. Classification and evaluation of photodermatoses. Dermatol Therapy 2003; 16:1–7.
24. Bruynzeel DP, Ferguson J, Anderson K, et al. Photopatch testing: a consensus methodology for Europe. J Eur Acad Dermatol Venereol 2004; 18:679–682.
25. Wilkinson DS. Photodermatitis due to tetrachlorosalicylanilide. Br J Dermatol 1961; 73:213–219.
26. Calnan CD, Harman RRM, Wells GC. Photodermatitis from soaps. Br Med J 1961; 2:1266.
27. Matthieu L, Meuleman L, Van Hecke E, et al. Contact and photocontact allergy to ketoprofen. The Belgium experience. Contact Dermatitis 2004; 50:238–241.
28. Neumann NJ, Hölzle E, Plewig G, et al. Photopatch testing: the 12-year experience of the German, Austrian, and Swiss photopatch test group. J Am Acad Dermatol 2000; 42:183–192.
29. Frain-Bell W, Gardiner J. Photocontact dermatitis due to quindoxin. Contact Dermatitis 1976; 1:256–257.
30. Scott KW, Dawson TAJ. Photocontact dermatitis arising from the presence of quindoxin in annual feeding stuffs. Br J Dermatol 1974; 90:543–546.
31. Schauder S, Schroder W, Geier J. Olaquindox-induced airborne photoallergic contact dermatitis followed by transient or persistent light reactions in 15 pig breeders. Contact Dermatitis 1996; 35(6):344–354.
32. Mark KA, Brancaccio RR, Soter NA, Cohen DE. Allergic and photoallergic contact dermatitis to plant and pesticide allergens. Arch Dermatol 1999; 135:67–70.
33. Feuerman EJ. Chromates as the cause of contact dermatitis in housewives. Dermatologica 1971; 143:292–297.
34. Tronnier H. Zur Lichtempfindlichkeit von Ekzematikern (unter besonderer Berücksichtigung des Chromatekzems). Arch Klin Exp Derm 1970; 237:494–506.
35. Burry JM, Kuchel R, Reid JG, Kirk J. Australian bush dermatitis: compositae dermatitis in South Australia. Med J Aust 1973; 1:110–116.
36. Epstein S. Role of dermal sensitivity in ragweed contact dermatitis. Arch Dermatol 1960; 82:48–55.
37. Thune PO, Solberg YJ. Photosensitivity and allergy to aromatic lichen acids, compositae oleoresins and other plant substances. Contact Dermatitis 1980; 6:81–87.
38. Ferguson J. Photosensitivity due to drugs. Photoderm Photoimmunol Photomed 2002; 18:262–269.
39. EMEA: http://www.emea.eu.int/pdfs/human/swp/039801en.pdf; FDA: http://www.fda.gov.cder/guidance/3640fnl.pdf.

40. Jacobs A, Brown PC, Conrad C, et al. CDER photosafety guidance for industry. Toxicol Pathol 2004; 32(suppl 2):17–18.
41. Fitzpatrick TB. The validity and practicality of sun-reactive skin types I through VI. Arch Dermatol 1988; 124:869–871.
42. LaDuca JR, Bouman PH, Gaspari AA. Nonsteroidal anti-inflammatory drug-induced pseudoporphyria: a case series. J Cutan Med Surg 2002; 6(4):320–326.
43. Maerker JM, Harm A, Foeldvari I, et al. Naproxen-induced pseudoporphyria. Hautarzt 2001; 52(11):1026–1029.
44. Sharp MT, Horn, TD. Pseudoporphyria induced by voriconazole. J Am Acad Dermatol 2005; 53(2):341–345.
45. Johnston GA. Thiazide-induced lichenoid photosensitivity. Clin Exp Dermatol 2002; 27(8):670–672.
46. Reed BR, Huff J, Jones SK, et al. Subacute cutaneous lupus erythematosus associated with hydrochlorothiazide therapy. Ann Intern Med 1985; 103:49–51.
47. Lowe G, Walker EM, Johnson BE, et al. Thiazide-induced photosensitivity, the use of bumetanide as alternative therapy: in vitro and in vivo studies. Br J Dermatol 1989; 121(suppl):58.
48. Burry JN, Lawrence JR. Phototoxic blisters from high frusemide dosage. Br J Dermatol 1976; 94:495–499.
49. Ferguson J. Phototoxicity due to fluoroquinolones. In: Hooper DC, Rubinstein E, eds. Quinolone Antimicrobial Agents. 3rd ed. Washington, D.C.: ASM Press, 2003:449–458.
50. Chalmers RTG, Muston HL, Srinivas V, et al. High incidence of amiodarone-induced photosensitivity in North-West England. Br J Dermatol 1982; 285:341.
51. Rappersberger K, Hönigsmann H, Ortel B, et al. Photosensitivity and hyperpigmentation in amiodarone-treated patients: incidence, time course, and recovery. J Invest Dermatol 1989; 93(2):201–209.
52. Collins P, Ferguson J. Narrow-band (TL-01) phototherapy: an effective preventative treatment for the photodermatoses. Br J Dermatol 1995; 132:956–963.
53. Yones SS, O'Donoghue NB, Palmer RA, et al. Persistent severe amiodarone-induced photosensitivity. Clin Exp Dermatol 2005; 30(5):500–502.
54. Ferguson J, Addo HA, Johnson BE, et al. Quinine induced photosensitivity: clinical and experimental studies. Br J Dermatol 1987; 117(5):631–640.
55. Metayer I, Balguerie X, Courville P, et al. Photodermatosis induced by hydroxychloroquine: 4 cases. Ann Dermatol Venereol 2001; 128(6–7):729–731.
56. Layton AM, Cunliffe J. Photosensitive eruptions to doxycycline—a dose related phenomenon. Br J Dermatol 1992; 127(suppl 30):31.
57. VA Cooperative No. 475 Group. Benefits and harms of doxycycline treatment for Gulf War veterans' illnesses: a randomized, double-blind, placebo-controlled trial. Ann Intern Med 2004; 141(2):85–94.
58. Carroll LA, Laumann AE. Doxycycline-induced photo-onycholysis. J. Drugs Dermatol 2003; 2(6):662–663.
59. Collins P, Ferguson J. Photodistributed nifedipine-induced facial telangiectasia. Br J Dermatol 1993; 129(5):630–633.
60. Asensio Sanchez VM, Carral Azor A, Garcia Pascual A. Verteporfin and photosensitivity in diabetic. Arch Soc Esp Oftalmol 2003; 78 (5):227–229.

15 | Cutaneous Porphyrias

Gillian M. Murphy
Department of Dermatology, Beaumont Hospital, Dublin, Ireland

Karl E. Anderson
Department of Internal Medicine, Division of Gastroenterology and Hepatology, University of Texas Medical Branch, Galveston, Texas, U.S.A.

- The porphyrias are each caused by specific enzyme deficiencies in heme biosynthesis.

- Patterns of elevated porphyrins and porphyrin precursors in urine stool and blood enable delineation of each porphyria type.

- Porphyria cutanea tarda is commonest in adults, treatment induces remission.

- Symptoms of erythropoietic protoporphyria usually stars in childhood.

- Bone marrow transplantation may induce cure in congenital erythropoietic porphyria.

- Diagnosis of acute porphyria is essential as avoidance of trigger factors for acute attacks may be lifesaving (an updated list of safe drugs is available at www.porphyria-europe.com/); treatment of acute attacks may be lifesaving.

- Genetic counseling should be provided with inherited porphyrias.

INTRODUCTION

The porphyrias are uncommon disorders due to deficiencies of enzymes in the metabolic pathway for synthesizing heme (Fig. 1). These enzyme deficiencies can lead to accumulation of pathway intermediates and either skin photosensitivity (caused by porphyrins in the cutaneous porphyrias) or neurological attacks (associated with increases in porphyrin precursors in the acute porphyrias). Intermediates accumulate first in either the bone marrow, where erythrocyte precursors actively synthesize heme for hemoglobin, or in liver, which produces large amounts of cytochrome P450 enzymes. On this basis, porphyrias are classified as either erythropoietic or hepatic (Table 1). Heme is also produced in other tissues for a variety of essential hemoproteins such as respiratory cytochromes, catalase and myoglobin.

The cutaneous manifestations of the porphyrias described in this chapter occur in both of the erythropoietic porphyrias and in three of the five hepatic porphyrias. When porphyrins absorb light at the Soret band region (400–410 nm), they enter an excited energy state and then release energy as fluorescence and by the formation of singlet oxygen and other

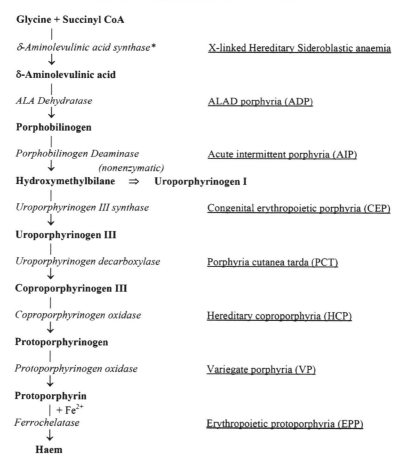

THE HAEM BIOSYNTHETIC PATHWAY

Glycine + Succinyl CoA

δ-Aminolevulinic acid synthase*   X-linked Hereditary Sideroblastic anaemia

δ-Aminolevulinic acid

ALA Dehydratase   ALAD porphyria (ADP)

Porphobilinogen

Porphobilinogen Deaminase   Acute intermittent porphyria (AIP)
      (nonenzymatic)

Hydroxymethylbilane   ⇒   Uroporphyrinogen I

Uroporphyrinogen III synthase   Congenital erythropoietic porphyria (CEP)

Uroporphyrinogen III

Uroporphyrinogen decarboxylase   Porphyria cutanea tarda (PCT)

Coproporphyrinogen III

Coproporphyrinogen oxidase   Hereditary coproporphyria (HCP)

Protoporphyrinogen

Protoporphyrinogen oxidase   Variegate porphyria (VP)

Protoporphyrin
      | + Fe^{2+}
Ferrochelatase   Erythropoietic protoporphyria (EPP)

Haem

FIGURE 1   The heme biosynthetic pathway. Enzymes catalyzing each step are indicated in italics, the products are in bold, and the diseases resulting from deficiencies in activity of each enzyme are underlined. Mutations of the erythroid form of δ-aminolevulinic acid synthase, encoded by a gene on the X-chromosome, are found in many cases of sideroblastic anemia. Deficiency of the ubiquitous enzyme, encoded by a gene on chromosome 3, has not been described. Induction of the ubiquitous enzyme, which is rate limiting in liver, and its feedback repression by the endproduct heme, play key roles in determining severity of the acute hepatic porphyrias.

TABLE 1 Classification of the Porphyrias

	Acute porphyrias	Cutaneous porphyrias
Hepatic porphyrias	ALAD porphyria Acute intermittent porphyria Hereditary coproporphyria Variegate porphyria	Porphyria cutanea tarda
Erythropoietic porphyrias		Congenital erythropoietic porphyria Erythropoietic protoporphyria

Abbreviation: ALAD, δ-aminolevulinic acid dehydratase.

oxygen species that can produce tissue damage. Neurological manifestations are important to recognize because they occur in two types of cutaneous porphyria, and are described briefly.

Porphyrins are tetrapyrroles, whereby four pyrroles form a large macrocycle. Heme (iron protoporphyrin) and other metalloporphyrins are formed by inserting a metal atom into the porphyrin macrocycle. Some porphyrins, including uroporphyrin, coproporphyrin and protoporphyrin have many conjugated double bonds, are reddish in color and can absorb visible light leading to generation of excited states. Most of the reduced porphyrin intermediates in the pathway (e.g., uroporphyrinogen, coproporphyrinogen) and heme are colorless, nonfluorescent and nonphotosensitizing.

The type of cellular damage depends on the solubility and tissue distribution of porphyrins. Two main patterns of skin damage are seen in the porphyrias. Excess amounts of water soluble uro- and coproporphyrins, which contain eight and four carboxyl groups, respectively, leads to chronic blistering of sun exposed skin, as seen in most of the cutaneous porphyrias. The quite different skin manifestations in erythropoietic protoporphyria (EPP), which consist of immediate burning sensation in the skin, sometimes followed by swelling, redness, purpura and erosions, are due to accumulation of protoporphyrin, which has only two carboxyl side chains, and is water-insoluble and lipophilic.

Patterns of individual porphyrins in plasma, erythrocytes, urine and stool and porphyrin precursors in urine help explain the clinical features of the porphyrias and allow the diagnosis of each to be made by biochemical methods (Tables 2, 3). Porphyrin abnormalities occur without

TABLE 2 Heme Pathway Intermediates and Their Derivatives that Accumulate and are Excreted in the Various Porphyrias

Porphyria	Erythrocytes	Plasma porphyrins	Urine	Feces
ADP	Zn protoporphyrin	NS[a]	ALA, coproporphyrin III	Coproporphyrin III
AIP	NS	NS	ALA, PBG, Uroporphyrin	NS
CEP	Uroporphyrin I, coproporphyrin I, Zn protoporphyrin	Marked increase (peak ~620 nm)[b]	Uroporphyrin I, coproporphyrin I	Coproporphyrin I
PCT	NS	Increased (peak ~620 nm)	Uroporphyrin, heptacarboxyl porphyrin	Isocoproporphyrin[c]
HEP	Zn protoporphyrin	Marked increase (peak ~620 nm)	Uroporphyrin, heptacarboxyl porphyrin	Isocoproporphyrin[c]
HCP	NS		ALA, PBG, coproporphyrin III	Coproporphyrin III
VP	NS	Increased (peak ~626 nm)	ALA, PBG, coproporphyrin III	Coproporphyrin III, protoporphyrin
EPP	Free protoporphyrin	Increased (peak ~635 nm)	NS	Protoporphyrin

Substantial increases that are diagnostically important are shown. With the exception of protoporphyrin, all porphyrins listed represent auto-oxidized derivatives of the corresponding porphyrinogens (reduced porphyrins) that are the actual pathway intermediates.
[a]Normal or not substantially increased.
[b] Fluorescence emission maximum of diluted plasma at neutral pH, which differentiates variegate porphyria and erythropoietic protoporphyria from other cutaneous porphyrias.
[c] Isocoproporphyrin is usually not the predominant fraction of fecal porphyrins in porphyria cutanea tarda and hepatoerythropoietic porphyria, but the increased amount is part of a complex pattern that is distinctive.
Abbreviations: ADP, δ-Aminolevulinic acid dehydratase porphyria; AIP, acute intermittent porphyria; ALA, δ-aminolevulinic acid; CEP, congenital erythropoietic porphyria; EPP, erythropoietic protoporphyria; HEP, hepatoerythropoietic porphyria; HCP, hereditary coproporphyria; PBG, porphobilinogen; PCT, porphyria cutanea tarda; VP, variegate porphyria.

TABLE 3   Diagnostic Evaluations for Cutaneous Porphyrias

Clinical features	Potential types of porphyria	First-line tests (for screening)	Second-line tests[a] (for confirmation)
Blistering lesions	PCT, VP, HCP, CEP, HEP	Plasma total[b,c] or	Plasma fluorescence scan[b,d]
		Urinary total porphyrins[b]	Fractionation of porphyrins if totals elevated
			Fecal and erythrocyte total porphyrins
			Urinary δ-aminolevulinic acid and porphobilinogen[e]
Nonblistering photosensitivity	EPP	Erythrocyte porphyrins[b] or	
		Plasma total porphyrins[c]	

Particularly when clinical features suggest the more common porphyrias, it is useful and most cost-effective to rely on a few first-line tests for screening.
[a]In addition to all screening tests listed.
[b]Screening tests that are sensitive for the uses shown.
[c]Screening tests that are specific for the uses shown.
[d]In some laboratories, plasma fluorescence scanning is used for screening, instead of measuring total plasma porphyrins.
[e]Elevation of these porphyrin precursors (especially porphobilinogen) is specific evidence for the acute porphyrias, of which two (hereditary coproporphyria and variegate porphyria) can cause blistering skin lesions.
Total urinary, fecal, and erythrocyte porphyrins are elevated nonspecifically in many medical conditions; determining patterns of the individual porphyrins (for example by HPLC separation) provide more specific information, but adds expense and is seldom necessary for screening.
Abbreviations: CEP, congenital erythropoietic porphyria; EPP, Erythropoietic protoporphyria; HCP, hereditary coproporphyria; HEP, hepatoerythropoietic porphyria; PCT, porphyria cutanea tarda; VP, variegate porphyria.

photosensitivity or neurological symptoms in many other conditions, such as sideroblastic and hemolytic anemias, iron deficiency, renal failure, hepatobiliary disease, and gastrointestinal hemorrhage. Rarely, as in some cases of sideroblastic anemia, there are associated photosensitivity features (1). A few conditions, such as lead poisoning and hereditary tyrosinemia type 1, are associated with increases in porphyrin precursors as well as porphyrins, particularly in erythrocytes, and urine.

Tests for porphyria should be carried out by a quality assured laboratory as missed diagnoses may be a consequence of false negative tests. False positive results and inconsequential abnormalities are also problematic. Measurement of plasma porphyrins or spectrofluorimetric scanning of diluted plasma at neutral pH will detect active cutaneous porphyrias and are useful for screening (2). Ethylene diamine tetra acetic acid (EDTA) plasma samples are more stable than serum samples. Cholestasis and some drugs can interfere with plasma fluorimetric assessment. Gene carriers with latent disease in family studies may be identified by measuring enzyme activity. However, DNA analysis is more reliable and becoming more widely used.

HISTORY OF THE PORPHYRIAS

The first documented reference to porphyria was in 1841 by Scherer. Acute porphyria was first described in Holland by Stokvis in 1889. In 1911, Günther described what we now term congenital erythropoietic porphyria (CEP). In 1912, Meyer-Betz injected himself with haematoporphyrin and became acutely photosensitive, thereby demonstrated that porphyrins can cause acute photosensitivity (3).

Acute intermittent porphyria was characterized by Waldenström in 1937, and variegate porphyria was recognized in South Africa in the 1940s and 1950s. In the 1950s, a massive outbreak of porphyria cutanea tarda (PCT) occurred in eastern Turkey (4), where an impoverished population consumed wheat that had been intended for planting and had been treated with the fungicide hexachlorobenzene. EPP, now known to be the third most common porphyria, was not clearly described until 1961.

In the 1970s and thereafter, specific enzyme deficiencies were recognized in the seven major types of porphyria, and subsequently the genes encoding these enzymes were cloned and sequenced. Multiple mutations have been identified in all porphyrias except the sporadic

TABLE 4 Defective Enzymes in Porphyrias

Porphyria	Defective enzyme	Chromosomal location
ALA dehydratase porphyria (ADP)	ALA dehydratase (ALAD)	9q34
Acute intermittent porphyria (AIP)	Porphobilinogen deaminase (PBGD)	11q23.3
Congenital erythropoietic porphyria (CEP)	Uroporphyrinogen III synthase (UROS)	10q25.3 → q26.3
Porphyria cutanea tarda (PCT)	Uroporphyrinogen decarboxylase (UROD)	1p34
Hepatoerythropoietic porphyria (HEP)		
Hereditary coproporphyria (HCP)	Coproporphyrinogen oxidase (CPO)	3q12.1
Variegate porphyria	Protoporphyrinogen oxidase (PPO)	1q22 → q23
Erythropoietic protoporphyria (EPP)	Ferrochelatase (FECH)	18q22

form of PCT (Fig. 1, Table 1). In addition, rare homozygous cases of the autosomal dominant porphyrias, and more complex cases with dual enzyme defects have been described.

PORPHYRIAS CAUSING BLISTERING SKIN LESIONS

Five types of porphyria can present with identical blistering skin lesions, but are readily differentiated by biochemical testing (Tables 1–3). Defective enzymes associated with these porphyrias have been identified (Fig. 1, Table 4). In three, namely PCT, variegate porphyria (VP) and hereditary coproporphyria (HCP) symptoms usually begin in adult life. HCP and VP can also cause acute neurological symptoms. Cutaneous manifestations of CEP and hepatoerythropoietic porphyria (HEP) are usually much more severe and mutilating and begin in early childhood. However, cases of CEP and HEP with less severe symptoms, sometimes beginning in adulthood, are also well documented.

PORPHYRIA CUTANEA TARDA

This is the most common and readily treated human porphyria. PCT is due to an acquired deficiency of Uroporphyrinogen decarboxylase (UROD) in the liver, although an inherited deficiency of this enzyme and other genetic factors sometimes contribute. This is an iron-related disease, which develops only with a normal or increased amount of hepatic iron.

Clinical Manifestations

Fluid-filled vesicles develop most commonly on the backs of the hands (Fig. 2), and also on the forearms, face, ears, neck, legs, and feet. These commonly rupture, leading to chronic, crusted lesions, and denuded areas that heal slowly and may become infected. The sun-exposed skin is also friable, and bullae or denudation of skin may result from minor trauma. Milia may precede or follow vesicle formation. Facial hypertrichosis and hyperpigmentation are particularly troubling in women (Fig. 3). Affected areas of skin sometimes become severely thickened, scarred and calcified. These findings have been termed *pseudoscleroderma*. Identical skin lesions can occur in VP and much less commonly in HCP. Skin findings in CEP and HEP resemble PCT but are usually much more severe and mutilating. Mild or moderate erythrocytosis is common in PCT, and is not well explained. Chronic lung disease from smoking may contribute.

A number of factors contribute to the development of PCT. These include alcohol use, smoking, estrogens, viral infections—particularly hepatitis C and less commonly HIV, and genetic factors such as mutations in the hemochromatosis gene (*HFE*) and inherited uroporphyrinogen decarboxylase (UROD) deficiency (5). Onset of symptoms at an earlier age may be noted in patients with genetic predisposing factors, such as an inherited partial deficiency of UROD or the C282Y/C282Y *HFE* genotype (6). Hepatitis C is especially prevalent among PCT patients in southern Europe and North America but in itself insufficient to cause PCT (7). Since the large outbreak of PCT in Turkey after hexachlorobenzene ingestion, individual cases and small outbreaks have been reported after exposure to other halogenated cyclic aromatic hydrocarbons, including di- and trichlorophenols and 2,3,7,8-tetrachlorodibenzo-*p*-dioxin (TCDD, dioxin) (8).

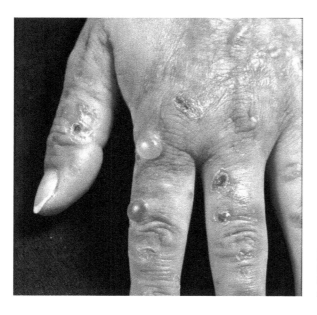

FIGURE 2 Blistering, erosions and scarring of the hand in porphyria cutanea tarda. *Source*: Courtesy of Herbert Hönigsmann, MD, Vienna, Austria.

Nonspecific liver abnormalities, such increased transaminases and gamma-glutamyltranspeptidase, are common. The long term risk for hepatocellular carcinoma is increased.

PCT may occur with other conditions predisposing to iron overload (9), and with diabetes mellitus. PCT occurs more commonly than expected in patients with cutaneous and systemic lupus erythematosus, precipitated by antimalarial therapy such as chloroquine which is porphyrogenic. Other immunological disorders such as scleroderma, and hematological malignancy are other recognized association (10). PCT that develop in patients with end-stage renal disease is usually more severe, sometimes with severe mutilation. In these patients, lack of urinary porphyrin excretion leads to much higher concentrations of porphyrins in plasma and the excess porphyrins are poorly dialyzable (11,12).

PATHOLOGY

Skin histopathology in PCT includes subepidermal blistering and deposition of periodic acid–Schiff-positive material around blood vessels and fine fibrillar material at the dermoepithelial

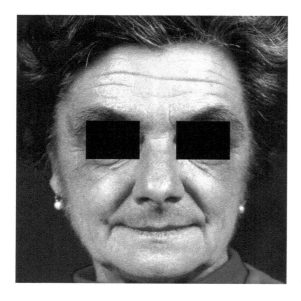

FIGURE 3 Hyperpigmentation and hypertrichosis in a woman with porphyria cutanea tarda. *Source*: Courtesy of Herbert Hönigsmann, MD, Vienna, Austria.

junction. Immunoglobulin G, other immunoglobulins, and complement are also deposited around dermal blood vessels and at the dermoepithelial junction. These histologic changes are found in other cutaneous porphyrias and are not diagnostic.

Liver tissue shows red fluorescence on exposure to long-wave ultraviolet light, reflecting accumulation of massive amounts of porphyrins. Microscopic, needle-like inclusions are fluorescent and birefringent; these are located in lysosomes. Paracrystalline inclusions are seen in mitochondria. Nonspecific liver histopathology includes necrosis, inflammation, increased iron, and increased fat.

Etiology and Pathogenesis

Hepatic UROD activity is <20% of normal in PCT; however, UROD protein level in the liver is normal. Iron does not directly inhibit UROD, but plays an essential porphyrinogenic role probably by promoting formation of reactive oxygen species that oxidize uroporphyrinogen to uroporphyrin and to a yet uncharacterized UROD inhibitor.

UROD is a dimeric enzyme that catalyzes the sequential, clockwise removal of the four carboxyl groups from the acetic acid side chains of uroporphyrinogen III (an octacarboxyl porphyrinogen) to form the four methyl groups of coproporphyrinogen III (a tetracarboxyl porphyrinogen). Substantial deficiency of this enzyme results in accumulation of uroporphyrinogen (isomers I and III), the intermediate substrates hepta-, hexa-, and pentacarboxyl porphyrinogens, and isocoproporphyrinogen. The latter is formed from pentacarboxyl porphyrinogen by coproporphyrinogen oxidase—a minor pathway that becomes accentuated when hepatic UROD is deficient. These excess porphyrinogens (reduced porphyrins) undergo nonenzymatic oxidation to the corresponding porphyrins (uro-, hepta-, hexa-, and pentacarboxyl porphyrins, and isocoproporphyrins). The excess porphyrins circulate from the liver to the skin, where sunlight exposure generates reactive oxygen species, activates the complement system, and produces lysosomal damage (13)

Susceptibility Factors in Human Porphyria Cutanea Tarda

The following factors can contribute to the development of all types of PCT, including the familial form (14).

1. *Iron and HFE mutations.* Serum ferritin levels are usually in the upper part of the normal range. Prevalence of the C282Y mutation of the HFE gene, which is the major cause of hemochromatosis in Caucasians, is increased in PCT, and ~10% of patients may be C282Y homozygotes, and tend to have more substantial increases in ferritin (15). In southern Europe, where the C282Y is less prevalent, the H63D mutation is more commonly associated (16). Murine models with disruption of one UROD allele [UROD(+/−)] and either one or two disrupted HFE alleles [HFE(+/−) or HFE(−/−)] provide insight into the roles of these mutations (17).

2. *UROD mutations.* Most patients (~80%) have no mutations of the UROD gene, and are said to have type 1 (sporadic) PCT. These patients have normal UROD activity in nonhepatic tissues such as erythrocytes and unaffected relatives. However, ~20% of PCT patients, who are said to have familial (type 2) PCT, are heterozygous for mutations that reduce UROD activity and immunoreactivity to ~50% of normal in all tissues (including erythrocytes). This partial deficiency of UROD is inherited as an autosomal dominant trait. Because penetrance is low, many patients with type 2 PCT have no family history of the disease. Many different mutations of the UROD gene have been identified in type 2 PCT (18). Type 3 PCT, which has not been clearly distinguished from type 1, describes the rare occurrence of PCT in more than one family member, but with normal erythrocyte UROD activity and no demonstrable UROD mutations.

3. *Hepatitis C.* The prevalence of hepatitis C in PCT ranges from 50% to 75% in many countries (14,19). How hepatitis C contributes to the development of PCT is poorly understood.

4. *HIV.* PCT is less commonly associated with HIV infection (20). The mechanism is unknown, but presumably is due to injury to hepatic tissue.

5. *Alcohol.* PCT has long been associated with excess alcohol use. Proposed mechanisms include generation of active oxygen species that contribute to oxidative damage,

mitochondrial injury, depletion of reduced glutathione and other antioxidant defenses, increased production of endotoxin, activation of Kupffer cells, and increased iron absorption.

6. *Smoking and cytochrome P450 enzymes.* Smoking is less extensively studied as a risk factor but is commonly associated with alcohol use in PCT (5,14). Smoking may contribute by increasing oxidative stress and inducing hepatic cytochrome P450 enzymes. The latter are thought to be important in oxidizing uroporphyrinogen to uroporphyrin, and generating a UROD inhibitor.

7. *Antioxidants.* Plasma ascorbate levels were reported to be substantially reduced in the majority of patients with PCT (21). Low levels of serum carotenoids further suggest that oxidant stress is important in PCT. Ascorbic acid deficiency can clearly contribute to uroporphyria in laboratory models.

8. *Estrogens.* These are commonly associated with PCT, especially in women (5,14).

Laboratory Evaluation and Diagnosis

Plasma and urinary porphyrins are substantially increased in clinically manifest PCT, and a predominance of uroporphyrin and heptacarboxyl porphyrin is considered diagnostic (Table 2). Measurement of total plasma porphyrins is perhaps most useful for screening, because urinary porphyrins are more subject to nonspecific increases especially in patients with liver dysfunction. A normal value excludes all porphyrias that produce blistering skin lesions. When increased, it is useful to determine the plasma fluorescence emission maximum at neutral pH, because a maximum near 620 nm is characteristic of PCT (as well as CEP and HCP) and, most importantly, excludes VP, which has a fluorescence maximum at or near 626 nm (22). Urinary δ-aminolevulinic acid (ALA) may be increased slightly in PCT, and PBG is normal.

After a diagnosis of PCT is established, the familial (type 2) form is distinguished from sporadic (type 1) PCT by finding decreased erythrocyte UROD activity, or more reliably by finding a disease-related *UROD* mutation.

Pseudoporphyria (also known as pseudo-PCT) is a poorly understood condition that presents with lesions that closely resemble PCT. Plasma porphyrins are not significantly increased in this condition, and there is no evidence that it is a disorder of porphyrin metabolism. Potentially photosensitizing drugs such as nonsteroidal antiinflammatory agents are sometimes implicated.

Treatment

Pseudoporphyria, VP, HCP, and even mild cases of CEP can produce similar cutaneous lesions but are unresponsive to treatment that is effective in PCT. Therefore, it is important to accurately establish the diagnosis biochemically. Liver imaging and a serum α-fetoprotein determination are advisable to exclude complicating hepatocellular carcinoma and to serve as a baseline for follow-up.

Patients should be evaluated for susceptibility factors including alcohol use, smoking, HCV and HIV infections, estrogen use, and *HFE* mutations (5,14), and should cease exposures to exogenous agents that have contributed. Although drugs that are associated with exacerbations of acute porphyrias are seldom reported to contribute to PCT, they should be avoided initially as a precaution. Familial and sporadic forms of PCT are treated in the same manner.

Phlebotomy and low-dose chloroquine (or hydroxychloroquine) are alternative therapies that if completed correctly almost always achieve a full remission. Prospective comparative treatment trials are lacking. Phlebotomy reduces body iron stores and liver iron content, and is considered the standard treatment at most centers. About 450 ml of blood can be removed at one-two-week intervals until the serum ferritin is below ~15 ng/mL, after which plasma porphyrin levels become normal. Hemoglobin or hematocrit levels should be followed to prevent symptomatic anemia. Continued phlebotomies are generally not needed, even if ferritin levels later return to normal. Porphyrin levels can be followed and treatment restarted if porphyrin levels begin to rise.

A low-dose regimen of chloroquine or hydroxychloroquine is most appropriate when phlebotomy is contraindicated or poorly tolerated. These 4-aminoquinoline antimalarial drugs concentrate in liver lysosomes and mitochondria, and may form complexes with and mobilize porphyrins, or possibly hepatic iron. A low-dose regimen (chloroquine 125 mg or hydroxychloroquine 100 mg—one half of a normal tablet—twice weekly until plasma or urine porphyrins are normalized) achieves a remission over several months with few side effects. Standard doses are likely to cause fever, malaise, nausea and transient acute hepatitis; therefore, they should be avoided. Low-dose chloroquine was reportedly not effective in patients homozygous for the *C282Y* mutation of the *HFE* gene (22). Infusions of desferrioxamine, an iron chelator, may be an alternative treatment approach when phlebotomy or antimalarials are contraindicated.

In general, treatment of hepatitis C should be delayed until after PCT is in remission. PCT is usually the more symptomatic of these conditions; its treatment has a higher response rate and is completed more quickly. Treatment of hepatitis C may be more effective after iron reduction. PCT sometimes presents during interferon-ribavirin treatment of hepatitis C, when treatment of PCT may be precluded by complications such as anemia.

Treatment of PCT is more difficult when associated with end-stage renal disease. Low volume phlebotomy (100–200 mL per treatment), combined with erythropoietin, are usually effective (23).

HEPATOERYTHROPOIETIC PORPHYRIA

This very rare disorder, in which excess porphyrins originate mostly from the liver, is the homozygous form of familial (type 2) PCT (24). In most cases, the clinical manifestations resemble CEP (see later discussion) rather the PCT. Blistering skin lesions, hypertrichosis, scarring, and red urine usually begin in infancy or childhood, and sclerodermoid skin changes are sometimes prominent (Fig. 4). Unusually mild cases have been described (25).

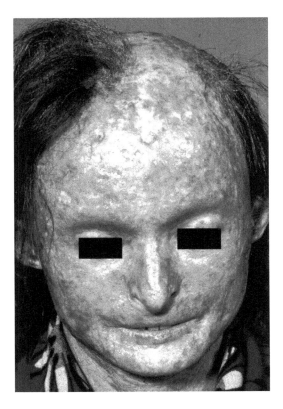

FIGURE 4 Sclerotic skin in a patient with hepatoerythropoietic porphyria. *Source*: Courtesy of Herbert Hönigsmann, MD, Vienna, Austria.

Etiology and Pathogenesis

Affected individuals are either homozygous or compound heterozygotes for UROD mutations. A variety of UROD mutations have been identified (24,25).

Laboratory Evaluation, Diagnosis and Treatment

HEP is recognized biochemically by predominant accumulation and excretion of uroporphyrin, heptacarboxyl porphyrin and isocoproporphyrins, hence resembling the profile of PCT. However, in contrast to PCT, increased erythrocyte zinc protoporphyrin is substantially increased. At least one genotype may be associated with predominant excretion of pentacarboxyl porphyrin (25).

Avoiding sunlight is important, as in CEP. Oral charcoal was helpful in a severe case associated with dyserythropoiesis. Phlebotomy has shown little or no benefit. Retrovirus-mediated gene transfer can correct porphyria in cell lines from patients with this disease, which suggests that gene therapy may be applicable in the future (26).

VARIEGATE PORPHYRIA AND HEREDITARY COPROPORPHYRIA

δ-Aminolevulinic acid dehydratase porphyria (ADP), acute intermittent porphyria (AIP), VP, and HCP are four types of hepatic porphyria that can present with acute neurological attacks (Table 1). Of note, only VP and HCP can present with blisters identical to those seen in PCT. AIP is most common of the four porphyrias, and ADP the least. AIP, HCP, and VP are autosomal dominant, whereas ADP autosomal recessive. All are heterogeneous at the molecular level.

VP is especially common among Caucasians of Dutch descent in South Africa, and almost all cases share the same protoporphyrinogen oxidase (PPO) mutation (R59W) (27). A founder effect also accounts for the very high prevalence of AIP in northern Sweden where almost all cases have the same porphobilinogen deaminase (PBGD) mutation (W198X). Very rare cases of homozygous AIP, HCP, and VP are manifested by severe neurological impairment early in life but not acute attacks (28). Homozygous cases of HCP and VP also have severe photosensitivity.

Neurological Manifestations

Symptoms of AIP are more common in women. The few documented cases of ADP have been mostly males. South African patients with VP have been reported recently to have milder and less frequent attacks than do patients with AIP, and these occur equally in males and females. Acute porphyric attacks may occur any time after puberty and are often precipitated by certain drugs, steroid hormones or dietary indiscretions. Abdominal pain is the most common symptom, and is usually severe, steady, and poorly localized. Other characteristic but nonspecific findings include tachycardia, hypertension, nausea, vomiting, constipation, bladder dysfunction and pain in the limbs, chest, head, and neck. Mental symptoms may include insomnia, agitation and hallucinations. Fever, abdominal tenderness and leukocytosis are usually not prominent.

Peripheral neuropathy occurs with some attacks and is a potentially life-threatening complication. Porphyric neuropathy is primarily motoric, but is often accompanied by paresthesia, dysesthesia, and loss of sensation. Muscle weakness usually affects the more proximal muscles of the upper extremities initially and may progress to quadraparesis and bulbar paralysis. This neuropathy begins with axonal degeneration rather than demyelinization. Cranial nerves may be affected. In addition to mental changes, central nervous system involvement may include seizures and the syndrome of inappropriate ADH secretion (SIADH).

Attacks may resolve within hours or days if the disease is recognized and treatment instituted early. Advanced motor neuropathy is usually associated with delayed diagnosis, but with treatment may improve over a period of several years. Chronic pain and depression have developed in some patients. AIP, HCP, and VP are commonly associated with mild

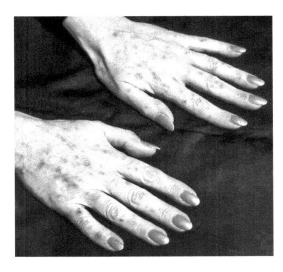

FIGURE 5 Erosions and hyperpigmentation in variegate porphyria. *Source*: Courtesy of Herbert Hönigsmann, MD, Vienna, Austria.

abnormalities in liver function, and the risks of cirrhosis and especially hepatocellular carcinoma (not associated with increases in serum α-fetoprotein) are increased (29). Additional long term risks include chronic hypertension and impaired renal function, which sometimes requires renal transplantation (30).

Cutaneous Manifestations

Blisters identical to those occurring in PCT occur commonly in VP (Fig. 5), much less commonly in HCP, and never in ADP and AIP. In HCP, hepatitis and other superimposed liver diseases may increase porphyrin retention and photosensitivity (31). Oral contraceptives may precipitate cutaneous manifestations of VP.

Etiology and Pathogenesis

As shown in Figure 1, ADP, AIP, HCP, and VP are due to deficiencies of the second, third, sixth and seventh enzymes of the heme biosynthetic pathway. ALAD is a zinc-containing, cytosolic enzyme consisting of eight identical subunits.

Coproporphyrinogen oxidase (CPO) is localized in the mitochondrial intermembrane space, is a dimer with a single active site, requires molecular oxygen, and is specific for the coproporphyrinogen III (not I) (32). Harderoporphyrinogen, a tricarboxyl porphyrinogen, is an intermediate in the two-step decarboxylation. Decarboxylation occurs first and more rapidly at the two position, and most of the harderoporphyrinogen formed is not released before being further decarboxylated at the four position to produce protoporphyrinogen IX(106). However, some CPO mutations associated with a variant form of HCP termed harderoporphyria impair substrate binding, and harderoporphyrinogen is prematurely released and excreted in excess amounts as harderoporphyrin (33).

PPO is a homodimer found in the inner mitochondrial membrane. It catalyzes the oxidation of protoporphyrinogen IX to protoporphyrin IX. Accumulation of protoporphyrinogen in VP may lead to inhibition of PBGD, which would account for increases in PBG, and formation of porphyrin–peptide conjugates, which may be present in plasma.

Multiple mutations have been found in each of these disorders. Certain drugs (e.g., barbiturates, phenytoin, metoclopramide, rifampin, and progesterone) increase the synthesis of heme and cytochrome P450 enzymes in the liver, which is associated with induction of ALAS1, the initial and most rate-limiting enzyme of the pathway in the liver. This causes the genetically deficient enzyme downstream form ALAS1 to become rate limiting. Restriction of calories and carbohydrate may favor induction of ALAS1 in liver via the peroxisome proliferator-activated receptor γ coactivator 1α (PGC-1α).

Formation of neurotoxic intermediates (perhaps ALA), and impaired formation of hemoproteins have been proposed as explanations for the neurologic symptoms.

Laboratory Findings and Diagnosis

A substantial increase in urinary PBG is a very specific indication that a patient has either AIP, HCP or VP (34). Increased PBG is usually accompanied by a less pronounced increase in ALA. Urinary coproporphyrin III are substantially increased in ADP, HCP, VP, and sometimes in AIP. ALA and PBG are generally increased for some time after (and probably before) an attack and increase further during the attack. Levels of these porphyrin precursors decrease more rapidly with recovery in HCP and VP than in AIP. Urinary porphyrins can remain elevated in HCP and VP after ALA and PBG return to normal.

Plasma porphyrins are normal or only slightly increased in ADP, AIP and most cases of HCP. In HCP patients with skin lesions plasma porphyrins are presumably substantially increased. Plasma porphyrins are commonly increased in VP. Fluorescence emission spectrum of plasma porphyrins at neutral pH is characteristic and can rapidly and reliably distinguish VP from other types of porphyria (Table 2). The emission peak is at or near 626 nm in VP, 620 nm in PCT, CEP, HCP, and (sometimes) AIP, and 634 nm in EPP (22). This fluorometric method is more effective than examination of fecal porphyrins for detecting asymptomatic VP (35).

Fecal porphyrins are normal or slightly increased in AIP, but substantially increased in HCP and VP. Fecal porphyrins consist almost entirely of coproporphyrin III in HCP, while approximately equal amounts of coproporphyrin III and protoporphyrin is the usual finding in VP. The ratio of fecal coproporphyrin III to coproporphyrin I is especially sensitive for detecting latent HCP heterozygotes (especially adults) (35). An increase in fecal "pseudo-pentacarboxyl porphyrin," a dicarboxyl porphyrin derived from protoporphyrin, is sometimes noted in VP. Increases in porphyrin precursors and porphyrins may be more severe in homozygous AIP, HCP, and VP, and are accompanied by substantial increases in erythrocyte zinc protoporphyrin.

Treatment and Prevention

Precipitating factors should be identified and removed whenever possible. Acute attacks often require hospitalization and treatment with narcotic analgesics, a phenothiazine for nausea and intravenous fluids for dehydration and electrolyte imbalances. Specific therapies, which act by repressing ALAS1, are carbohydrate loading and hemin (hematin or heme arginate). Early treatment with intravenous hemin is the most effective, and promptly reduces levels of ALA and PBG to normal and leads to more rapid recovery. Carbohydrate loading (usually intravenous glucose) can be used for mild attacks with mild pain and no paresis or hyponatremia. Cimetidine has been recommended for human acute porphyrias, but the mechanism is unclear and controlled observations are lacking. Treatment of seizures is problematic, since most anticonvulsants can exacerbate acute porphyrias. Liver transplantation was effective in a single case of severe AIP, but is still experimental. Long term control of hypertension may help prevent chronic renal impairment. Liver imaging is recommended yearly for early detection of hepatocellular carcinoma.

Symptoms can often be prevented by avoiding inciting factors. A list of safe and harmful drugs that is updated periodically is available from the European Porphyria Initiative (37). Pregnancy is usually well tolerated. Worsening symptoms during pregnancy are sometimes due to harmful drugs, such as metoclopramide, or reduced caloric intake due to hyperemesis gravidarum.

Consultation with a dietitian may be needed to address dietary indiscretions. GnRH analogues are used for preventing repeated attacks that are confined to the luteal phase of the menstrual cycle (37). Weekly or biweekly infusions of hemin are sometimes effective for preventing noncyclic attacks. The intravenous hemin product usually given in Europe is heme arginate, which is less thrombogenic than hematin (38).

No specific treatment is available for the chronic, blistering skin lesions, other than protection from sunlight.

TABLE 5 Congenital Erythropoietic Protoporphyria: Clinical Features

Cutaneous features	Other features and complications
Phototoxic burning on light exposure	Red urine (pink staining of nappy)
Blistering and scarring of light exposed sites	Brown-red teeth
Hypo and hyper-pigmentation	Scleromalacia, with perforation in severe cases
Hypertrichosis and scarring alopecia	Bone resorption
	Deformities of hands, feet and face
	Hemolytic anemia
	Splenomegaly ($\pm$ hypersplenism)
	Thrombocytopenia

CONGENITAL ERYTHROPOIETIC PORPHYRIA

CEP, also termed *Günther disease*, is a very rare autosomal recessive disease due to a deficiency of UROS. Mathias Petry, one of the original cases described by Günther, had severe skin lesions and mutilation and died at age 34.

Clinical Manifestations

Clinical features of CEP are summarized in Table 5. In most cases, reddish urine or pink staining of diapers by urine or meconium is observed shortly after birth. However, CEP can be recognized a cause of fetal loss, or intrauterine hemolytic anemia and nonimmune hydrops fetalis. Severe photosensitivity is usually noted soon after birth and may be worsened by phototherapy for hyperbilirubinemia (39). Skin friability, hypertrichosis, scarring, thickening, and areas of hypo- and hyperpigmentation and scarring alopecia are common, and usually much more severe than in PCT. In addition, phototoxic burning and blistering can lead to mutilation of light-exposed parts (Fig. 6), and even resorption of acral regions and the nose. Scleral and corneal damage (i.e., scleromalacia perforans) may occur. The teeth are characteristically red brown in color due to porphyrin deposition—an appearance termed *erythrodontia*—and

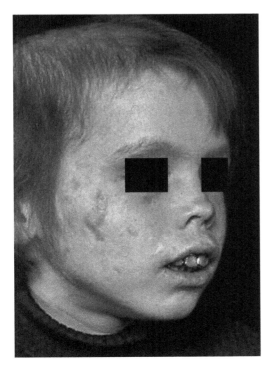

FIGURE 6 Scarring and stained teeth in congenital erythropoietic porphyria (Günthers disease).

fluoresce red with exposure to long-wave ultraviolet ligh (Fig. 6). Porphyrins are also deposited in bone. Expansion of the hyperplastic bone marrow contributes to bone demineralization; anemia is frequent, often hemolytic. Milder variants have been described with onset in adult life, often associated with thrombocytopenia or myelodysplasia (40,41).

Etiology and Pathogenesis

Many different mutations of the uroporphyrinogen III synthase (UROS) gene have been described. Studies correlating genotype and phenotype suggest a link between mutation type and disease severity (42). For example, a common mutation, C73R, is associated with less than 1% of normal enzyme activity; it has a severe phenotype (severe and mutilating photosensitivity, nonimmune hydrops fetalis, and/or transfusion dependency). Prenatal diagnosis is now possible. Late onset-CEP should prompt a search for underlying bone marrow malignancy (40,41).

UROS catalyzes inversion one of the terminal pyrrole rings (ring D) of hydroxymethylbilane (HMB), followed by rapid cyclization to form uroporphyrinogen III (Fig. 1). When the enzyme is deficient, HMB accumulates in bone marrow erythroid cells and cyclizes nonenzymatically and less rapidly, to form uroporphyrinogen I. The excess amounts of uroporphyrinogen I are metabolized by UROD to coproporphyrinogen I; the latter is not a substrate for CPO and therefore is not further metabolized. Both uroporphryinogen I and coproporphyrinogen I are autooxidized to the corresponding porphyrins, which are then found in circulating erythrocytes, plasma, urine and feces, and are photosensitizing.

Although UROS is markedly deficient in CEP, activity is sufficient to produce enough uroporphyrinogen III for heme formation. Heme production is actually increased in the bone marrow to compensate for ineffective erythropoiesis and hemolytic anemia. Intravascular hemolysis and increased splenic uptake of circulating erythrocytes may occur because the cells are damaged from the excess porphyrins or perhaps from a phototoxic mechanism.

Laboratory Evaluation and Diagnosis

CEP may is readily diagnosed by examination of porphyrins in urine, erythrocytes, plasma, and stool. Immediate fluorescence is evident on illumination of urine with a Wood's lamp, and is confirmed by marked increases in urinary porphyrins. Stable fluorescence of erythrocytes is evident on blood smears by fluorescence microscopy. A Wood's light is also useful to demonstrate fluorescence of the teeth, and in bone and other tissues post mortem.

Erythrocytes usually contain large amounts of uroporphyrin I, and to a lesser extent, excessive amounts of coproporphyrin I (Table 2). However, zinc protoporphyrin predominates in some cases, as in other autosomal recessive porphyrias. Urinary porphyrin excretion is markedly increased, consisting mostly of uroporphyrin I and coproporphyrin I. Plasma porphyrins are also markedly increased with a pattern similar to urine. Fecal porphyrins are markedly increased, with a predominance of coproporphyrin I.

Treatment

The severity of the disease determines how much light restriction should be advocated. Management of severely affected individuals with CEP means absolute avoidance of solar radiation of 360 to 500 nm for skin and eyes; scleromalacia perforans is an avoidable ocular complication. Other therapeutic measures are summarized in Table 6. Reduction of light exposure by wearing clothing, particularly hats, and gloves, greatly reduces damage to skin. Sunglasses excluding UV and visible light in the blue region should be worn to avoid conjunctival damage and scleromalacia perforans. Window glass and standard sunblocks are ineffective against visible light. Opaque sunblocks are effective but not usually acceptable other than in young children. Avoidance of outdoor activities is recommended and career guidance should advocate an indoor occupation.

TABLE 6 Approaches to Treatment of Congenital Erythropoietic Porphyria

Mechanism	Treatment	Current status
Reduce light exposure	Avoid sunlight, clothing, sunblocks.	Essential
Increase excretion of porphyrins	Oral superactivated charcoal	Sometimes effective
Reduce hemolysis	Splenectomy	Sometimes effective; may be temporary
Reduce bone marrow production of porphyrins	High level transfusion; may be combined with hydroxyurea	Temporary effect; may be complicated by iron overload, or viral infections
	Bone marrow transplantation	Effective; requires suitable donor

Bone marrow or stem cell transplantation is the most effective current treatment, and has resulted in marked reduction in porphyrin levels and photosensitivity (43,44). Gene therapy is being studied in laboratory models including cells from CEP patients (45).

ERYTHROPOIETIC PROTOPORPHYRIA

EPP is due to impairment in the final step in the heme biosynthetic pathway, which is catalyzed by the enzyme ferrochelatase (FECH). This is an autosomal dominant condition in most affected families, with considerable variation in penetrance

Clinical Manifestations

EPP is the third most common porphyria and the commonest childhood porphyria, with symptoms usually evident by age two years (46). Table 7 summarizes the clinical features in EPP (Fig. 7). Suspicion of EPP should be raised by the history of screaming or skin pain in a child on going outdoors. Neurological symptoms are absent, except in some patients with severe hepatic complications.

Protoporphyrin-containing gall stones may develop at an early age. Mild abnormalities of liver function may be detected in about 10% (3), and liver failure affects about 5%. Protoporphyric liver disease may be chronic, but can progress rapidly and be fatal. Recently, a variant form of EPP has been described in which FECH is not deficient and features of iron deficiency are prominent, implying that a genetic defect impairing iron availability for the final step in haem biosynthesis can cause EPP (47). Studies comparing hematological findings in these patients and those with known FECH mutations are needed.

Pathology

Histological evaluation shows thickening of the basement membrane of the dermal vasculature with an onion skin appearance due to repeated injury and repair. Complement activation also appears to be part of the injury associated with EPP as is histamine release from mast cells.

TABLE 7 Erythropoietic Protoporphyria: Cutaneous Features and Complications

Cutaneous features	Complications
Pain or burning in sunlight	Anemia
Erythema	Gallstones
Swelling	Liver failure
Purpura	
Sores on light exposed areas, mainly face	
Scarring (shallow, circular, or linear)	
Waxy thickening	

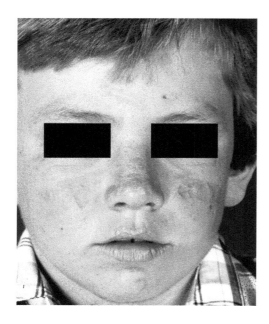

FIGURE 7 Typical scars on nose and cheeks with waxy thickening of facial skin in erythropoietic protoporphyria. *Source*: Courtesy of Herbert Hönigsmann, MD, Vienna, Austria.

Etiology and Pathogenesis

FECH is found in the mitochondrial inner membrane where it catalyzes the final step in heme synthesis, which is the insertion of ferrous iron (Fe^{2+}) into protoporphyrin IX (Fig. 1). This enzyme is specific for the reduced form of iron, but can utilize other metals such as Zn^{2+} and Co^{2+}. The enzyme has a rate-limiting role in erythroid cells in the bone marrow, which helps to explain protoporphyrin accumulation being almost entirely in erythroid cells in EPP.

It is well recognized that EPP is not always inherited as a dominant disease and that clinical expression does not occur in all affected family members. To date over 70 different FECH mutations have been identified in EPP patients (48). EPP is explained in most families by the combined presence of a disabling FECH mutation and a common, intronic polymorphism (IVS3-48T/C) affecting the other FECH allele, which leads to an aberrantly spliced mRNA that is degraded by a nonsense-mediated decay mechanism, such that the level of FECH mRNA is decreased (49). In rare families without this polymorphism, EPP is associated with inheritance of two FECH mutations and autosomal recessive inheritance. Therefore, it is now established that EPP is an autosomal dominant disease at the molecular level in most families, but that inheritance of two alleles associated with reduced FECH activity is required for sufficient erythroid accumulation of protoporphyrin to cause symptoms.

Protoporphyric liver disease is believed to result from delivery of excess protoporphyrin to the liver. Null mutations, result in a truncated protein, when heteroallelic with the IVS3-48T/C polymorphism, have been associated with risk for EPP-related liver disease. For example, amongst 89 patients with a null allele mutation, 18 developed liver disease, whereas all 19 patients with 16 missense mutations, which retain some enzyme activity, did not (50).

Similar to late-onset CEP, late-onset EPP can occur in patients who develop myelodysplasia or myeloproliferative disorders. It is thought to be due to an acquired somatic mutation of one FECH allele in bone marrow (51).

Laboratory Evaluation and Diagnosis

The diagnosis of EPP rests on finding substantially increased amounts protoporphyrin in erythrocytes, with free protoporphyrin rather than zinc protoporphyrin accounting for the increase (Table 3). Transient fluorescence of red cells by fluorescence microscopy reflects this increase. Formation of zinc protoporphyrin is apparently depends on normal FECH activity. In the variant form of EPP in which FECH activity is normal, erythrocytes contain increased amounts of both free and zinc protoporphyrin. Erythrocyte zinc protoporphyrin is also increased in many other conditions affecting erythrocytes, such as some homozygous porphyrias, iron deficiency, lead poisoning, anemia of chronic disease and hemolytic conditions (52).

A characteristic fluorescence peak (635 nm) is seen in plasma (diluted at neutral pH). The urine does not contain excess porphyrins. Stool protoporphyrin is variably increased.

Protoporphyrin levels and sensitivity to sunlight generally are stable for many years in the absence of liver disease, and precipitating factors that are important in the hepatic porphyrias seldom contribute. Assays for FECH require cells containing mitochondria. DNA studies are increasingly important, and will usually identify a disabling FECH mutation and the IVS3-48T/C polymorphism.

Early diagnosis of liver complications is important, and is evidenced by abnormal liver function tests, progressively increasing protoporphyrin levels in plasma and erythrocytes, decreases in fecal protoporphyrin and increased photosensitivity (53). If liver function is progressively abnormal, liver biopsy may be indicated, and reveals marked deposition of protoporphyrin in hepatocytes and bile canniculi, fluorescent inclusions, periportal fibrosis, and other features of cholestasis. Gallstones composed predominantly of protoporphyrin may cause cholecystitis or biliary obstruction.

Treatment

Similar to CEP, photoprotection is essential. Other specific therapeutic options are summarized in Table 8.

Patient follow up is advocated and erythrocyte and plasma porphyrin levels and liver function tests can be repeated at 6 to 12 month intervals. DNA studies are recommended, and the results facilitate genetic counseling. If patients need surgery, theatre personnel must be warned about the potential hazards of exposure of internal organs to prolonged visible light; severe burns to internal surfaces and wound dehiscence have been reported (54). Theatre lights should be filtered to reduce radiation of 380 to 420 nm.

Cholestyramine and activated charcoal should be considered in the management of hepatic complications of EPP. Other options include ursodeoxycholic acid, red blood cell transfusions, exchange transfusion, plasma exchange, and intravenous hemin to suppress

TABLE 8 Approaches to Treatment of Erythropoietic Protoporphyria

Mechanism	Treatment	Current status
Reduce light exposure or quench reactive oxygen species	β-Carotene	Possible efficacy
	Cysteine	Possible efficacy
	N-acetylcysteine	Not effective
	Narrowband UVB therapy	Protection factor of 8 is useful
Reduce tissue wheal and flare reaction	Antihistamines	Marginal efficacy
Interrupt enterohepatic circulation and increase excretion of protoporphyrin	Cholestyramine	Reserve for incipient liver disease
Reduce hemolysis or correct anemia	Splenectomy; transfusion	Sometimes effective; may be temporary
Correct liver failure	Liver transplantation	Liver disease likely to recur
Reduce bone marrow production of protoporphyrin	Bone marrow transplantation	Requires suitable donor

Note: Indicated in patients with liver failure or liver transplantation.

erythroid and hepatic protoporphyrin production. Liver transplantation may be necessary with more advanced disease (55). Acute neuropathy may occur with the very high porphyrin levels encountered with liver failure (56). Intermediate survival rates (up to five years follow up) after liver transplantation show survival rates comparable to the general transplant population. However, recurrent disease in the graft is likely. Bone marrow transplantation produced a remission of EPP in a patient with acute myelogenous leukemia (57). Sequential bone marrow transplantation was recently successful in preventing recurrence of protoporphyric liver disease (58), and it is likely that this option will be considered more often in the future. Studies mice suggest a potential future role for gene therapy in human protoporphyria (59).

ACKNOWLEDGMENTS

Preparation of this chapter was supported in part by grants from the US Food and Drug Administration Office of Orphan Product Development (FD-R-001459), the American Porphyria Foundation, and the National Center for Research Resources, National Institutes of Health (MO1 RR-00073).

REFERENCES

1. Lim H, Cooper D, Sassa S, Dosik H, Buchness MR, Soter N. Photosensitivity abnormal porphyrin profile and sideroblastic anemia. J Am Acad Dermatol 1992; 27 (2part 2):287–292.
2. Gibbs NK, Traynor N, Ferguson J. Biochemical diagnosis of the cutaneous porphyrias: five years experience of plasma spectro-fluorimetry. Br J Dermatol 1995; 133:18s
3. Murphy GM. Porphyria. In: Bolognia JL, Jorizzo JL, Rapini RP, eds. Dermatology. London: Mosby. 2003:679–689.
4. Schmid R. Cutaneous porphyria in turkey. N Eng J Med 1960; 263:397–839
5. Egger NG, Goeger DE, Payne DA, Miskovsky EP, Weinman SA, Anderson KE. Porphyria cutanea tarda: multiplicity of risk factors including HFE mutations, hepatitis C, and inherited uroporphyrinogen decarboxylase deficiency. Dig Dis Sci 2002; 47(2):419–426.
6. Brady JJ, Jackson HA, Roberts AG, et al. Co-inheritance of mutations in the uroporphyrinogen decarboxylase and hemochromatosis genes accelerates the onset of porphyria cutanea tarda. J Invest Dermatol 2000; 115(5):868–874.
7. O'Reilly FM, Darby C, Fogarty J, et al. Porphyrin metabolism in hepatitis C infection. Photodermatol Photoimmunol Photomed 1996; 12(1):31–33.
8. McConnell R, Anderson K, Russell W, et al. Angiosarcoma, porphyria cutanea tarda, and probable chloracne in a worker exposed to waste oil contaminated with 2,3,7,8-tetrachlorodibenzo-*p*-dioxin. Br J Ind Med 1993; 50:699–703
9. O'Reilly FM, Darby C, Fogarty J, et al. Screening of patients with iron overload to identify hemochromatosis and porphyria cutanea tarda. Arch Dermatol 1997; 133(9):1098–1101.
10. McKenna DB, Browne M, O'Donnell R, Murphy GM. Porphyria cutanea tarda and hematologic malignancy—a report of 4 cases. Photodermatol Photoimmunol Photomed 1997; 13(4):143–146.
11. Gibson GE, McGinnity E, McGrath P, et al. Cutaneous abnormalities and metabolic disturbance of porphyrins in patients on maintenance haemodialysis. Clin Exp Dermatol 1997; 22(3):124–127.
12. Anderson KE, Goeger DE, Carson RW, Lee S-MK, Stead RB. Erythropoietin for the treatment of porphyria cutanea tarda in a patient on long-term hemodialysis. N Engl J Med 1990; 322:315–317.
13. Lim HW. Pathophysiology of cutaneous lesions in porphyria. Sem Hematol 1989; 26:114–119.
14. Elder GH. Porphyria cutanea tarda and related disorders. In: Kadish KM, Smith K, Guilard R, eds. Porphyrin Handbook, Part II. Vol 14. San Diego: Academic Press, 2003:67–92. chapter 88.
15. Roberts AG, Whatley SD, Nicklin S, et al. The frequency of hemochromatosis-associated alleles is increased in British patients with sporadic porphyria cutanea tarda. Hepatology 1997; 25(1):159–161.
16. Dereure O, Aguilar-Martinez P, Bessis D, et al. HFE mutations and transferrin receptor polymorphism analysis in porphyria cutanea tarda: a prospective study of 36 cases from southern France. Br J Dermatol 2001; 144(3):533–539.
17. Philips JD, Jackson LK, Bunting M, et al. A mouse model of familial porphyria cutanea tarda. Proc Natl Acad Sci USA 2001; 98(1):259–264.
18. Anderson KE, Sassa S, Bishop DF, Desnick RJ. Disorders of heme biosynthesis: X-linked sideroblastic anemias and the porphyries. In: Scriver CR, Beaudet AL, Sly WS, Valle D, Childs B, Vogelstein B, eds. The Metabolic and Molecular Basis of Inherited Disease. 8th ed. Vol II. New York: McGraw-Hill, 2001:2991–3062, chapter 124.

19. Bulaj ZJ, Phillips JD, Ajioka RS, et al. Hemochromatosis genes and other factors contributing to the pathogenesis of porphyria cutanea tarda. Blood 2000; 95(5):1565–1571.
20. Wissel PS, Sordillo P, Anderson KE, Sassa S, Savillo RL, Kappas A. Porphyria cutanea tarda associated with the acquired immune deficiency syndrome. Am J Hematology 1987; 25:107–113.
21. Sinclair PR, Gorman G, Shedlofsky SI, et al. Ascorbic acid deficiency in porphyria cutanea tarda. J Lab Clin Med 1997; 130:197–201.
22. Poh-Fitzpatrick MB. A plasma porphyrin fluorescence marker for variegate porphyria. Arch Dermatol 1980; 116:543–547.
23. Shieh S, Cohen JL, Lim HW. Management of porphyria cutanea tarda in the setting of chronic renal failure: a case report and review. J Am Acad Dermatol 2000; 42(4):645–652.
24. Moran-Jimenez MJ, Ged C, Romana M, et al. Uroporphyrinogen decarboxylase: complete human gene sequence and molecular study of three families with hepatoerythropoietic porphyria. Am J Hum Genet 1996; 58(4):712–721.
25. Armstrong DK, Sharpe PC, Chambers CR, Whatley SD, Roberts AG, Elder GH. Hepatoerythropoietic porphyria: a missense mutation in the UROD gene is associated with mild disease and an unusual porphyrin excretion pattern. Br J Dermatol 2004; 151(4):920–923.
26. Fontanellas A, Mazurier F, Moreau-Gaudry F, Belloc F, Ged C, de Verneuil H. Correction of uroporphyrinogen decarboxylase deficiency (hepatoerythropoietic porphyria) in Epstein-Barr virus-transformed B- cell lines by retroviral-mediated gene transfer: fluorescence-based selection of transduced cells. Blood 1999; 94(2):465–474.
27. Meissner P, Hift RJ, Corrigall A. Variegate porphyria In: Kadish KM, Smith K, Guilard R, eds. Porphyrin Handbook, Part II. Vol 14. San Diego: Academic Press, 2003:93–120, chapter 89.
28. Solis C, Martinez-Bermejo A, Naidich TP, et al. Acute intermittent porphyria: studies of the severe homozygous dominant disease provides insights into the neurologic attacks in acute porphyrias. Arch Neurol 2004; 61(11):1764–1770.
29. Andant C, Puy H, Bogard C, et al. Hepatocellular carcinoma in patients with acute hepatic porphyria: frequency of occurrence and related factors. J Hepatol 2000; 32(6):933–939.
30. Andersson C, Wikberg A, Stegmayr B, Lithner F. Renal symptomatology in patients with acute intermittent porphyria. A population-based study. J Intern Med 2000; 248(4):319–325.
31. Barone GW, Gurley BJ, Anderson KE, Ketel BL, Abul-Ezz SR. The tolerability of newer immunosuppressive medications in a patient with acute intermittent porphyria. J Clin Pharmacol 2000; 41: 113–115.
32. Cacheux V, Martasek P, Fougerousse F, et al. Localization of the human coproporphyrinogen oxidase gene to chromosome band 3q12. Hum Genet 1994; 94:557–559.
33. Nordmann Y, Grandchamp B, De Verneuil H, Phung L, Cartigny B, Fontaine G. Harderoporphyria: a variant hereditary coproporphyria. J Clin Invest 1983; 72:1139–1149.
34. Anderson KE, Bloomer JR, Bonkovsky HL, et al. Recommendations for the diagnosis and treatment of the acute porphyrias. Ann Intern Med 2005; 142(6):439–450.
35. Hift RJ, Davidson BP, van der Hooft C, Meissner DM, Meissner PN. Plasma fluorescence scanning and fecal porphyrin analysis for the diagnosis of variegate porphyria: precise determination of sensitivity and specificity with detection of protoporphyrinogen oxidase mutations as a reference standard. Clin Chem 2004; 50(5):915–923.
36. (www.porphyria-europe.com/)
37. Anderson KE, Spitz IM, Bardin CW, Kappas A. A GnRH analogue prevents cyclical attacks of porphyria. Arch Int Med 1990; 150:1469–1474.
38. Timonen K, Mustajoki P, Tenhunen R, Lauharanta J. Effects of haem arginate on variegate porphyria. Br J Dermatol 1990; 123:381–387.
39. Murphy GM, Hawk JLM, Nicholson DC, et al. Congenital erythropoietic porphyria (Gunther's disease). Clin Exp Dermatology 1987; 12:61–65.
40. Murphy A, Gibson G, Elder GH, Otridge BA, Murphy GM. Adult-onset congenital erythropoietic porphyria (Gunther's disease) presenting with thrombocytopenia. J Roy Soc Med 1995; 88:357–358.
41. Kontos AP, Ozog D, Bichakjian C, Lim HW. Congenital erythropoietic porphyria associated with myelodysplasia presenting in a 72-year-old man: report of a case and review of the literature. Br J Dermatol 2003; 148(1):160–164.
42. Xu W, Warner CA, Desnick RJ. Congenital erythropoietic porphyria: Identification and expression of 10 mutations in the uroporphyrinogen III synthase gene. J Clin Invest 1995; 95:905–912.
43. Harada FA, Shwayder TA, Desnick RJ, Lim HW. Treatment of severe congenital erythropoietic porphyria by Bone marrow transplantation. J Am Acad Dermatol 2001; 45:279–282.
44. Dupuis-Girod S, Akkari V, Ged C, et al. Successful match-unrelated donor bone marrow transplantation for congenital erythropoietic porphyria (Gunther disease). Eur J Pediatr 2005; 164(2): 104–107. 2004, Nov 20.
45. Mazurier F, Geronimi F, Lamrissi-Garcia I, et al. Correction of deficient cd34(+) cells from peripheral blood after mobilization in a patient with congenital erythropoietic porphyria. Mol Ther 2001; 3(3):411–417.

46. Cox TM. Protoporphyria. In: Kadish KM, Smith K, Guilard R, eds. Porphyrin Handbook, Part II. vol 14. San Diego: Academic Press, 2003:121–149, chapter 90.

47. Wilson JHP, Edixhoven-Bosdijk A, Koole-Lesuis R, Kroos MJ, de Rooij FWM. A new variant or erythropoietic protoporphyria with normal ferrochelatase activity (abstract). Physiol Res 2003; 52:29S.

48. Stenson PD, Ball EV, Mort M, et al. Human Gene Mutation Database (HGMD): 2003 update. Hum Mutat 2003; 21(6):577–581.

49. Gouya L, Martin-Schmitt C, Robreau AM, et al. Contribution of a common single-nucleotide polymorphism to the genetic predisposition for erythropoietic protoporphyria. Am J Hum Genet 2006; 78(1):2–14. 2005 Nov 15.

50. Minder EI, Gouya L, Schneider-Yin X, Deybach JC. A genotype-phenotype correlation between null-allele mutations in the ferrochelatase gene and liver complication in patients with erythropoietic protoporphyria. Cell Mol Biol (Noisy-le-grand) 2002; 48(1):91–96.

51. Goodwin RG, Kell WJ, Laidler P, et al. Photosensitivity and acute liver injury in myeloproliferative disorder secondary to late-onset protoporphyria caused by deletion of a ferrochelatase gene inhematopoietic cells. Blood 2006; 107(1):60–62.

52. Hastka J, Lasserre JJ, Schwarzbeck A, Strauch M, Hehlmann R. Zinc protoporphyrin in anemia of chronic disorders. Blood 1993; 81:1200–1204.

53. Leone N, Marzano A, Cerutti E, et al. Liver transplantation for erythropoietic protoporphyria: report of a case with medium term follow-up. Digestive & Liver Disease 2000; 32:799–802.

54. Meerman L, Verwer R, Slooff MJ, et al Perioperative measures during liver transplantation for erythropoietic protoporphyria. Transplantation 1994; 57:155–158.

55. McGuire BM, Bonkovsky HL, Carithers RL, et al. Liver transplantation for erythropoietic protoporphyria liver disease. Liver Transpl 2005; 11(12):1590–1596.

56. Muley SA, Midani HA, Rank JM, Carithers R, Parry GJ. Neuropathy in erythropoietic protoporphyrias. Neurology 1998; 51(1):262–265.

57. Poh-Fitzpatrick MB, Wang X, Anderson KE, Bloomer JE, Bolwell B, Lichtin AE. Erythropoietic protoporphyria: altered phenotype after bone marrow transplantation for myelogenous leukemia in a patient heteroallelic for ferrochelatase gene mutations. J Amer Acad Dermatol 2002; 46:861–866.

58. Rand EB, Bunin N, Cochran W, Ruchelli E, Olthoff KM, Bloomer J. Sequential liver and bone marrow transplantation for treatment of erythropoietic protoporphyria. Pediatrics 2006 (Epub ahead of print).

59. Richard E, Robert E, Cario-Andre M, et al. Hematopoietic stem cell gene therapy of murine protoporphyria by methylguanine-DNA-methyltransferase-mediated in vivo drug selection. Gene Ther 2004; 11(22):1638–1647.

16 | Xeroderma Pigmentosum and Other DNA Repair-Deficient Photodermatoses

Mark Berneburg
Department of Dermatology, Eberhard Karls University, Tuebingen, Germany

Kenneth H. Kraemer
Basic Research Laboratory, Center for Cancer Research, National Cancer Institute, Bethesda, Maryland, U.S.A.

- Xeroderma pigmentosum (XP), Cockayne Syndrome (CS), and trichothiodystrophy (TTD): Rare autosomal recessive genodermatoses.

- XP: Photosensitivity, neuro-ophthalmological symptoms and a 1000-fold increased skin cancer risk.

- CS: Photosensitivity, growth and mental retardation, neuro-ophthalmological symptoms and progeria.

- TTD: Photosensitivity, growth and mental retardation, ichthyosis, and sulfur deficient hair.

- Heterogeneity and overlaps exist between XP, CS, and TTD.

- The diagnosis of these diseases is based on their clinical symptoms and is confirmed by cellular assays.

- Rigorous photoprotection is paramount in the care of DNA-repair deficient photodermatoses.

INTRODUCTION

Xeroderma pigmentosum (XP), Cockayne syndrome (CS), and trichothiodystrophy (TTD) are genodermatoses, characterized by deficiencies in DNA repair, basal transcription, or translesion synthesis. They have defective nucleotide excision repair (NER), a mechanism responsible for the repair of bulky forms of DNA damage such as sunlight induced DNA photoproducts, DNA cross-links, and alkylation damage. With an estimated prevalence on the order of one in a million in Western countries, these diseases are very rare. Consideration of the typical symptoms usually permits making the correct clinical diagnosis. Patients suspected of having one of these diseases can be referred to a center that specializes in their diagnosis and care. In recent years the underlying mechanisms as well as many of the genes involved have been identified. The understanding of mechanisms such as DNA repair, basal transcription, and translesion synthesis has helped to form a mechanistic explanation of symptoms of XP, TTD, and CS. These advances provide important insights into major physiological processes such as aging and carcinogenesis. NER, the central defect in most of these diseases, will be described in more detail.

NUCLEOTIDE EXCISION REPAIR

Patients suffering from XP, TTD, and CS are defective in the process of NER. This highly conserved mechanism repairs a multitude of DNA lesions (1–3). The repair of damage induced by UV-radiation is one of its central functions. The most prevalent lesions induced by UV are cyclobutane pyrimidine dimers (CPD). The 6-4 photoproducts (6-4PP) are less frequent but far more helix-distorting. This distortion of the DNA helix permits easier recognition of the 6-4PP by repair enzymes and is probably why 6-4PP are removed from the genome at a much faster rate than CPD.

Removal of DNA damage by NER can be carried out by two pathways, which differ mainly in damage recognition. Damage present in actively transcribed genes stalls the transcribing RNA polymerase at the site of the damage. This damage-polymerase complex leads to recruitment of the repair machinery that removes the damage and allows transcription to continue. The exact sequence, in particular the means of repair machinery recruitment of this so-called transcription coupled repair (TCR), is not entirely clear (4, 5). The regulation of the shift between transcription and repair is also not clear. However, it is known that a protein complex of 10 components of the basal transcription factor TFIIH are involved in DNA repair as well as in basal transcription, and the association of further proteins allows this core complex to carry out either of these two functions (6,7). Repair of DNA damage encountered by stalled RNA polymerase is very rapid. Within eight hours, TCR removes about 50% of CPD from actively transcribed genes. Cells from patients with mutations in most XP genes [except XPC and DDB2 (XPE)] have defects in TCR along with defects in global genome repair (GGR) as described below. Cells from CS patients are defective in TCR and have normal GGR.

GGR is a second form of repair that is carried out throughout the whole genome. GGR is slower than TCR. In this subpathway DDB2 recognizes the damage attracting a heterodimer of the XP-C protein and the human HR23B along with centrin 2. Cells from XP patients with defects in DDB2 (XPE) or XP-C are defective in GGR but not in TCR (8).

Following damage recognition, both processes converge (9). The XP-A/RPA protein complex binds to the damaged region and recruits the helicases XP-B and XP-D, which open the DNA helix. The XP-F and XP-G endonucleases incise the damaged strand of DNA on both sides of the lesion leaving a gap of about 21 to 29 nucleotides in length. This gap is filled in by DNA polymerases.

In addition to repair of UV damage, the NER system repairs bulky DNA damage such as that caused by carcinogens in cigarette smoke, by alkylating agents, and by DNA cross-linking agents. They have functions in the repair of oxidative DNA damage, basal transcription (10–12), as well as transcriptional regulation of genes in cellular metabolism (13,14). Furthermore, NER proteins are also involved in immunological processes (15–20). It appears likely that more processes will be identified employing components of NER. With this as background, the diseases XP, TTD, and CS will be described in further detail.

XERODERMA PIGMENTOSUM
Clinical Symptoms

XP is a rare autosomal recessive genetic disease with an estimated prevalence of $1:10^6$ in the United States and Europe and $1:10^5$ in Japan. XP is characterized by an approximately 1000-fold increased risk to develop skin cancer (1,21). The first symptoms of XP often manifest in early childhood (Table 1). Some infants or small children with XP experience severe acute sunburn reactions after a short exposure of the skin to sunlight. This reaction can persist for several weeks. However, approximately half of the XP patients do not have this acute sun sensitivity. They tan and freckle without burning. Many of these patients are in XP complementation group C. Freckling of the face of a child less than two years old is unusual in normal children and is an indication that the diagnosis of XP should be considered. With continued sun exposure freckling of sun-exposed skin continues to develop into the typical appearance of poikiloderma with hypo- and hyperpigmentation, atrophy, and telangiectasias. These pigmentary changes in addition to dry (xerotic) skin are reflected in the name of the disease (Fig. 1).

All XP patients are highly susceptible to development of sunlight-induced cancers of the skin and eyes. The median age of onset of skin cancers in XP patients is less than 10 years. This is a 50-year reduction in age of onset of first skin cancer as compared to the U.S. general population and is an indication of the importance of DNA repair in protection against skin cancer.

In some XP patients who do not have acute sun sensitivity, the early pigmentary changes might not be recognized, and the presence of skin cancers may be the first indication that the child has XP. Basal cell carcinoma (BCC) and squamous cell carcinoma (SCC) occur most frequently. The frequency of BCC, SCC, and malignant melanoma is elevated about 1000-fold. XP patients also have an increased frequency of internal cancers including central nervous

TABLE 1 Clinical Features of DNA Repair Deficient Photodermatoses Xeroderma Pigmentosum, Cockayne Syndrome, and Trichothiodystrophy

Symptoms	XP	CS	TTD
Skin photosensitivity	++	++	++
Skin pigmentary changes[a]	++	−	−
Skin telangiectasia	+	−	−
Ichthyosis	−	−	+
Skin cancer	++	−	−
Fragile hair with cysteine deficiency	−	−	++
Ocular changes[b]	+ (anterior eye)	+ (cataracts, retinal degeneration)	+ (congenital catatacts, nystagmus)
Hearing loss—progressive sensorineural deafness	+ or −	+	−
Mental retardation	+ (early loss of cerebral function)	++ (early loss of cerebellar function)	++
Neuropathology[c]	− or + (neuronal degeneration)	+ (dysmyelination)	+ (dysmyelination)
Growth retardation	− or +	++	++
Infections	−	+	+
Premature aging symptoms	+	++	+

[a]Pigmentary changes include poikiloderma with hypo- and hyperpigmentation.
[b]Ocular changes include conjunctival and corneal alterations in xeroderma pigmentosum (XP) and pigmentary retinal degeneration and cataracts in Cockayne syndrome (CS).
[c]Neurological changes in XP include microcephaly and are usually progressive and comprise reduction of deep tendon reflexes, peripheral neuropathy and loss of intellectual function. CS patients often have microcephaly, lack of myelination, and may have calcification of basal ganglia as well as other parts of the brain.
Abbreviations: −, absent; +, present; ++, markedly abnormal; CS, Cockayne syndrome; TTD, trichothiodystrophy; XP, xeroderma pigmentosum.

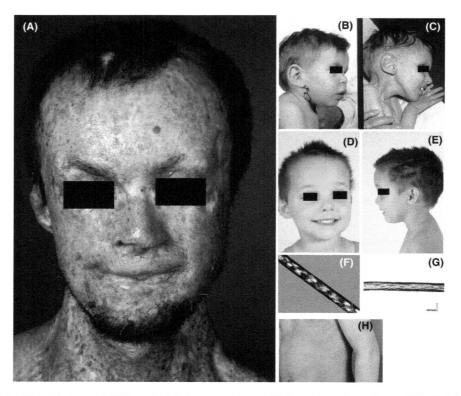

FIGURE 1 Clinical features of DNA repair deficiency syndromes. (**A**) Xeroderma pigmentosum (XP): Poikiloderma with hypo- and hyperpigmentation, telangiectasia, and scars after multiple excisions of cancers in a 29-year-old male patient with XP complementation group C. This patient developed the first skin symptoms at one year of age, the first skin tumor (squamous cell carcinoma) at the age of five and metastasis of a malignant melanoma at the age of 25. His whole facial skin was transplanted from the thigh region at the age of 18. (**B**) and (**C**) XP/Cockayne syndrome (CS) complex: Patient XP20BE with features of XP and CS and a defect in the XPG (ERCC5). (**B**) Age 18 months showing interspersed areas of XP-like increased and decreased pigmentation on his cheek. (**C**) Age six years showing typical CS cachexia, deep-set eyes, loss of subcutaneous tissue and XP-like pigmentation of his face and arm. *Source*: From Ref. 50. (**D**)–(**H**) Trichothiodystrophy (TTD): (**D**) and (**E**) Three-year old girl (TTD352BE) with short, brittle hair which is sparse and broken off at different lengths. She rarely has haircuts except to trim uneven areas. She is not sun sensitive. (**F**) Tiger tail appearance of hair with polarizing microscopy. (**G**) Irregular, undulating hair shaft with light microscopy [original magnifications (**F**) and (**G**), ×10]. (**H**) Marked ichthyosis in a five-year old male patient. *Source*: From Ref. 43.

system tumors (astrocytoma of brain or spinal cord, Schwanoma of the facial nerve) and lung cancers in patients who smoke.

All tissues that are exposed to sunlight may show abnormalities in XP patients. In addition to the skin, the eye and even the tip of the tongue can be involved. The eyes can have various inflammatory lesions such as conjunctival injection and pinguecula, sunlight induced keratitis, and corneal clouding. Many patients have dry eyes. The lids can develop symblepharon, ectropion or, in extreme cases, loss of lids. The lids and conjunctiva can develop BCC and SCC. The lips often show cheilitis. The tip of the tongue can show similar changes of telangiectasias, atrophy, and even SCC. In some parts of North Africa, XP is more common and children with tumors of the tip of the tongue should be considered as having XP until proven otherwise.

Early diagnosis before the development of skin tumors should be the goal. Interdisciplinary care in conjunction with dermatologists, ophthalmologists, and pediatricians is necessary.

Approximately 20% of XP patients show progressive neurological degeneration. The earliest signs of neurological involvement are often absence of deep tendon reflexes and high frequency sensorineural hearing loss. There is a tendency for the XP patients with neurological abnormalities to have a history of acute sun sensitivity in early life. The rate of progression of the neurological disease is variable. Patients develop loss of coordination, loss of ability to walk, intellectual deterioration, and difficulty swallowing. They eventually may develop quadraparesis. Magnetic resonance imaging of the brain shows enlarged ventricles due to loss of cerebral graymatter. The brain pathology shows primary neuronal degeneration without calcification.

Differential Diagnosis

XP has to be distinguished from the other DNA repair deficient photodermatoses such as CS and TTD (Table 1). Other diseases with increased photosensitivity in childhood, such as hydroa vacciniforme or erythropoietic porphyria (EP) have to be excluded (22). EP shows photosensitivity and poikiloderma followed by mutilations along with red fluorescence of teeth, erythrocytes, and urine. Unlike XP, patients suffering from EP describe pain during sun-exposure. Mutilations of EP patients do not come from tumors, but occur from phototoxic reactions of protoporphyrin IX generating apoptosis induced by reactive oxygen species. EP patients do not have an increased skin cancer risk.

Increased frequency of skin tumors may also point toward basal cell nevus syndrome (BCNS) (Goltz-Gorlin syndrome) caused by mutations in the patched (*PTCH*) gene (23,24). Clinically, BCNS can readily be distinguished from XP by the lack of poikiloderma and the presence of jaw cysts, palmar pits, abnormalities of the ribs and vertebrae, and calcification of the falx. BCNS patients do not have a high frequency of SCC or melanomas. Unlike XP patients, BCNS patients are hypersensitive to therapeutic X rays for treatment of skin or internal cancers and can develop hundreds of BCC in the field of X-ray treatment.

Epidermodysplasia verruciformis can also show poikiloderma and is characterized by multiple Bowenoid tumors originating from verrucae vulgaris containing human papilloma virus.

The rare diagnosis of dyschromatosis universalis hereditaria is particularly described to occur almost exclusively in Japanese patients and represents the most important differential diagnosis to the relatively frequent cases of XP-A. Patients with this disease suffer from dyschromia of the whole skin, with hyperpigmentation paralleled by mild xerosis cutis. In contrast to XP, UV-radiation is well tolerated, and an increased skin cancer risk does not exist.

Patients with Carney syndrome or leopard syndrome have multiple pigmented lesions without sun sensitivity. Unlike XP, the pigmentation of each lesion is more uniform and there is no hypopigmentation or telangiectasia.

Laboratory Diagnosis

The clinical diagnosis XP can be obtained by measuring post-UV cell survival and DNA repair capacity in cellular assays. For these assays, fibroblasts from the patient are generated from a skin biopsy and grown in the laboratory. For the survival, assay cells are placed in plates and exposed to increasing doses of UVC-radiation. Cell growth is assessed for several days. The growth of most cells after UV-exposure is greatly reduced compared to normal cells. XP variant cells have normal post-UV survival but are sensitized to post-UV cell killing by addition of caffeine. Another assay is unscheduled DNA synthesis (UDS), which is reduced in most XP patients with the exception of XP-variants (8). During the repair reaction necessary to restore the genomic integrity of the cell, radioactively labelled tritium is supplied in the medium. Radioactive incorporation into DNA, as assessed by autoradiography or scintillation counting, is directly proportional to the repair capacity, since in the last step of the repair reaction DNA polymerase incorporates nucleotides to fill the gap of excised damage-containing DNA. This repair reaction is reduced in fibroblasts derived from patients suffering from XP as compared to fibroblasts from normal donors. Specialized laboratories offer prenatal diagnosis for families with XP patients.

DNA Repair Genes

Complementation analysis revealed the presence of seven XP-subtypes (XP A to G), deficient in NER as well as a variant form with a deficiency in DNA polymerase eta (3,25). The genes defective in these complementation groups are cloned and designated according to the respective causative genes. The relationship between the defective genes and the clinical phenotypes is very complex (Fig. 2). Clinical symptoms in the different complementation groups are heterogeneous. XP group A is characterized by a defect in both TCR and GGR. This complementation group is most frequent in Japan. Most Japanese patients have the same splice site mutation due to a founder-effect. They have a particularly severe course with rapid neurological degeneration and reduced life expectancy. Remarkably, other patients with different mutations in the *XPA* gene may have minimal neurological abnormalities. XP complementation group B is extremely rare, with only six families described in the literature. Surprisingly, four families have the XP/CS complex, one has XP with mild neurological disease, and one has TTD. In Europe and northern Africa, XP-C represents the most frequent subgroup. Without sun protection, the clinical course of XP-C may be severe with multiple SCC, BCC, malignant melanoma, and internal tumors. These patients usually do not have acute sun sensitivity and do not have neurological abnormalities. As in other complementation groups, the high grade of consanguinity in affected families plays an important role. Patients with defects in the *XPD* gene have marked phenotypic heterogeneity. They may have only the skin disease of XP; XP with XP-type neurological disease, the XP/CS complex; TTD, combined TTD/XP; or cerebro-ocular-facial-skeletal syndrome. The phenotype appears to depend on the specific mutation in this gene that plays a role in NER and transcription. Patients with defects in the *XPG* gene may have only the skin disease of XP or may have XP/CS complex. XP-E and XP variant patients have skin disease without neurological abnormalities. XP-F patients may have mild disease or late onset of severe neurological degeneration.

Care and Management of Patients

Central to the care and management of patients is the strict avoidance of any exposure to UV-radiation. This does not categorically exclude outdoor activities. This would only deprive the already impaired young patients even more of possible spare time activities and endanger social development. Nevertheless, the skin has to be protected from UV by long sleeved

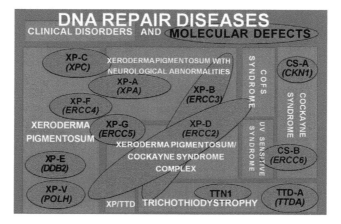

FIGURE 2   Relationship of clinical disorders to molecular defects in DNA repair diseases. Eight different clinical phenotypes are represented by red rectangular boxes. Twelve genes involved in DNA repair are indicated by gray ovals. The name of the complementation group is listed above the official name of the gene (in parentheses). The overlap of the ovals with the rectangles indicates that mutations in the indicated gene have been associated with the indicated phenotype. The diagram indicates that one clinical phenotype can be associated with defects in more than one gene and conversely, different defects in one gene may be associated with several different clinical phenotypes. *Abbreviations*: CS, Cockayne syndrome; TTD, trichothiodystrophy; XP, xeroderma pigmentosum. *Source*: From Ref. 51.

clothing covering the extremities to the wrists and heels. Since sports manufacturers included fashionable clothes designed with UV-protective textiles, it has become easier for patients to purchase practical and protective clothing. The head and facial area should be protected by hats, providing shade for nose and ears. Facial skin can additionally be protected by a visor mounted on the rim of a hat that holds a UV-protective screen, which allows good vision but complete filtration of UV-radiation. UV-protective films filtering at least 90% of the UV-spectrum should also cover all windows behind which XP patients live. This includes the house, kindergarten, school, work, as well as the cars in which the patients are transported. These films exist in formulations that do not stain or reduce the incoming visible light, thus allowing the presence in a room of light that does not visibly differ from nonprotected rooms.

In addition to these technical measures, sun-blocking lotions with highest possible UVB and UVA filters should be applied to the skin.

Effective chemoprevention of skin cancer by use of oral retinoids in XP patients has been demonstrated in a controlled study (26), however, there was considerable toxicity with the high doses used. Subsequent studies showed that some patients may respond to much lower doses. Local injections of interferon were shown to be effective in treating multiple melanoma in-situ lesions in one XP patient (27).

Experimental use of DNA repair proteins from algae or bacteria applied in topical formulations containing liposomes have recently been reported. This has been shown for two different repair proteins. Photolyase is an enzyme derived from the algae ancystis nidulans. This protein repairs some forms of UV-induced genomic DNA damage after activation by visible or UVA-radiation. Photolyase encapsulated in liposomes have been reported to exert immunoprotective effects (28). This enzyme is currently available in pharmacies in Germany, but has not been approved for use in the United States.

The second enzyme is a DNA glycosylase/AP lyase or T4 endonuclease V (T4endoV) that also repairs some forms of UV-induced genomic DNA damage (29). A randomized double-blind, placebo-controlled, international multicenter trial reported that application of T4endoV to the skin of patients with XP significantly reduced the incidence of actinic keratoses and BCC (30,31). As with photolyase, in this study T4endoV was encapsulated in liposomes and topically applied to the skin. The advantage of this enzyme is its activity without UV-radiation, since XP patients should not be exposed to UV-radiation at all. This enzyme has not yet been approved for use by the U.S. Food and Drug Administration.

The treatment of skin cancers utilizes the same methods as in people who do not have XP. However, the increased frequency of multiple primary neoplasms often necessitates multiple excisions. These may lead to extensive scarring and removal of large amounts of skin particularly in the face. Thus, methods to adequately remove cancers while sparing tissue are preferred. Biopsy followed by surgical excision or dessication and curettage is usually the first method of treatment. In vital areas such as near the eye or nose or with recurrent neoplasms of the face involving nerves, micrographic controlled surgery of tumors is often used. Standard cryotherapy is an effective and simple method of removal. XP patients with difficult to treat skin cancers or with internal cancers such as spinal cord or brain astrocytomas have been successfully treated with X-ray therapy. Surprisingly, in contrast to UV, the skin reaction to X-ray therapy in XP patients is usually normal (32).

In the past, before early diagnosis was possible, patients with XP had a markedly reduced life expectancy. They often died in early childhood by multiple tumors of the skin and eyes. With early detection, strict sun protection, and aggressive removal of early skin cancers, XP patients live much longer than in the past. However, the course of patients with progressive neurological degeneration does not appear to be altered by sun protection. Since XP is a recessive disorder, unless the patient marries a close relative, their children are usually genetically heterozygous and clinically indistinguishable from normal individuals.

COCKAYNE SYNDROME

Like XP, CS is an autosomal recessive genetic disease albeit with far lower prevalence (2,5,33). XP patients with neurological disease and CS patients share many of the same clinical features including marked skin sun sensitivity, microcephaly, progressive sensorineural hearing loss, short stature, and progressive neurological degeneration (34). Their cells are also hypersensitive to killing by UV-radiation and have defective DNA repair.

CS patients show a large variation with respect to severity of symptoms (Table 1). Characteristic features include typical bird-like face, with beaked nose and deep-set eyes, loss of subcutaneous fat, and prematurely aged appearance, which is why CS is considered to be a progeroid syndrome (Fig. 1). Further clinical symptoms include gait abnormalities, dental caries, and often cold hands and feet with blue discoloration. Particularly the combination of growth and mental retardation with photosensitivity should lead to the clinical differential diagnosis of CS or TTD. Neurological features of CS include dysmyelinisation of the white matter of the brain as opposed to primary neurodegeneration in XP, as well as calcification of basal ganglia, and other areas of the brain. Ocular changes seen in CS patients are cataracts and pigmentary retinal degeneration with neurological and ocular changes generally occurring later in the course of the disease. Clinical forms of CS can be divided into mild, moderate, and severe with reduction of life expectancy increasing from mild to severe.

There are two complementation groups in CS: CS-A and CS-B, but in addition to this, mutations in XP genes from complementation groups XP-B, XP-D, and XP-G can also lead to a combination of clinical symptoms of XP and CS (The XP/CS complex) (35,36). Cells from patients with CS are defective in transcription coupled DNA repair, although the exact function of CS-A and CS-B proteins has not been elucidated so far. Recent reports indicate that the CS-B protein may not only be involved in the repair of UV-induced DNA damage, but that it may also be involved in the repair of oxidative damage (10,11,37). In contrast to XP for which the DNA repair defect is presumed to be predominant, for CS as well as TTD an additionally subtle defect in basal transcription of genes has been hypothesized, which could be a possible reason why XP is characterized by an increased skin cancer risk but not CS or TTD (38). However, experimental data in support of this hypothesis only exists for TTD thus far.

As with XP, the clinical diagnosis is secured on the cellular level. For this, fibroblasts from patients are measured for their ability to recover from inhibition of RNA synthesis following UV-radiation. Although in normal cells the RNA synthesis has recovered within 24 hours, this is not the case in CS. For families with CS patients, prenatal diagnosis is available in specialized centers.

The care and management of patients with CS is difficult. Due to its photosensitivity, strict UV avoidance is indicated along with sun protection employing high protection factors in the UVA- and UVB-range.

TRICHOTHTIODYSTROPHY

TTD was termed by Price in 1980 (39,40) and like XP and CS, TTD is an autosomal recessive disease. The clinical features of TTD show great variation in form, expression, and severity. The large variety of clinical features was recently summarized by Itin et al. (41). Increased photosensitivity and DNA repair defect may be present, but there are also cases where they are absent. Clinical symptoms of TTD include a collodion membrane at birth and marked skin sun sensitivity (Table 1). Their hair is brittle with thin hair shafts that break upon minimal trauma. Stress factors such as fever and infections can lead to effluvium represented by episodes of hair loss followed by re-growth (41). Further clinical features of TTD are growth- and mental retardation, as well as ichthyosis (Fig. 1). Nail changes are features of TTD, and patients show a large variety of different neuro-ectodermal abnormalities affecting the hair, skin, nails, nerve system, and the eyes. The presence of brittle hair in combination with growth- and mental retardation under the third percentile possibly in combination with photosensitivity should lead to further diagnostic steps securing the diagnosis of TTD.

Most important diagnostic criterion are hair changes, caused by reduction of high sulphur matrix proteins and reduced cysteine content of the hairshaft matrix also underlying the fragility of the hair (18,42). As a hallmark of TTD, polarized light microscopy of TTD hair regularly reveals a pattern of light and dark areas of the hair leading to a typical "tiger tail" appearance in all hairs (43). Measurement of amino acid content of the hair by chromatography showing reduced content of cysteine-rich matrix proteins can be used to secure the diagnosis.

There are three different complementation groups of TTD. The majority of cases reveal mutations in the *XPD* gene and, in this complementation group, the site at which the nucleotide is mutated determines the phenotype of the disease (42,44,45). However, two patients have been reported that show the combination of TTD and XP features (46). The second group shows mutations in the *XPB* gene and has been described in only one kindred. Mutations in a newly discovered small protein component of the TFIIH complex, TTD-A, have been found to cause TTD in a few families. (47,48). A gene of unknown function on chromosome 7 (TTDN1) has been reported to be defective in some families with nonphotosensitive TTD (49).

In contrast to XP, patients with TTD are not characterized by an increased risk of skin cancer, although the causative mutations reside in the same gene. It has previously been demonstrated that, in addition to a repair defect, cells from XP patients also show alterations in immunosurveillance, whereas TTD cells do not exhibit this defect (15–18). This could help to explain the difference in skin cancer risk between the two syndromes. In addition to this, it is currently believed that the phenotype of TTD is also caused by subtle defects in basal transcription, which would make both CS and TTD transcription deficiency syndromes (38). Patients with TTD exhibit lower levels of ß-hemoglobin than normal individuals (13). This directly results in measurable decreases of simple clinical parameters. The mean corpuscular haemoglobin (MCH) as well as the mean cellular volume (MCV) of TTD-erythrocytes is significantly reduced. This finding not only supports the hypothesis that basal transcription is impaired but it also facilitates the diagnosis of TTD. Upon clinical suspicion of TTD, MCH, and MCV can be assessed in any clinical setting before more specialized tests are initiated.

As with CS, care and management of TTD patients is difficult. It is restricted to stringent photoprotective measures as described above in the case of photosensitivity and supportive measures to reduce handicaps by neuro-ectodermal symptoms. Scaling induced by ichthyosis can be improved by application of urea-containing lotions.

CONCLUSION

XP, CS, and TTD represent important model diseases for the pathogenesis of skin cancers as well as mechanisms underlying the process of aging. Therefore, by understanding underlying mechanisms it may not only be possible in the future to help these patients, but to also develop strategies that are also relevant to aging and carcinogenesis in the normal population.

On the clinical level, early diagnosis of DNA repair deficient photodermatoses is essential in order to allow early protective and supportive measures, which do help improve the quality of life and possibly also life expectancy.

REFERENCES

1. Berneburg M, Lehmann AR. Xeroderma pigmentosum and related disorders: defects in DNA repair and transcription. Adv Genet 2001; 43:71–102.
2. de Laat WL, Jaspers NG, Hoeijmakers JH. Molecular mechanism of nucleotide excision repair. Genes Dev 1999; 13:768–785.
3. Lehmann AR. Dual functions of DNA repair genes: molecular, cellular, and clinical implications. Bioessays 1998; 20:146–155.
4. van Hoffen A, Natarajan AT, Mayne LV, van Zeeland AA, Mullenders LH, Venema J. Deficient repair of the transcribed strand of active genes in Cockayne's syndrome cells. Nucleic Acids Res 1993; 21:5890–5895.
5. van Gool A, van der Horst E, Citterio E, Hoeijmakers JH. Cockayne syndrome: defective repair of transcription? EMBO J 1997; 16:4155–4162.
6. Schaeffer L, Moncollin V, Roy R, et al. The ERCC2/DNA repair protein is associated with the class II BTF2/TFIIH transcription factor. EMBO J 1994; 13:2388–2392.
7. Chang RD, Kornberg RD. Electron crystal structure of the transcription factor and DNA repair. Cell 2000; 102:609–613.
8. Lehmann AR. Nucleotide excision repair and the link with transcription. Trends Biochem Sci 1995; 20:402–405.

9. Wood RD. DNA damage recognition during nucleotide excision repair in mammalian. Biochimie 1999; 81:39–44.
10. Cooper T, Nouspikel SG, Clarkson SA, Leadon SA. Defective transcription-coupled repair of oxidative base damage. Science 1997; 275:990–993.
11. Le Page F, Kwoh A, Avrutskaya A, et al. Transcription-coupled repair of 8-oxoguanine: requirement for XPG, TFIIH and CSB. Cell 2000; 101:159–171.
12. Schaeffer L, Roy R, Humbert S, et al. DNA repair helicase: a component of BTF2 (TFIIH) basic transcription factor. Science 1993; 260:58–63.
13. Viprakasit V, Gibbons RJ, Broughton BC, et al. Mutations in the general transcription factor TFIIH result in TTD. Hum Mol Genet 2001; 10:2797–2802.
14. Keriel A, Stary A, Sarasin A, Rochette-Egly C, Egly JM. XPD mutations prevent TFIIH-dependent transactivation by nuclear receptors. Cell 2002; 109:125–135.
15. Norris PG, Limb GA, Hamblin AS, Hawk JL. Impairment of natural-killer-cell activity in xeroderma pigmentosum. N Engl J Med 1988; 319:1668–1669.
16. Norris PG, Limb GA, Hamblin AS, et al. Immune function, mutant frequency, and cancer risk in the DNA repair deficiency syndrome xeroderma pigmentosum. J Invest Dermatol 1990; 94:94–100.
17. Ahrens C, Grewe M, Berneburg M, et al. Photocarcinogenesis and inhibition of intercellular adhesion molecule 1 expression in cells of DNA-repair-defective individuals. Proc Natl Acad Sci USA 1997; 94:6837–6841.
18. Berneburg M, Clingen PH, Harcourt SA, et al. The cancer-free phenotype in trichothiodystrophy is unrelated to its repair defect. Cancer Res 2000; 60:431–438.
19. Vink AA, Shreedhar V, Roza L, Krutmann J, Kripke ML. Cellular target of UVB-induced DNA damage resulting in local suppression of contact hypersensitivity. J Photochem Photobiol B 1998; 44:107–111.
20. Shwarz A, Stander S, Berneburg M, et al. Interleukin-12 suppresses ultraviolet radiation-induced apoptosis by inducing DNA repair. Nat Cell Biol 2002; 4:26–31.
21. Kraemer KH, Levy DD, Parris CN, et al. Xeroderma pigmentosum and related disorders: examining the linkage. J Invest Dermatol 1994; 103:96–101.
22. Fritsch C, Bolsen K, Ruzicka T, Goerz G. Congenital erythropoietic porphyria. J Am Acad Dermatol 1997; 36:594–610.
23. Hahn H, Wicking C, Zaphiropoulous PG, et al. Mutations of the human homolog of Drosophila patched in the nevoid basal. Cell 85:841–851.
24. Johnson RL, Rothman AL, Xie J, et al. Human homolog of patched, a candidate gene for the basal cell nevus. Science 1996; 272:1668–1671.
25. Lehmann AR. The xeroderma pigmentosum group D (XPD) gene: one gene, two functions. Genes Dev 2001; 15:15–23.
26. Kraemer KH, Di Giovanna JJ, Moshell AN, Tarone RE, Peck GL. Prevention of skin cancer with oral 13-cis retinoic acid in xeroderma pigmentosum. N Engl J Med 1988; 318:1633–1637.
27. Turner M, Moshell A, Corbett D, et al. Clearing of melanoma-in-situ with intralesional interferon in a patient with xeroderma pigmentosum. Arch Dermatol 1994; 130:1491–1494.
28. Stege H, Roza L, Vink AA, et al. Enzyme plus Light therapy to repair immunosuppressive effects on human skin damaged by ultraviolet B-radiation. Proc Natl Acad Sci 2000; 97:1790–1795.
29. Kraemer KH, Di Giovanna J. Topical enzyme therapy for skin diseases? J Am Acad Dermatol 2002; 46:463–466.
30. Yarosh D, Alas LG, Yee V, et al. Pyrimidine dimer removal enhanced by DNA repair liposomes reduces the incidence of UV skin cancer in mice. Cancer Res 1992; 52:4227–4231.
31. Yarosh D, Klein J, O'Connor A, Hawk J, Rafal E, Wolf P. Effect of topically applied T4 endonuclease V in liposomes on skin cancer. Lancet 2001; 357:926–929.
32. Di Giovanna JJ, Patronas N, Katz D, Abangan D, Kraemer KH. Spinal cord astrocytoma in a patient with xeroderma pigmentosum: 9-year survival with radiation and isotretinoin therapy. J Cut Med Surg 1998; 2:153–158.
33. van Gool AJ, Citterio E, Rademakers S, et al. The Cockayne syndrome B protein, involved in transcription-coupled DNA repair. EMBO J 1997; 16:5955–5965.
34. Rapin I, Lindenbaum Y, Dickson DW, Kraemer KH, Robbins JH. Cockayne syndrome and xeroderma pigmentosum: DNA repair disorders with overlaps and paradoxes. Neurology 2000; 55:1442–1449.
35. Berneburg M, Lowe JE, Nardo T, et al. UV damage causes uncontrolled DNA breakage in cells from patients with combined features of XP-D and Cockayne syndrome. EMBO J 2000; 19:1157–1166.
36. Stefanini M, Fawcett H, Botta E, Nardo T, Lehmann AR. Genetic analysis of twenty-two patients with Cockayne syndrome. Hum Genet 1996; 97:418–423.
37. Nouspikel P, Lalle P, Leadon SA, Cooper PK, Clarkson SG. A common mutational pattern in Cockayne syndrome patients from xeroderma pigmentosum. Proc Natl Acad Sci USA 1997; 94:3116–3121.
38. Friedberg EC. Cockayne syndrome—a primary defect in DNA repair, transcription or both Bioessays 1996; 18:731–738.

39. Price VH, Odom RB, Ward WH, Jones FT. Trichothiodystrophy: sulfur-deficient brittle hair as a marker for a neuroectodermal symptom complex. Arch Dermatol 1980; 116:1375–1384.
40. Poissonnier M, Blanc A, Bat P. Genetic counseling in a case of neuro-ectodermosis: Vera Price Syndrome. J Genet Hum 1988; 36:361–365.
41. Itin PH, Sarasin A, Pittelkow M. Trichothiodystrophy: update on the sulfur-deficient brittle hair. J Am Acad Dermatol 2001; 44:891–920.
42. Botta E, Nardo T, Broughton BC, Marinoni S, Lehmann AR, Stefanini M. Analysis of mutations in the XPD gene in Italian patients with Cockayne Syndrome. Am J Hum Genet 1998; 63:1036–1048.
43. Liang C, Kraemer KH, Morris, A, et al. Characterization of tiger tail banding and hair shaft abnormalities in trichothiodystrophy. J Am Acad Dermatol 2005; 52:224–234.
44. Taylor EM, Broughton BC, Botta E. Xeroderma pigmentosum and trichothiodystrophy are associated with different mutations in the XPD (ERCC2) repair/transcription gene. Proc Natl Acad Sci USA 1997; 94:8658–8663.
45. Mariani E, Facchini A, Honorati AM, et al. Immune defects in families and patients with xeroderma pigmentosum and trichothiodystrophy. Clin Exp Immunol 1992; 88:376–382.
46. Broughton BC, Berneburg M, Fawcett H, et al. Two individuals with features of both xeroderma pigmentosum and trichothiodystrophy. Hum Mol Genet 2001; 10:2539–2547.
47. Vermeulen W, Bergmann E, Auriol J, et al. Sublimiting concentration of TFIIH transcription/DNA repair factor causes TTD-A. Nat Genet 2000; 26:307–313.
48. Giglia-Mari G, Coin F, Ranish JA, et al. A new, tenth subunit of TFIIH is responsible for the DNA repair syndrome trichothiodystrophy group A. Nat Genet 2004; 36:714–719.
49. Nakabayashi K, Amann D, Ren Y, et al. Identification of C7orf11 (TTDN1) gene mutations and genetic heterogeneity in non-photosensitive trichothiodystrophy. Am J Hum Genet 2005; 76:510–516.
50. Moriwaki S-I, Stefanini M, Lehmann AR, et al. DNA repair and ultraviolet mutagenesis in cells from a new patient with xeroderma pigmentosum group G and Cockayne syndrome resemble xeroderma pigmentosum cells. J Invest Dermatol 1996; 107:647–653.
51. Kraemer KH. From proteomics to disease. Nat Genet 2004; 36:677–678.

17 | Photoaggravated Dermatoses

Victoria P. Werth
Department of Dermatology, University of Pennsylvania, and Philadelphia V.A. Medical Center, Philadelphia, Pennsylvania, U.S.A.

Herbert Hönigsmann
Department of Dermatology, Medical University of Vienna, Vienna, Austria

- Atopic dermatitis can occasionally be exacerbated by ultraviolet radiation.

- Sunlight-induced erythema multiforme may actually reflect the fact that herpes may precipitate erythema multiforme.

- Antimalarials frequently can treat cutaneous lupus erythematosus and skin manifestations of dermatomyositis.

- Pellagra improves with a balanced, high-protein diet.

- There is a need for organized trials with the autoimmune blistering and connective tissue diseases.

PHOTOAGGRAVATED DERMATOSES

Photoaggravated dermatoses (or photoexacerbated skin diseases) represent a very heterogeneous group of conditions that share only one common feature: they can be induced or exacerbated by exposure to sunlight or to artificial therapeutic or cosmetic ultraviolet (UV) radiation (Table 1). It is important to recognize that these diseases are not true photodermatoses since they commonly develop without exposure to radiation. They are of diverse or unknown etiology and photoexacerbation occurs only in some, but not in all, of the affected subjects. In many instances, the role of light is clearly defined. In others, documentation of photosensitivity is poor and UV radiation may be one of several nonspecific factors that induce aggravation. In this chapter, a selection of common and important photoexacerbated diseases is discussed. Treatment is restriction of light exposure, use of high protection sunscreens, and appropriate treatment of the underlying disorder.

Acne

Acne aestivalis, first described by Hjorth et al. (1), is characterized by pruritic, 1 to 3 mm, pink or pale, dome-shaped papules occurring after sun exposure, usually on the face, neck, or trunk. Nieboer (2) further reported two such patients, describing the disorder as actinic superficial folliculitis, a predominantly follicular, pustular rash occurring several hours after sun exposure, but nonpruritic and affecting only the upper trunk and arms. Bacteriological, immunohistopathological, and photo-experimental investigations failed to reveal a cause for this sunlight-induced dermatosis. Verbov (3) described three additional patients with overlapping features of both acne aestivalis and actinic superficial folliculitis and proposed the unifying term actinic folliculitis. It was characterized by a pustular eruption appearing over the face, and sometimes the arms and upper chest, 4 to 24 hours after exposure to sunlight. The condition appears indeed to be a form of UV-exacerbated acne, for which high-protection-factor sunscreens, standard acne treatments, including topical retinoic acid, and topical and systemic antibiotics have not generally been helpful, although oral isotretinoin has been shown to be effective (4,5).

Darier's Disease

Several cases of photoaggravated Darier's disease have been reported (6). Baba and Yaoita (7) carried out provocation studies on the lesions of keratosis follicularis with UV radiation. Non-erythema-producing doses of UVB elicited the lesions in uninvolved skin sites in a 34-year-old man with this disease. The elicited lesions were compatible with those of keratosis follicularis both clinically and histopathologically. Similar irradiation with UVA produced no visible changes in the test area. Otley et al. performed an unblinded, controlled trial using UVB, UVA, or combination UVB/UVA phototherapy in patients with Darier's disease and reported that UVB irradiation was indeed capable of inducing lesions of Darier's disease, whereas UVA radiation alone and heat associated with phototherapy had no effect on the disease (8). We ourselves found massive worsening in two patients experimentally treated with psoralen and ultraviolet A (PUVA) (Fig. 1). Photoprotection by sunscreens and topical ascorbic acid may be helpful (8).

TABLE 1 Photoexacerbated Dermatoses

Acne	Atopic dermatitis
Darier's disease	Psoriasis
Transient acantholytic dermatosis	Lichen planus actinicus
Disseminated superficial actinic porokeratosis	Lupus erythematosus
Pellagra	Dermatomyositis
Herpes simplex	Bullous pemphigoid
Erythema multiforme	Pemphigus

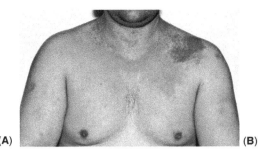 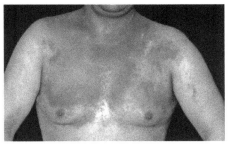

FIGURE 1   Darier's disease. (**A**) Before PUVA and (**B**) after PUVA.

Transient Acantholytic Dermatosis

Grover's disease is a nonimmune acantholytic dermatosis. The etiology and pathogenesis of Grover's disease is unknown. Factors that can trigger the disease include sweat, fever, heat, and sunlight. Some reports have hypothesized causation by poral occlusion of damaged eccrine intra-epidermal ducts, with spillage of sweat contents and focal acantholysis (9). Acantholysis is often not associated with the eccrine duct outflow tract. Different studies have shown the primary damage in the proteins of the desmosomal attachment plaque, such as desmoplakins I and II and plakoglobin (10,11).

It was first described by Grover in 1970 (12). The male-to-female ratio is at least 3:1 (13). Most reports are in older Caucasians, but there have been small numbers of cases reported from Japan and Korea (14). In some cases, it has been reported in association with other systemic diseases, such as both solid and hematological malignancies, human immunodeficiency virus infections, chronic renal failure, and hemodialysis (13,15,16). Grover reported statistically significant associations between transient acantholytic disease and asteatotic eczema, allergic contact dermatitis, atopic dermatitis, and irritation from adhesive tape (17). This suggests that nonspecific irritation can induce lesions.

Grover's disease is characterized by pruritic papules and vesicles, mainly distributed on the trunk. Some lesion can appear follicular, and plaques and bullous lesions have been noted. The lesions are typically located on the trunk and, to a lesser extent, the proximal extremities. Involvement of the face, scalp, and oral mucosa can occur, but palms and soles are typically spared (13). Localized variants have been reported and are more common in younger females (18). The disease lasts less than three months in most patients, but occasionally continues for two or three years, particularly in older patients. Seasonal recurrences can occur (19).

A history of initiation or exacerbation of lesions by sunlight has frequently been noted. Other reports have found exacerbation from tanning salon exposure and UVB (13).

Treatment includes topical and oral glucocorticoids and antibiotics. Oral and bath PUVA, as well as UVA1 phototherapy, have been successfully used (20–22). It is difficult to evaluate therapies because of the transient nature of this process.

Pellagra

Pellagra is a nutritional disorder due to nicotinic acid deficiency and is common in third-world countries with high malnutrition rates, where millet or maize is the principal nutrient in the diet (23). It can be seen in undernourished elderly people, chronic alcoholics, psychiatric and diabetic patients, or in individuals with gastrointestinal malabsorption or carcinoid tumors (24,25). Deficiency of niacin can occur with fever, thyrotoxicosis, and food faddism. Certain drugs such as isoniazid, pyrazinamide, ethionamide, 6-mercaptopurine, azathioprine, 5-fluorouracil, phenytoin, phenobarbital, sodium valproate, and chloramphenicol can cause this vitamin deficiency (26). Pellagra is a bilateral and symmetrical dermatosis affecting sun-exposed areas.

Clinical findings in pellagra include dermatitis, diarrhea, and dementia. The skin findings include intense red, scaly, and hyperpigmented plaques on sun-exposed areas, as well

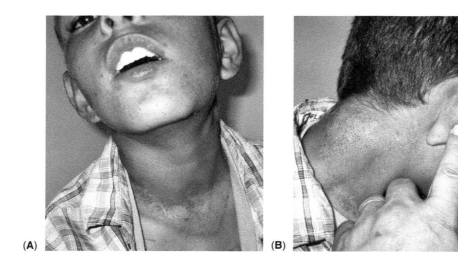

(A)   **(B)**

FIGURE 2   Pellagra. Photodistribution of lesions on (**A**) anterior chest; (**B**) posterior neck

as areas of heat, friction, or pressure (Fig. 2). The lesions can be edematous, with occasional vesicules or desquamation, and can have a burning sensation. Typical locations include involvement around the neck (Casal's necklace), which can extend towards the sternum, and follicular hyperkeratotic plugs can be present in a seborrheic distribution (Fig. 2A). Flexural areas can be macerated. Angular cheilitis, glossitis with papillary atrophy, a beefy tender tongue, and esophagitis are seen. The skin in long-standing lesions is thickened and hyperpigmented.

Treatment consists of a balanced, high-protein diet. Nicotinamide can be given 50 to 100 mg tid along with a vitamin B complex. Sunscreen and moisturizers are indicated.

Herpes Simplex and Other Viral Rashes

It is common knowledge that many patients experience herpes simplex eruptions after sun exposure, particularly while sun bathing, mountain hiking, or skiing in higher altitudes. The mechanism for viral activation by sunlight is unknown, but it may be possibly related to the fact that UVB radiation induces modulation of antigen presentation of herpes simplex virus (HSV) by Langerhans cells (27).

Several other nonspecific stimuli such as fever, hormonal changes (menses), or heat can trigger herpes lesions. Reports on sunlight-induced erythema multiforme (EM) may actually reflect the fact that herpes may precipitate EM (Fig. 3A). Relapsing gluteal herpes simplex is common in patients treated with narrowband UVB or PUVA. In a study from Japan with 4295 patients, sun-induced HSV-1 flare-up was reported by 10.4% of the total study population. However, this increased to 19.7% among patients diagnosed in July and August, to 28% among patients younger than 30 years diagnosed in July and August, and to 40% among patients younger than 30 years diagnosed in July and August with a recurrent infection (28). Also vaccinia, lymphogranuloma venereum, and varicella have all been recognized as having a photosensitivity component (29). In particular, varicella localizes in sun-exposed areas (30,31). Viral rashes occurring in sun-exposed areas are quite commonly misdiagnosed as drug eruptions or photodermatoses.

Erythema Multiforme

Photodistribution, that is, increased density or confluence of the lesions on skin exposed to light, is a common phenomenon of EM (32). However, cases of EM triggered by exposure to the sun are rare and have been reported as "photosensitive EM." Almost all patients had an otherwise normal tolerance to sunlight and eruptions developed only if HSV infection (32–34) or ingestion of drugs, such as carbanilides, phenylbutazone, aflaqualone, and antimalarials (35–37) had preceded the sun exposure (Fig. 3A and B).

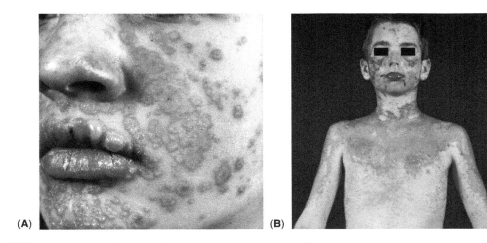

FIGURE 3 Erythema multiforme. (**A**) Herpes simplex-induced and (**B**) drug-induced.

The pathogenesis of photosensitive EM is unknown and could be a hypersensitivity reaction to a hypothetical photoproduct produced by UV radiation. In some cases, lesions could be provoked by phototesting with UVA and UVB below the normal limits for minimal erythemal doses (38).

In conclusion, photosensitive EM is very rare and may be secondary to HSV infection and drug intake as well as apparently idiopathic (38). Its differentiation from EM-like polymorphous light eruption may be very difficult and further studies are needed in order to assess diagnostic differential criteria, if any.

Atopic Dermatitis

A minority of patients with atopic eczema report mild to moderate, nonspecific exacerbation of their disease with marked pruritus and eczema in sun-exposed areas. Some may be sensitive to UV radiation on phototesting, but normal responses are the rule, thus allowing distinction from chronic actinic dermatitis. Frain-Bell and Scatchard (39) described patients with atopic dermatitis whose condition deteriorated during the summer by developing erythematous papules confined to light-exposed areas (Fig. 4). Phototests with UVA, UVB, and visible light did not reproduce such lesions. However, the majority of patients with atopic dermatitis will benefit from both sunlight and artificial UV irradiation. Thus, "photoaggravation" may sometimes be due to heat or humidity rather than a specific effect of sunlight.

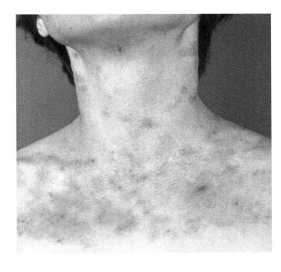

FIGURE 4 Atopic dermatitis. Photodistribution of lesions on neck, anterior chest.

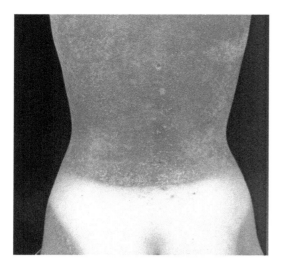

FIGURE 5 Photosensitive psoriasis. Back of patient showing clear involvement in photoexposed areas.

Psoriasis

Patients with psoriasis usually benefit from sunlight and UV phototherapy. However, some patients experience exacerbation of their disease after sun bathing, particularly, after sunburn (40–42) (Fig. 5). The exact incidence of this photosensitive form of psoriasis is not known and varies in the literature from 5.5% to 24%. In a questionnaire study encompassing 2000 patients in Sweden, the prevalence of photosensitivity was 5.5% (42). Forty-three percent of the light-sensitive patients had a history of polymorphous light eruption with secondary exacerbation of psoriasis lesions. Comparison between the photosensitive and the nonphotosensitive patients showed a statistically significant increase in type I skin, psoriasis affecting hands, heredity for photosensitivity, and advanced age in the photosensitive group. The investigators proposed that many patients developed polymorphous light eruption and secondarily psoriasis as a Koebner phenomenon (42). Interestingly, despite photosensitivity, in our experience and in that of others such patients can be successfully treated with photochemotherapy (43). In summary, photosensitivity is well recognized but poorly defined in psoriasis. Many patients probably have polymorphous light eruption, other light sensitivity (44,45), or fair skin to explain the subsequent development of psoriatic lesions as a Koebner phenomenon.

Lichen Planus Actinicus

Actinic lichen planus (LP) is a rare variant of LP that affects mainly Middle Eastern children and teenagers (46,47). The lesions occur on sun-exposed skin, usually the face, and have three clinical types: annular, dyschromic, and hyperpigmented (Fig. 6). The dyschromic type presents as discrete and confluent whitish papules and the pigmented types consists of hypermelanotic patches. Lesions can occur on sun-protected skin and buccal mucosa (48,49), but not the nails (50). Lesions are not pruritic and are not induced by trauma (50).

Sunlight is a major precipitating cause, with lesions occurring in the spring and summer, with residual hyperpigmentation in the winter. The minimal erythema dose (MED) was performed in one case, and was normal (51).

Treatment includes topical or intralesional steroids, antimalarials, and sunscreen (52).

Lupus Erythematosus

There are clearly both environmental and genetic factors in the pathogenesis of cutaneous lupus erythematosus (CLE) (53–55). Sunlight exposure, the anti-Ro antibody, HLA type, and polymorphisms in complement molecules, and tumor necrosis factor-alpha (TNF-α) have all been correlated with the presence of the subacute CLE (SCLE) subset (56–60). The pathogenesis of CLE is complex, with a role for UV light-induced apoptosis, potential delayed clearance of

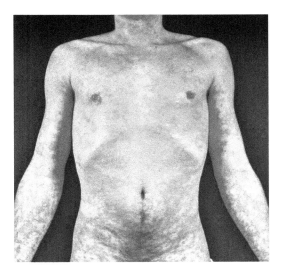

FIGURE 6 Lichen planus actinicus.

apoptotic debris, antigen presentation with documented interferon (IFN)-alpha producing plasmacytoid dendritic cells in the skin, subsequent T-cell and autoantibody responses, and a complex pro-inflammatory cascade that includes induction of chemokines, cytokines, and adhesion molecules that bring CD4+ T-cells into the skin (61).

Lupus Erythematosus-Specific Skin Lesions

Skin manifestations of LE include chronic CLE, subacute CLE, and acute CLE (62). Since systemic evaluation and treatment are often indicated, it is important to confirm the clinical suspicion of CLE with a skin biopsy. Chronic CLE includes a number of entities that can be found as skin disease alone or in association with systemic lupus erythematosus (SLE). In one study, 10% of SLE patients had discoid LE (DLE) as their first manifestation of LE, and thus patients, in addition to a baseline assessment for SLE activity, also need to be followed to assure that significant SLE does not develop (63).

Chronic Cutaneous Lupus Erythematosus

DLE can occur as a localized process, commonly above the neck in photoexposed areas. Lesions of DLE can be erythematous, raised, indurated papules, or plaques. The lesions may have adherent, keratotic scale, with or without a carpet tack sign, follicular plugging, and telangiectasias. Atrophic scarring as well as dyspigmentation may occur in older lesions, and involvement of the scalp frequently results in permanent scarring alopecia. Hypertrophic LE, seen in 2% of CLE, shows a keratotic thicker plaque than is typical of DLE. There is no particular different prognostic or therapeutic significance to this diagnosis beyond that of DLE. Lupus profundus includes firm, deep subcutaneous nodules that atrophy over time. There may be overlying skin surface changes typical of DLE. Another subcategory of chronic CLE is tumid or papulomucinous LE. This is a particularly photosensitive variant of chronic CLE that is not typically associated with the presence of lupus serologies or SLE (64).

Subacute Cutaneous Lupus Erythematosus

SCLE was first described as a distinct subset in 1979 (65). It can present as papulosquamous, psoriasiform plaques and annular-polycyclic plaques, with either form seen in about 50% of these patients, and some patients have features of both presentations. Some patients with SCLE also have vesiculobullous lesions, often located at the periphery of annular SCLE lesions. There are also some patients who develop EM or toxic epidermal necrolysis (TEN)-like skin lesions in association with their SCLE lesions (66). Patients with SCLE are photosensitive, with lesions commonly located on the extensor arms, shoulders, V of the neck, back, and less commonly the face (Fig. 7A and B). SCLE lesions typically heal without

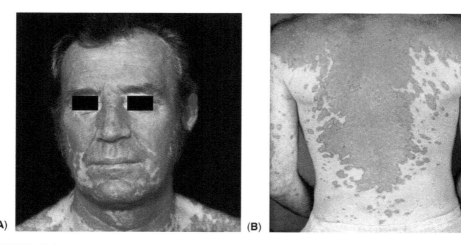

FIGURE 7 Subacute cutaneous lupus erythematosus: (**A**) face and (**B**) back.

scarring, but may have postinflammatory hypopigmentation and telangiectasias. About 50% of patients meet criteria for SLE, and patients with SCLE frequently have high titers of anti-SSA and anti-SSB antibodies in their serum (60). SCLE, a disease seen primarily in Caucasian females, is associated with the ancestral haplotype HLA-B8, DR3, and an increased disease association with the $-308A$ TNF-α promoter polymorphism has been found (54,57,67). These patients have a lower incidence of renal or central nervous system disease, and the more typical systemic symptoms that can be seen in up to 50% include arthritis/arthralgias, fever/malaise, and myalgias. Drug-induced SCLE is frequent, and the list of implicated medications is growing (68,69).

Acute Cutaneous Lupus Erythematosus
Acute CLE can clinically present as the typical malar erythema, but other manifestations include widespread morbilliform or exanthematous eruption in a photodistribution, sparing the knuckles, and bullous or TEN-like acute CLE skin lesions. The lack of targeting of the metacarpal phalangeal (MCP), proximal interphalangeal (PIP), and distal interphalangeal (DIP) joints can help distinguish LE from dermatomyositis (DM). The malar erythema can be either patch or plaque-like, and there is a tendency to spare the nalolabial folds, as opposed to DM, which can sometimes be in the differential diagnosis. Unusual presentations seen in acute CLE skin lesions also include involvement of the lips and periorbital edema. The bullous LE subset seen in acute CLE is a subepidermal blistering process. The criteria normally utilized for making the diagnosis include the diagnosis of SLE based on the American Rheumatologic Association (ARA) criteria, vesicles and bullae arising on, but not limited to, sun-exposed skin, routine histopathological findings consistent with dermatitis herpetiformis, and a direct immunofluorescence revealing IgG and/or IgM and often IgA and C3 at the dermal–epidermal junction (70,71). Sera from such patients often contain autoantibodies that react with the epidermolysis bullosa acquisita antigen, type VII collagen (70). However, some patients do have immunoreactants to the epidermal side of 1 M NaCl split skin as well as other autoantibodies in their sera (71,72).

Skin lesions found to be associated with a worse prognosis include photosensitivity, alopecia, oral ulcers, and Raynaud's phenomenon (73). Photosensitivity is a clinical observation that is not specific to CLE. If a biopsy is obtained from sun-induced skin lesions, and if the photosensitivity is due to the presence of LE, then the biopsy would show a lupus-specific skin lesion.

Phototesting in Cutaneous Lupus Erythematosus
UV light is a well-established trigger of CLE (74–78), and SCLE is one of the more photosensitive skin lesions in CLE (79). Skin lesions often occur in a photodistributed pattern and are more common in summer (65,80). Photoprovocation studies employing artificial sources

of UVA (320–400 nm), UVB (290–320 nm), and visible light show a large variability in the reported results, with the percentages of SCLE patients showing photoprovocation ranging from 50% to 100% in response to UV radiation (81–88). The variation can be partially explained by differences in light sources and filters, UV doses and dosing schedules, size of the testing area, and site of testing (85). In one study, phototesting showed induction of CLE lesions in 63% of patients with SCLE, in 72% of tumid LE cases, in 60% of SLE cases, and in 45% of CCLE cases (14). Of those with UV-induced lesions, 53% were induced by a combination of UVB and UVA, 34% by UVA alone, and 42% by UVB alone (81).

There is no significant difference between the MED of CLE patients and control populations (81,85,88).

Therapy of Cutaneous Lupus Erythematosus

Treatment of CLE includes sun avoidance, sunblocking garments, and sunscreens. There is evidence that sunscreens containing Mexoryl are more effective at inhibiting broad-spectrum UVA and UVB phototesting-induced CLE lesions than non-Mexoryl containing sunscreen (89). Topical glucocorticoids and topical calcineurin inhibitors (pimecrolimus and tacrolimus) are helpful for limited disease or as adjunctive to systemic therapy. Antimalarials (Tables 2 and 3), immunosuppressives, thalidomide, dapsone, retinoids, and clofazamine can be helpful for more extensive or scarring disease (90). Glucocorticoids are occasionally used for short-term treatment if a patient has rapidly progressing scarring lesions or extensive involvement. Low-dose UVA1 (5 J/cm^2) has been reported to be beneficial (80). Recently, a validated index to measure CLE activity and damage has been developed (91). This will hopefully facilitate trials of therapies for CLE, and there is clearly a need for organized therapeutic trials (92).

Dermatomyositis

There are increased apoptotic cells in lesional DM skin (93). Exposure of normal keratinocytes in vivo and in vitro to UVB induces DNA damage and apoptosis (94,95), but it is unclear whether there is an increased susceptibility to UV or whether in fact there are cytotoxic effects from CD4+ T-cells in the skin or from keratinocyte or T-cell derived inflammatory cytokines. Adhesion molecules and chemokines are upregulated by UV light, which can bring inflammatory cells into the skin. There are clearly genetic risk factors for DM, and Caucasian females are at a much-increased risk of having cutaneous findings of DM (96).

TABLE 2 Treatment of Cutaneous Lupus Erythematosus

Sun and heat avoidance
Avoid or stop potentially triggering drugs, especially in SCLE
Sunscreens
UVB SPF-30 or greater
Avobenzone (Parsol® 1789)
Inorganic sunscreens (TiO$_2$ and ZnO)
Sunscreens containing Mexoryl® SX and Mexoryl® XL
Sunscreens containing Tinosorb® S and Tinosorb® M
Topical and intralesional steroids
Topical calcineurin inhibitors (pimecrolimus and tacrolimus)
Antimalarials
Hydroxychloroquine (<6.5 mg/kg/day)
Combination hydroxychloroquine and quinacrine (100 mg/day)
Combination chloroquine (<3.5 mg/kg/day) and quinacrine
Dapsone (start at 50 mg/day and titrate up to 150 mg/day as tolerated)
Retinoids (1 mg/kg/day), usually for rapid control but not long-term therapy
Thalidomide (100 mg/day until responds, then gradually decrease to as little as 25 mg every three days)
Methotrexate, CellCept, and azathioprine
Corticosteroids (for acute skin disease only)

Abbreviations: SCLE, subacute cutaneous lupus erythematosus; SPF, sun protection factor.

TABLE 3   Approach to Use of Antimalarials

Begin plaquenil (usually 300–400 mg/day, depending on weight)
Wait 6–8 wk for effect
If lupus still active, add quinacrine 100 mg/day
Taper quinacrine as tolerated after disease controlled
If still not controlled, switch from plaquenil to chloroquine
Try to stop antimalarials in winter

In Europe, the prevalence of DM increases with decreasing geographical latitude (97). One study found the relative prevalence of DM correlated with surface UV irradiance and there was a strong correlation to the amount of anti-Mi-2 autoantibodies (98).

The distribution of skin lesions in DM suggests that photoinduction is important (99,100). Common skin changes include an erythematous, often violaceous eruption on the face, particularly in the periorbital area (heliotrope pattern), sun-exposed areas of the face, anterior chest, upper back and shoulders, posterior neck, scalp, and over the joints on the hands, elbows, knees, and malleolus (Fig. 8). Skin biopsy show perivascular inflammation consisting of CD4+ T-cells and B-cells, as well as vasculopathy. DM patients can have autoantibodies directed against conformational epitopes on cytoplasmic and nuclear components (101). These include autoantibodies that bind to and inhibit the function of aminoacyl-transfer RNA synthetases (anti-synthetases), seen in both DM and polymyositis, and those that react with Mi-2, a 240 kDa SNF2-superfamily helicase associated with the nucleosome remodeling and deacetylase complex, seen only in DM.

DM can be associated with an underlying malignancy, and the increased risk of malignancy is present for at least five years after initial diagnosis (102). Patients should obtain baseline and regular screening for malignancy during that time (103). Frequently associated malignancies include lung, ovarian, pancreatic, stomach, colorectal, and non-Hodgkins lymphoma (104). There are patients who have amyopathic or hypomyopathic forms of DM (105,106). Patients should always be screened with pulmonary function tests (PFTs) for occult interstitial lung disease, in addition to the usual screening for underlying malignancy. If PFTs are abnormal, then chest X ray and high-resolution CAT scan should be obtained.

Studies have detected sunlight-induced exacerbation of cutaneous DM (107,108). One study suggested that the MED to UVB radiation was decreased in DM (108).

Therapy must be directed at the manifestation of DM present. Patients with muscle and skin disease must be treated with steroids and, for resistant disease, adjunctive immunosuppressive therapies. Patients with interstitial lung disease frequently require cyclophosphamide. Cutaneous findings of DM can be treated with antimalarials, either hydroxychloroquine or chloroquine, and if that is not effective, then quinacrine is added, as described in the lupus erythematosus section (109,110). Resistant patients can benefit from additional treatment

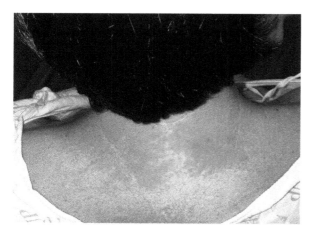

FIGURE 8   Dermatomyositis.

with azathioprine, mycophenolate mofetil, or methotrexate (111). There have been recent case reports and small case series reporting the efficacy of Rituximab in some patients (112).

Bullous Pemphigoid

One study suggested that activation of transcription of the bullous pemphigoid (BP) antigen gene seen after UV radiation is a potential mechanism of exacerbation of BP by UV (113). The exact mechanism of UV induction is unknown.

BP is a nonscarring bullous disease that presents with tense blisters, often in a flexural distribution. It can be generalized or localized, and blister formation may preceed or be accompanied by an urticarial or eczematous eruption.

It has been noted for years that BP can be induced or exacerbated with UV irradiation (114,115). There are reports of exacerbations by UVB, UVA, and PUVA (116,117).

The therapy of BP includes glucocorticoids. Some reports suggest that mild disease can be treated with topical steroids, topical tacrolimus, tetracycline and niacinamide, dapsone, or sulfapyridine (118,119). Severe disease usually requires systemic glucocorticoids, usually at a dose of 0.75 mg/kg/day, although individual patients may respond to lower doses. One large study found topical steroids worked and minimized side effects in moderate to severe disease (118). Some patients require adjunctive therapy with immunosuppressives such as azathioprine, methotrexate, mycophenolate mofetil, or in very unresponsive disease cyclophosphamide. Very resistant patients may benefit from plasmapheresis in combination with glucocorticoids and immunosuppressives or from intravenous immunoglobulin (120).

Pemphigus

The etiology of the photoexacerbation of pemphigus is unclear. There appears to be enhanced binding of pemphigus autoantibodies to keratinocyte membrane after in vivo UV light exposure, suggesting that UV exposure of the epidermis may uncover increased Dsg1 and Dsg3 epitopes, which then become available to pathogenic autoantibodies. There is also increased acantholysis of keratinocytes noted with UV (121–123). In addition, adhesion signals transmitted by binding of pemphigus antibodies may be modulated by additional as yet undefined factors enhanced by UV irradiation (124). Pro-inflammatory cytokines such as IL-1, IL-8, TNFα, and granulocyte macrophage colony stimulating factor are increased in skin after UV radiation and could play a role in recruitment of inflammatory cells to skin and in acantholysis (125–128).

Clinically, lesions can present with erosions or flaccid blisters (Fig. 9). One epidemiological study linked sunlight and air temperature to disease activity in pemphigus vulgaris (129). It has been noted for years that pemphigus erythematosus, pemphigus foliaceus, and pemphigus vulgaris can be induced with UV, including UVB and PUVA irradiation (121,124,130–135). In one patient, irradiation with two MEDs of UVB induced pemphigus lesions at 24 hours (132).

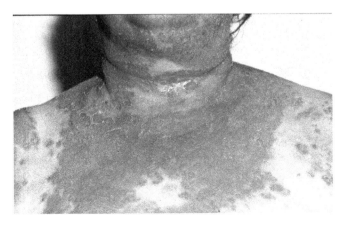

FIGURE 9 Pemphigus vulgaris.

Treatment of pemphigus vulgaris normally includes a combination of glucocorticoids and an immunosuppressive, such as azathioprine, methotrexate, or mycophenolate mofetil. Severe unresponsive disease or patients who may not tolerate glucocorticoids sometimes require adjunctive therapy with intravenous immunoglobulin, plasmapheresis, or more potent immunosuppressives like cyclophosphamide or chlorambucil. For more mild disease or patients who are steroid-dependent, tetracycline or dapsone may provide additional benefit (136,137). Rituximab, TNFα inhibitors, and photopheresis have been anecdotally reported to be of benefit. There is a need for validated activity indices, standardized definitions, and multicenter trials to systematically evaluate therapies in pemphigus.

REFERENCES

1. Hjorth N, Sjolin KE, Sylvest B, et al. Acne aestivalis—mallorca acne. Acta Derm Venereol 1972; 52:61–63.
2. Nieboer C. Actinic superficial folliculitis; a new entity? Br J Dermatol 1985; 112:603–606.
3. Verbov J. Actinic folliculitis. Br J Dermatol 1985; 113:630–631.
4. Norris PG, Hawk JL. Actinic folliculitis—response to isotretinoin. Clin Exp Dermatol 1989; 14:69–71.
5. Veysey EC, George S. Actinic folliculitis. Clin Exp Dermatol 2005; 30:659–661.
6. Kimoto M, Akiyama M, Matsuo I. Darier's disease restricted to sun-exposed areas. Clin Exp Dermatol 2004; 29:37–39.
7. Baba T, Yaoita H. UV radiation and keratosis follicularis. Arch Dermatol 1984; 120:1484–1487.
8. Heo EP, Park SH, Yoon TJ, et al. Induction of Darier's disease by repeated irradiation by ultraviolet B; protection by sunscreen and topical ascorbic acid. J Dermatol 2002; 29:455–458.
9. Antley CM, Carrington PR, Mrak RE, et al. Grover's disease (transient acantholytic dermatosis): relationship of acantholysis to acrosynringia. J Cutan Pathol 1998; 25:545–549.
10. Hashimoto K, Moiin A, Chang MW, et al. Sudoriferous acrosyringeal acantholytic disease: a subset of Grover's disease. J Cutan Pathol 1996; 23:151–164.
11. Hashimoto K, Fujiwara K, Harada M, et al. Junctional proteins of keratinocytes in Grover's disease, Hailey–Hailey's disease, and Darier's disease. J Dermatol 1995; 22:159–170.
12. Grover RW. Transient acantholytic dermatosis. Arch Dermatol 1970; 101:426–434.
13. Davis MD, Dinneen AM, Landa N, et al. Grover's disease: clinicopathologic review of 72 cases. Mayo Clin Proc 1999; 74:229–234.
14. Kato N, Furuya K. Two cases of transient acantholytic dermatosis—with the analysis of 20 cases reported in Japan. Nippon Hifuka Gakkai Zasshi 1991; 101:453–460.
15. Rockley PF, Bergfeld WF, Tomecki KJ, et al. Myelodysplastic syndrome and transient acantholytic dermatosis. Cleve Clin J Med 1990; 57:575–577.
16. Casanova JM, Pujol RM, Taberner R, et al. Grover's disease in patients with chronic renal failure receiving hemodialysis: clinicopathologic review of 4 cases. J Am Acad Dermatol 1999; 41:1029–1033.
17. Parsons JM. Transient acantholytic dermatosis (Grover's disease): a global perspective. J Am Acad Dermatol 1996; 35:653–666.
18. Gudi VS, Edwards S, White MI. Localized transient acantholytic dermatosis in a patient with left hemiparesis. Acta Derm Venereol 2004; 84:232.
19. Chalet M, Grover R, Ackerman AB. Transient acantholytic dermatosis: a reevaluation. Arch Dermatol 1977; 113:431–435.
20. Paul BS, Arndt KA. Response to transient acantholytic dermatosis to photochemotherapy. Arch Dermatol 1984; 120:121–122.
21. Lüftl M, Degitz K, Plewig G, et al. Bath psoralen-UV-A therapy for persistent Grover disease. Arch Dermatol 1999; 135:606–607.
22. Breuckmann F, Appelhans C, Altmeyer P. Medium-dose ultraviolet A1 phototherapy in transient acantholytic dermatosis. J Am Acad Dermatol 2005; 52:169–170.
23. Malfait P, Moren A, Dillon JC, et al. An outbreak of pellagra related to changes in dietary niacin among Mozambican refugees in Malawi. Int J Epidemiol 1993; 22:504–511.
24. Stratigos JD, Katsambas A. Pellagra: a still existing disease? Br J Dermatol 1977; 96:99–106.
25. Lu JY, Yu CL, Wu MZ. Pellagra in an immunocompetent patient with cytomegalovirus colitis. Am J Gastroenterol 2001; 96:932–934.
26. Gillman MA, Sandy KR. Nicotinic acid deficiency induced by sodium valproate. S Afr Med J 1984; 65:986.
27. van der Molen RG, Out-Luiting C, Claas FH, et al. Ultraviolet-B radiation induces modulation of antigen presentation of herpes simplex virus by human epidermal cells. Hum Immunol 2001; 62:589–597.

28. Ichihashi M, Nagai H, Matsunaga K. Sunlight is an important causative factor of recurrent herpes simplex. Cutis 2004; 74:14–18.
29. Pace BF, Owens DW. Photosensitivity eruption following smallpox vaccination. Cutis 1969; 5: 850–853.
30. Castrow FF, Wolf JE Jr. Photolocalized varicella. Arch Dermatol 1973; 107:628.
31. Gilchrest B, Baden HP. Photodistribution of viral exanthems. Pediatrics 1974; 54:136–138.
32. Huff C, Weston WL. The photodistribution of erythema multiforme. Arch Dermatol 1980; 116:477.
33. Galosi A, Plewig G, Hölzle E, et al. Light-induced postherpetic erythema exsudativum multiforme [German]. Hautarzt 1986; 37:494–498.
34. Wolf P, Soyer HP, Fink-Puches R, et al. Recurrent post-herpetic erythema multiforme mimicking polymorphic light and juvenile spring eruption: report of two cases in young boys. Br J Dermatol 1994; 131:364–367.
35. Shiohara T, Chiba M, Tanaka Y, et al. Drug-induced, photosensitive, erythema multiforme-like eruption: possible role for cell adhesion molecules in a flare induced by Rhus dermatitis. J Am Acad Dermatol 1990; 22:647–650.
36. Ortel B, Sivayathorn A, Hönigsmann H. An unusual combination of phototoxicity and Stevens–Johnson syndrome due to antimalarial therapy. Dermatologica 1989; 178:39–42.
37. Leroy D, Le Maitre M, Deschamps P. Photosensitive erythema multiforme apparently induced by phenylbutazone. Photodermatology 1985; 2:176–177.
38. Calzavara Pinton PG, Venturini M, Capezzera R, et al. Photosensitive erythema multiforme and erythema multiforme-like polymorphous light eruption. Photodermatol Photoimmunol Photomed 2003; 19:157–159.
39. Frain-Bell W, Scatchard M. The association of photosensitivity and atopy in the child. Br J Dermatol 1971; 85:105–110.
40. Farber EM, Bright RD, Nall ML. Psoriasis. A questionnaire survey of 2,144 patients. Arch Dermatol 1968; 98:248–259.
41. Doyle JA. Photosensitive psoriasis. Australas J Dermatol 1984; 25:54–58.
42. Ros AM. Photosensitive psoriasis. Sem Dermatol 1992; 11:267–268.
43. Ros AM, Eklund G. Photosensitive psoriasis. An epidemiologic study. J Am Acad Dermatol 1987; 17:752–758.
44. Zalla MJ, Muller SA. The coexistence of psoriasis with lupus erythematosus and other photosensitive disorders. Acta Derm Venereol Supplementum 1996; 195:1–15.
45. Sahoo B, Kumar B. The coexistence of photosensitive psoriasis with chronic actinic dermatitis. Dermatology 2002; 204:77–79.
46. Denguezli M, Nouira R, Jomaa B. Actinic lichen planus: an anatomical study of 10 Tunisian cases. Ann Dermatol Venereol 1994; 121:543–546.
47. Salman SM, Kibbi AG, Zaynoun S. Actinic lichen planus: clinicopathologic study of 16 patients. J Am Acad Dermatol 1989; 20:226–231.
48. Dostrovsky A, Sagher F. Lichen planus in subtropical countries. Arch Dermatol Syphilol 1949; 59:308–328.
49. Dilaimy M. Lichen planus subtropicus. Arch Dermatol 1976; 112:1251–1253.
50. Isaacson D, Turner ML, Elgart ML. Summertime actinic lichenoid eruption (lichen planus actinicus). J Am Acad Dermatol 1981; 4:404–411.
51. Skowron F, Grezard P, Merle P, et al. Erythematosus actinic lich planus: a new clinical form associated with oral erosive lichen planus and chronic active hepatits B. Br J Dermatol 2002; 147:1032–1034.
52. Zanca A. Lichen planus actinicus. Int J Dermatol 1978; 17:506–508.
53. Millard TP, Kondeatis E, Cox A, et al. A candidate gene analysis of three related photosensitivity disorders: cutaneous lupus erythematosus, polymorphic light eruption and actinic prurigo. Br J Dermatol 2001; 145:229–236.
54. Werth VP, Zhang W, Dortzbach K, et al. Association of a promoter polymorphism of TNFalpha with subacute cutaneous lupus erythematosus and distinct photoregulation of transcription. J Invest Dermatol 2000; 115:726–730.
55. Werth VP, Bashir M, Zhang W. Photosensitivity in rheumatic diseases. J Investig Dermatol Symp Proc 2004; 9:54–63.
56. Racila DM, Sontheimer CJ, Sheffield A, et al. Homozygous single nucleotide polymorphism of the complement C1QA gene is associated with decreased levels of C1q in patients with subacute cutaneous lupus erythematosus. Lupus 2003; 12:124–132.
57. Sontheimer RD, Maddison PJ, Reichlin M, et al. Serologic and HLA associations in subacute cutaneous lupus erythematosus, a clinical subset of lupus erythematosus. Ann Intern Med 1982; 97:664–671.
58. Lacour JP. Lupus and sun. Revue de Medecine Interne 1996; 17:196–199.
59. Watson RM, Talwar P, Alexander E, et al. Subacute cutaneous lupus erythematosus-immunogenetic associations. J Autoimmun 1991, 4, 73–85.

60. Lee LA, Roberts CM, Frank MB, et al. The autoantibody response to Ro/SSA in cutaneous lupus erythematosus. Arch Dermatol 1994, 130, 1262–1268.
61. Meller S, Winterberg F, et al. Ultraviolet radiation-induced injury, chemokines, and leukocyte recruitment: an amplification cycle triggering cutaneous lupus erythematosus. Arthritis Rheum 2005, 52, 1504–1516.
62. Sontheimer RD. The lexicon of cutaneous lupus erythematosus-A review and personal perspective on the nomenclature and classification of the cutaneous manifestations of lupus erythematosus. Lupus 1997, 6, 84–95.
63. Yell JA, Mbuagbaw J, Burge SM. Cutaneous manifestations of systemic lupus erythematosus . Br J Dermatol 1996, 135, 355–362.
64. Kuhn A, Sonntag M, Richter-Hintz D, et al. Phototesting in lupus erythematosus tumidus-review of 60 patients. Photochem Photobiol 2001, 73, 532–536.
65. Sontheimer RD, Thomas JR, Gilliam JN. Subacute cutaneous lupus erythematosus: a cutaneous marker for a distinct lupus erythematosus subset. Arch Dermatol 1979; 115:1409–1415.
66. Perera GK, Black MM, McGibbon DH. Bullous subacute cutaneous lupus erythematosus. Clin Exp Dermatol 2004; 29:265–267.
67. Provost TT, Watson R. Anti-Ro(SS-A) HLA-DR3-positive women: the interrelationship between some ANA negative, SS, SCLE, and NLE mothers and SS/LE overlap female patients. J Invest Dermatol 1993; 100:14S–20S.
68. Reed BR, Huff JC, Jones SK, et al. Subacute cutaneous lupus erythematosus associated with hydrochlorothiazide therapy. Ann Intern Med 1985; 103:49–51.
69. Shapiro M, Sosis AC, Junkins-Hopkins JM, et al. Lupus eyrthematosus induced by medications, ultraviolet radiation, and other exogenous agents: a review, with special focus on the development of subacute cutaneous lupus erythematosus in a genetically predisposed individual. Int J Dermatol 2004; 43:87–94.
70. Gammon WR, Briggaman RA. Bullous SLE: a phenotypically distinctive but immunologically heterogeneous bullous disorder. J Invest Dermatol 1993; 100:28S–34S.
71. Yell JA, Allen J, Wojnarowska F, et al. Bullous systemic lupus erythematosus: revised criteria for diagnosis. Br J Dermatol 1995; 132:921–928.
72. Chan LS, Lapiere JC, Chen M, et al. Bullous systemic lupus erythematosus with autoantibodies recognizing multiple skin basement membrane components, bullous pemphigoid antigen 1, laminin-5, laminin-6, and type VII collagen. Arch Dermatol 1999; 135:569–573.
73. Parodi A, Massone C, Cacciapuoti M, et al. Measuring the activity of the disease in patients with cutaneous lupus erythematosus. Br J Dermatol 2000; 142:457–460.
74. Cripps DJ, Rankin J. Action spectra of lupus erythematosus and experimental imunofluorescence. Arch Dermatol 1973; 107:563–567.
75. Epstein JH, Tuffanelli D, Dubois EL. Light sensitivity and lupus erythematosus. Arch Dermatol 1965; 91:483–485.
76. Wysenbeek AJ, Block DA, Fries JF. Prevalence and expression of photosensitivity in systemic lupus erythematosus. Ann Rheum Dis 1989; 48:461–463.
77. Haga HJ, Brun JG, Rekvig OP, et al. Seasonal variations in activity of systemic lupus erythematosus in a subarctic region. Lupus 1999; 8:269–273.
78. Amit M, Molad Y, Kiss S, et al. Seasonal variations in manifestations and activity of systemic lupus erythematosus. Br J Rheumatol 1997; 36:449–452.
79. Lee LA, Farris AD. Photosensitivity diseases: cutaneous lupus erythematosus. J Investig Dermatol Symp Proc 1999; 4:73–78.
80. Parodi A, Caproni M, Cardinali C, et al. Clinical, histological and immunopathological features of 58 patients with subacute cutaneous lupus erythematosus. A review by the Italian group of immunodermatology. Dermatology 2000; 200:6–10.
81. Lehmann P, Hölzle E, Kind P, et al. Experimental reproduction of skin lesions in lupus erythematosus by UVA and UVB radiation. J Am Acad Dermatol 1990; 22:181–187.
82. Wolska H, Blaszczyk M, Jablonska S. Phototests in patients with various forms of lupus erythematosus. Int J Dermatol 1989; 28:98–103.
83. van Weelden H, Velthuis PJ, Baart de la Faille H. Light-induced skin lesions in lupus erythematosus: photobiological studies. Arch Dermatol Res 1989; 281:470–474.
84. Walchner M, Messer G, Kind P. Phototesting and photoprotection in LE. Lupus 1997; 6: 167–174.
85. Sanders CJ, van Weelden H, Kazzaz GA, et al. Photosensitivity in patients with lupus erythematosus: a clinical and photobiological study of 100 patients using a prolonged phototest protocol. Br J Dermatol 2003; 149:131–137.
86. Hasan T, Nyberg F, Stephansson E, et al. Photosensitivity in lupus erythematosus, UV photoprovocation results compared with history of photosensitivity and clinical findings. Br J Dermatol 1997; 136:699–705.

87. Leenutaphong V, Boonchai W. Phototesting in oriental patients with lupus erythematosus. Photodermatol Photoimmunol Photomed 1999; 15:7–12.

88. Kuhn A, Sonntag M, Richter-Hintz D, et al. Phototesting in lupus erythematosus: a 15-year experience. J Am Acad Dermatol 2001; 45:86–95.

89. Stege H, Budde MA, Grether-Beck S, et al. Evaluation of the capacity of sunscreens to photoprotect lupus erythematosus patients by employing the photoprovocation test. Photodermatol Photoimmunol Photomed 2000; 16:256–259.

90. Callen JP. Update on the management of cutaneous lupus erythematosus. Br J Dermatol 2004; 151:731–736.

91. Albrecht J, Taylor L, Berlin JA, et al. The CLASI (cutaneous LE disease area and severity index): an outcome instrument for cutaneous lupus erythematosus. J Invest Dermatol 2005; 125:889–894.

92. Heath M, Raugi GJ. Evidence-based evaluation of immunomodulatory therapy for the cutaneous manifestations of lupus. Adv Dermatol 2004; 20:257–291.

93. Pablos JL, Santiago B, Galindo M, et al. Keratinocyte apoptosis and p53 expression in cutaneous lupus and dermatomyositis. J Pathol 1999; 188:63–68.

94. Coates PJ, Save V, Ansari B, et al. Demonstration of DNA damage/repair in individual cells using in situ end labelling: association of p53 with sites of DNA damage. J Pathol 1995; 176:19-26.

95. Schwarz A, Bhardwaj R, Aragane Y, et al. Ultraviolet-B-induced apoptosis of keratinocytes: evidence for partial involvement of tumor necrosis factor-alpha in the formation of sunburn cells. J Invest Dermatol 1995; 104:922–927.

96. Werth VP, Callen JP, Ang G, et al. Associations of tumor necrosis factor-α (TNFα) and HLA polymorphisms with adult dermatomyositis: implications for a unique pathogenesis. J Invest Dermatol 2002; 119:617–620.

97. Hengstman GD, van Venrooij WJ, Vencovsky J, et al. The relative prevalence of dermatomyositis and polymyositis in Europe exhibits a latitudinal gradient. Ann Rheum Dis 2000; 59:141–142.

98. Okada S, Weatherhead E, Targoff IN, et al. Global surface ultraviolet radiation intensity may modulate the clinical and immunologic expression of autoimmune muscle disease. Arthritis Rheum 2003; 48:2285–2293.

99. Sontheimer RD. Photoimmunology of lupus erythematosus and dermatomyositis: a speculative review. Photochem Photobiol 1996; 63:583–594.

100. Cheong WK, Hughes GR, Norris PG, et al. Cutaneous photosensitivity in dermatomyositis. Br J Dermatol 1994; 131:205–208.

101. Miller FW. Myositis-specific autoantibodies: touchstones for understanding the inflammatory myopathies. JAMA 1993; 270:1846–1849.

102. Sigurgeirsson B, Lindelof B, Edhag O, et al. Risk of malignancy in patients with dermatomyositis or polymyositis. N Engl J Med 1992; 326:363–367.

103. Callen JP. When and how should the patient with dermatomyositis or amyopathic dermatomyositis be assessed for possible cancer? Arch Dermatol 2002; 138:969–971.

104. Hill CL, Zhang Y, Sigurgeirsson B, et al. Frequency of specific cancer types in dermatomyositis and polymyositis: a population-based study. Lancet 2001; 357:96–100.

105. Euwer R, Sontheimer R. Amyopathic dermatomyositis (dermatomyositis sine myositis). Presentation of six new cases and review of the literature. J Am Acad Dermatol 1991; 24:959–966.

106. Sontheimer RD. Would a new name hasten the acceptance of amyopathic dermatomyositis (dermatomyositis sine myositis) as a distinctive subset within the idiopathic inflammatory dermatomyopathies spectrum of clinical illness? J Am Acad Dermatol 2002; 46:626–636.

107. Everett MA, Curtis AC. Dermatomyositis: a review of 19 cases in adolescents and children. Arch Int Med 1957; 100:70–76.

108. Dourmishev L, Meffert H, Piazena H. Dermatomyositis: comparative studies of cutaneous photosensitivity in lupus erythematosus and normal subjects. Photodermatol Photoimmunol Photomed 2004; 20:230–234.

109. Sontheimer RD. The management of dermatomyositis:current treatment options. Exp Opin Pharmacother 2004; 5:1083–1099.

110. Ang GC, Werth VP. Combination antimalarials in the treatment of cutaneous dermatomyositis: a retrospective study. Arch Dermatol 2005; 141:855–859.

111. Edge JC, Outland JD, Dempsey JR, et al. Mycophenolate mofetil as an effective corticosteroid-sparing therapy for recalcitrant dermatomyositis. Arch Dermatol 2006; 142:65–69.

112. Levine TD. Rituximab in the treatment of dermatomyositis: an open-label pilot study. Arthritis Rheum 2005; 52:601–607.

113. Kayashima K, Koji T, Nozawa M, et al. Activation of bullous pemphigoid antigen gene in mouse ear epidermis by ultraviolet radiation. Cell Biochem Funct 1998; 16:107–116.

114. Person JR, Rogers III RS. Bullous pemphigoid and psoriasis; does subclinical bullous pemphigoid exist? Br J Dermatol 1976; 95:535–540.

115. Thomsen K, Schmidt H. PUVA-induced bullous pemphigoid. Br J Dermatol 1976; 95:568–569.

116. Perl S, Rappersberger K, Fodinger D, et al. Bullous pemphigoid induced by PUVA therapy. Dermatol 1996; 193:245–247.
117. Pfau A, Hohenleutner U, Hohenleutner S, et al. UV-A-provoked localized bullous pemphigoid. Acta Derm Venereol 1994; 74:314–316.
118. Joly P, Roujeau JC, Benichou J, et al. A comparison of oral and topical corticosteroids in patients with bullous pemphigoid. N Engl J Med 2002; 346:321–327.
119. Wojnarowska F, Kirtschig G, Highet A, et al. Guidelines for the management of bullous pemphigoid. Br J Dermatol 2002; 147:214–221.
120. Kirtschig G, Khumalo NP. Management of bullous pemphigoid. Recommendations for immunomodulatory treatments. Am J Clin Dermatol 2004; 5:319–326.
121. Cram DL, Fukuyama K. Immunohistochemistry of ultraviolet-induced pemphigus and pemphigoid lesions. Arch Dermatol 1972; 106:819–824.
122. Gschnait F, Pehamberger H, Holubar K. Pemphigus acantholysis in tissue culture: studies on photoinduction. Acta Derm Venereol 1978; 58:237–239.
123. Reis VM, Toledo RP, Lopez A, et al. UVB-induced acantholysis in endemic pemphigus foliaceus (fogo selvagem) and pemphigus vulgaris. J Am Acad Dermatol 2000; 42:571–576.
124. Kano Y, Shimosegawa M, Mizukawa Y, et al. Pemphigus foliaceus induced by exposure to sunlight. Dermatol 2000; 201:132–138.
125. Oxholm A, Oxholm P, Staberg B, et al. Immunohistological detection of interleukin 1-like molecules and tumor necrosis factor in human epidermis. Br J Dermatol 1988; 118:369–377.
126. Felician C, Toto P, Amerio P, et al. In vivo and in vitro expression of interleukin-1alpha and tumor necrosis factor-alpha are involved in acantholysis. J Invest Dermatol 2000; 114:71–77.
127. Werth VP, Zhang W. Wavelength-specific synergy between ultraviolet radiation and interleukin-1 alpha in the regulation of matrix-related genes: mechanistic role for tumor necrosis factor-alpha. J Invest Dermatol 1999; 113:196–201.
128. Köck A, Schwarz T, Kirnbauer R, et al. Human keratinocytes are a source for tumor necrosis factor alpha: evidence for synthesis and release upon stimulation with endotoxin or ultraviolet light. J Exp Med 1990; 172:1609–1614.
129. Kyriakis KP, Vareltzidis AG, Tosca AD. Environmental factors influencing the biologic behavior of patterns of pemphigus vulgaris: epidemiologic approach. Int J Dermatol 1995; 34:181–185.
130. Cram DL, Winkelmann RK. Ultraviolet-induced acantholysis in pemphigus. Arch Dermatol 1965; 92:7–13.
131. Jacobs SE. Pemphigus erythematosus and ultraviolet light. Arch Dermatol 1965; 91:139–141.
132. Muramatsu T, Iida T, Ko T, et al. Pemphigus vulgaris exacerbated by exposure to sunlight. J Dermatol 1996; 23:559–563.
133. Fryer EJ, Lebwohl M. Pemphigus vulgaris after initiation of psoralen and UVA therapy for psoriasis. J Am Acad Dermatol 1994; 30:651–653.
134. Aghassi D, Dover JS. Pemphigus foliaceus induced by psoralen-UV-A. Arch Dermatol 1998; 134:1300–1301.
135. Deschamps P, Pedailles S, Michel M, et al. Photo-induction of lesions in a patient with pemphigus erythematosus. Photodermatology 1984; 1:38–41.
136. Bystryn JC, Rudolph JL. Pemphigus. Lancet 2005; 366:61–73.
137. Werth VP, Fivenson D, Pandya A, et al. Multicenter randomized placebo-controlled clinical trial of dapsone as a glucocorticoid-sparing agent in maintenance phase pemphigus vulgaris. J Invest Dermatol 2005 [abstr]; 125:1088.

18 | Photoprotection

Henry W. Lim
Department of Dermatology, Henry Ford Hospital, Detroit, Michigan, U.S.A.

Herbert Hönigsmann
Department of Dermatology, Medical University of Vienna, Vienna, Austria

- There are several new photostable broad-spectrum UV filters that are available in many parts of the world except in the United States.

- Sun protection factor is a reflection of UVB protection of sunscreen; harmonization of UVA protection is ongoing.

- Photoprotectiveness of garment is rated by ultraviolet protection factor (UPF); UPF is becoming more widely used.

- Developments in the glass industry have resulted in the availability of glass that has significant UV filtering properties up to 380 nm.

- Several non-UV filter, topical and systemic photoprotective agents have been identified; larger studies are needed for most.

- These developments are of great benefit to our patients in reducing the acute and chronic effects of sun exposure.

INTRODUCTION

Acute and chronic exposures to sunlight are known to produce a range of deleterious effects including edema, sunburn, photoaging, photoimmunosuppression, and photocarcino-genesis. As such, the use of photoprotective measures has long been advocated by the dermatologic and general medical communities. Photoprotection includes the avoidance of sunlight during the peak UVB hours (10 AM to 4 PM), the use of sunscreen on exposed areas, wearing of a hat, protective clothing, and sunglasses.

In Asian cultures, especially among women, fair and unblemished skin is highly valued. Therefore, in Asian countries, many of which are in the tropical or subtropical area, photoprotection is used to minimize tanning and dispigmentation.

ASSESSMENT OF PHOTOPROTECTION
Sun Protection Factor

The concept of sun protection factor (SPF) was developed by Franz Greiter in 1962, and adopted by the U.S. Food and Drug Administration (FDA) in 1978 (1,2). Currently, this is a universally accepted method to measure the protectiveness of sunscreen. SPF is the ratio of the minimal erythema dose (MED) of sunscreen-protected skin over the MED of the sunscreen-unprotected skin. For this assessment, solar-simulated radiation light source is used and sunscreen is applied at a concentration of 2 mg/cm^2. Because the end point of this assessment is cutaneous erythema, SPF is a reflection predominately of the biologic effect of UVB. SPF is not designed to measure the protectiveness of against UVA; in fact, it is known that the SPF of a product does not correlate with its UVA protectiveness. Furthermore, at the tested concentration of 2 mg/cm^2, it requires approximately one ounce (30 mL) of sunscreen to cover the entire body surface. It is now known that in actual use, most consumers do not use sunscreen at this concentration. In fact, the overall median application concentration has been found to be only 0.5 mg/cm^2. This results in significantly lower "in use" of SPF as compared to the labeled SPF (3,4).

The U.S. FDA requires that for any sunscreen to be labeled as "water resistant" and "very water resistant," the product would have to maintain its labeled SPF following 2 × 20 minutes of water emersion, and 4 × 20 minutes water emersion, respectively (5).

UVA Protection Factor

Currently, there is no worldwide standard that has been accepted by all countries (see Chap. 19). For example, in vitro methods are use in Australia, the United Kingdom, and Germany, and an in vivo method is used in Japan and several Asian countries. At the time of this writing, the U.S. FDA has not recommended any UVA protection assessment method to be used for sunscreens marketed in the United States.

In February 2005, the regulatory body governing the establishment of German industrial standards (Deutsche Industrienorm, DIN) introduced the new DIN Method 67502, entitled "Characterization of UVA protection of dermal sun care products by measuring the transmittance with regards to the sun protection factor," also known as the UVA balance method. The DIN will probably be adopted by the European Commission as the standard (6–8).

The objective of this new method is to balance the level of UVA protection provided by a sunscreen with the level of UVB protection it provides, therefore addressing some of the limitations of other standards. For example, according to the Australian standard, the level of UVA protection may remain constant regardless of the level of UVB protection provided. In other words, an SPF 4 sun care product could provide the same level of UVA protection as SPF 15 and SPF 30 products, and still in compliance with that standard.

The first step in the assessement of the UVA balance is the calculation of in vitro SPF, taking into account the erythemal action spectrum. This value is then adjusted to the corresponding SPF that is stated on the label. Based on this result, an in vitro UVA/persistent pigmentation darkening (PPD) protection factor can be calculated. The UVA balance represents the ratio of the in vitro UVA/PPD protection factor (UVA) and the in vivo UVB protection, reflected as the labeled SPF value (7,8). In the DIN Method 67502, no limits for UVA/UVB balance are given (6).

Immune Protection Factor

It is known that SPF, with erythema as its end point, is a poor predictor of immunosuppression (9). As such, the concept of immune protection factor (IPF) has been developed (10). The principle of IPF is to assess the ability of sunscreen to prevent the immunosuppression induced by solar-simulated radiation. However, there are a variety of methods used, all are quite laborious and time consuming to perform. It is likely that it will be many years before the IPF is used as part of the labeling of commercial products.

Ultraviolet Protection Factor

This is a standard that was first developed in Australia in 1996 (11). It is now widely used in Australia, the European Union, and the United States. Ultraviolet protection factor (UPF) is an in vitro measurement of relative amount of UV that penetrates a fabric, resulting in cutaneous erythema; the latter is derived from the erythemal action spectrum (12). The importance of using the erythemal action spectrum data is that a fabric that allows a greater portion of UVB to be transmitted will receive a UPF value that is lower than a fabric that allows less UVB to penetrate, even though both fabrics may transmit the same amount of radiation.

TOPICAL UV FILTERS
Regulations

In the United States, sunscreens are regulated as over-the-counter medications by the FDA (5). In order for a new UV filter to be included in the monograph, a New Drug Application (NDA) needs to be made, a process that may take years. Similar regulations are also in place in Australia and Japan. In 2002, the FDA instituted a second application process, the Time and Extend Application (TEA) (13). The TEA process indicates that if a sunscreen has been marketed and sold for a minimum of five years in a foreign country, data generated in that country can be used for the application.

In the European Union, South America, Asia, and Africa, sunscreens are regulated as cosmetics resulting in a simpler and more expeditious approval process.

UV FILTERS APPROVED IN THE UNITED STATES

The list of UV filters included in the latest version (1999) of FDA sunscreen monograph is shown in Table 1.

New UV Filters

Through the TEA process, there are currently three UVB filters and two broad-spectrum UV filters that are undergoing the approval by the U.S. FDA. These filters are isoamyl *p*-methoxycinnamate [U.S. adopted name (USAN): amiloxate], 4-methylbenzylidene camphor (USAN: enzacamene), ethylhexyl triazone (USAN: octyl triazone), methylene-bis-benzotriazolyl tetramethylbutyl-phenol (Tinosorb® M; USAN: bisoctrizole), and *bis*-ethylhexyloxyphenol methoxyphenyl triazine (Tinosorb® S; USAN: bemotrizinol). In addition, a UVA filter, terephthalidene dicamphor sulfonic acid (Mexoryl® SX; USAN: ecamsule) was approved by the US FDA through the NDA in July, 2006 (14,15).

UV filters that are available in the European countries are listed in Table 2.

Sunscreen Use in Children

Regular use of sunscreen with an average SPF of 7.5 for the first 18 years of life could reduce the lifetime incidence of nonmelanoma skin cancer by 78% (16). It should be emphasized, however, that UV exposure occurs throughout life, with men over 40 years of age receiving the most exposure (17,18). Therefore, sunscreen should be used by children as well as adults.

TABLE 1 UV Filters Listed in the U.S. Food and Drug Administration Sunscreen Monograph

USAN[a]	INCI name	λ_{max} (nm); or absorption range	Comment
Organic absorbers: UVB filters			
PABA derivatives			
Aminobenzoic acid (PABA)	PABA	283	Stains clothing Not widely used
Padimate O	Ethylhexyl dimethyl PABA	311	Most commonly used PABA derivative Photolabile
Cinnamates			
Octinoxate	Ethylhexyl methoxycinnamate	311	Most widely used UVB filter Photolabile
Cinoxate	Cinoxate	289	
Salicylates			
Octisalate	Ethylhexyl salicylate	307	Weak UVB absorbers
Homosalate	Homosalate	306	Improves photostabiltiy of other filters
Trolamine salicylate	TEA salicylate	260–355	Weak UVB absorbers Good substantivity—used in water-resistant sunscreens and hair-care products
Others			
Octocrylene	Octocrylene	303	Photostable Improves photostability of photolabile filters
Ensulizole	Phenylbenzimidazole sulfonic acid	310	Water-soluble Enhances SPF of the final product
Organic absorbers: UVA filters			
Benzophenones			
Oxybenzone	Benzophenone-3	288,325	Most commonly used UVA filter Most common cause of photoallergic contact dermatitis to UV filters Photolabile
Sulisobenzone	Benzophenone-4	366	
Dioxybenzone	Benzophenone-8	352	
Others			
Avobenzone	Butyl methoxydibenzoylmethane	360	Photolabile Enhances the photodegradation of octinoxate
Meradimate	Menthyl anthranilate	340	A weak UVA filter
Inorganic Absorbers			
Titanium dioxide	Titanium dioxide	See below[b]	No report of sentitization reaction
Zinc oxide	Zinc oxide	See below[b]	Photostable; used to enhance photostability of the final product Micronized zinc oxide has better UVA1 protection compared to micorfine titanium dioxide

(Continued)

TABLE 1 UV Filters Listed in the U.S. Food and Drug Administration Sunscreen Monograph (*Continued*)

USAN[a]	INCI name	λ_max (nm); or absorption range	Comment
			Micronized zinc oxide has lower refractive index compared to micorfine titanium dioxide, hence appears less white Commonly coated with dimethicone or silica to maintain their effectiveness as sunscreen

[a]USAN, United States Adopted Name; this is the name used by the FDA in the listing.
[b]λ_max ranges from visible to UVA to UVB range, depending on the particle size. As the pigment is micronized (10–50 nm in diameter), λ_max shifts towards UVB.
Abbreviations: INCI, International nomenclature of cosmetic ingredients; PABA, *para*-Aminobenzoic acid; SPF, sun protection factor; TEA, the time and extend application.
Source: From Refs. 4, 5.

Because of the concern about percutaneous absorption of sunscreens, the 1999 FDA sunscreen monograph recommends that the use of sunscreens in children under the age of six months should be decided by their physicians (5). For this group of patients, it would be prudent to use other means of photoprotection; and sunscreens could be used on an infrequent basis on the exposed areas.

Photostability of UV Filters

All UV filters, especially avobenzone, octinoxate, and padimante O, are photolabile (Table 3) (19). In the past few years, however, many sunscreen manufactures have been able to combine

TABLE 2 UV Filters Available in Europe

para-Aminobenzoic acid (PABA)[a]
Benzophenone-3 (oxybenzone)[a]
Benzophenone-4 (sulisobenzone)[a]
Benzylidene camphor
Benzylidene camphor sulfonic acid
bis-Ethylhexyloxyphenol methoxyphenol triazine (bemotrizinol; Tinosorb®S)
Bisymidazylate
Butyl methoxydibenzoylmethane (avobenzone; Parsol® 1789)[a]
Camphor benzalkonium methosulfate
Diethylamino hydroxybenzoyl hexyl benzoate
Diethylhexyl butamido triazone
Dimethicodiethylbenzal malonate
Drometrizole trisiloxane (silatriazole; Mexoryl®XL)
Ethoxylated ethyl 4-aminobenzoic acid (PEG-25 PABA)
Ethylhexyl methoxycinnamate (octinoxate; octyl methoxycinnamate)[a]
Ethylhexyl dimethyl PABA (padimate O; octyl dimethyl PABA)[a]
Ethylhexyl salicylate (octisalate; octyl salicylate)[a]
Homosalate (homomenthyl salicylate)[a]
Isoamyl p-methoxycinnamate (amiloxate)
4-Methylbenzylidene camphor (enzacamene)
Methylene bis- benzotriazolyl tetramethylbutylphenol (bisoctrizole; Tinosorb®M)
Octocrylene[a]
Octyl triazone
Phenylbenzimidazole sulfonic acid (ensulizole)[a]
Polyacrylamidomethyl benzylidene camphor
Terephthalylidene dicamphor sulphonic acid (ecamsule; Mexoryl®SX)
Titanium dioxide[a]
Zinc oxide[a]

[a]Approved in the United States.
Source: From Ref. 15.

TABLE 3 Photostability of UV Filters

Photolabile filters (USAN/INCI/trade name)	Filters/agent frequently added to enhance photostability of the final product (USAN/INCI/trade name)
UVB filters Octinoxate (ethylhexyl methoxycinnamate) Padimate O (ethylhexyl dimethyl PABA)	*UVB filters* Enzacamene (4-methylbenzylidene camphor)[a] Homosalate (homosalate) Octisalate (ethylhexyl salicylate) Octocrylene (octocrylene)
UVA filters Avobenzone (butyl methoxydibenzoylmethane; Parsol® 1789)	*UVA filter* Oxybenzone (benzophenone-3) *Broad-spectrum UVB–UVA filter* *bis*-Ethylhexyloxyphenol methoxyphenol triazine (bemotrizinol; Tinosorb® S) Methylene-bis-benzotriazolyl tetramethylbutylphenol (biscotrizole; Tinosorb® M) Titanium dioxide (microfine) Zinc oxide (micronized) *Not a UV filter* Diethylhexyl 2,6-naphthalate

[a]Undergoing U.S. Food and Drug Administration Time and Extend Application approval process.
Abbreviations: INCI, International nomenclature of cosmetic ingredients; PABA, *para*-aminobenzoic acid; USAN, United States adopted name.

these photolabile filters with other filters, which resulted in final products that are photostable. Agents that are frequently used to increase the photostability are listed in Table 3 (4,20).

Photostable filters have also been developed. Four are available in many parts of the world: methylene-bis-benzotriazolyl tetramethylbutyl-phenol (bisoctrizole; Tinosorb® M), bis-ethylhexyloxyphenol methoxyphenyl triazine (bemotrizinol; Tinosorb® S), terephthalidene dicamphor sulfonic acid (ecamsule; Mexoryl® SX), and drometrizole trisiloxane (silatriazole; Mexoryl® XL). As of 2006, all except silatriazole are undergoing the approval processes in the United States, and ecamsule has now been approved.

Sunscreen Use and Vitamin D

This topic has been extensively reviewed (21,22). The action spectrum for synthesis of vitamin D_3 in the epidermis is in the UVB range; such synthesis occurs at suberythemogenic doses of UVB. Therefore, for many individuals, incidental sun exposure, along with balanced diet, is sufficient to maintain sufficient vitamin D level. However, for individuals with a higher risk of vitamin D insufficiency, such as elderly individuals who are home bound and dark-skinned individuals who work mostly indoors, oral vitamin D_3 supplementation is recommended. Because the action spectrum for vitamin D photosynthesis and cutaneous photocarcinogenesis cannot be separated, and because the public health message should be delivered in a simple, clear, and understandable fashion, it is prudent not to advise the general public to use sun exposure as a means of achieving sufficient vitamin D level.

CLOTHING

UV protectiveness of clothing is assessed by the UPF. This is an in vitro measurement combining the UV transmission data with two weighing factors, solar spectral irradiance and erythema effectiveness at each UV wavelength. The latter accounts for the fact that UPF is a better reflection of the protectiveness of fabrics against UVB than UVA (23).

Although UPF value could be measured for all swatches of fabrics, different guidelines are used in different parts of the world to have a lable-UPF for a given garment. These include the Australian Standard AS/NZS 4399; the standard commonly used in the United States, ASTM D6603-00; British Standard EN 13758-1:2002; and European Standard EN 13758-2 (11,24–26). The variations among these standards include the requirement for the

TABLE 4 UV-Protection Classification of Garments

Label	Label-UPF
Good protection	15–24
Very good protection	25–39
Excellent protection	40–50+

Abbreviation: UPF, ultraviolet protection factor.

TABLE 5 Factors Affecting Sun-Protectiveness of Garments

Style of garment
Number of layers
Fabric thickness
Type of fibers (polyester > wool > silk > nylon > cotton, rayon)
Laundering
Wetness
Optical whitening agents
UV absorbers
Stretching

body parts that the garment is to cover, and the ways that the fabric must be prepared for testing (number of launderings, hours of in vitro UV exposure), and the minimum UPF value that is required to be classified as sun-protective clothing. For example, both AS/NZS 4399 and ASTM D6603-00 require a lable-UPF value of 15 or above, whereas EN 13758-2 requires UPF of greater than 40 for a garment to be labeled as sun-protective. ASTM D-6603 requires that fabrics be subjected to 40 launderings and many hours of UV exposure prior to testing. UV-protection classification of garment is shown in Table 4.

As recently reviewed, there are several factors that affect the sun protectiveness of clothing (Table 5) (12). The style of the garment dictates the body parts that would be covered. Double layer fabrics, such as frequently used on the shoulder area, would provide better protection compared to single layer. Thickness of the fabric also correlates with sun protectiveness. The type of fibers used in fabrics contributes to the UPF (27). Polyester is the best UV absorber, followed by wool, silk, and nylon. Cotton and rayon, which are cellulose fibers, have the poorest UV absorption. Laundering garments made from cotton, rayon, or linen will result in an increase in their UPF because of shrinkage, causing a decrease in the fabric porosity. UPF is decreased when the garment is wet as more UV would be able to be transmitted. Optical whitening agents are widely incorporated in many laundry detergents in the United States and Europe. These agents absorbed UV radiation at 360 nm and convert it to visible light wavelength of 430 nm; the emission of visible light from the fabric makes the fabric look "brighter." Therefore, optical brightening agents would result in decreased UV transmission through the fabric. In addition, UV absorbers can be added to the fabrics during the manufacturing process, resulting in an increase in the UPF. UV absorbers are also available in some laundry detergents, rise-cycle fabric softeners, or as a dedicated laundry additive (11). Stretching of the fabric would decrease the UPF by increasing the porosity of the fabric.

GLASS

This topic has been recently reviewed (28). Glass is high quality silica sand mixed with other materials such as salt cake, limestone, dolomite, feldspar, soda ash, and cullet (cullet is broken glass) (29). As shown in Table 6, with recent developments, there are many types of glass that have very good UV protection (up to 380 nm). It should be noted that most types of glass have UV transmission at wavelengths beyond 380 nm; it is because, although technologies are available to develop coatings that could absorb up to 400 nm without significantly

TABLE 6   Type of Glass

Type	T_{vis}	T_{UV}	Comment
Clear glass	>90%	>72%	
Tinted/heat-absorbing glass	62%	40%	Absorbs 40–50% of solar energy.
Reflective glass	19%	17%	Mirror-like appearance. Used in commercial buildings.
Low-emissivity glass	71%	20%	Reduces loss of generated heat, and minimizes solar heat gain. Used in residential and commercial buildings.
Laminated glass	79%	<1%	Two pieces of glass are bound to a plastic interlayer to prevent fragments from falling free if broken. Reduces sound transmission. Used for car windshield, and in airports, museums, and large public spaces.
UV-blocking coated glass	80%	<1%	UV coating blocks >98% of UV (up to 380 nm)
Spectrally selective and UV-blocking insulating glass	69%	<1%	Reduces heat loss/gain Blocks >99% of UV (up to 380 nm)

Abbreviations: T_{UV}, transmission in the UV range (assessed from 300–380 nm); T_{vis}, transmission in the visible light range (assessed from 400–780 nm).
Source: From Ref. 28; Adapted from Guardian Industries Corp. (Auburn Hills, Michigan, U.S.A.).

affecting the transmission of visible light, presently, application of such technologies would increase the production cost that would prohibit the economic viability of such a product.

All windshields of cars are made of laminated glass, which allows <1% of UV (300–380 nm) to pass through. However, side and rear windows are usually made from nonlaminated glass; therefore, a higher level of UVA can pass through those windows (28). It has been demonstrated that when the arm is placed near a nonlaminated clear car window for 30 minutes, an exposure of 5 J/cm² of UVA could be achieved, which is sufficient to induce cutaneous eruption in patients with severe photosensitivity (30). If a laminated gray window glass were used instead, at least 50 hours of UV exposure would be required to induce lesions in these patients. After-market tinting of side and rear car windows has become popular; in the United States, after-market tinting must comply with the federally-mandated visible light transmittance of at least 70% for automobile windshields, except for the top 4 inches (31). Although the minimum allowable transmittance levels for side and rear windows are determined by each state in the United States, most states do not allow tinting with less than 35% visible light transmittance.

OTHERS
Sunless Tanning Agents

Preparations containing dihydroxy acetone (DHA) are now widely used as artificial tanning agents. DHA was first recognized as a skin-coloring agent in the 1920s. DHA reacts with basic amino acids in keratinized stratum cormeum to form yellow brown pigments called melanoidins (32). Because the pigments bind covalently to stratum cormeum, the color does not wash off easily until the stratum cormeum is shed-off in three to seven days. DHA is considered to be safe and is approved by the FDA as a cosmetic agent. Because melanoidins absorb primarily in the visible and UVA range, topical application of DHA results in SPF of only 1.6 to 2.3 (33). Sunless tanning products use DHA in concentrations ranging from 1% to 15%; most drug store products are in the 3% to 5% range (34).

Bronzers are water-soluble dyes, commonly prepared as moistures or powders that can be applied to the skin. They do easily wash off and, therefore, can only function as a cover up.

Antioxidants

Because UV radiation induces oxidative stress on the skin, antioxidants have been widely used as a photoprotective measure. Topical antioxidants are poor UV absorbers; therefore, they are commonly used in combination with UV filters in sunscreen products. Antioxidants can be administered orally or topically. Combination of high doses of oral antioxidants, L-ascorbic acid (vitamin C, 3 gm/day), and alpha tocopherol (vitamin E, 2 gm/day) for 50 days resulted in an increase in the MED to solar-simulated radiation; no increase was noted for patients treated with either of the antioxidants alone (4,35). However, in healthy individuals, six months of daily oral supplementation with 400 IU of vitamin E did not result in any protection to UV-induced skin damage (36). Another antioxidant, beta-carotene (120–180 mg/day), is known to diminish the photosensitivity in erythropoietic protoporphyria (37). In mice, topical tocopherol (vitamin E) or topical L-ascorbic acid (vitamin C) could suppress the induction of UV-induced inflammation, prevent photoimmunosuppression, and decrease UV-induced photocarcinogenesis (38,39).

Another potent antioxidant that has been widely studied is (–)-epigallocatechin-3-gallate, a polyphenol in green tea (40,41). Topical application of green tea extracts have been reported to decrease inflammation, carcinogenesis, and immunosuppression. It has been estimated that the above effect can be achieved with 10 caps of green tea a day, a relatively large amount of ingestion. Over-the-counter capsules containing green tea extracts are now available. Topically, green tea polyphenols do not function as effective UVB filter, as they have an absorption maximum at 273 nm (42).

DNA Excision Repair Enzyme and Photolyase

T4 endonuclease V is a DNA excision repair enzyme that repair cyclobutane pyrimidine dimers formed following predominantly UVB exposure. Topical application of T4N5 liposomes for one year in patients with xeroderma pigmentosum resulted in decreased formation of new actinic kertoses and basil cell carcinomas, as compared to the controlled group (43). Investigations are ongoing on the effect of this novel preparation as chemoprevention of skin cancers in otherwise healthy individual.

Photolyase, which specifically converts cyclobutane dimers into their original DNA structure after exposure to photoreactivating light, might also offer additional protection as sunscreen component to reverse harm caused by sun (44). There exist only limited data on its action in humans, and more research is needed to see if photolyase works with all degrees of sunburn and whether it can reduce risk of skin cancer.

Polypodium Leucotomos

Polypodium leucotomos is an extract from a fern plant grown in Central America. Oral and topical forms of this compound have been shown to be photoprotective against UVB and PUVA-induced phototoxicity, to increase immediate pigment-darkening dose, MED, minimal phototoxic dose, and minimal melanogenic dose. It has antioxidant and anti-inflammatory property. Because *P. leucotomos* has SPF of only 3 to 8, it is thought that the above biologic properties are independent from its property as a UV filter (45). Although studies have been done in human subjects, a larger study is needed. It is available in the United States and in many parts of the world as an over-the-counter vitamin supplement.

Miscellaneous Agents

Other agents that have been reported to have photoprotective properties are listed in Table 7 (4).

CONCLUSION

In the past 20 years, significant advances have been achieved in the area of photoprotection. There are several new photostable broad-spectrum UV filters that are available. Understanding and labeling of photoprotectiveness of clothing have improved very significantly. Developments in the glass industry have resulted in the availability of glass that has significant UV filtering properties up to 380 nm. In addition, several other topical and systemic photoprotective agents have been identified, all functioning by mechanism(s) that is separate from

TABLE 7 Other Agents with Photoprotective Property

Agent	Source	Comment
N-Acetylcysteine	Synthetic	Increase of glutathione level (endogenous antioxidant)
Butyrated hydroxytoluene	Preservatives, additives	Synthetic antioxidant
Cadmium chloride	Synthetic	Induction of metallothionein
Caffeic acid and ferulic acid	Plants and vegetables	Antioxidant and radial scavenging
Calcitriol (1,25-dihydroxyvitamin D3)	Kidneys	Induction of metallothionein (scavenger of free radicals)
Celecoxib	Synthetic	Cyclooxygenase 2 inhibitor
Cistus	Mediteranian shrubs	Free radical scavenging
2-Furildioxime (FDO)	Synthetic	Iron chelator
Isoflavone metabolites		Protection against UV-induced inflammation and immunosuppression
Genistein	Soybean	
Equol	Red clover	
Isoflavones	Plants	Antioxidants
Melatonin	Synthetic	Antioxidant
Plant oligosaccharides		Prevention of UVB-induced systemic immunosuppression
Xyloglucans	Tamarind seeds	
Aloe poly/oligosaccharide	Aloe barbadensis	
Omega-3 polyunsaturated fatty acid	Fish oil	Decrease of sunburn cell formation, anti-inflammation
Zinc		Antioxidant

Source: Modified from Ref. 4.

filtration of the UV radiation. Taken together, these developments are of great benefit to our patients in reducing the acute and chronic effects of sun exposure.

REFERENCES

1. Editorial. Von der Fettcreme zur Sonnenpflege. Parfümerie und Kosmetik 1999; 11/12:16–18.
2. Department of Health, Education and Welfare, Food and Drug Administration. Sunscreen drug products for over-the-counter human use. Federal Register 1978; 43:38206–38269.
3. Azurdia RM, Pagliaro JA, Diffey BL, Rhodes LE. Sunscreen application by photosensitive patients is inadequate for protection. Br J Dermatol 1999; 140:255–258.
4. Kullavanijaya P, Lim HW. Photoprotection. J Am Acad Dermatol 2005; 52:937–958.
5. Department of Health and Human Services, Food and Drug Administration. Sunscreen drug products for over-the-counter human use; final monograph. Federal Register 1999; 64:27666–27693.
6. Characterization of UVA protection of dermal suncare products by measuring the transmittance with regard to the sun protection factor. DIN 67502, Deutsches Institut für Normung e.V., Berlin February 2005.
7. Gers-Barlag H, Wendel V, Klette E, Wolber R, Wittern KP. UVA balance—The accurate and skin relevant assessment of the UVA protection of sunscreens. 7th Joint ASCC NZCSS Australasian Conference Auckland, New Zealand, 2004.
8. Dippe R, Klette E, Mann T, Wittern K-P, Gers-Barlag H. Comparison of four different in vitro test methods to assess the UVA protection performance of sunscreen products. SÖFW-J 2005; 131:1–6.
9. Kelly DA, Young AR, McGregor JM, Seed PT, Potten CS, Walker SL. Sensitivity to sunburn is associated with susceptibility to ultraviolet radiation-induced suppression of cutaneous cell-mediated immunity. J Exp Med 2000; 191:561–566.
10. Fourtanier A, Moyal D, Maccario J, et al. Measurement of sunscreen immune protection factors in humans: a consensus paper. J Invest Dermatol 2005; 125:403–409.
11. Standards Association of Australia. Standard AS/NZS 4399: sun protective clothing: evaluation and classification. Homebush, Australia: Australian/New Zealand Standards, 1996. http://www.saiglobal.com (accessed May 22, 2006).
12. Hatch KL, Osterwalder U. Garments as solar ultraviolet radiation screening materials. Dermatol Clin 2006; 24(1):85–100.
13. Department of Health and Human Services, Food and Drug Administration. Additional criteria and procedures for classifying over-the-counter drugs as generally recognized as safe and effective and not misbranded. Federal Register 2002; 67:3060–3076.

14. Department of Health And Human Services, Food and Drug Administration. Over-the-counter drug products; safety and efficacy review; additional sunscreen ingredients, [Docket No. 2005 N–0446], Federal Register 2005; 70(232):Notices 72449.

15. Tuchinda C, Lim HW, Osterwalder U, Rougier A. Novel emerging sunscreen technologies. Dermatol Clinics 2006; 24:105–117.

16. Stern RS, Weinstein MC, Baker RS. Risk reduction for nonmelanoma skin cancer with childhood sunscreen use. Arch Dermatol 1986; 122:537–545.

17. Godar DE, Wengraitis SP, Shreffler J, Sliney DH. UV doses of Americans. Photochem Photobiol 2001; 73:621–629.

18. Godar DE, Urbach F, Gasparro FP, van der Leun JC. UV doses of young adults. Photochem Photobiol 2003; 77:452–457.

19. Maier H, Schauberger G, Brunnhofer H, Hönigsmann H. Change of ultraviolet absorbance of sunscreens by exposure to solar-stimulated radiation. J Invest Dermatol 2001; 117:256–263.

20. Chatelain E, Gabard B. Photostabilization of butyl methoxydibenzoylmethane (Avobenzone) and ethylhexyl methoxycinnamate by bis-ethylhexyloxyphenol methoxyphenyl triazine (Tinosorb S), a new UV broadband filter. Photochem Photobiol 2001; 74:401–406.

21. Lim, HW, Gilchrest BA, Cooper KD, et al. Sunlight, tanning booths, and vitamin D. J Am Acad Dermatol 2005; 52:868–876.

22. Wolpowitz D, Gilchrest BA. The vitamin D questions: how much do you need and how should you get it? J Am Acad Dermatol 2006; 54:301–317.

23. Georgouras KE, Stanford DG, Pailthorpe MT. Sun protective clothing in Australia and the Australian/New Zealand standard: an overview. Australas J Dermatol 1997; 38(suppl 1):S79–S82.

24. American Society for Testing and Materials (ASTM International). Standard D 6603-00, Standard guide for labeling of UV-protective textiles. In: Bailey SJ, Baldwin NC, McElrone EK, et al., eds. ASTM standards. Vol. 7:03. 2004:1187–1191. Available from: http://www.astm.org (accessed May 22, 2006).

25. British Standards Institute. BS EN 13758-1:2002. Textiles. Solar UV protective properties. Method of test for apparel fabrics. Available from: http://www.bsonline.bsi-global.com (accessed May 22, 2006).

26. European Committee for Standardization. Standard EN 13758-2: textiles—solar UV-protective properties. Part 2: classification and marking of apparel. Available from: http://www.cenorm.be (accessed May 22, 2006).

27. Crews PC, Kachman S, Beyer AG. Influences on UVR transmission of undyed woven fabrics. Textile Chemist Colorist 1999; 31:17–26.

28. Tuchinda C, Srivannaboon S, Lim HW. Photoprotection by window glass, automobile glass and sunglasses. J Am Acad Dermatol 2006; 54:845–854.

29. National Glass Association. General information on glass. Available from: http://www.glass.org/indres/info.htm (accessed May 21, 2006).

30. Hampton PJ, Farr PM, Diffey BL, Lloyd JJ. Implication for photosensitive patients of ultraviolet A exposure in vehicles. Br J Dermatol 2004; 151:873–876.

31. LaMotte J, Ridder W III, Yeung K, De Land P. Effect of aftermarket automobile window tinting films on driver vision. Hum Factors 2000; 42:327–336.

32. Fu JM, Dusza SW, Halpern AC. Sunless tanning. J Am Acad Dermatol 2004; 50:706–713.

33. Faurschou A, Janjua NR, Wulf HC. Sun protection effect of dihydroxyacetone. Arch Dermatol 2004; 140(7):886–887.

34. Wikipedia: Dihydroxyacetone. Available from: http://en.wikipedia.org/wiki/Dihydroxyacetone (accessed May 3, 2006).

35. Fuchs J, Kern H. Modulation of UV-light-induced skin inflammation by D-alpha-tocopherol and L-ascorbic acid: a clinical study using solar simulated radiation. Free Radic Biol Med 1998; 25:1006–1012.

36. Werninghaus K, Meydani M, Bhawan J, Margolis R, Blumberg JB, Gilchrest BA. Evaluation of the photoprotective effect of oral vitamin E supplementation. Arch Dermatol 1994; 130:1257–1261.

37. Mathews-Roth MM. Carotenoid functions in photoprotection and cancer prevention. J Environ Pathol Toxicol Oncol 1990; 10:181–192.

38. Krol ES, Kramer-Stickland KA, Liebler DC. Photoprotective actions of topically applied vitamin E. Drug Metab Rev 2000; 32:413–420.

39. Darr D, Dunston S, Faust H, Pinnell S. Effectiveness of antioxidants (vitamin C and E) with and without sunscreens as topical photoprotectants. Acta Derm Venereol 1996; 76:264–268.

40. Katiyar SK, Challa A, McCormick TS, Cooper KD, Mukhtar H. Prevention of UVB-induced immunosuppression in mice by the green tea polyphenol (-)-epigallocatechin-3-gallate may be associated with alterations in IL-10 and IL-12 production. Carcinogenesis 1999; 20:2117–2124.

41. Katiyar SK, Elmets CA. Green tea polyphenolic antioxidants and skin photoprotection (Review). Int J Oncol 2001; 18:1307–1313.

42. Elmets CA, Singh D, Tubesing K, Matsui M, Katiyar S, Mukhtar H. Cutaneous photoprotection from ultraviolet injury by green tea polyphenols. J Am Acad Dermatol 2001; 44:425–432.

43. Yarosh D, Klein J, O'Connor A, et al. Effect of topically applied T4 endonucleaseV in liposomes on skin cancer in xeroderma pigmentosum: a randomised study. Lancet 2002; 357:926–929.
44. Decome L, De Meo M, Geffard A, Doucet O, Dumenil G, Botta A. Evaluation of photolyase (Photosome) repair activity in human keratinocytes after a single dose of ultraviolet B irradiation using the comet assay. J Photochem Photobiol B 2005; 79:101–108.
45. Middelkamp-Hup MA, Pathak MA, Parrado C, et al. Oral Polypodium leucotomos extract decreases ultraviolet-induced damage of human skin. J Am Acad Dermatol 2004; 51:910–918.

19 | Novel Developments in Photoprotection: Part I

Uli Osterwalder
Ciba Specialty Chemicals, Basel, Switzerland

Henry W. Lim
Department of Dermatology, Henry Ford Hospital, Detroit, Michigan, U.S.A.

- Clothing is the ideal sunscreen, except when it is not suitable (e.g., face, hands, and at the beach).

- Sunscreen's major function is historically the prevention of erythema; there is now an international method to determine the sun protection factor.

- Uniform protection over the whole UVB- and UVA-range is the ultimate goal in photoprotection.

- Progress in topical and systemic products for radical scavenging and DNA repair may become an important supplement to the photoprotection strategy.

- Sunscreens become better and better in UVA protection. Various new broad-spectrum and UVA protection actives are now available.

- Standards for UV protection raise the level of photoprotection.

- Various standards to assess UVA protection are already established in certain countries or are under discussion; international harmonization attempts are ongoing.

MODALITIES OF PHOTOPROTECTION
Preventing UV Radiation from Reaching the Skin

Sunscreens were originally developed to protect the skin from sunburn, which is caused predominantly by UVB. The need for UVA protection began to be recognized about 15 to 20 years ago. In 1991, a UVA conference was held in San Antonio, Texas. Brian Diffey then said:

> We do not yet know the importance of UVA with regard to photoaging…and…skin cancer…. It would seem prudent, therefore, to encourage the development of sunscreens which absorb more or less uniformly throughout the UV spectrum.
>
> *Diffey* (1)

While UVA has long been known to induce pigment darkening and tanning, the understanding of the other biologic effects of UVA was just emerging in 1991; these effects are now well-recognized. These include oxidative damage to the DNA and cell membrane, photoaging, photoimmunosuppression, and phtotocarcinogenesis (see Chaps 5–8). Ninety-five percent of the UV radiation reaching the surface of the earth is UVA, which is a long wave UV that penetrates well into the mid-dermis. There is relatively little fluctuation of UVA throughout the day and in different seasons of the year (2). Therefore, it is now recognized that it is equally important to develop UV filters to protect against the deleterious effects of UVB, as well as those of UVA (3).

UV Protection by Topical Sunscreens

Topically applied sunscreens are widely used and come in various forms, as creams, lotions, sprays, sticks, gels, mousse, etc. Whereas their benefit in preventing sunburn, actinic keratoses and squamous cell carcinomas is undisputed, their role in prevention of other forms of skin cancer is still controversial (4,5). It has been suggested by some authors (6) that sunscreens with higher sun protection factor (SPF) may encourage people to stay for a longer time in the sun, and thus lead to an increased exposure of UVA radiation, which would cause more harmful effects for the skin. It should be emphasized that sunscreens should not be considered and used as the only means of photoprotection, but should be regarded as a part of a sensible photoprotection strategy, which includes sun avoidance during the peak UVB hours (10 AM to 4 PM), wearing photoprotective clothings, wide-brimmed hat, and sunglasses. In this chapter, some of the new developments in photoprotection will be reviewed.

UV Protection by Clothings

Using clothing to protect one's skin from damaging ultraviolet radiation while out-of-doors is not a new concept or practice. What is relatively new is the interest in (*i*) developing methods to quantify sun protection performance of fabrics, (*ii*) understanding how to engineer sun protection performance into fabrics, (*iii*) establishing procedures for labeling garments with sun protection information, and (*iv*) providing understandable guidelines to individuals about how to select garments (those labeled and not labeled for sun protection performance) for wearing out-of-doors on summer days. Hatch and Osterwalder (7) have recently reviewed the subject.

The focus in this chapter is to compare and contrast the use of fabric and topical sunscreens for sun protection effectiveness. Textiles may be regarded as the ideal sunscreen when compared with topical products and their ability to prevent sunburn. Over the last decade, the UV transmission of textiles has been quantified and standardized in Australia, Europe, and the United States. UV protection afforded by textile is rated using ultraviolet protection factor (UPF), which is an in vitro measurement that assesses the relative amount of UV that penetrates a fabric. Although the UPF is heavily influenced by UVB, in contrast to the issue of UVA transmission with sunscreens, all fabrics do attenuate radiation in the UVA and the visible range (7,8).

However, the common belief that clothings protect the skin reliably from sunburn and other sun-induced damages is not generally correct. Any textile transmits a certain amount of UV radiation. Fabric UPFs values can certainly be as high as, or higher than, that of

TABLE 1 Comparison of Garments and Sunscreens as Photoprotective Measure

Comparison factor	Sunscreens	Garments
Cost	≥US $1 per one full body application	Use of "regular" garments does not have an additional cost unless dedicated UV absorber is purchased and applied Labeled UV protective clothing is costly
Replacement frequency	Need to be purchased regularly	Garments keep their protective property over years (depends on wear)
UV protection testing method	Sunscreen SPF testing is complex and costly because it is an in vivo test	Fabrics are easier to test because UPF is an in vitro test
Long-lasting/photostability	Reapplication every two hours Some UV filters are photolabile	Garments keep their protective property over the whole day
Area of protection	Can easily be applied on regularly sun-exposed areas (e.g., face, neck, dorsum of hands, etc.)	Not practical to cover face and dorsum of hands with garments
Even and sufficient application	Require an even application to avoid having areas of inadequate protection People tend to under-use sunscreens so the protection stated on the product may not be realized	All garment covered areas benefit from photoprotection
Timing of application	Should be applied 20 to 30 minutes prior to sun-exposure Some "instant" protection is available now	Could be put on at the last minute
Water proofness-staying power on the skin	Even "very water resistant" sunscreens can be rubbed off or washed off	UPF values may decrease (or increase in some cases) when the fabric is wet, but it is never washed off

Abbreviations: SPF, sun protection factor; UPF, ultraviolet protection factor.

topical sunscreens. For example, cotton T-shirts have UPF of five to nine, cotton, linen, and rayon have UPF of <15, whereas denim has UPF of 1700 (7). The major disadvantage of using garments as sun-screening materials is probably that most garments do not come labeled with an UPF value. In general, the amount of light transmitted through the fabric when it is held to a visible light source would give a rough estimation of the UPF values; therefore, consumers can make reasonable judgments about relative sun protection performance of a fabric. In the past few years, laundry additive that increased the UPF values by up to four-folds have become available (9). Application of broad-spectrum sunscreens along with garment is part of the proper photoprotection strategy. Each option has its advantages and disadvantages as outlined in Table 1.

Radical Scavenging in the Skin

Even the best sunscreen or sunproof clothing still let pass some UV radiation. Since UVR induces reactive oxygen species (ROS) in the skin, radical scavenging by antioxidants is part of a good photoprotection strategy. Antioxidants can be administered systemically or topically. Oral ingestion of vitamins E and C, carotenoids, and polyphenols, for example, from green tea, is commonly done (10). A recent study evaluated the effects of topical application of 47 different substances (drugs, plant extracts, plant ingredients, and polysaccharides) on UV radiation-induced lipid peroxidation (11). Amantadine, bufexamac, tryptophan, melatonin, propranolol, and hyaluronic acid were found to have antioxidative property, whereas pro-oxidative effects were shown with ascorbic acid. Buckwheat extract, extracts of St. John's Wort, melissa, and sage significantly reduced the level of radiation-induced lipid peroxidation. The authors concluded that the administration of antioxidants in cosmetic formulations or sunscreens might be helpful for the protection of the human skin against UV-induced damage. In vivo experiments with antioxidants should follow to allow in vitro–in vivo correlation and clinical interpretation of the data.

Helping the Repair of DNA and Cell Damage

Besides topical UV protection and radical scavenging, there is a third part of photoprotection strategy that becomes increasingly more important. DNA is constantly damaged and repaired by repair enzymes. The small protein T4 endonuclease V recognizes the major form of DNA damage produced by UVB, which is the cyclobutane pyrimidine (CPD) (12). In a randomized clinical study of the effects of liposomal T4 endonuclease V in patients with xeroderma pigmentosum, the rate of formation of actinic keratoses and basal cell carcinoma was reduced by 68% and 30%, respectively, compared to the control group (13). In another example, people with a polymorphism in the DNA repair gene 8-oxo-guanine glycosylase (OGG1) have an increased risk of skin cancer. Yarosh et al. (14) found that the cells with this variant polymorphism have an increased sensitivity of about 20% to a broad range of cytotoxic agents. The DNA deficits caused by immunosuppressive drugs or the OGG1 polymorphism can be overcome by the delivery of DNA repair enzymes in liposomes. The data suggest that deficits in DNA repair, even if they are not as severe as in the case of XP, may contribute to increased rates of cancer, and that topical therapy with DNA repair enzymes may be a promising avenue for after-sun protection.

IMPROVEMENTS IN TOPICAL SUNSCREENS—NEW DEVELOPMENTS AROUND CONVENTIONAL UV ABSORBERS
Stabilization

Photolabile UVA filter, butyl methoxydibenzoylmethane (BMBM; avobenzone; Parsol® 1789) can be stabilized by combining it with other UV filters, such as octocrylene, 4-methylbenzylidene camphor (MBC), or *bis*-ethylhexyloxyphenol methoxyphenyl triazine (BEMT) (15), or with an agent which is not a UV filter, diethylhexyl 2,6-naphthalate (DEHN, Corapan TQ) (16). The presence of other UV filters reduce the number of photons absorbed by avobenzone and facilitate the transfer of absorbed energy from avobenzone to the other UV filters, hence minimizing the photodegradation of avobenzone. Energy transfer from avobenzone to DEHN is probably the mechanism responsible for the photostabilizing effect of the latter.

Encapsulation

The efficacy and safety aspect of UV absorbers has also been addressed by reducing skin penetration via encapsulation of UV absorbers within a silica shell of 1 μm in diameter [e.g., Eusolex® UV Pearls™ containing octinoxate (ethylhexyl methoxycinnamate)] (17). With this technique, the organic filter is entrapped in the capsule, decreasing the probability of allergic, photoallergic, or irritant contact dermatitis. Furthermore, it would prevent the incompatibility among sunscreen ingredients. The drawback of this technology is that it is rather expensive, and thus only a few sunscreen manufacturers have incorporated it so far.

Micronization

The microfine inorganic pigments TiO_2 and ZnO have been improved considerably to allow the easier incorporation into formulations and to become cosmetically better accepted, but some limitations still remain (18). Micronization to primary particle sizes of <20 nm results in less scattering of visible light, hence minimizing the whitening effect. However, as the particle size is decreased, the peak of the absorption spectrum shifts to the shorter wavelength, decreasing the absorption in the UVA range. Microfine ZnO has a more uniform but weaker absorption at the 290 to 380 nm than microfine TiO_2.

Upon exposure of TiO_2 and ZnO to UV, photocatalytic process takes place, resulting in the generation of ROS. To minimize the photocatalysis, inorganic filters are frequently coated with aluminum oxide. In order to optimize formulating properties, a coating of dimethicone or silica may be added. A new development is the coating of TiO_2 with <1% of manganese (19) (Optisol®, Oxonica Healthcare, Oxfordshire, U.K.). There are two effects of the coating: The production of radicals resulting from the electron elevation to the conduction band is suppressed, and the extinction spectrum is changed towards higher extinction in the UVA-range, resulting in better absorption in the UVA range. First products containing Optisol® are available since 2006.

A method to boost the efficacy of current filter systems is the incorporation of nonabsorbing particles that refract UV radiation, thus leading to a longer pathway that the UV would have to travel through the sunscreen film before reaching the epidermis (20). One such product is SunSpheres® (Rohm and Hass, Philadelphia, Pennsylvania, U.S.A.), a styrene/acrylates copolymer, which is a non-UV absorbing material. Products containing SunSpheres® are available in the U.S. market (Nivea Vital, Dove, Yves Saint Laurent, etc.). Film-forming agents may lead to better spreading of the product on the skin, resulting in a final product that is more efficient for a given amount of UV filter.

NEW SUNSCREEN ACTIVES FOR SUNSCREENS
Strategy for Photostable Broad-Spectrum

Sunscreen manufacturers have four basic requirements on sunscreen actives, which all must be fulfilled by the existing and new ingredients before they can be incorporated in a final product.

- Efficacy
- Safety
- Registration
- Patent freedom

In this chapter, the focus will be to demonstrate how the efficacy of new sunscreen actives is achieved. A more comprehensive view on this topic has been published (21).

Efficacy
Besides an efficient UV absorption, photostability and solubility as described earlier, there are other important parameters regarding efficacy that need to be considered. The UV absorber substance must be compatible with all other ingredients in a formulation; there should be no discoloration of skin and hair, no staining of textiles, and no odor. For water resistant claim, the UV absorber should be insoluble in water. And last but not least, the cost of UV filter, hence the final product, should be affordable to the general consumers.

Safety
Sunscreen actives should have no adverse effect on humans and environment. Although direct comparison with a new pharmaceutical drug is not appropriate, the development of a new sunscreen active for global use is highly demanding. The toxicological studies required for a global registration are listed in Table 2 (22).

Registration
In order to exploit the full economic potential of a UV filter, UV absorber manufacturers aim for global registration. In the European Union, South America, Asia, and Africa, where sunscreens are regulated as cosmetics, approval is possible within one to two years of filing. In Australia, Japan and, the United States, where sunscreens are regulated as over-the-counter medications, the approval process normally takes longer. In the U.S., until 2002, approval of all new UV filters need to go through the New Drug Application (NDA) process, with clinical studies to be done in the U.S. At the time of this writing, a UVA filter, terephthalidene dicamphor sulfonic acid (TDSA; ecamsule; Mexoryl® SX), is undergoing the United States Food and Drug Administration (FDA) approval through this process.

In 2002, the U.S. FDA initiated an additional approval process, the Time and Extend Application (TEA) (23). The TEA process indicates that after a minimum of five years of foreign marketing experience in the same country, a new sunscreen active can be submitted

TABLE 2 Typical International Safety Dossier
of a New Sunscreen

Acute oral and dermal toxicity
Dermal, ocular irritation, and skin sensitization
Photo-irritation and photo-sensitization
Subchronic oral and topical toxicity
Chronic toxicity
Fertility, early embryonic development
Embryofetal toxicity and peri-/postnatal toxicity
In vitro and in vivo percutaneous absorption
Topical and oral pharmacokinetic and metabolism
In vitro and in vivo genetic toxicity
Carcinogenicity
Photo-carcinogenicity
Safety and efficacy in man

Source: Adapted from Ref. 22.

for application for registration with the FDA. If the FDA deems the UV filter is acceptable to be considered for inclusion in the Sunscreen Monograph, efficacy and safety data then have to be submitted. As of 2006, three UVB filters and two broad-spectrum UV filters that are widely used outside the U.S. have received the status of "eligibility to enter the Sunscreen Monograph" through the TEA process (24). These are listed subsequently:

UVB filters

- Isoamyl p-methoxycinnamate (IMC). US adopted name (USAN): amiloxate.
- 4-Methylbenzylidene camphor (MBC). USAN: enzacamene.
- Ethylhexyl triazone (EHT). USAN: octyl triazone.

Broad-spectrum UV filters

- Methylene-bis-benzotriazolyl tetramethylbutyl-phenol (MBBT; Tinosorb® M). USAN: bisoctrizole.
- Bis-ethylhexyloxyphenol methyoxyphenyl triazene (BEMT) (Tinosorb® S). USAN: bemotrizinol.

Patent Freedom

Patenting of sunscreen actives and their applications deserve special attention (21). Some UV filters are patented for the exclusive use of certain sunscreen companies. As a consequence, the UV filter manufacturers/suppliers have to make sure that as soon as the identity of a new ingredient becomes known, "all" measures have to be taken, for example, publication of combinations of that novel ingredient with other sunscreen actives and other important compounds, such as emollients, emulsifiers, or thickeners. Patent freedom means the free use of sunscreen actives by any sunscreen manufacturer, that is, any infringement of any third party patent rights must be avoided.

Chemistry/Actives

Over the last 5 to 10 years, a number of photostable UV filters that cover UVA or both the UVB and UVA range have been developed and approved in the European Union (25) (Fig. 1). In 2006, three of these new ingredients, Mexoryl® SX, Tinosorb® M, and Tinosorb® S, are at various stages of approval process by the U.S. FDA.

- Approved in 1993, TDSA (ecamsule; Mexoryl® SX) was the first photostable UVA filter. It is water-soluble, that is, will be in the water phase of an emulsion system and can thus act synergistically together with filters in the oil-phase. The TDSA is also used together with stabilized avobenzone and UVB filters to give equal coverage of UVB and UVA.

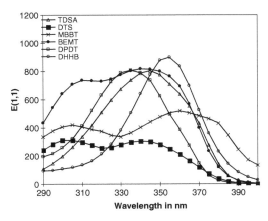

TDSA (Ecamsule; Mexoryl ®SX). 1993
UVA, photostable, soluble in aqueous
phase (Exclusive to L'Oreal sunscreens)

DTS (Silatriazole; Mexoryl ®XL). 1998
Broad-spectrum, photostable, soluble in oil-
phase (Exclusive to L'Oreal sunscreens)

MBBT (Bisoctrizole, Tinosorb ®M). 2000
Broad-spectrum, photostable, microfine
particles dispersed in aqueous phase

BEMT (Bemotrizinol, Tinosorb ®S). 2000
Broad-spectrum, photostable, soluble in oil-
phase

DPDT (no USAN, Neoheliopan ®AP). 2000
UVA, photostable, soluble in aqueous
phase

DHHB (no USAN, Uvinul ®A plus) 2005
UVA, photostable, soluble in oil-phase

FIGURE 1 Possibilities of covering the UVA range with new UV filters available in Europe. *Abbreviations*: BEMT, bis-ethylhexyloxyphenol methoxyphenyl triazine; DTS, drometrizole trisiloxane; DPDT, disodium phenyl dibenzimidazole tetrasulfonate; DNHB, diethylamino hydroxybenzoyl hexylbenzoate; MBBT, methylene-bis-benzotriazolyl tetramethylbutyl-phenol; TDSA, terephthalidene dicamphor sulfonic acid; USAN, United States Adopted Name.

- Approved in 1998, drometrizole trisiloxane (DTS; silatriazole; Mexoryl® XL) was the first photostable broad-spectrum filter. Siloxane groups were added to the benzotriazole chromophore for better water resistance.
- Approved in 2000, MBBT (bisoctrizole; Tinosorb® M) is a photostable broad-spectrum UV filter with strong absorption both in UVB and UVA. Its unique feature is that it comes as microfine organic particles. Hence, it is not only absorbing UV radiation, but also scattering and reflecting it. The microfine organic particles are dispersed in the water phase, leading to a synergistic effect together with oil-soluble filters.
- Approved in 2000, disodium phenyl dibenzimidazole tetrasulfonate (DPDT; Neo Heliopan® AP) is a new water-soluble UVA filter. Similarly to TDSA and MBBT, it should show synergistic effects together with filters in the oil phase.
- Approved in 2000, BEMT (bemotrizinol; Tinosorb® S) is a photostable broad-spectrum filter that is oil-soluble. Similar to other photostable UV filters that have strong absorbance in UVA and UVB range, number and amount of other UV filters can be reduced in a given product that contains bemotrizinol.

Approved in 2005, diethylamino hydroxylbenzoyl hexyl benzoate (DHHB; Uvinul® A Plus) is a replacement of avobenzone as an oil-soluble UVA filter. Unlike avobenzone, DHHB is photostable.

Designing Oil-Soluble Broad-Spectrum UV Filter
Chemistry for Photostability in Broad-Spectrum/UVA Protection
The UV absorbers are widely used to protect polymers (e.g., plastics, fibers, and coatings) against photo-degradation. Numerous investigations have demonstrated that photostability is of key importance to the filters in order to provide long-term protection of polymer substrates (e.g., no degradation after several years of Florida outdoor testing). In general, UV absorbers with an intramolecular hydrogen bond exhibit very efficient radiation-free energy transformation processes, resulting in inherent photostability. For polymer applications, the following UV stabilizer technologies have been subsequently developed, and listed in the order of year of introduction:

- Methyl salicylates (1960) → o-hydroxybenzophenones (1965–1970) → 2-(2-hydroxyaryl)-benzotriazoles (1975–1990) → 2-(2-hydroxyaryl)-1,3,5-triazines (since 1995).

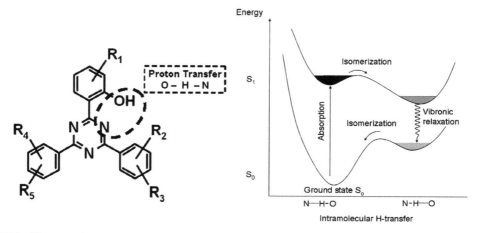

FIGURE 2 The general structure of hydroxyphenyltriazines. A model for the conversion of absorbed UV-energy to heat by extremely fast photo-tautomerism (about 10^{-12} sec).

Presently, hydroxyphenyltriazines (HPTs; Fig. 2) represent the most advanced class of UV absorbers for the photoprotection of all kind of polymer substrates (26–28). Owing to their molecular structure, HPTs exhibit a UV absorption spectrum with two distinctive peaks (29). This is due to the presence of two electronic transitions with strong dipole moments, both of which are polarized perpendicular to each other (shown in Fig. 3). In order to obtain broad-spectrum absorbance, OH and OR substituents at the three phenyl groups have to be introduced and positioned as follows (Fig. 3): Two ortho-OH groups are required for efficient energy dissipation via intramolecular hydrogen bridges. In order to obtain strong absorption in the UVA, the para-positions of the two respective phenyl moieties should be substituted by OR, resulting in a bis-resorcinyl triazine chromophor (R=alkyl). The remaining phenyl group attached to the triazine is leading to UVB absorption. It can be demonstrated that maximal "full spectrum" performance is achieved with OR located in the para-position.

Without solubilizing substituents, HPTs are nearly insoluble in cosmetic oils. They exhibit the typical properties of pigments (e.g., high melting points). In order to increase solubility in oil phases, the structure of this UV filter has to be modified accordingly. The introduction of two 2-ethyl-hexyl groups (Fig. 3) results in the formation of BEMT, a new oil-soluble UV filter with true broad-spectrum performance.

In general, the photostability of a UV filter depends on how well the molecule is able to release the absorbed energy to the environment in form of heat. BEMT contains two intramolecular hydrogen bonds (O-H-N), which lead to an excited state intramolecular proton transfer (photo-tautomerism) after photoexcitation (Fig. 2). This results in rapid radiationless

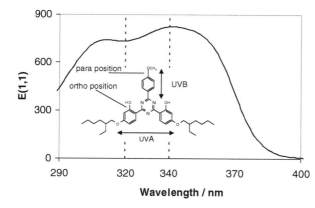

FIGURE 3 Molecular structure and UV-absorption spectrum of bemotrizinol, measured in EtOH, normalized extinction (1 cm, 1%) E(1,1) max = 820 (342 nm). *Arrows* indicate the directions of the UVA and UVB transitions.

TABLE 3 New class of UV Filter Vs. Conventional Categories

	Physical form	
Chemistry	Soluble	Insoluble
Organic	Traditional UV filters, for example octinoxate, oxybenzone, and avobenzone	Bisoctrizole (Tinosorb M)
Inorganic	NA	Traditional microfine UV filters Titanium dioxide, Zinc oxide

Abbreviation: NA, not available.

conversion that ensures that the UV radiation, efficiently absorbed by the filter, is almost quantitatively transformed into harmless vibrational energy (i.e., heat). The entire photo-tautomeric cycle only lasts about 10^{-12} seconds, leaving no time for undesirable side reactions (e.g., formation of triplet states and generation of singlet oxygen or radicals). This mechanism, which has been elucidated only recently (30), explains well why BEMT is photostable (>95% recovery of parent BEMT is observed analytically after exposure to 50 minimal erythema dose (MED) of solar simulated UV). Figure 2 illustrates the role of the intramolecular hydrogen bridge in the quantitative conversion of UV radiation to vibrational energy (31).

A New Class of Sunscreen Actives—Microfine Organic Particles

A new class of UV absorber has been developed by Ciba Specialty Chemicals (Basel, Switzerland). For the first time, organic UV absorbers come as microfine particles, thus combining the typical properties of organic filters (strong absorbance) with those of particulate UV filters (scattering and reflection) (32). The organic molecules used have an inherent extraordinary photostability. The result is a highly efficient sunscreen due to its triple action: UV absorption, light scattering, and light reflection. The new class is combining the best features of both conventional classes of UV filters. The properties of this new class of UV filter are compared with those of conventional filters in Table 3.

MBBT (bisoctrizole; Tinosorb® M) is the first representative of this new class of UV absorber (Figs. 4 and 5). It is an aqueous dispersion containing 50% of colorless organic microfine particles with a size below 200 nm. The small particles are stabilized in their size by a surfactant.

Safety of the New UV Absorbers

All new UV absorbers underwent the scrutiny of the European approval process, hence they can all be considered safe. In case some safety concerns should occur, the European Commission asks the Scientific Committee of Cosmetic Products (SCCP) to re-evaluate the safety data. Thus, it is possible that a certain filter can be delisted. In the United States, the FDA first asks the TEA

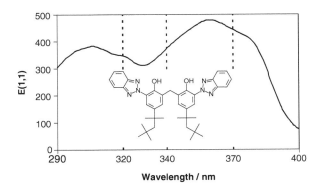

FIGURE 4 Bisoctrizole, the first microfine organic particle UV filter.

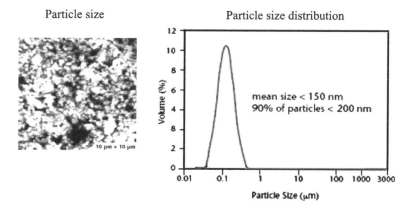

Particle size   Particle size distribution

FIGURE 5 Particle size distribution of bisoctrizole.

process for the five-year marketing experience abroad, that is, the clinical evidence that a UV filter does not show any adverse effects. The next step is the submission of the safety package containing additional preclinical long-term dermal cancer and photo-cocarcinogenicity studies; safety data are evaluated prior to approval (33,34).

The 500 Dalton Rule

In the development of UV absorbers over the last decades, besides the new developments, such as encapsulation, polymers, and microfine pigments, there was also a general development of the new sunscreen actives towards higher molecular weight filters. The "500 Dalton rule," known from the development of transdermal drugs, can be seen as a common denominator. The 500 Dalton rule for the skin penetration of chemical compounds and drugs states that when topical dermatological therapy or percutaneous systemic therapy is the objective, the development of new innovative compounds should be restricted to molecular weights of under 500 Dalton (35). Conversely, one may postulate a 500 Dalton rule for the development of sunscreen actives, which says that the development of new innovative compounds should be restricted to molecular weight of over 500 Dalton, when UV filtering on, rather than in, the skin is the objective. As shown in Figure 6, the development over the past 50 years is clearly heading in that direction. However, it should be noted that the 500 Dalton rule is neither a necessity nor a sufficient condition for the safety of a new sunscreen active.

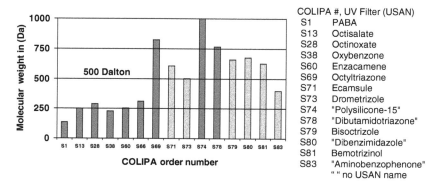

FIGURE 6 The 500 Dalton rule. A trend towards molecular weight of more than 500 Daltons in the development of oil-soluble UV filters in the last 50 years. *Abbreviations*: COLIPA, European Cosmetic, Toiletry, and Perfumery Association; USAN, United States Adopted Name.

EMERGING SUNSCREEN ASSESSMENT METHODS AND STANDARDS

Sunscreen assessment methods and standards assure transparency among products, and thus also lead to better photoprotection. Over the last decades the average SPF of sunscreens has steadily increased. While there have been significant awareness and concerns on the importance of UVA protection by sunscreens, there has not been a worldwide consensus on the methods of assessment of UVA protection. The United Kingdom is a good example that the introduction of a UVA standard (the Boots Star Rating in 1992 as a measure of the UVA/UVB ratio) leads to significantly better UVA protection (36).

Understanding Sun Protection Factor

Historically, the sole purpose of sunscreens was to prevent sunburn. The SPF is the ratio between the minimal dose that produces perceptible erythema on the skin (i.e., MED) in the presence or absence of $2 \, mg/cm^2$ of sunscreen, using solar-simulated radiation as a light source (37). However, the actual protection provided by a sunscreen is a dynamic process; therefore, it is also important to choose a representation of the sunscreen beyond the static view commonly seen.

The exposure time is the most important influence factor for any effect of UV radiation. This is best illustrated in Figure 7, inspired by the Australian Standard document (38). For individuals with skin phototype 1 to 2, one MED is reached within about 10 minutes without sunscreen (i.e., SPF 1). With SPF 15 and SPF 30 sunscreens, the time to reach one MED is prolonged accordingly to 150 and 300 min. However, in a proper photoprotection strategy, sunscreen is not used to reach one MED. In contrast, sunscreen should be used to stay well below one MED. The example in Figure 7 shows that a two-hour exposure of a person with skin phototype 1 leads to 80%, 40%, or 20% of a MED if a sunscreen of SPF 15, 30, or 60 (labeled 50+) is applied, respectively. It should be noted that the example shown in Figure 7 is based on the assumption that the UV filters are photostable, and the sunscreens are applied at a concentration of $2 \, mg/cm^2$ (the worldwide standard used in SPF testing). Many of the currently used UV filters do degrade following UV exposure (39). In actual use, consumers apply on average $0.5 \, mg/cm^2$ of sunscreens (40). Some exposed sites are frequently missed, and with regular or outdoor activities, sunscreens are rubbed off, or washed off with water and sweat exposure. Furthermore, sunscreens with the same SPF frequently have different UVA protection factor; therefore, a high SPF sunscreen may not necessarily provide good UVA protection (3). It is for these reasons that sunscreens should be used as one of the measures to minimize the acute and chronic effects of UV exposure in daily and recreational outdoor activities; they should not be advocated to encourage unnecessary sun exposure.

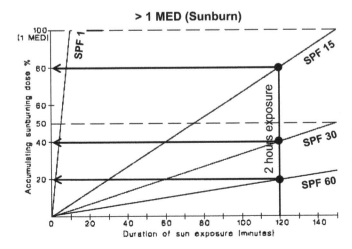

FIGURE 7 Dynamics of the UV dose reaching the skin through sunscreens over time. The example shows the minimal erythema dose received by skin phototype 1 or 2 with the assumption that the sunscreen is photostable, and sunscreens are applied at a concentration of $2 \, mg/cm^2$. *Abbreviations*: MED, minimal erythema dose; SPF, sun protection factor.

TABLE 4   Selected Methods for the Assessment of UVA Protection by Sunscreens that are Currently in Discussion

	Type of method	Reference
In vivo	UVA-PF via erythema	(44)
	PPD (Japanese Standard)	(45,46)
	Others	
In vitro	Australian Standard	(47)
	Critical wavelength	(49)
	UVA/UVB ratio, Boots star rating	(49,50)
	UVA-balance	(51,52)
	Harmonized in vitro UVA method (PPD, COLIPA)	(53)
	Others	
In silico	Computer simulation based on spectral data of UV filters and sunscreen film model	(54–57)

UVA Standards for Sunscreens

UVA and broad-spectrum claims are very common in modern sun protection products. The introduction of the SPF began in the 1950s (41). It took several decades to gain global acceptance and public understanding of this concept. A consensus on the method for UVA assessment would also be highly desirable since this would provide the same criterion for all companies and eventually result in better product quality and increased understanding by consumers and the general public. To date, health authorities and regulatory agencies worldwide still have not yet come to an agreement on a generally acceptable UVA assessment method (2). There are several in vivo and in vitro methods available, and there is also the possibility to assess the performance of a sunscreen by computer simulation, that is, in silico (Table 4).

In Vivo Determination of UVA Protection

A first attempt to determine the "right" degree of UVA protection came from the United States by Urbach around 1990 (42,43). The SPF was seen as the only measure for UV damage. According to that reasoning, a UVA-protection factor (UVA-PF) of 20% of the SPF is always sufficient to avoid any erythema from UVA radiation. The ratio of damage (erythema) from the UVB and UVA components in sunlight over a day is 80% from UVB and 20% from UVA. Of the 20% due to UVA (320–400 nm), 62% of the damage risk has been ascribed to the shorter UVA2 wavelengths (320–340 nm). The UVA-PF is determined similarly to the SPF by causing erythema, but by applying UVA radiation instead of solar-simulated UVR, first described by Cole (44).

The sunscreen manufacturer, L'Oreal, developed another in vivo method to assess UVA protection (45). The persistent pigment darkening (PPD) method is based on the ability of sunscreen to protect against the development of PPD, which is the result of a chemical reaction of melanin following within hours of exposure to UVA radiation. The PPD method, with its classification of PA+, PA + +, PA+++, became the Japanese Standard in 1995 (46), and is widely used in many countries in Asia. In France, there is an initiative to combine SPF and UVA-PF (assessed by pigment darkening method) to a broad-spectrum pass/fail criterion SPF/UVA-PF < 3.

In Vitro Determination of UVA Protection

In 1993, the Australian/New Zealand Standard was established (47). This standard sets an absolute transmittance limit of 10% in the UV range of 320 to 360 nm for any product to make "broad spectrum" claim. "Broad spectrum" product must have a SPF of not less than four. An analysis of the data of about 50 sunscreen samples revealed that fulfilling the Australian Standard corresponds to the a UVA-PF (PPD) of 4 ± 1 (48).

Diffey was the first to describe two relative in vitro methods based on simple transmittance measurement on a UV/VIS transparent substrate. The two methods are referred to as the UVA/UVB ratio and the critical wavelength (49).

The sunscreen manufacturer and retailer Boots in the United Kingdom developed and enforced the *Boots Star Rating System* based on Diffey's ratio of the mean absorbance in the UVA over the mean absorbance in the UVB (49). In 2005, the original four-star rating system was revised to include a fifth-star, defined by a UVA/UVB ratio >0.91 (50). Today, this rating comes closest to uniform UV protection, but does not take into account photostability.

Only recently the UVA-balance has been developed (51). In 2005, it became an official German industry standard DIN 67502 (52). In this method, an in vitro UVA-PF, analogous to PPD, is determined from spectral transmittance data. The in vitro SPF is calculated, and the whole spectral curve is adjusted to the in vivo SPF by a correction factor. This new curve is then used to calculate the in vitro UVA-PF value. This method takes into account the photostability of the UV filters at least partially by considering the SPF.

All other in vitro methods have a common limitation in not taking into account the photostability of UVA absorbers. With photolabile UV filters (e.g., unstabilized avobenzone), these methods can lead to an overestimation of the UVA protection capability.

A comparison of the in vitro methods discussed earlier regarding their ability to discriminate sunscreens providing different degrees of UVA protection revealed the following ranking of the methods (48).

1. UVA-balance (UVA/UVB ratio that partially takes into account photostability).
2. UVA/UVB ratio (UVA protection proportional to UVB protection, different levels/star rating).
3. Australian UVA Standard (absolute limit leads to relatively low UVA protection at high SPF).
4. Critical wavelength (370 nm limit provides only relatively low UVA protection).

The latest attempt to address this issue is discussed in a task force of the European Cosmetic, Toiletry, and Perfumery Association (COLIPA) (53). It is anticipated that in 2006, an improved UVA-balance with an irradiation step prior to the transmittance measurement should become the official recommendation. The UVA-PF value determined by the UVA balance (52) is used to determine a preirradiation dose. The actual UVA-PF is then determined from the spectral data of the preirradiated sample using the same (SPF) correction factor as before.

Australia and Japan have established their own official standards, whereas the European Union and the United States have not. There is a good probability that we will see a consolidation of all this efforts and worldwide harmonization in the near future. In 2006, the European Union issued a recommendation "on the efficacy of sunscreen products and the claims made relating thereto," stating that the UVA-PF should be at least 1/3 of the SPF (54).

In Silico Determination of UVA Protection

Only recently yet another approach to determine the performance of a sunscreen, referred to as in silico (Table 4), has become precise enough to be considered seriously. The SPF as well as any UVA parameter can be calculated from the extinction spectrum of the UV filters in the sunscreen and an assumption about the nonhomogenous sunscreen film that is formed on the skin (55,56). The in vitro SPF is determined by calculating the transmittance spectrum of the sunscreen and taking into account the nonuniform sunscreen film together with the known solar spectrum. The latest more sophisticated version also takes into account the photoinstability of certain UV filter combinations (e.g., avobenzone with octinoxate) as well as the distribution of the UV filters between oil and water phase that may lead to a synergistic effect (57,58). Figure 8 shows the progress in UVA protection on sample calculations of four SPF 30 sunscreens: (*i*) a "UVB sunscreen," (*ii*) a sunscreen fulfilling Australian Standard, (*iii*) a sunscreen fulfilling the German UVA-balance (33% threshold), and (*iv*) a sunscreen that achieves five-star rating in the United Kingdom. Note that all four sunscreens provide exactly the same protection against erythema, since they are all SPF 30.

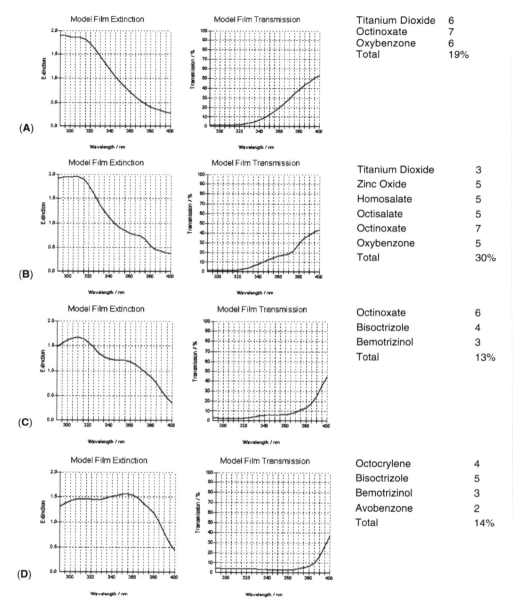

FIGURE 8 Progress in UVA protection. Sample calculations of four SPF 30 sunscreens with different degrees of UVA protection: (**A**) a "UVB sunscreen," (**B**) a sunscreen fulfilling Australian Standard, (**C**) a sunscreen fulfilling the German UVA-balance (33% threshold), and (**D**) a sunscreen that achieves 5-star rating. *Abbreviations*: PPD, persistent pigment darkening; SPF, sun protection factor.

Sample Calculation

In silico results	A	B	C	D
SPF	31	31	31	31
UVA-PF (PPD)	6	7	14	26
UVA PF/SPF	0.19	0.23	0.45 ($<$1/3)	0.84 ($>$1/3)
AUS STD	FAIL	PASS	PASS	PASS
Critical wavelength (nm)	369	373	379	381
UVA/UVB ratio	0.45	0.46	0.66	0.90
UVA balance (DIN 67502)	11	14	34	99

CONCLUSION

In addition to sun avoidance and sunproof clothing, topical sunscreens remain an important part of any photoprotection strategy. Topical and systemic products that act as antioxidants or help the repair of the skin become valuable supplements in photoprotection. Stimulated by the new requirements towards better UV protection, seven new UV absorbers have been developed and approved in Europe over the last few years. These new filters give the formulators new possibilities to cover the whole UV range from 290 to 400 nm, and also to use less filter due to the boosting effect of the new UVA and broad-spectrum filters. However, only three of them, ecamsule, bisoctrizole, and bemotrizinol are currently under review by the FDA for approval in the U.S. The full potential of the new sunscreen actives can only be exploited when proper standards for the assessment of UVA protection are being established. After the introduction of such standards in Australia, Japan, United Kingdom, and Germany, UVA protection increased significantly in these countries. European harmonization is under way; eventually, the assessment of UVA protection should be harmonized globally.

REFERENCES

1. Diffey BL. The need for sunscreens with broad spectrum protection. In: Urbach F. ed. Biological Responses to Ultraviolet A Radiation. A Symposium on UVA Radiation. San Antonio, TX, June 1991. Overland Park, KS: Valdenmar Publication Co., 1992:321–328.
2. Lim HW, Naylor M, Hönigsmann H, et al. American Academy of Dermatology Consensus Conference on UVA protection of sunscreens: summary and recommendations. J Am Acad Dermatol 2001; 44:505–508.
3. Fourtanier A, Moyal D, Maccario J, et al. Measurement of sunscreen immune protection factors in humans: a consensus paper. J Invest Dermatol 2005; 125:403–409.
4. Thompson SC, Jolley D, Marks R. Reduction of solar keratoses by regular sunscreen use. N Engl J Med 1993; 329:1147–1151.
5. Green A, Williams G, Neale R, et al. Daily sunscreen application and beta-carotene supplementation in prevention of basal-cell and squamous-cell carcinomas of the skin: a randomised controlled trial. Lancet 1999; 354:723–729.
6. Autier P, Doré JF, Négrier S, et al. Sunscreen use and duration of sun exposure: a double-blind, randomized trial, J Natl Cancer Inst 1999; 91:1304.
7. Hatch KL, Osterwalder U. Garments as ultraviolet radiation screening materials. Dermatol Clin 2006; 24:85–100.
8. Hoffmann K, Laperre J, Avermaete A, Altmeyer P, Gambichler T. Defined UV protection by apparel textiles. Arch Dermatol 2001; 137:1089–1094.
9. Wang SQ, Kopf AW, Marx J, Bogdan A, Polsky D, Bart RS. Reduction of ultraviolet transmission through cotton T-shirt fabrics with low ultraviolet protection by various laundering methods and dyeing: clinical implications. J Am Acad Dermatol 2001; 44:767–774.
10. Stahl W, Mukhtar H, Afaq F, Sies H. Vitamins and polyphenols in systemic photoprotection. In: Gilchrest BA, Krutmann J, eds. Skin Aging. Berlin, Heidelberg, Germany: Springer-Verlag, 2006:113–120.
11. Trommer H, Neubert RH. Screening for new antioxidative compounds for topical administration using skin lipid model systems. J Pharm Pharm Sci 2005; 15;8(3):494–506.
12. Krutmann J, Yarosh Daniel. Modern photoprotection of human skin. In: Gilchrest BA, Krutmann J, eds. Skin Aging. Berlin, Heidelberg, Germany: Springer-Verlag, 2006:103–112.
13. Yaros D, Klien J, O'Connor A, Hawk J, Rafal E, Wolf P. Effect of topically applied T4 endonuclease V in liposomes on skin cancer in xeroderma pigmentosum: a randomised study. Lancet 2001; 357:926–929.
14. Yarosh DB, Canning MT, Teicher D, Brown DA. After sun reversal of DNA damage: enhancing skin repair. Mutat Res 2005; 571(1–2):57–64. Epub 2005 Jan 26.
15. Chatelain E, Gabard B. Photostabilization of butyl methoxydibenzoylmethane (avobenzone) and ethylhexyl methoxycinnamate by bis-ethylhexyloxyphenol methoxyphenyl triazine (Tinosorb S), a new UV broadband filter. J Photochem Photobiol 2001; 74:401–406.
16. Bonda C, Steinberg DC. A new photostabilizer for full spectrum sunscreens. Cosmet Toiletries 2000; 115(6): 37–45.
17. Patent MERCK AG WO 00/09652, 2000, Silica-Mikrocapsules filled with functional molecules.
18. Schlossmann D, Shao Y. Inorganic ultraviolet filters. In: Shaath N, ed. Sunscreens: Regulations and Commercial Development. Cosmetic Science and Technology Series. 3rd edn. Vol. 28. Chap. 14. Boca Raton, FL: Taylor & Francis Group, 2005.
19. Wakefield G, Lipscomb S, Holland E, Knowland J. The effects of manganese doping on UVA absorption and free radical generation of micronised titanium dioxide and its consequences for the

photostability of UVA absorbing organic sunscreen components. Photochem Photobiol Sci 2004; 3(7):648–652. Epub 2004 May 21.

20. Mufti J, Cernasov D, Macchio R. New Technologies in Topical Delivery Systems, HAPPI, March 2002

21. Herzog B, D Hueglin, Osterwalder U. New sunscreen actives. Chapter 16 In: Shaath N, ed. Sunscreens: Regulations and Commercial Development. Cosmetic Science and Technology Series. 3rd edn. Vol. 28. Chap. 16. Boca Raton, FL: Taylor & Francis Group, 2005.

22. Nohynek G, Schaefer H. Benefit and risk of organic ultraviolet filters. Regul Toxicol Pharm 2001; 33:1–15.

23. Food and Drug Administration, Additional Criteria and Procedures for, Classifying Over-the-Counter Drugs as, Generally Recognized as Safe and, Effective and Not Misbranded, 21 CFR Part 330, [Docket No. 96 N–0277], RIN 0910–AA01, Federal Register/Vol. 67, No. 15/Wednesday, January 23, 2002/Rules and Regulations, 3060-3076.

24. Food and Drug Administration Over-the-Counter Drug Products; Safety and Efficacy Review; Additional Sunscreen Ingredients, [Docket No. 2005 N–0446], Federal Register/Vol. 70, No. 232/ Monday, December 5, 2005/Notices 72449.

25. Tuchinda C, Lim HW, Osterwalder U, Rougier A. Novel emerging sunscreen technologies. Dermatol Clinics 2006; 24:105–117.

26. Rabek JF. Photostabilization of Polymers, Principles and Applications. London: Elsevier Applied Science Publishers, 1990.

27. Gugumus F. In: Gächter R, Müller H, eds. Kunststoff-Additive. Munich, Germany: C. Hanser Verlag, 1989.

28. Waiblinger F, Fluegge AP, Keck J, Stein M, Kramer HEA, Leppard D. Irradiation-dependent equilibrium between open and closed form of UV absorbers of the 2-(2-Hydroxyphenyl)-1,3,5-triazine type. Res Chem Intermed 2001; 27:5–20.

29. Hueglin D, Herzog B, Mongiat S. Hydroxyphenyltriazines: a new generation of cosmetic UV filters with superior photoprotection. Oral presentation at 22nd IFSCC, Edinburgh, 23–26 September 2002.

30. Keck J, Roessler M, Schroeder C, et al. Ultraviolet absorbers of the 2-(2-hydroxyaryl)-1,3,5-triazine class and their methoxy derivatives: fluorescence spectroscopy and X-ray structure analysis. J Phys Chem B 1998; 102(36):6975–6985.

31. Otterstedt J-EA. Photostability and molecular structure. J Chem Phys 1973; 58(12):5716–5725.

32. Osterwalder U, Luther H, Herzog B. UV-A Protection with a new class of UV Absorber, 47. SEPAWA Kongress, Proceedings 2000; 153–164.

33. Learn DB, Sambuco CP, Forbes PD, Hoberman AM, Plautz JR, Osterwalder U. Twelve-month topical study to determine the influence of bisoctrizole (Tinosorb® M-active) on photocarcinogenesis in hairless mice. Biannual meeting, European Society of Photobiology, 3–8 September 2005.

34. Learn DB, Sambuco CP, Forbes PD, Hoberman AM, Plautz JR, Osterwalder U. Twelve-month topical study to determine the influence of bemotrizinol (Tinosorb® S) on photocarcinogenesis in hairless mice. Biannual meeting, European Society of Photobiology, 3–8 September 2005.

35. Bos JD, Meinardi MM: The 500 Dalton rule for the skin penetration of chemical compounds and drugs. Exp Dermatol 2000; 9(3):165–169.

36. Brown MW. UVA Protection, Sunscreen Conference. London: 2001, 11–12 June.

37. United States Food and Drug Administration, HHS. Sunscreen drug products for over-the-counter human use; final monograph. Final rule. Fed Regist 1999; 64(98):27, 666-27, 693.

38. Australian/New Zealand Standard™, Sunscreen products—Evaluation and classification, Originated in Australia as AS 2604—1983, Previous edition AS/NZS 2604:1997, Fifth edition 1998.

39. Maier H, Schauberger G, Brunnhofer K, Honigsmann H. Change of ultraviolet absorbance of sunscreens by exposure to solar-simulated radiation. J Invest Dermatol 2001; 117:256–262.

40. Kullavanijaya P, Lim HW. Photoprotection. J Am Acad Dermatol 2005; 52:937–958.

41. Schulze R. Einige Versuche und Bemerkungen zum Problem der handelsüblichen Lichtschutzmittel, Parfum und Kosmet 1956; 37:310.

42. Urbach F. Ultraviolet A transmission by modern sunscreens: is there a real risk? Photodermatol Photoimmunol Photomed 1992–1993; 9(6):237–241.

43. Agin PP, Cole CA, Corbet C, et al. Balancing UV-A and UV-B protection in sunscreen products: proportionality, quantitative measurement of efficacy, and clear communication to consumers. In: Shaath N, ed. Sunscreens: Regulations and Commercial Development. Cosmetic Science and Technology Series. 3rd edn. Vol. 28. Chap. 40. Boca Raton, FL: Taylor & Francis Group, 2005.

44. Cole C. Multicenter evaluation of sunscreen UVA protectiveness with the protection Factor A test method. J Am Acad Dermatol 1994; 30:729–736.

45. Chardon A, Moyal D, Horseau C. Persistent pigment-darkening response as a method for evaluation of ultraviolet A protection assays. In: Lowe NJ, Shaath, NA, Pathak MA, eds. Sunscreens: Development, Evaluation, and Regulatory Aspects. 2nd ed. New York: Marcel Dekker Inc., 1997:559–582.

46. JCIA Measurement Standard for UVA Protection Efficacy. Japan Cosmetic Industry Association—JCIA, 9-14, Toranomon 2-Chome, Minato-Ku Tokyo, 1995:105.

47. Australian/New Zealand Standard, AS/NZS 2604: 1993.

48. Osterwalder U, Baschong W, Herzog B. Broad Spectrum UV protection and its assessment. Australian Society of Cosmetic Chemists, 39th Annual Conference, Brisbane, Queensland, 17–20 March 2005.
49. Diffey BL. A method for broad spectrum classification of sunscreens. Int J Cosm Sci 1994; 16:47–52.
50. The Revised Guidelines to the Practical Measurement of UVA : UVB Ratios According to The Boots Star Rating System, The Boots CO PLC, 2004.
51. Gers-Barlag H, Wendel V, Klette E, Wolber R, Wittern KP. UVA Balance The Accurate and Skin Relevant Assessment of the UVA Protection of Sunscreens, 7th Joint ASCC NZCSS Australasian Conference Auckland, New Zealand, 2004.
52. Characterization of UVA protection of dermal suncare products by measuring the transmittance with regard to the sun protection factor, DIN 67502, Deutsches Institut für Normung e.V., Berlin, February 2005.
53. Gers-Barlag H. Harmonized in vitro UVA Method, Sunscreen Conference "2010—A Sun Odysee," London, 8/9 June 2005.
54. Commission Recommendation on Efficacy of Sunscreen Products and the Claims Made Relating Thereto. Official J Eur Union 2006; 49:39–43.
55. Herzog B, Mendrok C, Mongiat S, Mueller S, Osterwalder U. The Sunscreen simulator: a formulator's tool to predict SPF and UVA parameters. SÖFW J 2003; 129(7):25–36.
56. Ferrero L, Pissavini M, Marguerie S, Zastrow L. Efficiency of a continuous height distribution model of sunscreen film geometry to predict a realistic sun protection factor. J Cosmet Sci 2003; 54:463–481.
57. Herzog B, Müller S, Neuenschwander A, Deshayes C, Acker S, Osterwalder U. Improved Simulation of Sun Protection Factors and UVA-Parameters—A Useful Tool for the Development of Sunscreen Formulations, accepted as oral presentation at 24th IFSCC Congress, Osaka, Japan, 16–19 October 2006.
58. Ciba Specialty Chemicals, Ciba® Sunscreen Simulator, www.cibasc.com/sunscreensimulator.

20 | Novel Developments in Photoprotection: Part II

André Rougier and Sophie Seite
La Roche-Posay Pharmaceutical Laboratories, Asnières, France

Henry W. Lim
Department of Dermatology, Henry Ford Hospital, Detroit, Michigan, U.S.A.

- SPF is a reflection of UVB protection.

- No consensus has been reached on the standardized way to assess UVA protection factor (UVA-PF).

INTRODUCTION

I n vitro and in vivo studies provide a body of evidence that adequate protection of the skin against ultraviolet (UV)-induced damages requires photostable broad-spectrum sunscreens with a proper level of UVA protection. The need is not restricted to products for sunbathers for whom the main concern is acute effects of UVB. The increased use of UVA sources over the last decade in the treatment of dermatoses and in artificial tanning has resulted in the increased focus on the cutaneous damage likely to be caused by UVA radiation.

Solar radiation reaching the surface of the earth, and thereby the surface of our skin, contains infrared, visible, and UV radiation (UVR). Of major interest to dermatologists is the UVR segment of the radiation, as it is almost exclusively the cause of skin disorders arising from sun exposure. The UVR component of sunlight reaching the surface of the earth is composed of radiation with wavelengths of 280 to 400 nm and accounts for 10% of the total energy emitted by the sun.

There are three types of UVR, based on their wavelength: (*i*) UVA (320–400 nm), (*ii*) UVB (290–320 nm), and (*iii*) UVC (200–290 nm). Shorter wavelengths of radiation are more energetic and potentially more destructive than longer wavelengths. Fortunately, UVC, the shortest wavelength in the UV spectrum, is completely absorbed by the gases in the atmosphere. Therefore, UVR reaching the skin consists only of UVB and UVA (Fig. 1).

UVB is the next shortest wavelength. It reaches the earth in relatively small amounts (about 5%), but is very efficient in producing biological response. UVA is lower in energy than UVB; nevertheless, UVA is 20 times more abundant than UVB. UVA can be further subdivided into UVA1 (400–340 nm) and UVA2 (340–320 nm) (Fig. 2).

The extent of an individual's exposure to UVR varies widely depending on a multiplicity of factors, such as weather, hour of the day, season, pollution, humidity, temperature, and also geographic factors, such as altitude and latitude. These can be summarized as follows.

1. In temperate climate, the quantity of UV reaching the skin first depends on seasons: UVB exposure is much greater in summer than in winter.
2. There is greater exposure for both UVA and UVB with decreasing latitude.
3. The quantity of UVR increases by 4% every 1000 feet above sea level. Indeed, as the atmospheric layer traveled by the UVR is thinner, the filtration effect is reduced.
4. The time of the day also plays an important part: UVB is strongest between 10 AM and 4 PM, especially around mid-day, whereas UVA follows the variation of visible light.
5. Finally, several environmental factors contribute to influence UV exposure. UV can be modified according to the nature of terrain, which induces different reflection of the

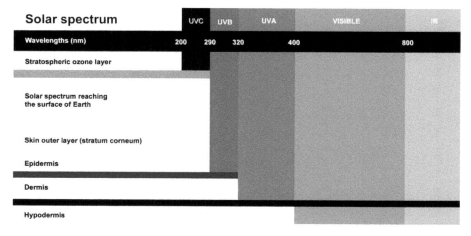

FIGURE 1 Penetration of ultraviolet into the skin.

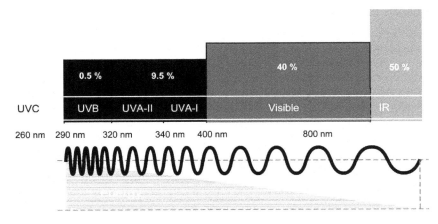

FIGURE 2 Electromagnetic radiation at the surface of the earth.

radiation. UVB is almost entirely filtered by clouds, whereas UVA is not. Glass filters UVB and UVA2, but not the longer wavelength UVA1 (1).

UVB are far more sensitive to the above factors than UVA. Consequently, there is more consistent exposure of the skin to UVA throughout the day when compared with UVB (2,3). As wavelength increases, there is a corresponding percentage increase in the depth of penetration of UVR (Fig. 1). UVB penetrates the epidermis and is almost fully absorbed in upper dermis, whereas one-quarter of the UVA reaches as far as the mid-dermis.

UVA EFFECTS

The visible damaging effects of UVA only appear after years of exposure. Thus, it has been demonstrated that UVA plays a major role in premature aging of the skin. In addition, it is now well established that UVA has a significant role in DNA damage, photoimmunosuppression, and induction of various photodermatoses. UVA is by far the most common action spectrum for drug-induced photosensitivity. In the past few years, significant advances on UVA protection has been achieved due to the development of potent UVA filters and the use of novel combination of filters (4).

EVALUATION OF SUN-PROTECTION FACTORS AND UVA-PROTECTION FACTOR

The classical approach to assess the protective efficacy of a sunscreen product is the worldwide harmonized method of the determination of sun protection factor (SPF), which is based on the evaluation of solar-simulated radiation (SSR)-induced erythema, that is, predominantly UVB-induced sunburn reaction. SPF is the ratio of UVR dose producing minimal erythema dose in sunscreen-protected versus unprotected skin area, using the product at a concentration of 2 mg/cm^2 (5). It is a reflection of predominantly the biological effect of UVB; SPF is not an assessment of UVA protection. Despite the availability of several reliable methods, no consensus has been reached in the United States and in the European Union on the method(s) to be used for assessment of UVA protection (6). At present, persistent pigment darkening (PPD) method, which evaluates the stable portion of pigment darkening of the skin following UVA irradiation, is probably the most widely used one (6,7). This method has been approved by the Japanese authorities as the official method to measure UVA protection (8).

In 2001, an in vitro UVA protection assessment method was published, which was proposed as a candidate for the future harmonized UVA protection measurement (9). The method combines the merits of in vitro as well as in vivo determinations by combining the results of in vivo SPF with in vitro UV (290–400 nm) transmission measurement.

SUNSCREEN FILTERS PHOTOSTABILITY

Photostability is the ability to resist the influence of UVR, visible light, and heat. Development of photostable sunscreens is extremely important to preserve the UV-protective capacity and to prevent the reactive intermediates of photo-unstable filter substances behaving as photo-oxidants, when coming into direct contact with the skin.

The filter that was in a lower state (ground state) turns to higher energy state (excited state) by absorbing the energy of an UV photon. From excited state, different relaxation processes may occur.

1. The excited state molecule may simply return to its ground state while releasing the absorbed energy to the environment as heat. Then the filter fully recovers its ability to absorb UVR photon again and again. This filter is considered as photostable.
2. Structural transformation or degradation may take place whereby the filter loses, more or less rapidly, its UV-absorbing capacity, and hence its protective potency. The filter is considered to be photo-unstable.
3. The excited molecule can interact with other molecules in its micro-environment, such as other ingredients contained in sunscreen product, ambient oxygen, or skin biomolecules (proteins, lipids, etc.), and thus lead to the production of undesirable reactive species. The filter is considered to be photoreactive.

Indeed, photostability is an essential requirement to protect against UVA-induced effects, such as photoaging and genotoxicity (10,11); a photo-unstable formulation is not as protective as the photostable one in the prevention of molecular events associated with photoaging and genotoxicity (12–14).

BROAD-SPECTRUM SUNSCREENS

The novel filters (4,15) of the broad-spectrum sunscreens used in the different studies presented in this chapter are the following.

UVA Filters

Terephtalylidene Dicamphor Sulfonic Acid (ecamsule, Mexoryl® SX)
It is a strong short UVA photostable absorber, which absorbs UVR between 290 and 390 nm with a peak at 345 nm (Fig. 3). Mexoryl® SX was patented by L'Oréal in 1982 and approved by the European Economic Community (EEC) in 1991.

Drometriazole Trisiloxane (silatriazole, Mexoryl® XL)
This was first introduced in the European Academy of Dermatology and Venereology meeting in 1998. It is the first broad UV filter against UVA and UVB spectrum (Fig. 4). Mexoryl® XL

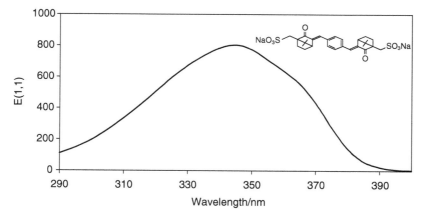

FIGURE 3   The structure and absorption spectrum of Mexoryl® SX.

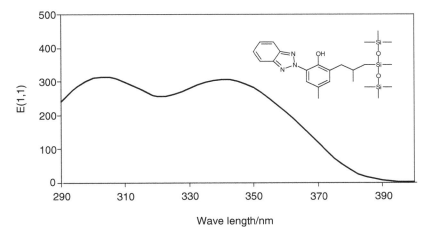

FIGURE 4 The structure and absorption spectrum of Mexoryl XL.

belongs to the photostable group of the hydroxybenzotriazole. Its structure composes of two different chemical groups: hydroxyphenylbenzotriazol, which provides photostable UVA and UVB absorption, and short siloxan chain, which provides liposolubility of the molecule. Mexoryl® XL has two absorption spectra in UVB and UVA range (290–320 nm, λ_{max} 303 nm and 320–360 nm, λ_{max} 344 nm). By combining the lipophilic Mexoryl® XL with hydrophilic Mexoryl® SX, a high level of photoprotection can be achieved (9). Since 1999, the combination of Mexoryl® SX and Mexoryl® XL has been used in the Anthélios product line of La Roche-Posay.

Butyl Methoxydibenzoylmethane (avobenzone, Parsol® 1789)
Avobenzone is a broad UVA absorber; however, its drawback is photo-instability. The photo-instability of avobenzone can be avoided by combining it with octocrylene or 4-methylbenzylidene camphor (L'Oreal patents US5576354 and US5587150). The rationale for the photostabilizing property of this combination is that in the presence of either one of these filters, there would be less photons directly affecting the avobenzone.

UVB Filters
Butyl Methoxydibenzoylmethane (Octocrylene, Uvinul 539R) and 4-Methylbenzylidene Camphor (Eusolex 6300)
These UVB filters prevent the photo-induced degradation of avobenzone, thus avoiding any loss in the long-UVA absorbing properties of the final product.

BIOLOGICAL EFFECTS OF UVA, AND UVA PROTECTION BY SUNSCREENS
Protection of Cell Nucleus

The comet assay is a simple and visual technique for measuring DNA breakage. It has been extensively used both to characterize genotoxins and to analyze DNA repair following phototoxic effects of UV (16,17).

Following UV SSR, keratinocytes whose DNA is impaired (fragmented) show a "comet shape." Comets can be observed very early after irradiation without any sign of cell toxicity. The amount of comets produced and the length of trail can be measured by image analysis and recorded. These parameters reflect the size and number of DNA fragments and thus the degree of photodamages.

When the same experiment is performed in the presence of Mexoryl® SX in the culture medium, comet induction is almost abrogated (18).

In contrast to UVB, UVA mainly impairs nuclear DNA by producing reactive oxygen species (ROS), triggering genotoxic reaction. Moreover, the comet test is more easily detected in melanocytes than in unpigmented cells; therefore, melanocytes are considered to be the target cell for UV, especially UVA radiation (19). An in vitro study of two SPF 7 sunscreens

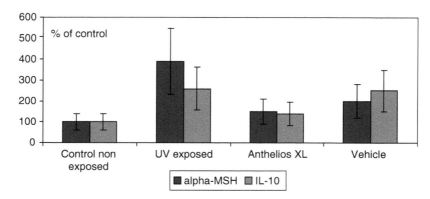

FIGURE 5 Production of α-melanocyte-stimulating hormone and interleukin-10 in skin blisters fluids 24 hours after ultraviolet irradiation. *Abbreviations*: α-MSH, α-melanocyte-stimulating hormone; UV, ultraviolet; IL-10, interleukin-10.

with different UVA protection factor (UVA-PF) (7 vs. 3, assessed by PPD method) was performed; the effect of these sunscreens on the UVA-induced genotoxicity in melocyte cell culture was assessed by the comet assay. The results showed that only the broad-spectrum sunscreen with an UVA-PF of 7 was able to prevent photo-oxidative damage (18).

It is known that increased p53 protein in nucleus of cells occurs following UV exposure. Therefore, determination of p53 accumulation can be used as a marker for detection of UV-induced cell damage and as an endpoint to evaluate sunscreen efficacy (20,21). In human subjects, sunscreen with UVA-PF of 14 was more protective in preventing the accumulation of p53 compared with sunscreen with low UVA-PF of 6, although both had the same SPF of 25.

Protection of the Immune System

It is well established that exposure to UVR can result in immunosuppression (22). Although the precise chromophore for the photoimmunosuppression is not known, urocanic acid (UCA) has been considered as a possible candidate. UCA is located in the epidermis and its peak of absorption spectrum is at 277 nm. On absorption of photons, *trans*-UCA is isomerized to *cis*-form, the latter has been implicated in UVR-induced immunosuppression and photocarcinogenesis (3).

Photoproduction of *cis*-UCA in human skin exposed to UVB + UVA radiation has been used to compare the protection of sunscreens having the same SPF of 60 but different UVA-PF (12 vs. 3) (23). Similar to the genotoxicity and p53 studies, product with higher UVA-PF was more efficient in preventing *cis*-UCA production than sunscreen with lower UVA-PF.

A high SPF and a high UVA-PF sunscreen (SPF > 60, UVA-PF 28; Anthelios XL, containing octocrylene, Mexoryl® SX, Mexoryl® XL, avobenzone, and TiO$_2$) was found to prevent the suppression of delayed type hypersensitivity response in human following six days of sun exposure (24).

In a subsequent study, the protective effect of the same broad-spectrum sunscreen on the UV-induced production of immunosuppressive mediators, interleukin-10 (IL-10), and α-melanocyte-stimulating hormone (α-MSH) was investigated in suction blister fluids (25). The results showed that IL-10 and α-MSH expressions were significantly upregulated in UV-irradiated skin both at the protein and at the mRNA level. Pretreatment with the broad-spectrum sunscreen resulted in decreased expression of both IL-10 and α-MSH (Fig. 5).

CLINICAL EFFECTS OF UVA AND PROTECTION BY SUNSCREENS
Protection Against Photosensitizations

Besides the direct actions of UVA radiation on the immune system, photosensitization reactions also occur, which can be induced by skin contact with certain compounds. Photosensitization by exogenous agents covers two large types of clinical scenarios, photoxicity and photoallergy. These two types of reaction may be differentiated according to their etiology and their clinical characteristics.

It should be noted that the vast majority of phototoxins and photoallergens have their action spectra in the UVA range (26). The phototoxins include psoralens, porphyrins, tars, antibiotics, (cyclins), and nonsteriodal anti-inflammatory substances. The photoallergens include perfumes, UV filters, agents of vegetable origin, antibiotics, and nonsteriodal anti-inflammatory substances. The most susceptible anatomical regions are, of course, those most exposed to the sun: (*i*) the ears, (*ii*) nose, (*iii*) cheeks, (*iv*) upper chest, (*v*) nape of the neck, (*vi*) lateral neck, (*vii*) extensor forearms, and (*viii*) dorsum of hands.

In a study in human subjects, a broad-spectrum sunscreen with SPF >60, UVA-PF 28 (Anthelios XL 50$^+$, containing octocrylene, Mexoryl$^®$ SX, Mexoryl$^®$ XL, avobenzone, and TiO$_2$) has been shown to be protective against UVA-induced phototoxicity in subjects taking oral doxycycline or limecycline (27). In a study presented as a poster, the same broad-spectrum sunscreen was reported to be protective against UV-induced erythema in patients using topical chlorpromazine or topical benzoyl peroxide (28). Recently, the usage of Anthelios XL 50$^+$ has also been verified for targeted skin protection in patients treated during summer by Roaccutane$^®$ caps (Roche) for cystic acne or rosacea. This experiment clearly showed that the use of a high SPF sunscreen with UVA-PF of 28, together with good co-operation of patients resulted in trouble-free treatment by systemic retinoids even in summer (29).

Protection Against Photo-Induced Dermatoses
Polymorphous Light Eruption
Polymorphous light eruption (PLE) is one of the most frequent photodermatoses with an estimated incidence of approximately 3% to 17%. Moreover, photoprovocation testing has revealed that 75% of PLE patients are sensitive to either UVB + UVA or to UVA alone (30). Photoprotection, including the use of broad-spectrum sunscreen, is an integral part of the management of PLE (31).

Three different sunscreens with high SPFs, 35, 60, and 75, but different UVA-PFs of 3 to 28, were compared for their ability to prevent the development of skin lesions in PLE patients (32). The sunscreen with SPF 50$^+$ and UVA-PF 28 (Anthelios XL 50$^+$: containing octocrylene, Mexoryl$^®$ SX, Mexoryl$^®$ XL, avobenzone, and TiO$_2$) protected the development of PLE in all patients, whereas sunscreens with high SPFs of 35, 60, and 75; but low UVA-PF values of 3 to 5 protected only 23% to 45% of the patients. In addition, effective prevention of clinically apparent skin lesions was associated with complete inhibition of UVA-induced expression of ICAM-1 mRNA. Of interest, all three tested products had avobenzone as a UVA filter. However, the one with the highest UVA-PF also had Mexoryl$^®$ SX and Mexoryl$^®$ XL, indicating that the type of UV filters used is critical for the efficacy of a given sunscreen to provide photoprotection. This observation further supports the concept that PLE represents an abnormal response of human skin towards UV, including UVA radiation that results in an increased expression of pro-inflammatory molecules such as ICAM-1.

Lupus Erythematosus
Lupus erythematosus (LE) is an autoimmune disease that is triggered and exacerbated by UVR. As a consequence, photoprotection is one of the measures in the management of these patients (33).

Eleven patients with LE were repeatedly exposed to UVA; the ability of sunscreens with high SPFs of 35 to 75 but different UVA-PF of 3 to 28 was studied. Similar to results observed in PLE, high UVA-PF 28 sunscreen (Anthelios XL 50$^+$) prevented the development of lesions in all patients, whereas those with lower UVA-PF only partially did so (34). High UVA-PF product also prevented the increased expression of ICAM-1 associated with development of lesions (34).

Solar Urticaria
Solar urticaria (SU) is a rare photosensitive disorder. Within 5 to 10 minutes of sun exposure, patients experience itching, erythema, and patchy or confluent whealing. Chronically exposed skin (face and arms) is generally less susceptible to be involved than areas normally covered. Action spectrum ranges from UVB to UVA and to visible range. Management of SU is challenging.

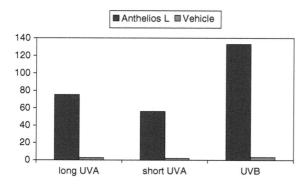

FIGURE 6 Solar urticaria protection factors (SUPFs) in each triggering spectral band [SUPF = minimal urticarial dose with sunscreen or vehicle/MUD unprotected]. *Abbreviations*: SUPF, solar urticaria protection factor; MUD, minimal urticarial dose.

The protective effect of a high SPF and high UVA-PF product (SPF 60, UVA-PF 12; Anthelios L containing Eusolex 6300, Mexoryl® SX, avobenzone, and TiO$_2$) was assessed in SU patients ($n = 10$) following 1000 W Xenon arc solar simulator exposure (35). The minimal urticarial dose (MUD) on unprotected area was determined for each patient and for each triggering spectral band (UVA1: 360 nm, UVA2: 335 nm, and UVB: 310 nm) by clinical assessment of erythema and swelling in the early minutes following each UV exposure. MUD on protected area was then measured for each triggering spectral band following application (2 mg/cm^2) of either the broad-spectrum sunscreen or its vehicle and SU protecting factor (SUPF), which was determined by dividing the MUD value obtained with the sunscreen or its vehicle by the MUD value obtained without any product. Results showed that the SUPFs of the vehicle were 2.7, 2, and 3.3, respectively, in the long UVA, short UVA, and UVB range, whereas these SUPFs were of 75, 56, and 133 on the broad-spectrum sunscreen-treated areas (Fig. 6).

Therefore, these experiments confirmed that the different parts of the UV spectrum could elicit SU. Moreover, it was found that most of the patients react to very low doses of UV, particularly in the UVA domain, confirming the extreme skin sensitivity of this photodermatosis. The results also indicate that the use of broad-spectrum sunscreens with highly efficient UV filters can be considered as an option in the management of patients with SU with action spectra in the UV range. For those with visible light sensitivity, physical agents such as opaque clothings are the only available external photoprotective measure at this time.

Melasma

Melasma or chloasma is a pigmentary disorder, which typically appears on the face and occurs most frequently in women with a skin phototype III or higher (36). Clinically, melasma is characterized by the appearance of hyperpigmentation that develops on the forehead, cheeks, and chin and is classified as medium, moderate, or severe. Melasma can develop as a result of pregnancy or taking oral contraceptives, but it can also occur spontaneously. It can affect up to 50% to 70% of pregnant women, often motivating the request for a therapeutic solution (37). It can be the result of a combination of several factors: (*i*) genetic and ethnic (determining phototype), (*ii*) hormonal, and (*iii*) environmental (exposure to UVB and UVA) (38). Treatment is difficult. Removing factors that trigger the condition, such as exposure to the sun, tanning beds, or exogenous estrogen treatments constitutes useful measures.

The effect of a high SPF and high UVA-PF sunscreen (SPF50$^+$, UVA-PF 28; Anthelios XL containing octocrylene, Mexoryl® SX, Mexoryl® XL, avobenzone and TiO$_2$) was assessed in the course of a 12-month clinical trial carried out on 200 pregnant individuals (39). The results showed that out of the 185 patients who completed the study, only five new cases of melasma were observed, that is, an occurrence of 2.7%, which is much lower than the 53% previously observed in comparable conditions and same geographical area. It is also worth noting that within six months, a clinical improvement was observed in 8 out of the 12 subjects who were affected by a pre-existing melasma that had been observed at the time of their visit for inclusion in the study.

Colorimetric measurements showed that, at the end of their pregnancy, the parturient's skin was significantly lightened (increase in parameter L^* in 38.4% of the cases) and significantly less pigmented (reduction in parameter b^* in 50.3% of the cases), thus giving a significantly lighter skin color [increase of individual tripology angle (ITA) in 68.6% of the cases] compared to their visit at the beginning of the study. These observations demonstrate the benefits of external broad-spectrum sunscreen in preventing and even improving this dermatosis.

Daily Photoprotection and Photoaging

The aging processes of the skin involve two clinically and biologically independent processes that occur simultaneously: chronological aging (intrinsic aging), which affects the skin by slow and irreversible tissue degradation, and photoaging (extrinsic aging), which results from repeated exposure to UVRs. In areas exposed to sun, skin damages resulting from photoaging are added to degenerations of tissues resulting from chronological aging. Photoaging leads to marked cutaneous alterations, clinically characterized by wrinkles, roughness, mottled dyspigmentation, telangectasia, and a variety of benign and malignant neoplasms. Both UVB and UVA have been implicated in the pathophysiology of photoaging, the former by its direct DNA-damaging effect and the latter through the generation of ROS (40).

During UVA-induced oxidative process and free radicals production, part of the energy is released in the form of photons, a process termed chemiluminescence. These photons can be detected and amplified by a photomultiplier. This allows for the quantification of oxidative stress and protection afforded by topically applied formulations. The oxidative stress induced by a single suberythemal dose of UVA (320–400 nm, 1 J/cm^2) has been assessed by means of chemiluminescence; the effect of a day cream with photoprotection (SPF 15, UVA-PF 12; Hydraphase XL, containing octocrylene, Mexoryl® SX, Mexoryl® XL, avobenzone) was evaluated (41). The results showed that the day cream leads to a decrease of about 75% and 40% of chemiluminescence when compared with untreated or placebo-treated skin. These results suggest that the use of a cream with both UVB and UVA protection can possibly prevent the deleterious effects of free radicals induced by daily exposure to suberythemal doses of UV.

Induction of matrix metalloproteinases (MMPs) following UVR exposure is known to play an important role in photoaging (40). A study was done to evaluate the effect of broad-spectrum sunscreen in this process. Buttock skin of 10 healthy subjects was exposed to 100 J/cm^2 UVA1 irradiation (340–400 nm). This dose was previously shown to induce MMP-1 expression. Application of an SPF50$^+$, UVA-PF 28 product (Anthelios XL, containing octocrylene, Mexoryl® SX, Mexoryl® XL, avobenzone, and TiO$_2$) 20 minutes prior to exposure to 100 J/cm^2 of UVA1 resulted in the suppression of UVA1-induced expression of ICAM1 and MMP-1 (Fig. 7) (42).

UVA is known to be involved in the development of pigmented skin lesions associated with skin aging. The effect of a broad-spectrum sunscreen (SPF 15, UVA-PF 12; Hydraphase XL, containing octocrylene, Mexoryl® SX, Mexoryl® XL, avobenzone) was evaluated in a bilateral comparison study, using vehicle as a control. Twenty healthy women were exposed on the neckline three times a week for three months to suberythemal doses of UVA (20, 25, and 30 J/cm^2, respectively, for the first, second, and third month). Evaluation of skin pigmentation was performed monthly by visual examination and by using a chromameter (Minolta CR 200). Clinically and following Wood's lamp examination, pigmentation was found to be more intense on the vehicle-treated side. Moreover, clinical examination of actinic lentigines indicated that the pigmentation of these lesions was not changed on the vehicle-treated side, whereas it was significantly decreased on the daily cream-protected side (Fig. 8) (43). It thus appears that the use of a day cream containing broad-spectrum filters in chronic UVA exposure conditions not only offers an efficient protection on the induction of pigmentation, but also allows a lightening of pre-existing pigmented lesions.

Broad-spectrum sunscreens containing Mexoryl® with a high SPF and UVA-PF is protective against the deleterious effects of UV light radiation in vitro and in patients with photodermatoses, and in processes associated with photoaging.

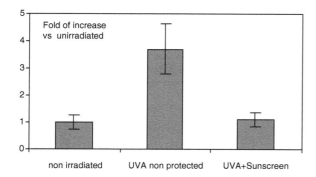

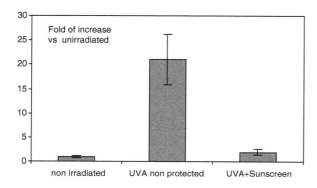

FIGURE 7 Intercellular adhesion molecule 1 (ICAM-1) and matrix metalloproteinase-1 (MMP-1) expression in skin biopsies following a single UVA-1 irradiation ($100 \, J/cm^2$) in broad-spectrum sunscreen protected and nonprotected areas.

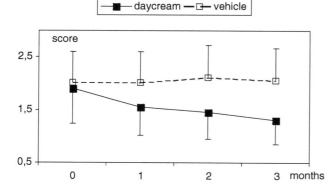

FIGURE 8 Evolution of pigmented lesions following chronic UVA irradiation on nonprotected skin and skin protected by a daily cream with photoprotection.

CONCLUSION

The ideal sun-protection product should have good UVB and UVA filters, and the filters must remain effective throughout the duration of long exposure time. Therefore, the ideal sunscreen product should thus fulfill the following criteria:

1. well tolerated
2. cosmetically pleasant
3. nontoxic or allergenic, nonphototoxic, or photoallergenic
4. equally effective against UVA and UVB
5. photostable
6. water resistant
7. high SPF.

TABLE 1 EEC Rules for Sunscreen Products Labelling

Labeled category	Labelled sun protection factor	Measured sun protection factor [measured in accordance with the principles recommended in point 10 (a)]	Recommended minimum UVA protection factor [measured in accordance with principles recommended in point 10 (b)]	Recommended minimum critical wavelength [measured in accordance with principles recommended in point 10 (c)]
Low protection	6	6–9.9	1/3 of labelled sun protection factor	370 nm
	10	10–14.9		
Medium protection	15	15–19.9		
	20	20–24.9		
	25	25–29.9		
High production	30	30–49.9		
	50	50–59.9		
Very high protection	50+	60≤		

In recent years, novel and highly efficient sunscreens that fulfill the above criteria have been developed (4). Daily practice of sensible photoprotection, including the use of broadspectrum sunscreen, should help to prevent the acute and chronic side effects of sun exposure.

According to the very recent European Commission (EEC) guidelines (44), the minimum degree of protection provided by sunscreen products should be as follows:

1. a UVB protection of SPF 6.
2. a UVA PF of 1/3 of the SPF, as obtained by the *persistent pigment darkening method* (PPD).
3. a critical wavelength of 370 nm.

The new EEC rules for sunscreen labelling are presented in Table 1.

REFERENCES

1. Tuchinda C, Srivannaboon S, Lim HW. Photoprotection by window glass, automobile glass and sunglasses. J Am Acad Dermatol 2006; 54:845–854.
2. Godar DE. UV Doses Worldwide. Photochem Photobiol 2005; 81:736–749.
3. Kullavanijaya P, Lim HW. Photoprotection. J Am Acad Dermatol 2005; 52(6):937–958.
4. Tuchinda C, Lim HW, Osterwalder U, Rougier A. Novel emerging sunscreens technologies. Dermatol Clin 2006; 24:105–117.
5. Collaborative development of a sun protection factor test method: a proposed European standard. Int J Cosm Sci 1996; 18:203–218.
6. Lim HW, Naylor M, Hönigsmann H et al. American Academy of Dermatology Consensus Conference on UVA Protection of Sunscreens: Summary and Recommendations. J Am Acad Dermatol 2001; 44:505–508.
7. Moyal D, Chardon A, Kollias N. UVA protection efficacy of sunscreens can be determined by the persistent pigment darkening (PPD) method (Part 2). Photodermatol Photoimmun Photomed 2000; 16:250–255.
8. Japan Cosmetic Industry Association (JCIA). Measurements standard for UVA protection efficacy. Tokyo, Japan, 1996.
9. Wendel V, Klette E, Wittern KP, Gers-Barlag H. A new in vitro test method to assess the UVA protection performance of sun care products. SÖFW 2001; 127:12–31.
10. Diffey BL, Stokes RP, Forestier S, Mazillier C, Richard A, Rougier A. Suncare product photostability: a key parameter for more realistic in vitro efficacy evaluation. Part I: In vitro efficacy assessment. In: Rougier A, Schaefer H, eds. Protection of the Skin Against Ultraviolet Radiations. Paris, France: John Libbey Eurotext, 1998:137–142.
11. Forestier S, Mazillier C, Richard A, Rougier A. Suncare product photostability: a key parameter for more realistic in vitro efficacy evaluation. Part II: chromatographic analysis. In: Rougier A, Schaefer H, eds. Protection of the Skin Against Ultraviolet Radiations. Paris, France: John Libbey Eurotext, 1998:143–148.
12. Gaspar LR. Evaluation of the photostability of different UV filters combinations in a sunscreen. Int J Pharm 2006; 307(2):123–128.

13. Marrot L, Belaidi JP, Meunier JR. Comet assay combined with p53 detection as a sensitive approach for DNA photoprotection assessment in vitro. Mutat Res 2005; 571(1–2):175–184.
14. Marrot L, Belaidi JP, Lejeune F, Meunier JR, Asselineau D, Bernerd. Photostability of sunscreen products influences the efficiency of protection with regard to UV-induced genotoxic or photoageing-related endpoints. Br J Dermatol 2004; 151(6):1234–1244.
15. Bouillon C. Recent advances in sun protection. J. Dermatol Sci 2000; 23(suppl 1):S57–S61.
16. Collins AR, Ai-guo M, Duthie SJ. The kinetics of repair of oxidative DNA damage (strand breaks and oxidized pyrimidines) in human cells. Mutation Res 1995; 336:69–77.
17. Alapetite C, Moustacchi E, Wachter T, Sage E. Use of alkaline comet assay to detect DNA repair deficiencies in human fibroblasts exposed to UVC, UVB, UVA, and gama rays. Int J Radiat Biol 1996; 69:359–369.
18. Fourtanier A, Bernerd F, Bouillon C. Protection of skin biological targets by different types of sunscreens. Photoderm Photoimmunol Photomed 2006; 22:22–32.
19. Marrot L, Belaidi JP, Meunier JR. The human melanocyte as a particular target for UVA radiation and an endpoint for photoprotection assessment. Photochem Photobiol 1999; 69:686–693.
20. Marrot L, Belaidi JP, Chaubo C, et al. An in vitro strategy to evaluate the phototoxicity of solar UV at the molecular and cellular level: application to photoprotection assessment. Eur J Dermatol 1998; 8:403–412.
21. Marrot L, Belaidi JP, Meunier JR. Comet assay combined with p53 detection as a sensitive approach for DNA protection assessment in vitro. Exp Dermatol 2002; 11 (suppl 1):33–36.
22. Schwarz T. Mechanism of UV induced immunosuppression. Keio J Med 2005; 54:163–171.
23. Krien P, Moyal D, Rougier A. Influence of highprotective sunscreens on the photoisomerization of urocanic acid in human skin. In: Rougier A, Schaefer H eds. Protection of the Skin Against Ultraviolet Radiations. Paris, France: John Libbey Eurotext, 1998:183–187.
24. Moyal D, Duteil C, Queille-Roussel C, Ortonne JP, Hourseau C, Rougier A. Prevention of solar induced immunosuppression by highly protective broadspectrum sunscreen. Eur J Dermatol 2002; 12:XII–XIV.
25. Schiller M, Brzoska T, Böhm M. Solar-simulated ultraviolet radiation-induced upregulation of the melanocortin-1 receptor, proopiomelanocortin, and $\propto$ -melanocyte-stimulating hormone in human epidermis in vivo. J Invest Dermatol 2004; 122:468–476.
26. Gould JW, Mercurio MG, Elmets CA. Cutaneous photosensitivity diseases induced by exogenous agents. J Am Acad Dermatol 1995; 33:551–576.
27. Duteil L, Queille-Roussel, Rougier A, Richard A, Ortonne JP. High protective effect of a broad-spectrum sunscreen against tetracycline phototoxicity. Eur J Dermatol 2002; 12:X–XI.
28. Duteil L, Quelle-Roussel C, Rougier A, Ortonne JP.High protective effect of UVA filter reinforced sunscreens against phototoxicity of chlorpromazine and benzoyl peroxide. Poster AAD annual meeting. 1998.
29. Zelenkova H, Stracenska J, Richard A, Rougier A. Protective effect of a broadspectrum UVA-UVB sunscreen in the retinoid therapy during summer season. Poster EADV Annual Meeting, 2002.
30. Hawk J, Lim HW. Photodermatoses. In: Bolognia JL, Jorizzo JL, Rapini RP, eds. Dermatology. 1st ed. London: Mosby, 2003:1365–1384.
31. Hönigsmann H. Polymorphous light eruption. In: Lim HW, Soter NA, eds. Clinical Photomedicine. New York: Marcel Dekker, 1993:167–180.
32. Stege H, Budde M, Grether-Beck S, et al. Sunscreens with high SPF values are not equivalent in protection from UVA induced polymorphous light eruption. Eur J Dermatol 2002; 12:IV–VI.
33. Costner MI, Sontheimer RD. Lupus erythematosus. In: Freedberg IM, Eisen AZ, Wolf K, Austen KF, Goldsmith LA, Katz SI, eds. Fitzpatrick's Dermatology in General Medicine. New York: McGraw-Hill, 2003:1677–1693.
34. Stege H, Budde MA, Grether-Beck S, Richard A, Rougier A, Krutmann J. Evaluation of the capacity of sunscreens to photoprotect lupus erythematosus patients by employing the photoprovocation test. Eur J Dermatol 2002; 12:VII–IX.
35. Peyron JL, Raison-Peyron N, Meynadier J, Moyal D, Rougier A, Hourseau C. Prevention of solar urticaria using a broadspectrum sunscreen and determination of solar urticaria protection factor (SUPF). In: Rougier A, Schaefer H, eds:Protection of the Skin Against Ultraviolet Radiations. Paris, France: John Libbey Eurotext, 1998:201–205.
36. Halder RM, Nandedkar MA, Neal KW. Pigmentary disorders in ethnic skin. Dermatol Clin 2003; 21:617–628.
37. Muzaffar F, Hussain J, Haroo H.S. Physiologic skin changes during pregnancy: a study of 140 cases. Int J Dermatol 1998; 37(6):429–431.
38. Perez ML. The stepwise approach to the treatment of melasma. Cutis 2005; 75(4):217–222.
39. Lahkdar H, Zouhair K, Khadir K, Essari A, Richard A, Seite S and Rougier A. Evaluation of the effectiveness of an external broad-spectrum sunscreen in the prevention of chloasma in pregnant women. JEADV. In press.
40. Chung J, Cho S, Kang S. Why does the skin age? In: Rigel DS, Weiss RA, Lim, HW, Dover JS, eds. Photoaging. New York: Marcel Dekker, Inc., 2004:1–13.

41. Rougier A, Richard A. In vivo determination of the skin protection capacity of a day-cream by means of ICL-S. Eur J Dermatol 2002; 12:XIX–XX.
42. Rougier A, Krutmann J. Unpublished data.
43. Duteil L, Queille-Roussel C, Rougier A, Richard A, Ortonne JP. Chronic UVA exposure: protective effect on skin induced pigmentation by a daily use of a day care cream containing broad band sunscreen. Eur J Dermatol 2002; 12:XVII–XVIII.
44. The Commission of the European Communities. Commission recommendation on the efficacy of sunscreen products and the claims made. Official J Eur Union 2006; 265:3943.

21 | Public Education in Photoprotection

Cheryl Rosen
Division of Dermatology, Toronto Western Hospital, University of Toronto, Toronto, Ontario, Canada

Mark Naylor
University of Oklahoma, Tulsa, Oklahoma, U.S.A.

- Public education about sun protection/skin cancer prevention is very important.

- Improvement in knowledge in sun protection/skin cancer prevention does not equal change in attitude or behavior.

- Programs should be ongoing, and include coordinated multilevel approaches that use different strategies for different target populations within the population as a whole.

- Programs need to be evaluated for their effectiveness, and adapted to improve effectiveness if possible.

- Environmental change (e.g. increased provision of shade) and policy change (e.g. at workplaces, day care centres, schools) at the community level enable an individual to change their sun protection behavior.

INTRODUCTION

Because of the etiologic relationship between sun exposure and skin cancer, a vast array of efforts have been made to increase the public's awareness of the risks of sun exposure. Programs have attempted to increase the public's knowledge about the risks of sun exposure, to modify attitudes toward tanning and prolonged sun exposure and to change sun-protective behaviors. The behaviors that are generally recommended to decrease sun exposure include limiting the time spent in the sun, particularly during times of peak ultraviolet (UV) irradiance, use of protective clothing, use of sunglasses, and seeking shade when outdoors. Use of sunscreens with both UVB and UVA coverage is also recommended.

A great deal of material has been developed and distributed to the public both on a small-scale and on a large community-wide or country-wide basis. In 1998, an issue of Clinics in Dermatology published reviews on prevention programs from many countries (1–11).

Different countries have established programs, often as collaborations between different health-related organizations. Australia, with very high rates of skin cancer, has been a leader in public education in photoprotection (12). The SunSmart program of the Cancer Council Victoria, Australia, has been named the "World Health Organization Collaborating Center for the Promotion of Sun Protection" (13).

The Centers for Disease Control and Prevention in the United States in conjunction with the United States Department of Health and Human Services had developed a program called Choose Your Cover, which was a five-year skin cancer prevention and education campaign. This program was aimed at young people and focused on having fun outdoors while using a variety of methods to protect the skin, including seeking shade, wearing clothing, sunglasses and a hat, and using sunscreen. Although this campaign has concluded, the material that was developed is available on the internet (14).

The evaluation of programs for effectiveness is very important. The Centers for Disease Control and Prevention in the United States evaluated published studies to determine which programs were supported by sufficient evidence to be recommended (15). It was determined that the only programs that had sufficient evidence to recommend them were educational and policy approaches in primary schools and in recreational or tourism sites. Studies done in primary schools and recreational or tourism sites provided sufficient evidence of improving the use of sun-protective clothing, including hats. Other behavioral endpoints were not found to have been affected in reported studies (15).

However, because there is insufficient evidence to recommend a particular strategy does not mean that the strategy has been proven to be ineffective (16). Many programs have not been evaluated. Much research remains to be done on which programs are the most effective.

Programs which have been designed and implemented in one location can be adapted for use by another area and the influence of the adapted programs on sun-protective behavior can then be evaluated. Programs can evolve based on information learned during an evaluation process.

A review paper examining primary prevention in Australia and in other countries (17) focused on the prevalence of prevention activities and not on the outcomes of these activities. The sun-protective behaviors of children, adolescents, and adults were studied. Although sunscreen use is generally not recommended as the first method of protection, it was found to be the most frequently used method in children. Hats and clothing were used much less frequently. Not surprisingly, the sun-protective behavior of children was dependent on the advice of parents. Sunscreen use was used most commonly by adolescents as well. Although adolescents may have fairly good knowledge of the need for sun protection, their behavior may not reflect this knowledge (18).

An educational program was presented to one group of students in Sweden, with another group acting as the control (18). Although the knowledge of the risks of sun exposure increased at a post-test three months after the intervention, attitudes toward sun protection and tanning did not change. These authors utilized the transtheoretical model of behavior change that has been applied in health promotion and disease prevention. It is postulated that people move through five discrete stages, from (*i*) precontemplation to (*ii*) contemplation to (*iii*) preparation to (*iv*) action, and (*v*) maintenance, when changing behavior (19). This model has also been used in other sun-protection programs (20). Another model of behavior is termed the theory of reasoned action [for review, see (21)]. Behaviors that are under volitional control are determined by intention, which is the result of the attitude toward the behavior and the subjective perception of norms surrounding the behavior. The social-cognitive theories of attitude and behavior change propose that people actively make decisions whose attitudes are based on knowledge and beliefs about the benefits and negative aspects of the particular behavior (12). Attempts to change behavior are affected by social and environmental factors. Health promotion programs are often based on theoretical models of human behavior.

Positive attitudes toward tanning continue (22) and this remains a major difficulty in changing sun-protective behavior . In Australia, attitudes towards tanning appeared to have changed in the 1990s, with a preference for a light tan or no tan, when compared with a deep tan (23). However, it later appeared that this changed attitude was becoming less popular and that further ongoing public education would be required (23). The Canadian National Survey on sun exposure and protective behaviors, conducted in 1996, revealed that 35% of adult Canadians surveyed wanted to get a tan (24). In a survey of American teenagers published in 2002, 75.3% preferred tanned skin (25).

After surveying knowledge, attitudes, and behaviors of children, adolescents, and adults, Stanton et al. (17) recommend the development of an ongoing "coordinated multilevel approach to increase sun protection that uses a range of strategies." Messages are required within the overall strategy that specifically target particular groups, such as adolescents (17). The Australian SunSmart program is an example of a comprehensive health promotion strategy, which has developed over many years.

PROGRAMS

Melia et al. (26) evaluated primary prevention programs in the U.K., particularly those studies investigating changes in behavior. Of note, the patterns of sun exposure and the lower incidence and mortality of skin cancer in the U.K. may affect the design and messages of prevention programs. Mass media programs may have increased knowledge of the risks of overexposure to the sun, but positive attitudes to tanning persisted (26). A "Suncool" program in schools which involved a booklet, a video, and other information handouts resulted in an increase in knowledge at four months, but behavior in groups of children exposed to the program did not differ from those who were not (26).

Schools

A number of programs have been developed for schools.

The Cancer Council Australia began a national program for schools in 1998. Schools that implement the sun-protection policies become accredited SunSmart schools. Accredited schools have written sun-protection policies, relating to educational curriculum, student and staff behavior, and the school environment (27). Sun protection is to be taught to students of all ages. Schools must work to increase the amount of shade available and to reschedule outdoor activities to avoid peak UV exposure times. Students are required to wear wide-brimmed hats or hats which cover the back of the neck. In 2001, the National Skin Cancer Steering Committee Secondary Schools Working Group on behalf of the Cancer Council Australia published "UV risk reduction: a planning guide for secondary schools" (28). The CDC published guidelines for school programs for skin cancer prevention (29). There are seven guidelines put forward for schools to use.

- Guideline 1: Policy development to decrease UV exposure.
- Guideline 2: Environmental change. This guideline suggests physical and social environmental conditions that support sun protection.
- Guideline 3: Education.
- Guideline 4: Family involvement.
- Guideline 5: Professional development for school administrators and teachers.
- Guideline 6: School health services.

■ Guideline 7: Periodic evaluation of whether schools are implementing and continuing to follow the guidelines.

These guidelines can be adapted to help establish sun-protection programs in a variety of settings.

Recreation Areas

Outdoor recreation areas for children and adults appear to be natural targets for sun awareness intervention. The supervisors of the facilities are able to provide educational material to the people attending the centers. People working at the facilities, such as camp counselors, lifeguards, and coaches can receive training sessions concerning sun-protection methods.

A number of programs have been carried out at swimming pools. A multicomponent intervention to reduce children's radiation (UVR) exposure during swimming classes was designed (30). Forty-eight swimming classes ($n = 169$ children, mean age = 7) were randomly assigned to either the intervention or the control condition. The six-week intervention included a UVR reduction curriculum presented at poolside by aquatics instructors and home-based activities for children and their parents. Apart from an increased use of hats, there was no difference between the control swim classes and those that received the sun protection intervention (30).

The Pool Cool program in Hawaii and Massachusetts was a randomized trial which consisted of a six-week intervention effort involving lifeguards/swimming instructors at pools in both states (31). The aquatic staff at the control group of swimming pools received instruction on injury prevention, whereas those at the intervention group of pools received education about sun protection, a curriculum to teach to their swimming students along with interactive activities for the students and their parents. Sunscreen dispensers and signs with sun-protection tips were provided and the staff received hats and sunscreen as incentives for teaching the sun-protection lessons and for completing the surveys (31). The aquatic staff in the interactive group had fewer sunburns and sun-protection policies improved significantly compared to the control group, but overall sun-protection behaviors were no different at the two groups of swimming pools. The post-test survey was at six to eight weeks. The children enrolled in these swim classes were also studied, along with their parents (32). Statistically significant increases were seen in the children's use of sunscreen, shade-seeking behavior, and "overall sun-protection habits" when compared with the control group. Parents of the involved children were also noted to have an increase in their overall sun protection habits (32). More recently, the Pool Cool program has continued to expand to more swimming pools across the United States. Strategies to best result in implementation, maintenance, and sustainability of the Pool Cool program are being studied (33).

Health Care Practitioners and Medical Students

The role of physicians, nurses, and medical students in skin cancer prevention has been studied. In 1999, Guenther and Gooderham (34) developed a program about sun protection for grade four children, to be delivered by medical students. This program is the culmination of a week of dermatology teaching to the medical students. At the end of the week of teaching, the medical students had increased their knowledge about skin cancer and sun protection, and their intent to adopt sun-protective measures increased (34). One year later, the medical students were surveyed and were found to have retained the knowledge from the previous course and had had 50% fewer sunburns during the past summer (35). However, the perception of the attractiveness of tanned skin persisted among the medical students (35). The grade four children were interviewed before, immediately after, and one month after the teaching session. An intention to increase sun-protection behaviors was noted and knowledge about sun protection increased (36). When parents were involved in the learning activities of their children, fewer children were reported to have sunburns over the summer vacation (37).

Primary care physicians do not counsel their patients concerning skin cancer prevention as frequently as they discuss other preventive measures (38). Skin cancer prevention education and counseling was performed at 2.3% of visits to American primary care physicians ($n = 439$) when compared with review of breast self-examination at 13% of visits, diet at 25.3%, nutrition at 5.7%, and tobacco at 17.9% of visits. One reason for this was thought to be a lack of knowledge of the area. For this reason, a two-hour curriculum on skin cancer prevention, counseling and screening was developed and provided to a group of physicians (39). Following this course, physicians were surveyed and found to significantly increase how often they discussed skin cancer prevention with their patients. This was confirmed by exit interviews with patients. However, this study is limited by the small number of participating physicians ($n = 22$) (39).

Workplace

Outdoor workers can be in the sun for prolonged periods of time. Complete avoidance of sun exposure is not possible due to the nature of the occupation. Policies, education, and procedures at the workplace can lead to increased sun protection. Planning to allow maximum use of available shade and use of sun-protection equipment such as protective clothing, hats with broad brims, sunscreen, and sunglasses can decrease the exposure of outdoor workers to the sun.

A randomized controlled trial investigated the effect of a week long intervention on the knowledge, attitudes, and behaviors of outdoor electrical workers in Australia (40). Twelve workplace sites were randomized to receive the intervention. The intervention consisted of an education session (a 30-minute lecture about skin cancer in Australia, the increased risk of developing skin cancer in outdoor workers, and methods of skin protection) and a skin screening session. Although the knowledge level of the intervention group increased significantly compared to the control group, and the use of sun-protective behaviors increased, attitudes (including the perceived benefit of having a tan) toward sun exposure did not change (40).

A program entitled Project SunWise was presented to the San Diego United States Postal Service. This program offered free wide brim hats, free sunscreen, reminders to use sunscreen and to wear hats as well as education on sun safety (41). Although baseline data reveal that these outdoor workers do not protect themselves well against sun exposure, the results of the intervention are not yet published (42).

An Israeli study examined a graded intensity program that led to an increase in sun protective behaviors over the 20-month study period (43). An education session stressed the risks of skin cancer related to sun exposure and methods of sun protection. The complete and partial intervention groups were given hats, sunscreens, and sunglasses. The complete intervention group had the education session repeated one year after the first session. The minimal group had only one education session eight months prior to the end of the study. At the end of the study, the two groups with greater intervention had increased their use of sunscreen (increased by 82% and 52%). There was also a decrease in the amount of sun-exposed skin in the group with the greatest intervention (43). In a follow-up study, sun-protection behavior remained higher in those employees who had received the education session (44). Regulations instituted by the employer after the initial study was finished were more effective in those who had received the education sessions (44).

A randomized trial was conducted to determine whether a sun-protection program (Go SunSmart) could be effective at high altitude skin resorts (45). Twenty-six different skin resorts were randomized to receive the program, which was comprehensive in its scope. Details of the program components are noted within the published report. A 14% reduction in the number of sunburns obtained while skiing or snowboarding during the winter of the study was found at the resorts that received the Go SunSmart program.

Community-Wide Interventions

The SafeSun Project conducted in New Hampshire was a community-wide multicomponent intervention, from 1995 until 1997, which measured children's sun-protection behavior at beaches as the outcome (46). Ten towns were randomized to receive the intervention. Schools, day-care centers, doctors' offices, and beaches were sites where sun-protective programs occurred. Children were observed at the beach in the summer of 1995 and then again in 1997. In the towns with the active intervention, the proportion of children using at least some sun protection increased significantly. Increased protection was due primarily to an increase in sunscreen use, while the use of shade and protective clothing remained low (46).

Another multicomponent, community-based study, The Falmouth Safe Skin Project, was conducted in Falmouth, Massachusetts from 1994 to 1997 (47). This study involved an advisory board from the community, with multiple target audiences including newborns and their parents and children from infancy through elementary school. Parents at hospitals after the birth of a baby, at childcare centers, at schools received information about sun protection. Children at summer camps received instruction from their counselors. Sun-protection materials were widely available. Local media was involved. Data were obtained by self-report surveys by parents. Knowledge about sun protection was increased in the community. The incidence of painful sunburns in children decreased. In children less than six years old, 18.6% had had a painful sunburn at baseline, whereas only 3.2% had a painful sunburn in 1997. The use of sunscreen increased but the use of protective clothing did not.

The Australian SunSmart program continues as an active advocate for sun protection in Australia. The 20-year review of the program provides interesting insights into the successes and difficulties of health promotion programs (12).

PUBLIC EDUCATION AND PHOTOPROTECTION

The risk of skin cancer is not uniformly the same in the population, as the risk factors for skin cancer are known to be number of nevi, blue eyes, fair hair, inability to tan, a family history of skin cancer, place of residence, and others outlined elsewhere in this book. The risk is lower for people with darker skin, but is not nonexistent. In fact, the thickness of melanoma at the time of diagnosis in blacks and Hispanic people in Florida is greater than that of white people (48). Using the California Cancer Registry as a data source, a statistically significant 1.8% increase per year in the incidence of invasive melanoma was found in Hispanic men between 1988 and 2001 (49). A similar but not significant increase was found in Hispanic women during the same time period. Tumors that were greater than 1.5 mm at the time of diagnosis increased by 11.6% per year in Hispanic men and 8.9% per year in Hispanic women (49). Melanoma is not uncommon in Californian Hispanics, occurring at a comparable incidence to Hodgkin's disease. Skin cancer prevention campaigns can address the need for different messages for different populations.

The message concerning sun protection can be delivered at several levels. An individual can be reached by their physician, their school, and their workplace. Community-based programming is received by the individual who decides whether it is a message that is important to them.

Targeting messages to a specific audience may be required for further public education programming. Research has shown that there are gender differences in the beliefs of young American adults concerning sunscreen use (21). Teenagers have been a difficult group to reach with the standard sun-protection messages (12).

Community-based intervention is not only public health messages delivered through the mass media or by pamphlets distributed at various locations. Environmental change, enabling people to more readily change their behavior, is extremely important. An example from Australia is the removal of sales tax from sun-protection products (23). Governmental and nongovernmental agencies interested in skin cancer prevention have worked toward changes in policy. Municipalities may develop shade guidelines for new or existing buildings. Tree planting and maintenance can be made municipal or school board priorities. Policies to protect outdoor workers can be put in place. By working with school boards, sun awareness and skin cancer prevention can become part of the school science or health curriculum.

RECENT CONTROVERSY

Vitamin D, which is produced in the skin by exposure of a precursor molecule to UVB radiation, has long been known to be involved in bone health and the prevention of rickets. The role of vitamin D and/or UVR in the epidemiology of a variety of diseases is being examined. For this reason, some are questioning the current sun protection messages (50). This is an issue that must be followed carefully.

REFERENCES

1. Zaitz C, Campbell I, Santos OL. Sun education in Brazil. Clin Dermatol 1998; 16(4):533–534.
2. Schulz EJ. Sun education in South Africa. Clin Dermatol 1998; 16(4): 531–533.
3. Rivers JK. Sun education in Canada. Clin Dermatol 1998; 16(4):530–531.
4. Marks R. Sun education in Australia. Clin Dermatol 1998; 16(4):528–530.
5. Kim ST. Sun education in Korea. Clin Dermatol 1998; 16(4):526–527.
6. Katsambas AD, Katoulis AC, Varotsos C. Sun education in Greece. Clin Dermatol 1998; 16(4): 525–526.
7. Graham-Brown RA. Sun education in the United Kingdom. Clin Dermatol 1998; 16(4):523–525.
8. Goihman-Yahr M. Sun education in Venezuela. Clin Dermatol 1998; 16(4):522–523.
9. George AO. Sun education in Africa: Nigeria and West African subregion. Clin Dermatol 1998; 16(4):520–521.
10. Brenner S, Wohl Y, Landau M. Sun education in Israel. Clin Dermatol 1998; 16(4):518–520.
11. Barnes L. Sun education in Ireland. Clin Dermatol 1998; 16(4):517–518.
12. Montague M, Borland R, Sinclair C. Slip! Slop! Slap! and SunSmart 1980–2000: skin cancer control and 20 years of population-based campaigning. Health Educ Behav 2001; 28(3):290–305.
13. www.sunsmart.com.au, accessed August 2006.
14. www.cdc.gov/chooseyourcover/, accessed August 2006.
15. Saraiya M, Glanz K, Briss P, et al. Preventing skin cancer: findings of the task force on community preventive services on reducing exposure to ultraviolet light. MMWR Recomm Rep 2003; 52(RR-15): 1–12.
16. Glanz K, Halpern AC, Saraiya M. Behavioral and community interventions to prevent skin cancer: what works? Arch Dermatol 2006; 142(3):356–360.
17. Stanton WR, Janda M, Baade PD, et al. Primary prevention of skin cancer: a review of sun protection in Australia and internationally. Health Promot Int 2004; 19(3):369–378.
18. Kristjansson S, Helgason AR, Mansson-Brahme E, et al. 'You and your skin': a short-duration presentation of skin cancer prevention for teenagers. Health Educ Res 2003; 18(1):88–97.
19. Prochaska JO, Velicer WF. The transtheoretical model of health behavior change. Am J Health Promot 1997; 12(1):38–48.
20. Weinstock MA, Rossi JS. The Rhode island Sun Smart Project: a scientific approach to skin cancer prevention. Clin Dermatol 1998; 16(4):411–413.
21. Abroms L, Jorgensen CM, Southwell BG, et al. Gender differences in young adults' beliefs about sunscreen use. Health Educ Behav 2003; 30(1):29–43.
22. Alberg AJ, Herbst RM, Genkinger JM, et al. Knowledge attitudes and behaviors toward skin cancer in Maryland youths. J Adolesc Health 2002; 31(4):372–377.
23. Marks R. Two decades of the public health approach to skin cancer control in Australia: why, how and where are we now? Australas J Dermatol 1999; 40(1):1–5.
24. Shoveller JA, Lovato CY, Peters L, et al. Canadian national survey on sun exposure & protective behaviours: adults at leisure. Cancer Prev Control 1998; 2(3):111–116.
25. Geller AC, Colditz G, Oliveria S, et al. Use of sunscreen, sunburning rates and tanning bed use among more than 10,000 US children and adolescents. Pediatrics 2002; 109(6):1009–1014.
26. Melia J, Pendry L, Eiser JR, et al. Evaluation of primary prevention initiatives for skin cancer: a review from a UK perspective. Br J Dermatol 2000; 143(4):701–708.
27. www.cancer.org.au, accessed August 2006.
28. National Skin Cancer Steering Committee S.S.W.G. UV Risk Reduction: A Planning Guide for Secondary School Communities. East Sydney: Cancer Council Australia, 2001.
29. Glanz K Saraiya M Wechsler H. Guidelines for school programs to prevent skin cancer. MMWR Recomm Rep 2002; 51(RR-4):1–18.
30. Mayer JA, Slymen DJ, Eckhardt L, et al. Reducing ultraviolet radiation exposure in children. Prev Med 1997; 26(4):516–522.
31. Geller AC, Glanz K, Shigaki D, et al. Impact of skin cancer prevention on outdoor aquatics staff: the Pool Cool program in Hawaii and Massachusetts. Prev Med 2001; 33(3):155–161.
32. Glanz K, Geller AC, Shigaki D, et al. A randomized trial of skin cancer prevention in aquatics settings: the Pool Cool program. Health Psychol 2002; 21(6):579–587.
33. Glanz K, Steffen A, Elliott T, et al. Diffusion of an effective skin cancer prevention program: design, theoretical foundations and first-year implementation. Health Psychol 2005; 24(5):477–487.
34. Gooderham MJ, Guenther L. Impact of a sun awareness curriculum on medical students' knowledge attitudes and behaviour. J Cutan Med Surg 1999; 3(4):182–187.

35. Liu KE, Barankin B, Howard J, et al. One-year follow-up on the impact of a sun awareness curriculum on medical students' knowledge, attitudes and behavior. J Cutan Med Surg 2001; 5(3):193–200.
36. Gooderham MJ, Guenther L. Sun and the skin: evaluation of a sun awareness program for elementary school students. J Cutan Med Surg 1999; 3(5):230–235.
37. Barankin B, Liu K, Howard J, et al. Effects of a sun protection program targeting elementary school children and their parents. J Cutan Med Surg 2001; 5(1):2–7.
38. Oliveria SA, Christos PJ, Marghoob AA, et al. Skin cancer screening and prevention in the primary care setting: national ambulatory medical care survey 1997. J Gen Intern Med 2002; 16(5):297–301.
39. Mikkilineni R, Weinstock MA, Goldstein MG, et al. The impact of the basic skin cancer triage curriculum on provider's skin cancer control practices. J Gen Intern Med 2001; 16(5):302–307.
40. Girgis A, Sanson-Fisher RW, Watson A. A workplace intervention for increasing outdoor workers' use of solar protection. Am J Public Health 1994; 84(1):77–81.
41. www.public health.sdsu.edu/communitymain/php.
42. Pichon LC, Mayer JA, Slymen DJ, et al. Ethnoracial differences among outdoor workers in key sun-safety behaviors. Am J Prev Med 2005; 28(4):374–378.
43. Azizi E, Flint P, Sadetzki S, et al. A graded work site intervention program to improve sun protection and skin cancer awareness in outdoor workers in Israel. Cancer Causes Control 2000; 11(6):513–521.
44. Shani E, Rachkovsky E, Bahar-Fuchs A, et al. The role of health education versus safety regulations in generating skin cancer preventive behavior among outdoor workers in Israel: an exploratory photo-survey. Health Promot Int 2000; 15:333–339.
45. Buller DB, Andersen PA, Walkosz BJ, et al. Randomized trial testing a worksite sun protection program in an outdoor recreation industry. Health Educ Behav 2005; 32(4):514–535.
46. Dietrich AJ, Olson AL, Sox CH, et al. Persistent increase in children's sun protection in a randomized controlled community trial. Prev Med 2000; 31(5):569–574.
47. Miller DR, Geller AC, Wood MC, et al. The Falmouth Safe Skin Project: evaluation of a community program to promote sun protection in youth. Health Educ Behav 1999; 26(3):369–384.
48. Hu S, Soza-Vento RM, Parker DF, et al. Comparison of stage at diagnosis of melanoma among Hispanic, black and white patients in Miami-Dade County Florida. Arch Dermatol 2006; 142(6): 704–708.
49. Cockburn MG, Zadnick J, Deapen D. Developing epidemic of melanoma in the Hispanic population of California. Cancer 2006; 106(5):1162–1168.
50. Lucas RM, Repacholi MH, McMichael AJ. Is the current public health message on UV exposure correct? Bull World Health Organ 2006; 84(6):485–491.

22 | Phototherapy with UVB: Broadband and Narrowband

Michael Zanolli
Division of Dermatology, Vanderbilt University Medical Center, Vanderbilt University, Nashville, Tennessee, U.S.A.

Peter M. Farr
Department of Dermatology, Royal Victoria Infirmary, Newcastle upon Tyne, England, U.K.

- UVB continues to be a vital therapeutic option for treatment of skin diseases.

- The most effective wavelength for treatment of psoriasis is within the UVB range of ultraviolet light.

- The minimal erythema dose is important to determine for the most effective and efficient use of UVB, especially with NBUVB.

- UVB effects can be enhanced with topical or systemic therapy when used in combination treatment regimens.

- Diseases other than psoriasis can be effectively treated with UVB.

INTRODUCTION

The application of ultraviolet (UV) light B for the treatment of skin diseases illustrates the application of a natural process based on observation of its beneficial effect, followed by further investigation and refinement of the delivery for practical use. The healing qualities of terrestrial sunlight have been known for centuries. Sunlight has not only therapeutic effects on inflammatory dermatosis such as psoriasis and eczematous dermatitis, especially the UVB range of the UV light spectrum, but has essential functions which are adaptive for life on our Earth.

This chapter is concerned with the application of UVB wavelengths and the medical therapeutic effect on skin conditions and diseases. The discussion will include basic photobiology of the dosage and delivery of the various modalities incorporating UVB wavelengths, and in what circumstances this therapeutic intervention may be most beneficial. It is the opinion of the authors that the delivery of UVB radiation is not some obscure undefined attempt at hopeful healing, but should be approached as delivery of a dose of radiation containing a therapeutic window and based on current photobiologic principles and insight. Previous decades have provided the basis for artificial sources of UVB to be used for medical purposes, and we should continue its advancement by applying available technology in conjunction with an enhanced insight into the photobiology of the skin and the cutaneous immune system.

SOURCES OF UVB
Different Lamp Types

Sources used for whole body UVB phototherapy are now mainly fluorescent lamps, although metal halide lamps may also be used for whole body use. Localized delivery of UVB wavelengths utilizes a xenon gas or a filamentous light source. Three broad types of fluorescent lamp are available in addition to xenon gas sources of UV light:

1. Standard broadband (BB) UVB lamps (Fig. 1). These lamps, such as the TL-12 (Philips) or FS40 (Westinghouse) are the archetypal BB lamps used for many years in phototherapy of psoriasis. They have a broad spectral emission, with a significant component (5.5%) at wavelengths less than 290 nm. With increased understanding of the wavelength-response for clearance of psoriasis and subsequent clinical trials, it is clear that these lamps are not the most efficient treatment sources currently available. Their usage is likely to be limited, and with time may become obsolete, at least for treatment of skin disorders.

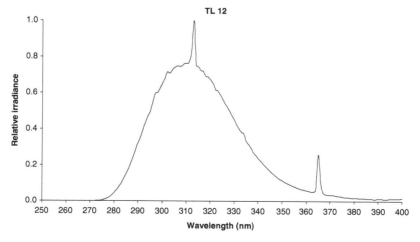

FIGURE 1   The emission spectrum of a conventional broadband UVB fluorescent lamp (TL-12).

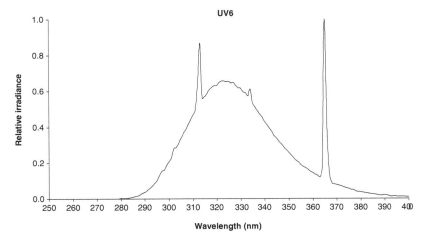

FIGURE 2 The emission spectrum of a selective broadband UVB fluorescent lamp (UV6).

2. Selective BBUVB lamps (Fig. 2) (1). These lamps, such as the UV6 (Sylvania) have been available for many years. They also have a broad spectral emission, but with a significantly smaller component (0.5%) at wavelengths less than 290 nm.
3. Narrowband (NB) UVB lamps (Fig. 3). The NBUVB lamp (TL-01, Philips) was introduced in 1988, specifically to treat psoriasis (2). Unlike conventional fluorescent lamps, it has a relatively narrow emission, with 87% at 311 ± 2 nm and only 0.1% at wavelengths less than 290 nm. The TL-01 lamp is now used widely in the United Kingdom, continental Europe, and increasingly in the United States (3,4).
4. In addition to fluorescent lamps, which allow exposure of large areas of skin, a 308 nm excimer laser has been used to treat individual plaques of psoriasis (5). Recently, nonlaser 308 nm xenon chloride lamps have been developed (6). These can achieve high irradiant values in the region of 50 mW/cm^2 over a relatively wide area of 512 cm^2.

Lamp Spectra

The lamp spectra is shown in the Figures 1–3.

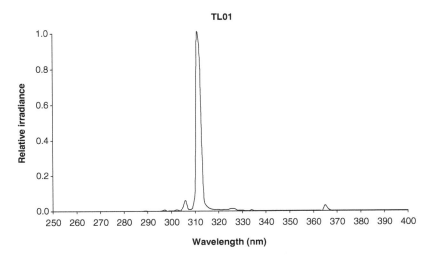

FIGURE 3 The emission spectrum of a narrowband UVB fluorescent lamp (TL-01).

UVB PHOTOTHERAPY—PSORIASIS
Action Spectrum for Clearance of Psoriasis

It is the potential for developing erythema in nonlesional skin, which limits the dose of UVB that can be used for each treatment (7), lesional psoriasis being relatively resistant to developing erythema. The erythemal sensitivity of normal skin varies considerably within the UVB waveband, and this needs to be taken into account when investigating the relative efficacy of one wavelength for treating psoriasis compared with another. It is appropriate, therefore, to compare response to different wavelengths (or lamps) using doses that are equivalent in terms of the minimal erythema dose (MED).

Although it is often stated that wavelengths around 311 to 313 nm are the most effective at clearing psoriasis, there is only limited evidence to support this assertion. In their early studies of the UV wavelengths effective in clearing psoriasis, Fischer et al. (8) examined the efficacy of discrete wavelengths from 254 to 405 nm. They demonstrated that radiation at 313 nm was effective, particularly at higher doses. However, the investigators did not compare 313 nm with other wavebands within the UVB region.

Parrish and Jaenicke (1) in their pioneering work on the action spectrum for clearance of psoriasis studied the response to different wavelengths: 254, 280, 290, 296, 300, 304, and 313 nm. They irradiated small areas of lesional skin on a daily basis, using various multiples of the MED. No clearance of psoriasis was found with wavelengths of 290 nm or less at suberythemal doses within the plaques of psoriasis. Clearance was achieved at wavelengths of between 296 and 313 nm without producing an observable erythema, with some suggestion of a better response at 313 nm. However, only four patients were studied, and they were subsequently found to have relatively treatment-resistant psoriasis.

It seems reasonable to conclude that wavelengths less than 290 nm, although highly erythemogenic, are not effective at clearing psoriasis unless marked erythema is produced at the treatment site, and that within the remainder of the UVB waveband (290–320 nm), there is as yet insufficient evidence of differential efficacy (9). This information can be used to predict the efficacy of different lamp types at treating psoriasis.

A conventional BBUVB lamp (such as the TL-12) emits 5.5% of its output at less than 290 nm, compared with around 0.5% for a selective UVB lamp (such as the UV6), and 0.1% for a NB lamp (TL-01) (4). When the lamps' spectra are weighted according to the erythema action spectrum (10), the contribution to erythema from clinically ineffective radiation <290 nm is 21.8% (TL-12), 6.9% (UV6), and 2.3% (TL-01).

A "phototherapy index," based on the Parrish and Jaenicke (1) action spectrum, gives the predicted efficacy of different lamp types at treating psoriasis (11). An index <1 indicated that doses greater than the MED would be required to clear psoriasis, whereas an index >1 indicated that clearance could be achieved with suberythemal doses. For minimal erythema treatment doses, the calculated phototherapy indices were 0.6 (conventional BB), 1.3 (selective BB) and 1.5 (NB) (11).

Minimal Erythema Dose

The MED is the designation for the production of pink erythema in response to delivery of UV light. The utility of determining the MED is generally under-realized by those physicians who treat patients having an inflammatory skin disease with any of the forms of UVB. Various wavelengths of the UV light spectrum can produce erythema, and the wavelengths most efficient at producing erythema are in the UVC range. UVA can also produce erythema if given at high enough doses.

The determination of the MED from UVB wavelengths, whether BB or NB, has the most therapeutic significance when incorporated into protocols that base dosing of UVB on the MED. It is important to recognize that the skin does not have to turn pink or red to have a therapeutic benefit from UVB phototherapy (12). It has been a longstanding observation, however, that production of erythema within a plaque of psoriasis from any wavelength may cause a clearing of the inflammatory skin disease (1). As a balance between the therapeutic benefit and side effects of UV light, the best dose for whole body treatment should be below the

TABLE 1 Suggested Dosage for UVB Minimal Erythema Dose

	Skin types I–III	Skin types IV–VI
A.	20 mJ/cm^2	40 mJ/cm^2
B.	30 mJ/cm^2	50 mJ/cm^2
C.	40 mJ/cm^2	60 mJ/cm^2
D.	50 mJ/cm^2	70 mJ/cm^2
E.	60 mJ/cm^2	80 mJ/cm^2
F.	80 mJ/cm^2	100 mJ/cm^2

burning threshold to reduce unwanted symptoms, but be aggressive enough to limit the number of treatments and increase the efficacy.

The determination of a MED is dependent upon proper dosimetry of the phototherapy device and wavelength used. The measurement of the dose must be matched to the wavelength because if a photometer has optics designed for a broad spectrum of UVB, it will give an inaccurate reading if applied to a set of lamps used to deliver NBUVB. The measurement of the MED actually determines the dose–response to the UVB light delivered. The desired end point is pink erythema with discernable edges. Table 1 provides the parameters for delivery of graduated doses for BBUVB, whereas Table 2 provides the parameters for NBUVB doses. The location of the body for testing of the MED should be the lateral hip or upper buttocks areas. The MED will vary on different areas of the body if UVB hardening has occurred on the forearm or sun-exposed areas, thus over-estimating the effects on more sun-protected regions of the skin (13). The real benefit of having a known dose of BBUVB or NBUVB producing erythema is to more accurately estimate the dose with the least risk of a sunburn reaction. This will allow the selection of a more accurate dose with the best therapeutic response for delivery of whole body UVB or NBUVB, with fluorescent lamps and with localized delivery of UVB to the affected skin.

Application of localized doses of UV to selected sites of involvement has been used more frequently due to the availability of systems such as the excimer laser or high-fluence UVB limited wavelength delivery. The MED is an essential part of the determination of dose since the protocols developed thus far for targeted UVB treatment of inflammatory skin disease depends upon using multiples of the MED to the site of active disease, most commonly psoriasis (14). By utilizing the MED, the clinician has at least a defined parameter to proceed with the treatment. Further refinement of the selection of the best dose for targeted therapy of psoriasis will depend on more experience and dose–response prospective studies. Currently, a multiple of four to six times the MED is used for the extremities and a multiple of two to four times the MED is used for plaques of psoriasis on the trunk.

Treatment Regimens

Whole Body Treatment of Psoriasis (Table 3)

The application of UVB therapy is most often utilized for psoriasis. The treatment protocols for other inflammatory skin diseases differ from psoriasis, and are addressed in a separate section of this chapter. UVB has been a central part of treatment of psoriasis since the use of hot quartz lamp in early Goeckerman and Ingram therapy (15,16). The hot quartz lamp has a discontinuous emissions spectrum and high potential for sunburn reactions. Both treatment regimens

TABLE 2 Suggested Dosage for Narrowband-UVB Minimal Erythema Dose

	Skin types I–III	Skin types IV–VI
A.	200 mJ/cm^2	600 mJ/cm^2
B.	400 mJ/cm^2	800 mJ/cm^2
C.	600 mJ/cm^2	1000 mJ/cm^2
D.	800 mJ/cm^2	1200 mJ/cm^2
E.	1000 mJ/cm^2	1400 mJ/cm^2
F.	1200 mJ/cm^2	1600 mJ/cm^2

TABLE 3 Whole Body Approach to UVB Treatment of Psoriasis
(Broadband and Narrowband)

General principles for UVB total body treatment for psoriasis
   MED versus Fitzpatrick skin type to determine starting dose
   Starting dose of 50–70% of MED
   Frequency of 3 or 4 times/wk
   Increase the dose by 10–25% of the MED each treatment
   Modification of the dose dependent upon clinical response

Abbreviation: MED, minimal erythema dose.

were very effective and produced long remissions when done properly and to the point of clearing.

The main problems associated with the two previous therapies are the intensive specialized nursing time and the duration of the daily treatments. These are best delivered in a Dermatology inpatient hospital service with seven day a week therapy. Very few centers are able to deliver true Goeckerman or Ingram therapies, and they have been modified to be more convenient and more conducive to outpatient therapy. Modification of the treatment regimens occurred with the advancement of the delivery of UVB with fluorescent lamps and moved to the outpatient setting or Day Care Center (17). Nonetheless, daily treatment is the best approach, but the time off required from work and/or away from family, coupled with the excessive expense of the treatment, led to a decline in its utilization. In the 1980s and 1990s, more and more emphasis was placed on office-based delivery of UV therapy including photochemotherapy with psoralen and UVA light (PUVA).

The next step in advancement of UVB treatment of psoriasis has been the advent of a reduced potential for erythema, which was the most frequent limiting side effect for completion of a course of treatment. The use of lamps with emissions in an NB wavelength helped maximize the therapeutic effects of UVB, although not containing a significant amount of wavelengths less than 300 nm, which will cause a phototoxic effect on the skin due to direct immediate injury. The uses of lamps or devices, which have either NB or limited wavelengths within the UVB region, are the current UV treatment of choice for psoriasis in an office setting. BBUVB can be used very effectively and is still very prevalent in the United States as the treatment modality for physicians who have had the availability of UVB equipment prior to the year 2000. Currently, however, the great majority of UVB treatment devices being sold to Dermatologists are NBUVB, at least in North America (personal survey of UVB device manufacturers in 2005).

There are actually very few accepted protocols for treatment of psoriasis, whether with BBUVB or NBUVB. The one variable that can be utilized and at least gives an anchoring data point is the MED. The most accurate and reliable protocols for delivery of UVB depend on obtaining a MED prior to therapy. The initial dose of UVB light can then be determined. Subsequent doses of UV light are most commonly calculated as an increase based on a percentage of the initial MED. The alternative is to estimate a safe starting dose of UVB based on the Fitzpatrick skin type (18).

An example of the use of the MED as a starting point with a conservative protocol is: if a patient has a determination of an MED for NBUVB at 600 mj/cm^2, the first dose may be 300 mj/cm^2 or 50% of the MED. A common factor by which to increase the dose is 10% of the MED. This simple calculation by the phototherapy technician would yield a second dose of $300 + 60 = 360$ mj/cm^2. The third dose, if no redness occurs over a two-day time span, would be $360 + 60 = 420$ mj/cm^2. Please note that due to the wider spectrum of the BBUVB lamp and the dosimetry used to measure the flux of the lamp, the dosages for BBUVB are dramatically different than for NBUVB.

The frequency of treatments is another variable parameter at different phototherapy centers. In general, the frequency of the traditional BBUVB treatment is five times per week. The advent of NBUVB has brought with it attempts to make this mode of therapy as accessible as possible. Studies comparing treatment rates of five times per week versus three times per week demonstrated a slight difference, but it was not statistically significant (19). This information, coupled with the attempt to minimize travel and time away from work, have led many centers to schedule NBUVB treatments three times per week. It should be noted that less than three times per week usually does not bring about the induction of a sufficient initial response or progressive clearing and the treatment series would be inadequate. In general, the frequency of treatment using NBUVB is either three or four times per week (scheduled Monday, Wednesday, Friday or Monday, Tuesday, Thursday, Friday).

A third major consideration of a regimen for treatment with either BBUVB or NBUVB is the monitoring of the progress by the phototherapy technician and the physician. Progress should be apparent from the first week onward. If the treatment's aggressiveness is too modest, no improvement will be appreciated and an increase in the dose increment should be implemented. Conversely, modification of the advancement of the dose or even a reduction of the dose should occur, if the patient displays redness or reports redness between treatments. If a patient is still red 48 hours following the previous treatment, whether from BBUVB or NBUVB, the treatment should be postponed and the patient re-evaluated in 24 to 48 hours. The need for monitoring of the patient and adjustment of the treatment schedules point toward the invaluable function of the phototherapy technician and the benefits of having the phototherapy center within or in close proximity to the general clinic or a location easily accessible by the clinician.

With any sort of longitudinal treatment regimens, such as treatments with UVB, a treatment flow sheet is essential for documentation and determination of the next dose. Documents such as consent forms, flow sheets, guidelines for treatment schedules, and dosage of either BBUVB or NBUVB are available in a manual and can be modified by the attending physician, depending on the individual response of each patient (18).

Localized UVB Treatment for Psoriasis (Table 4)

The use of NBUVB for total body treatment has been an advancement for outpatient phototherapy for psoriasis. Application of existing technology in the form of the excimer laser at 308 nm for the localized treatment of psoriasis was used and found to be beneficial (5,14). There are major differences in the treatment with localized UVB to the areas of psoriasis as compared to the whole body UVB treatment. The most important of which is the dosing schedule being adapted for use and undergoing development over the past few years (20). The overall approach is for high dose localized treatment limited to the areas of resistant psoriasis. This treatment schedule is dependent upon obtaining the MED for the wavelength and delivery system used. There are still clinical modifications necessary to have determination of the best multiple of the MED for which area of the body, but the extremities tolerate four to six times the MED within plaques of psoriasis with some crusting and blistering to be expected. The benefit of just treating the resistant psoriasis is to spare the clinically uninvolved skin the dose of the UV light and thus the potential for long-term UVB injury. Other more recent devices have been developed for treatment of localized areas in addition to the laser light, such as a xenon gas light source emitting light at 308 nm, but with asynchronous light and a filamentous light source with a spectrum of UVB from 300 to 320 nm as the peak emission. The spot size for the laser delivery of UVB light is small at 1.8 cm^2 as is the device with the filamentous light source manufactured by Theralight^{TM}. The hand held Excelite^{TM} system has variable sized ports up to 8 cm^2, which has more utility in certain circumstances. Due to the high doses used and the therapeutic effects on the psoriasis skin, the average treatment course of localized UVB consists of 6 to 10 treatments. Prospective studies regarding the use

TABLE 4 Localized Approach to UVB Treatment of Psoriasis

General Principles for UVB Localized Treatment of Psoriasis
  MED necessary
  Multiples of the MED used for treatment
  Fewer treatments needed
  Local side effects expected
  Frequency of once or twice a week
  Modification of the dose dependent upon clinical response

Abbreviation: MED, minimal erythema dose.

of high dose localized UVB have reported fewer number of treatments and longer remission times than with conventional total body NBUVB therapy (21).

Acute

The most obvious potential side effect of UVB phototherapy is the development of erythema or "sunburn." A degree of erythema is to be expected from time to time during a course of phototherapy, as treatment regimes frequently employ dose increments until erythema is achieved. The dose–response curve for erythema is steep and appears identical for both BB and NBUVB lamps (22); a risk of unpleasant burning is apparent at doses greater than the MED. The time-course of erythema is also identical for NB and BB lamps, peaking at around 12 hours. There is no published evidence to support the stated view that NB lamps have less burning potential than other sources. Because of the time-course of UVB erythema, treatments are not normally given more frequently than once daily.

A curious but infrequent side effect of NBUVB phototherapy of psoriasis is lesional blistering. The blisters are painful, often multiple, and not necessarily associated with erythema. It has been suggested that they may be due to excessive apoptosis induced by UVB within the plaque of psoriasis (23). An in depth discussion of the acute effects of UV radiation on the skin can be found in chapter 6 of this textbook.

Risk of Skin Malignancy With UVB Phototherapy

Although an increased risk of skin malignancy, particularly nonmelanoma skin cancer is predicted with UVB phototherapy, epidemiologic studies to date have failed to show any consistent significant risk (24). This may be due partly to the small size of the study populations and often relatively short follow-up. However, another factor may be that the BBUVB lamps available at the time of these studies were of insufficient efficacy to be used repeatedly as monotherapy for large numbers of patients and, therefore, cumulative UVB doses have remained relatively small. With the development of more effective sources, particularly NBUVB lamps, phototherapy is increasingly being used as a first-line treatment for patients with moderate psoriasis, and individual patients are likely, as was the case with PUVA, to have repeated courses of treatment and accumulate high lifetime UVB doses. A further point of concern is the possibility that NBUVB lamps may be more carcinogenic than the BB lamps they have largely replaced. Young (25) summarized data from murine studies (26–28) as indicating that NBUVB may be two to three times more carcinogenic per MED than BBUVB. It was suggested (25) that any increased cancer risk would be negated by the increased efficacy of NBUVB. However, although clinical trials have shown that NBUVB is more effective than BBUVB, the actual differences in response to treatment are relatively small. Therefore, the relative risk of NBUVB phototherapy compared to BB will remain uncertain until long-term follow-up studies become available, as was the case with psoralen photochemotherapy (29). Presently available follow-up data (30,31) is of too short duration to be definitive.

Another method of predicting risks of nonmelanoma skin cancer from UVB phototherapy is to extrapolate from murine phototumorigenesis models. Diffey (32) has estimated that eight annual whole body treatment courses, each of 25 exposures, would increase the relative risk of skin cancer compared with a nontreated individual by a factor of 1.2. This model presents an estimate of average risk that will clearly be modified by skin type and other susceptibility factors, and makes an assumption that TL-01 radiation is no more carcinogenic than sunlight for the same erythemal exposure. Nevertheless, in the absence of epidemiologic data, this sort of modeling may allow explanation to patients of potential risks of repeated courses of phototherapy.

Topical

The combination of topical therapies used in the treatment of psoriasis and UVB is so common, it is considered routine. Insight must be utilized, however, because the chemical composition of certain topical agents may either alter the effects of the dose of UVB on the skin, or the chemicals in the topical agent may be altered. The most salient example of a common topical chemical used in the treatment of psoriasis and alteration of the dose of UVB is salicylic acid. It is common for a patient to use some sort of keratolytic agent to reduce scale thickness overlying plaques of psoriasis. The use of a lotion or cream containing salicylic acid may be unknown to the phototherapist or clinician, unless specifically inquired about. The problem with concomitant use of salicylic acid and UVB is its significant photoabsorbant properties in the UVB spectrum. Salicyclic acid has been used just for this property in some sunscreens. Thus, the amount of UVB, whether BBUVB or NBUVB, actually reaching the epidermis would be much lower than the delivered dose. The result would be an inadequate response due to under treatment, or a variable response from one treatment to another depending upon the presence of the topical lotion on any particular day. Unexpected phototoxic reactions may occur in that instance. The problem can be avoided if the salicyclic acid is applied after the delivery of UVB.

Topical therapy immediately preceding the delivery of UVB should be consistent, and used to enhance the therapeutic effect by promoting better penetration of the UV radiation into the skin or by the combination of a different therapeutic effect of the topical medications. As part of the standard protocol for delivery of UVB light in a referral center or a practitioner's office, a petroleum-based topical agent should be used prior to treatment on the area of psoriasis. Simple mineral oil will suffice and does not have additives that may alter the desired effects. The purpose for standard use of mineral oil is to help decrease the air-keratin interfaces through which the light must travel prior to entering the stratum granulosum and then the lower epidermis. This is especially important for treatment of psoriatic plaques having the appearance of a white micaceous scale on their surface. Each time light passes from the air and hits the surface of the keratin of a scale, a small portion of that light is reflected leaving less energy to penetrate the skin. Saturating the top layer of the plaque of psoriasis with mineral oil, or other petrolatum product, will reduce this reflectance and thereby increase the percentage of delivered light that will actually reach the site of action.

Traditionally, the combination of UVB with tar and anthralin under occlusion has been used with great success for treating psoriasis. The Goeckerman therapy uses crude coal tar from 2% to 5%, and the Ingram method uses increasing concentrations of anthralin paste over the plaques of psoriasis in combination with UVB. These two treatments have been mentioned earlier in the chapter and require specialized facilities and using care to execute (22).

The main categories of other topical psoriasis therapy can all be used in conjunction with UVB phototherapy. They are: corticosteroids, topical calcipotriene, topical retinoids, and topical calcineurin inhibitors. The basic principles of combining a topical agent with UVB apply to all these classes of medication. If the mechanism of action of any of the topical agents can help promote less scaling and a thinning of the plaque of psoriasis, the induction and effect of the UVB will be enhanced.

Certain combinations of topical therapy with UVB are worth special comment. Calcipotriene can cause an alteration in the MED (33) and should not be used immediately prior to UV therapy. However, the combination of calcipotriene twice a day with only two days of UVB per week were equal to the treatment with UVB alone three days per week (34). Likewise, the topical retinoid tazaratene, when used with UVB, was more effective in a shorter time period and using a lower total dose than UVB treatment alone or UVB plus the vehicle of the gel used for tazorotene (35). Recently, application of the topical anti-inflammatory calcineurin inhibitors for treatment of specialized locations, such as eyelids and body folds, has become more prevalent. Small body surface areas (BSAs) and limited use in areas not routinely exposed to UV light would be the most prudent course of utilization due to in vitro cell culture inhibition of UV-induced DNA repair (36). Widespread and large BSA use of these agents in combination with UVB needs further investigation.

Systemic

Patient selection is important when considering the combination of a systemic agent and the various modalities of therapeutic UVB. Various systemic agents effective for psoriasis treatment have appreciable immunosuppressive effects, which have to be considered when adding another form of therapy with known direct effects on the skin's immune mechanisms and a potential increased risk of skin cancers. Of course, these effects and resultant changes in the balance of the cytokine environment are some of the primary reasons for the effects when treating a patient with psoriasis vulgaris. Specifically, patients who require suppression of their immune regulation because of organ transplantation have a higher incidence of skin cancer formation and UVB needs to be used with caution. Patients who have an increased risk of developing skin cancer, such as long-term PUVA patients or individuals with a history of multiple nonmelanoma skin malignancies, should not have the combination of cyclosporine and UVB. Even if caution is warranted, there are systemic agents used in combination with UVB, which enhance the overall response and may help to reduce the overall total dose and number of treatments necessary for adequate response.

The combination therapy with the most evidence of an enhanced therapeutic effect is systemic retinoid plus UVB light (37–39). To maximize the effectiveness of this combination treatment, the systemic retinoid should be initiated two weeks prior to the start of UVB treatment. This allows the retinoid to have effects on the psoriatic plaques, including a decrease in the thickness and a decrease in surface scaling (40). This combination has comparable efficacy, although demonstrating a reduction in the number of UVB treatments and total dose of irradiation required when compared to UVB alone. The systemic retinoid may be added to a treatment course already in progress, but a reduction or holding of the UVB dose should be established for two weeks while the retinoid effect on the skin is realized. This caution is recommended to avoid unexpected phototoxic reactions after the addition of the retinoid. When used in combination with UVB, the dose of the retinoid may be reduced as compared to a monotherapy dose schedule (41).

UVB can be combined with other systemic agents, including the new generation of protein and antibody immune modifiers. However, well-controlled long-term data for the use of this particular combination are not yet available. In contrast, the success of using the combination of methotrexate and UVB has been established (42). An uncommon potential problem with the use of methotrexate and UVB is a severe reaction to a phototoxic side effect in a patient who has had a previous sunburn or redness from UVB or sunlight. Cyclosporin is a very effective agent as a monotherapy and has been used to help decrease the activity of psoriasis as a short-term agent followed by maintenance with UVB modalities (43). Long-term use of this combination has a high theoretical risk of a marked increased incidence of nonmelanoma skin cancer with UVB and a reported increased risk with PUVA (44).

Home UVB

The utilization of home delivery of UVB therapy, particularly NBUVB is increasing. Two important parameters must be kept in mind when considering the option of home light therapy. First, UVB home units are not designed for tanning. A home unit for treatment of psoriasis and other inflammatory skin diseases is a medical device only available by prescription. There exists misconceptions by some physicians on the general nature of UV delivery systems, and tanning parlor operators may at times misrepresent the efficacy of the UVA units they use for tanning and make claims for treatment of skin diseases. A home UVB device should be used as medical device for treatment of skin disease under the supervision of a Dermatologist.

Secondly, patient selection is vitally important for the best results and to decrease the potential misuse of the home unit. Not every patient is a good candidate for home UVB therapy just as not every patient should receive a TNF alpha inhibitor for treatment of psoriasis. Characteristics most consistent with the proper use and prescription of home units for patients with psoriasis are compliance, demonstrated efficacy to BBUVB or NBUVB previously, and no relative contraindications for use of UVB whether in the office or home. Those patients selected for home UVB therapy need to be able to follow the instructions given to them by the physician and/or phototherapy technician. It is also preferable to require such patients to keep a log of the treatments as is done in an office or treatment center.

Even though a thoughtful process should be undertaken when considering a patient for home phototherapy, many patients prefer the convenience and time-saving aspects of a home unit (45). With the advent of home unit utilization and the NBUVB wavelengths used in the Tl-01 Lamp, a pilot study of a relatively small number of subjects had good results and was compliant with the protocols (46). There is a need, however, to further explore the degree of actual compliance and effectiveness of home NBUVB when not delivered by trained personnel (47).

The notion that the use of commercial tanning parlors could be used for patients when travel and time to the office or center is inconvenient or not possible has been entertained. Tanning lamps with 99.3% of UVA output do not show any statistical benefit over a control of commercial florescent lamps for home or office use (48). Even with the application of tanning lamps with 4.7% of UVB, which has some therapeutic effect on psoriasis, the variability and inconsistency of the delivery and monitoring of the output of lamps make the use of tanning facilities substandard as a medical treatment (49).

Treatment regimens associated with home NBUVB therapy have not been standardized. As a practical matter, the measurement of MED and treatment based on the MED is not feasible. Therefore, assignment of a Fitzpatrick skin type and calculation of a starting dose based on the irradiance of the unit (easily obtained from the manufacturer) is the usual approach to the protocol. Maintenance of therapy is dependent upon the judgment of the clinician and can be done during the winter months at once a week frequency. A vacation from treatment with artificial sources of UVB is usually given during the summer months.

UVB PHOTOTHERAPY—OTHER DISORDERS

The application of UVB phototherapy for other skin diseases and conditions has been a natural development and extension of the use of phototherapy for psoriasis. The observation of the efficacy for selected diseases, and in some cases prospective clinical trials, has been the basis for considering UVB phototherapy as an accepted practice and therapeutic option. The case studies and isolated reports of the beneficial effects for a particular inflammatory skin disorder or a T-cell proliferative diseases are many. The degree of prospective controlled trials regarding diseases other than psoriasis are few compared to the list of diseases reported as responding to UVB phototherapy. The advent of NBUVB over the past 10 years can serve as a model for how reporting of studies and experiences lead to the induction of a therapy into the accepted practice of dermatology. Hundreds of reports relating the application of NBUVB to other dermatoses have been critically reviewed (50). Less than five percent of the reviewed articles met the stringent criteria of a consistent adequate protocol with a sample size and control group incorporated into the experience enabling interpretation of the reported results with a high degree of confidence. Part of this dilemma is the frequency of the diseases being treated with UVB does not provide a large sample size or an adequate cohorts of patients able to participate in a prospective study. Thus, many of the reports on efficacy are of a small sample size and accumulated over time rather than a coordinated clinical trial.

There is a definite list of skin disorders, which have both the common experience and consistently favorable response coupled with reliable data to form a basis for treatment with UVB therapy, whether BBUVB or NBUVB (Table 5). Other inflammatory disorders certainly can have a favorable response to treatment with UVB, but the implementation of a treatment plan depends upon the individual established protocols extrapolated from other

TABLE 5   List of UVB Responsive Dermatosis

Atopic Dermatitis
Vitiligo
CTCL
PMLE
Pruritus
Other
Lichen Planus
Granuloma Annulare
Acquired Perforating Disorders
Urticaria

Abbreviations: CTCL, cutaneous T cell lymphoma; PMLE, polymorphous light eruption.

diseases or from personal experience. In general, the application of UVB for disorders other than psoriasis is based upon suberythemogenic doses of BB or NB UVB. Progression and frequency of the treatment are based upon the clinical response and a physician's previous experience for the less frequently treated disorders. Short discussion regarding the application of UVB therapy to diseases with the strongest foundation of evidence and experience follow.

Atopic Dermatitis (Atopic Eczema)

Use of UVB therapy for atopic dermatitis can be a very helpful addition to the treatment approach (51). Phototherapy treatment is especially relevant to those children and adolescents who have been maintained on topical corticosteroids with a high degree of BSA involvement. One of the difficulties relevant to the treatment of atopic dermatitis with broad-spectrum UVB lamps is the inclusion of more erythemogenic wavelengths below 300 nm. There is a variable response to low wavelength UVB on the skin of atopic patients, which may result in uneven erythema. The erythema and/or smarting reaction is a common concern and a limiting factor for treatment with BBUVB. Open prospective studies (52,53) showed improvement of eczema with NBUVB, and this was confirmed in a randomized trial comparing NBUVB, BBUVA, and "placebo" visible light (54). The treatment protocol for atopic dermatitis treated with NBUVB is usually twice a week, but up to three times a week can be done. Treatment protocols adopted at various centers are generally based upon selection of the Fitzpatrick skin type. Precautions and concerns are necessary to help modify the occurrence of other acute side effects of UVB therapy, such as provocation of herpes simplex in an atopic individual. Other forms of phototherapy, including UVA1, may also be used to treat eczema effectively (see Chapter 23) (55).

Vitiligo

Vitiligo was the most frequently NBUVB treated disease, excluding psoriasis, reported in a review of the experience of a major U.S. phototherapy referral center (56). Many types of phototherapy have been used to treat vitiligo, such as PUVA, topical PUVA, BBUVB, and NBUVB (57). The application of UVB therapeutic modalities remain a mainstay of treatment due to their simplicity and recently the additional availability of localized delivery systems to treat the affected areas of depigmentation (58). The localized delivery systems have the advantage of only treating diseased skin and also offers less potential for development of acute and long-term side effects. A bilateral comparison trial showed a clear therapeutic benefit of the use of standard delivery of NBUVB versus the control side (59,60). A critical review of the reports for treatment of vitiligo with phototherapy options in comparison trials concluded the efficacy, benefit/risk profile, and cost of NBUVB made it the primary choice for photo (chemo)therapeutic options for the disease (50).

The approach to treatment with NBUVB for vitiligo is to treat the patient as if they had type I Fitzpatrick response to UV. Therapy is usually two to three times weekly with initiation of the dose at either 50% to 70% of the average NBUVB MED for type I skin, which is reported as 400 mj/cm^2 (61). The usual number of treatments as compared to atopic dermatitis is high and the treatment course may last years as long as there is continued gradual improvement.

Cutaneous T Cell Lymphoma

Phototherapy of various modalities has been used to treat early stage cutaneous T cell lymphoma (CTCL) with good response. PUVA therapy has been used with high rates of clearance for early stage CTCL (62). More recent investigations and experience helps define the role of NBUVB for treatment of stage IA and IB CTCL specifically (63). Comparison trials of the use of psoralen combined with UVB and NBUVB versus NBUVB alone have been done to add insight into the patient selection and therapeutic response for early stage CTCL (64).

The duration of remission is an important concern for any modality of treatment for CTCL. The induction of a remission whether partial or complete can be obtained with phototherapy in stages IA, IB, and in IIA in the majority of the cases. The maintenance of response has been associated with the use of PUVA as the best modality of phototherapy, but now there is more experience with the use of NBUVB. Longer termed longitudinal studies are needed for confidence in the maintenance of the response.

Polymorphous Light Eruption

UV light has been utilized to treat various forms of photosensitivity disorders, including polymorphous light eruption (PMLE) (65). The approach to treatment of PMLE with UVB has been to gradually increase a suberythemogenic dose to induce a tolerance to UVB, prior to the spring and summer seasons. This approach is termed hardening and helps permit normal amounts of natural sunlight with less activation of the PMLE in affected individuals. A prospective comparison trial of PUVA versus NBUVB in individuals with PMLE showed both to be highly effective in preventing symptoms of the disease (66). The optimal approach to treatment of PMLE with UVB requires the determination of an MED to start treatment at a tolerable dose of UVB between 50% and 70% of the MED, followed by gradual increase of 10% of the MED or as tolerated by the patient.

Pruritus

Pruritus can be induced as a sign of internal disease or as an associated symptom of an inflammatory skin disease. Examples of pruritus as a symptom of a skin disease include atopic dermatitis, contact dermatitis, lichen planus, psoriasis, among many others. The use of UVB light in this type of circumstance is directed at treatment of the underlying dermatologic disease. Treatment of pruritus related as a symptom of chronic renal failure, polycythemia vera, lymphoma, or other internal causes of pruritus has been accepted as an effective treatment (67).

The application of BBUVB for treatment of pruritus associated with renal disease is expected to provide significant relief from the symptom and has been recognized as more effective than placebo over 25 years ago (68). Various protocols to treat pruritus associated with the underlying disease both with using MED or estimating a skin type is available (18,67). In either method used, it is apparent a suberythemogenic dose of UVB or NBUVB is adequate for response at a frequency of twice a week.

Other

There are various other inflammatory disorders reported to be responsive to BBUVB or NBUVB. These include lichen planus, granuloma annulare, acquired perforating disorders, and urticaria. As more experience and clinical data is available regarding the expected response and protocols which best treat each of the disorders, the clinician may apply the same principles regarding suberythemogenic BB or NBUVB as with other nonpsoriasis diseases. These disorders are included in the review of NBUVB treatment of skin disease beyond psoriasis (50).

REFERENCES

1. Parrish JA, Jaenicke KF. Action spectrum for phototherapy of psoriasis. J Invest Dermatol 1981; 76(5):359–362.
2. van Weelden H, De La Faille HB, Young E, van der Leun JC. A new development in UVB phototherapy of psoriasis. Br J Dermatol 1988; 119(1):11–19.
3. Zanolli M. Phototherapy treatment of psoriasis today. J Am Acad Dermatol 2003; 49(suppl 2): S78–S86.
4. Ibbotson SH, Bilsland D, Cox NH, et al. An update and guidance on narrowband ultraviolet B phototherapy: a British Photodermatology Group Workshop Report. Br J Dermatol 2004; 151(2):283–297.
5. Bonis B, Kemeny L, Dobozy A, et al. 308 nm UVB excimer laser for psoriasis. Lancet 1997; 350:1522.
6. Aubin F, Vigan M, Puzenat E, et al. Evaluation of a novel 308-nm monochromatic excimer light delivery system in dermatology: a pilot study in different chronic localized dermatoses. Br J Dermatol 2005; 152(1):99–103.

7. Speight EL, Farr PM. Erythemal and therapeutic response of psoriasis to PUVA using high-dose UVA. Br J Dermatol 1994; 131(5):667–672.
8. Fischer T, Alsins J, Berne B. Ultraviolet-action spectrum and evaluation of ultraviolet lamps for psoriasis healing. Int J Dermatol 1984; 23(10):633–637.
9. Farr PM, Diffey BL. Action spectrum for healing of psoriasis. Photodermatol Photoimmunol Photomed 2006; 22(1):52.
10. McKinlay AF, Diffey BL. A reference action spectrum for ultraviolet induced erythema in human skin. CIE J 1987; 6(1):17–22.
11. Diffey BL, Farr PM. An appraisal of ultraviolet lamps used for the phototherapy of psoriasis. Br J Dermatol 1987; 117(1):49–56.
12. Hofer A, Fink-Puches R, Kerl H, Wolf P. Comparison of phototherapy with near vs. far erythemogenic doses of narrow band ultraviolet B in patients with psoriasis. Br J Dermatol 1998; 138: 96–100.
13. Olson RL, Sayre RM, Everett MA. Effects of anatomic location and time on ultraviolet erythema. Arch Dermatol 1996; 93:211–215.
14. Asawanonda P, Anderson RR, Chang Y, Taylor CR. 308 nm excimer laser for the treatment of psoriasis: a dose-response study. Arch Dermatol 2000; 136(5):619–624.
15. Goeckerman WH. The treatment of psoriasis. Northwest Med 1925; 24:229–231.
16. Ingram JT. The approach to psoriasis. Br Med J 1953; 2:591–594.
17. Mentor A, Cram DL. The Goeckerman regimen in two psoriasis day care centers. Arch Dermatol 1968; 98:178–182.
18. Zanolli M, Feldman SR, eds. In: Phototherapy Treatment Protocols for Psoriasis and Other Phototherapy Responsive Dermatosis. 2nd ed. London: Taylor and Francis Press, 2005.
19. Dawe RS, Wainright NJ, Cameron H, Ferguson J. Narrowband ultraviolet B phototherapy for chronic plaque psoriasis: three times or five times weekly treatment? Br J Dermatol 1998; 138:833–839.
20. Trehan M, Taylor CR. High dose 308 nm excimer laser for the treatment of psoriasis. J Am Acad Dermatol 2002; 46:732–737.
21. Feldman SR, Mellem BG, Housman TS, et al. Efficacy of the 308 nm excimer laser for treatment of psoriasis: Results of a multicenter study. J Am Acad Dermatol 2002; 46:900–906.
22. Das S, Lloyd JJ, Farr PM. Similar dose-response and persistence of erythema with broad-band and narrow-band ultraviolet B lamps. J Invest Dermatol 2001; 117(5):1318–1321.
23. Calzavara-Pinton PG, Zane C, Candiago E, et al. Blisters on psoriatic lesions treated with TL-01 lamps. Dermatology 2000; 200(2):115–119.
24. Lee E, Koo J, Berger T. UVB phototherapy and skin cancer risk: a review of the literature. Int J Dermatol 2005; 44(5):355–360.
25. Young A. Carcinogenicity of UVB phototherapy assessed. Lancet 1995; 345:1431–1432.
26. Flindt-Hansen H, McFadden N, Eeg-Larsen T, et al. Effect of a new narrow-band UVB lamp on photocarcinogenesis in mice. Acta Derm Venereol 1991; 71(3):245–248.
27. Wulf HC, Hansen AB, Bech-Thomsen N. Differences in narrow-band ultraviolet B and broad-spectrum ultraviolet photocarcinogenesis in lightly pigmented hairless mice. Photodermatol Photoimmunol Photomed 1994; 10(5):192–197.
28. Gibbs NK, Traynor NJ, MacKie RM, et al. The phototumorigenic potential of broad-band (270–350 nm) and narrow-band (311–313 nm) phototherapy sources cannot be predicted by their edematogenic potential in hairless mouse skin. J Invest Dermatol 1995; 104(3):359–363.
29. Stern RS, Lange R. Non-melanoma skin cancer occurring in patients treated with PUVA five to ten years after first treatment. J Invest Dermatol 1988; 91(2):120–124.
30. Weischer M, Blum A, Eberhard F, et al. No evidence for increased skin cancer risk in psoriasis patients treated with broadband or narrowband UVB phototherapy: a first retrospective study. Acta Derm Venereol 2004; 84(5):370–374.
31. Man I, Crombie IK, Dawe RS, et al. The photocarcinogenic risk of narrowband UVB (TL-01) phototherapy: early follow-up data. Br J Dermatol 2005; 152(4):755–757.
32. Diffey BL. Factors affecting the choice of a ceiling on the number of exposures with TL01 ultraviolet B phototherapy. Br J Dermatol 2003; 149(2):428–430.
33. Lebwohl M, Quijije J, Gillard J, et al. Topical calcipotriol is degraded by ultraviolet light. J Invest Dermatol 2003; 121(3):594–595.
34. Ramsay CA, Schwartz BE, Lowson D, et al. Calcipotriene cream combined with twice weekly broad band UVB phototherapy: a safe, effective and UVB sparing antipsoriatic combination therapy. The Canadian Calcipotriol and UVB Study Group. Dermatology 2000; 200:17–24.
35. Koo J, Lowe N, Lew-Kaya D, et al. Tazarotene plus UVB in the treatment of psoriasis. J Am Acad Dermatol 2000; 43:821–828.
36. Yarosh DB, Pena AV, Nay SL, et al. Calcineurin inhibitors decrease DNA repair and apoptosis in human keratinocytes following ultraviolet B irradiation. J Invest Dermatol 2005; 125(5): 1020–1025.

37. Fritsch PO, Höningsmann H, Jaschke E, et al. Augmentation of oral methoxsalen photochemotherapy with an oral retinoic acid derivative. J Invest Dermatol 1978; 70:178–182.

38. Iest J, Boer J. Combined treatment of psoriasis with acetretin and UVB phototherapy compared with acetretin alone and UVB alone. Br J Dermatol 1989; 120:665–670.

39. Green C, Lakshmipathi T, Johnson BE, Ferguson J. A comparison of the efficacy and relapse rates of NBUVB (TL-01) monotherapy vs etretinate (re-TL-01) vs etretinate PUVA (re-PUVA) in the treatment of psoriasis patients. Br J Dermatol 1992; 127:5–9.

40. Lowe N, Prystowsky JH, Bourget T, et al. Acetretin plus UVB therapy for psoriasis: Comparisons with placebo plus UVB and acetretin alone. J Am Acad Dermatol 1991; 24:591–594.

41. Lebwohl M, Drake L, Menter A, et al. Consensus conference: acitretin in combination with UVB or PUVA in the treatment of psoriasis. J Am Acad Dermatol 2001; 45(4):544–553.

42. Paul BS, Monitaz K, Stern RS, et al. Combined methotrexate ultraviolet B therapy in the treatment of psoriasis. Am Acad Dermatol 1982; 7:758–762.

43. Koo J, Bandow G, Feldman SR. The art and practice of UVB phototherapy for the treatment of psoriasis. In: Weinstein GD, Gottlieb AB, eds. Therapy of Moderate to Severe Psoriasis. New York: Marcel Dekker Inc., 2003.

44. Oxholm A, Thomsen K, Menne T. Squamous cell carcinomas in relation to cyclosporine therapy of non malignant skin disorders. Acta Derm Venereol (Stock) 1989; 69:89–90.

45. Feldman SR, Clark A, Reboussin DM, Feischer AB. An assessment of potential problems of home phototherapy treatment of psoriasis. Cutis 1996; 58(1):71–73.

46. Cameron H, Yule S, Moseley H, et al. Taking treatment to the patient: development of a home TL-01 ultraviolet B phototherapy service. Br J Dermatol 2002; 147(5):957–965.

47. Koek MB, Buskiens E, Bruijnzeel-Koomen CA, Sigurdsson V. Home ultraviolet B phototherapy for psoriasis: discrepancy between literature, guidelines, general opinions and actual use. Results of a literature review, a web search, and a questionnaire among dermatologists. Br J Dermatol 2006; 154(4):701–711.

48. Turner RJ, Walshaw D, Diffey BL, Farr PM. A controlled study of ultraviolet A sunbed treatment of psoriasis. Br J Dermatol 2000; 143(5):919–920.

49. Su J, Pearce DJ, Feldman SR. The role of commercial tanning beds and ultraviolet A light in the treatment of psoriasis. J Dermatolog Treat 2005; 16(5–6):324–326.

50. Gambichler T, Bruechkmann F, Altmeyer P, Kreuter A. NBUVB in skin conditions beyond psoriasis. J Amer Acad Dermatol 2005; 52:660–670.

51. Jekler J, Larkö O. UVB phototherapy of atopic dermatitis. Br J Dermatol 1988; 119:697–705.

52. George SA, Sisland DJ, Johnson BE, Ferguson J. Narrowband (TL-pq) UVB air conditioned phototherapy for chronic severe adult atopic dermatitis. Br J Dermatol 1993; 128:49–56.

53. Hudson-Peacock MJ, Diffey BL, Farr PM. Narrow-band UVB phototherapy for severe atopic dermatitis. Br J Dermatol 1996; 135(2):332.

54. Reynolds NJ, Franklin V, Gray JC, et al. Narrow-band ultraviolet B and broad-band ultraviolet A phototherapy in adult atopic eczema: a randomised controlled trial. Lancet 2001; 357: 2012–2016.

55. Krutmann J. Phototherapy for atopic dermatitis. Clin Exp Dermatol 2000; 25(7):552–558.

56. Yashar SS, Gielczyk R, Scherschum L, Lim HW. Narrow band ultraviolet B treatment for vitiligo, pruruitus, and inflammatory dematoses. Phot dermatol Photimmunol Photomed 2003; 19:164–168.

57. Njoo MD, Spuls PI, Bos JD, et al. Nonsurgical repigmentation therapies in vitligo: meta analysis of the literature. Arch Dermatol 1998; 134:1532–1540.

58. Asawanonda P, Charoenloap M, Korkij W. Treatment of localized vitiligo with targeted broadband UVB pototherapy: a pilot study. Photodermatol Photoimmunol Photomed 2006; 22:133–136.

59. Hamzavi I, Jain H, McLean D, et al. Parametric modeling of narrowband UV-B phototherapy for vitiligo using a novel quantitative tool: the vitiligo area scoring index. Arch Dermatol 2004; 140:677–683.

60. El-Mofty M, Mostafa W, Esmat S, et al. Narrow band ultraviolet B 311 nm in the treatment of vitiligo: two right-left comparison studies. Photodermatol Photimmunol Photomed 2006; 22:6–11.

61. Schershuon L, Kim JJ, Lin HW. Narrow Band ultraviolet B is a useful and well tolerated treatment for vitiligo. J Amer Acad Dermatol 2001; 44:999–1003.

62. Herrmann JJ, Roenigk HH Jr, Honigsmann H. Ultraviolet radiation for treament of cutaneous T-cell lymphoma. Hematology and Oncology Clinics of North America 1995; 9:1077–1088.

63. Gathers RC, Scherschum L, Malick F, et al. Narrowband UVB phototherapy for early-stage mycosis fungoides. J Am Acad Dermatol 2002; 47(2):191–197.

64. El Mofty M, El-Arourty M, Salonas, M, et al. Narrow band UVB (311), psoralen UVB (311), and PUVA therapy in the treatment of early stage mycosis fungoides: a right left comparative study. Photodermatol Photoimmunol Photomed 2005; 21:281–286.

65. Millard TP, Hhawk JL. Photosensitivity disorders: cause, effect, and management. Am J Clin Dermatol 2002; 3:339–346.

66. Bisland D, George SA, Gibbs NK, et al. A comparison of narrow band phototherapy (TL-01) and photochemotherapy (PUVA) in the management of polymorphic light eruption. Br J Dermatol 1993; 129:708–712.
67. Rivard J, Lim HW. Ultraviolet phototherapy for pruritus. Dermatologic Therapy 2005; 18:344–354.
68. Gilchrest BA, Rowe JW, Brown RS, et al. Ultraviolet phototherapy of uremic pruritus: long term results and possible mechanism of action. Annual of Int Med 1979; 91:17–21.

23 | Ultraviolet-A1 and Visible Light Therapy

Jean Krutmann
Department of Dermatology and Environmental Medicine, Institut für Umweltmedizinische Forschung (IUF), Heinrich-Heine University, Düsseldorf, Germany

Akimichi Morita
Department of Geriatric and Environmental Dermatology, Nagoya City University Graduate School of Medical Sciences, Nagoya, Japan

- UVA-1 phototherapy currently represents an investigational treatment form that was originally elaborated and tested for its efficacy for atopic dermatitis.

- The efficacy of UVA-1 in atopic dermatitis is confirmed by several studies. Doses of $130 \, J/cm^2$ have been used, but more recently medium- and low-dose regimens are being explored. UVA-1 has not yet been compared directly with the standard phototherapies for atopic dermatitis (narrowband UVB or Psoralen plus UVA).

- UVA-1 therapy appears promising in localized scleroderma, however, controlled comparative studies needed. Its efficacy is probably based on increased collagenase expression in treated skin.

- UVA-1 therapy was reported to be beneficial in several other dermatoses, including systemic sclerosis, chronic sclerodermoid GvHD, urticaria pigmentosa, and cutaneous T cell lymphoma. However, these indications require confirmation in larger patient series.

- Studies indicate that UVA-1 may be also an effective treatment for psoriasis in HIV+ patients but not in HIV− patients and that UVA-1, unlike UVB, does not activate HIV in human skin.

- Visible light therapy of atopic dermatitis showed some effect in one study. However, these single center study results have not yet been confirmed by other groups.

INTRODUCTION

I n 1981, Mutzhas et al. (1) reported the development of an irradiation device, which almost exclusively emitted in the long-wave ultraviolet (UV) A range, that is, UVA-1 (340–400 nm). The combination of a metal halide lamp with a novel filtering system offered, for the first time, the unique possibility to expose human skin to high doses of UVA-1 radiation without causing a sunburn reaction. Soon thereafter, UVA-1 irradiation devices proved to be useful in photoprovocation testing for patients with UVA-sensitive photodermatoses, in particular polymorphic light eruption. It took, however, more than a decade before the therapeutic potential of these novel irradiation devices was recognized and systematically exploited. In 1992, Krutmann and Schöpf (2) reported that exposure to high doses of UVA-1 radiation was beneficial for patients with severe acute atopic dermatitis. These observations prompted a continually growing interest in the therapeutic use of UVA-1 radiation. As a consequence, there is now a substantial body of literature to suggest that for selected indications UVA-1 phototherapy is superior to conventional phototherapeutic modalities (3). A major difference between UVA-1 and UVB or UVA/UVB radiation is given by the fact that with UVA-1 phototherapy it has been possible to achieve therapeutic responses by penetrating deep into the dermis without the usual side effects caused by less penetrating UVB and UVB-like wavelengths in the UVA-2 region (4). In addition, UVA-1 radiation has some unique immunomodulatory features indicating that, under appropriate circumstances, it might prove superior even when compared with psoralen plus UVA (PUVA) therapy (5). UVA-1 phototherapy was used first to treat patients with atopic dermatitis, but it has since been found to be efficacious in several other skin diseases, such as localized and systemic scleroderma, in which other therapeutic options are limited. This development has been fostered by studies, in which the photobiological and molecular basis of UVA-1 phototherapy was analyzed. Currently, the indications for UVA-1 phototherapy fall into four major categories: (*i*) T-cell-mediated skin diseases, (*ii*) mast cell-mediated skin diseases, (*iii*) connective tissue diseases, and (*iv*) phototherapy in HIV positive patients (Table 1).

UVA-1 AND VISIBLE LIGHT THERAPY FOR T-CELL-MEDIATED SKIN DISEASES

In vitro studies have demonstrated that UVA-1 radiation is a potent inducer of apoptosis in human T lymphocytes (6). At a molecular level, UVA-1 radiation-induced apoptosis differs from apoptosis observed in UVB-irradiated or PUVA-treated cells because it is mediated through a pathway that does not require protein synthesis. This so-called preprogrammed cell death or early apoptosis appears to be highly specific for UVA-1 radiation and is mediated through the generation of singlet oxygen. The in vivo relevance of these in vitro findings is suggested by the observation that UVA-1 phototherapy of patients with atopic dermatitis resulted in apoptosis of skin-infiltrating T-helper cells (7). The appearance of apoptotic

TABLE 1   Indications for UVA-1 Therapy

Indication	Type of study	Comment
Atopic dermatitis	Several open studies, one multicenter trial	Established indication
Urticaria pigmentosa	Two open studies	Promising results, "long-lasting effects" controlled study lacking
Localized scleroderma	Two open studies	Very promising, "breakthrough" controlled comparative studies needed
Systemic sclerosis	One open study	Very promising, "breakthrough", controlled comparative studies needed
CTCL	Two open studies, one comparative study	Promising multicenter trial ongoing
Psoriasis/HIV +	One open study	Very promising, "therapy of choice" larger studies required
Psoriasis/HIV−	Case report	Disappointing
Alopecia areata	Unpublished study	Not effective
Solar urticaria	Several cases	Not effective
Lichen planus	Several cases	Not effective

Abbreviation: CTCL, cutaneous T-cell lymphoma.

T cells was then followed by their depletion from lesional skin, a reduction in the in situ expression of the pro-inflammatory T-cell-derived cytokine interferon-γ, and clearing of atopic eczema (8,9). Therefore, it is now generally believed that UVA-1 radiation-induced T-helper cell apoptosis constitutes the basis of UVA-1 phototherapy in patients with atopic dermatitis. As a clinical consequence, UVA-1 phototherapy has been extended to the treatment of other T-cell-mediated skin diseases including cutaneous T-cell lymphoma (CTCL) (10).

UVA-1 and Visible Light for Atopic Dermatitis

The therapeutic efficacy of UVA-1 radiation in the management of patients with atopic dermatitis was first evaluated in an open study in patients with acute, severe exacerbations (11). They were exposed daily to 130 J/cm^2 at an irradiation intensity of 70 mW/s for 15 consecutive days (Fig. 1). Therapeutic effectiveness was assessed by a clinical scoring system as well as by monitoring serum levels of eosinophil cationic protein (12,13). The latter represents a laboratory parameter that can be measured objectively and which has been shown to correlate well with disease activity. In that study, UVA-1 phototherapy was found to be highly efficient in promptly inducing clinical improvement. This was associated with a concomitant reduction in elevated serum levels of eosinophil cationic protein. Patients treated with UVA-1 were compared to subjects who had been treated with UVA/UVB phototherapy, which at that time was considered the best phototherapy for atopic dermatitis available. Significant differences were observed in favor of UVA-1 phototherapy, indicating that UVA-1 phototherapy was the phototherapy of choice for patients with severe atopic dermatitis.

During the subsequent years, there have been numerous reports confirming these original observations (14–16). It should be noted that in their pilot study, Krutmann et al. (11) employed UVA-1 phototherapy as a monotherapy, thereby suggesting that it might represent a therapeutic alternative to the gold standard in the treatment of severe atopic dermatitis, glucocorticosteroids. Indeed, a direct comparison of UVA-1 phototherapy with a standardized topical glucocorticosteroid treatment revealed that for the treatment of patients with severe, exacerbated atopic dermatitis UVA-1 phototherapy was at least equivalent to topical glucocorticosteroids (17). To date, this study is also the only one to provide a multicenter evaluation of the therapeutic efficacy of UVA-1

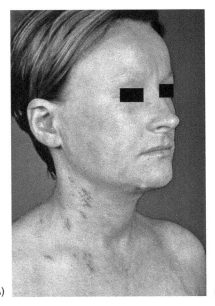 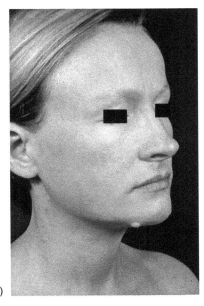

(A)   **(B)**

FIGURE 1   Patient with acute, severe atopic dermatitis before (**A**) and after (**B**) 15 exposures to 130 J/cm^2 UVA-1.

phototherapy by studying a larger number of patients with severe atopic dermatitis ($n = 53$) in a controlled randomized fashion. Patients were treated with UVA-1 ($10 \times 130\,\text{J/cm}^2$), UVA/UVB (minimal erythema dose-dependent), or topical fluocortolone. After 10 treatments, patients in all three groups had improved, but improvement was significantly greater in UVA-1 irradiated or fluocortolone-treated patients compared to UVA/UVB phototherapy. Significant reductions in serum levels of eosinophil cationic protein were only observed after glucocorticosteroid or UVA-1 therapy. The multicenter trial thus confirmed the original observation that UVA-1 phototherapy was of great benefit for patients with severe atopic dermatitis.

Local UVA-1 phototherapy appears to be an interesting option in the management of patients with chronic vesicular dyshidrotic hand eczema. In an open pilot study, palms and backs of hands of 12 patients with an acute exacerbation of their disease were exposed to 15 UVA-1 irradiations with a dose of $40\,\text{J/cm}^2$ per day over a period of three weeks. After one week, all but one patient reported a marked relief of itch. After the third week, significant clinical improvement was noted in 10 out of 12 patients (18).

It has recently been shown that wavelengths within the visible range can be effectively used to treat patients with atopic hand and foot eczema (19). This development was prompted by the observation that UVA-1 phototherapy-induced apoptosis in house dust-mite specific T-cells, which had been cloned from lesional skin of patients with atopic eczema, is mediated through the generation of singlet oxygen. This reactive oxygen species, however, cannot only be generated by wavelengths in the UV, but in particular in the near visible range (Soret band, 405 nm). A UV-free partial body irradiation device with an emission maximum between 400 and 450 nm has, therefore, been developed and found to induce prompt and long-lasting improvement in patients with atopic hand and foot eczema (Fig. 2). In marked contrast to UV radiation, which is a complete carcinogen, visible radiation does not increase the risk for skin cancer, and UV-free phototherapy might, therefore, be well suited for the treatment of children and young adults, who represent the vast majority of patients with atopic dermatitis. Further studies are clearly required to confirm these preliminary results in independent studies and to assess the efficacy of UV-free phototherapy for generalized forms of atopic dermatitis.

There is currently a debate whether the therapeutic efficacy of UVA-1 for this indication is dose-dependent. Recent studies indicate that similar to a high-dose regimen with

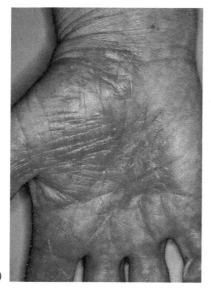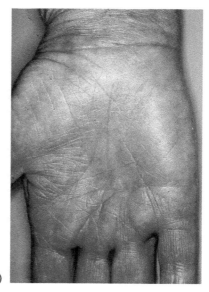

(A)   **(B)**

FIGURE 2   Patient with atopic hand eczema before (**A**) and after (**B**) UV-free phototherapy.

130 J/cm^2, a medium UVA-1 dosage schedule is superior to UVA/UVB (14). Also, therapeutic efficacy within the UVA-1 range seems to be dose-dependent, because irradiations with 50 J/cm^2 were superior to a low-dose regimen (20 J/cm^2) (20). Very recently, a high-dose protocol (130 J/cm^2 was found to be superior to a medium-dose regimen (50 J/cm^2), which again was more efficient than a low-dose schedule (20 J/cm^2). Thus, the use of low doses of UVA-1 does not offer any advantage over conventional phototherapeutic modalities such as UVA/UVB or 311 nm UVB and should, therefore, be discouraged. In contrast, medium- and high-dose UVA-1 are clearly superior to conventional phototherapy, but for achieving an optimal therapeutic response, a high-dose regimen with 130 J/cm^2 seems to be necessary.

UVA-1 for Cutaneous T-Cell Lymphoma

CTCL is a neoplasm of helper T-cells that initially manifests in the skin. The most common form is mycosis fungoides. Helper T-cells in mycosis fungoides are located intra-epidermally and below the epidermis as band-like dermal infiltrates. Topical treatment of patch and plaque CTCL thus requires modalities capable of penetrating into the dermis. For stage IA and IB CTCL, the treatment of choice is PUVA therapy, which, similar to UVA-1 radiation, induces T-cell apoptosis (21). From a theoretical point of view, UVA-1 phototherapy is an alternative to PUVA for this indication because UVA-1 radiation reaches deeper layers of the dermis at higher intensities compared with PUVA and UVA-1 phototherapy avoids the unwanted side effects resulting from the photosensitizer, 8-methoxypsoralen.

Plettenberg et al. (10) used UVA-1 phototherapy as a monotherapy in three patients with histologically proven CTCL, stages IA and IB. For whole-body UVA-1 irradiations, patients were exposed to 130 J/cm^2 ($n = 2$) or 60 J/cm^2 ($n = 1$) UVA-1 radiation daily (Fig. 2). In each of the three patients, skin lesions began to resolve after only a few UVA-1 radiation exposures. Complete clearance was observed between 16 and 20 exposures, regardless of whether the high- or medium-dose regimen was used. These clinical data were corroborated by histological evaluation. In all three patients, histological features of mycosis fungoides were present prior to therapy, whereas after UVA-1 phototherapy, the epidermis looked almost normal and only a few lymphocytic infiltrates were left in the dermis. In a second study, 10 patients with early stages of CTCL were treated with daily doses of 100 J/cm^2 UVA-1. In 10 out of 10 patients, complete remissions were observed after a total of 20 to 25 exposures (22). In a recent comparative study, CTCL patients were randomly assigned to either UVA-1 ($n = 10$) or PUVA ($n = 10$) therapy (23). Again, UVA-1 phototherapy was found to be efficient in the treatment of early stages of CTCL, and no significant differences in favor of PUVA therapy were observed.

The current mainstay for the treatment of stage IA-to IB-CTCL is PUVA therapy. From a practical point of view, UVA-1 phototherapy has significant advantages over PUVA because unwanted side effects resulting from the systemic application of the photosensitizer are completely avoided. Therefore, an international (Düsseldorf, Vienna, Brescia, Muenster, Nagoya, and Heidelberg) multicenter trial has been initiated to compare the efficacy of UVA-1 and PUVA therapy for early stages of CTCL in a controlled study. This trial will also provide information about the duration of remission-free intervals that can be achieved with UVA-1 phototherapy. The UVA-1 dose being used in this study is in the medium rather than the high-dose range and has been extrapolated from in vitro studies (24). In these experiments, neoplastic T-cells were shown to be significantly more sensitive to UVA-1 radiation-induced apoptosis when compared with normal T-cells. This is in line with the previous notion that exposure to 60 J/cm^2 UVA-1 was equally effective to a 130 J/cm^2 UVA-1 regimen for patients with CTCL. The optimal dose for treating CTCL patients might thus differ from the one to be used for atopic dermatitis patients.

UVA-1 for Urticaria Pigmentosa

Induction of apoptosis in skin-infiltrating cells and their subsequent depletion from skin is thought to represent the major mechanisms of action of UVA-1 phototherapy for yet another indication, urticaria pigmentosa. In initial studies, skin sections from patients before and after UVA-1 therapy were assessed for effects on mast cells by histochemical and immunohistochemical techniques (25). It was found that UVA-1 phototherapy reduced the density of dermal mast cells and that this decrease was closely linked to significant clinical improvement. These studies indicated that changes in the number, and possibly function, of dermal mast cells may contribute to the clinical effects of this treatment. It was, therefore, not surprising to learn that UVA-1 therapy proved to be of benefit for patients suffering from cutaneous mastocytosis. In a pilot study, four adult patients with severe generalized urticaria pigmentosa were treated with a high-dose UVA-1 regimen, which was used as a monotherapy (26). UVA-1 phototherapy was given once daily five times per week for two consecutive weeks. The initial dose was 60 J/cm^2 UVA-1; subsequently, the daily dose was 130 J/cm^2 UVA-1 per body half. In all patients, UVA-1 therapy induced a prompt improvement of cutaneous symptoms, which was reflected by a reduction of increased histamine in 24-hour urine to normal levels. In addition to skin symptoms, two patients presented with systemic manifestations of urticaria pigmentosa such as diarrhea and migraine. After 10 treatments, relief from systemic symptoms was noted and elevated serum serotonin was reduced to normal in both patients. No relapse occurred in any of the patients for more than two years after cessation of UVA-1 therapy. This is in contrast to PUVA therapy for urticaria pigmentosa, which is characterized by recurrence after five to eight months. The long-lasting effectiveness of UVA-1 for urticaria pigmentosa has recently been confirmed in a second study (27). In total, 15 patients with urticaria pigmentosa were treated using a high-dose UVA-1 regimen. Of the patients, 14 of 15 showed a prompt response to UVA-1 phototherapy and were free of cutaneous and/or systemic symptoms after cessation of phototherapy. A two-year follow-up of these patients revealed that eight months after phototherapy, 100% of UVA-1- treated patients were still in full remission. Remission free intervals of one year were observed for 70% and of 18 months for 40% of these patients.

Differences in the recurrence rate between UVA-1- and PUVA-treated urticaria pigmentosa patients might be explained by the fact that UVA-1 therapy is associated with a reduction in numbers of dermal mast cells, which has not been observed after PUVA therapy (28,29,15). This hypothesis is supported by recent in vivo studies that demonstrate a significant decrease in the number of dermal mast cells in UVA-1-, but not in PUVA-treated, patients. By employing a double-staining technique, it could also be demonstrated that lesional skin of patients with urticaria pigmentosa constitutively contained a low percentage of apoptotic mast cells and that this percentage was significantly increased by UVA-1 phototherapy (27). In contrast, PUVA therapy did not cause mast cell apoptosis. Taken together, these studies indicate that UVA-1 phototherapy, by virtue of its capacity to induce apoptosis in skin-infiltrating mast cells, is capable of depleting these cells from the skin of urticaria pigmentosa patients. As a consequence, therapeutic responses to UVA-1 phototherapy are long-lasting and, therefore, UVA-1 phototherapy has the potential to replace PUVA as the therapy of choice for urticaria pigmentosa patients.

UVA-1 for Connective Tissue Disease

Patients with localized scleroderma develop one or multiple, circumscribed, ivory-white, indurated plaques, which may be up to 20 cm in diameter and are frequently surrounded by an inflammatory halo known as the lilac ring (30). Although the disease has a self-limited course, sclerosis of skin lesions may cause significant morbidity and discomfort. It is possible that sclerotic skin lesions lead to muscle atrophy and thereby disfiguration of the trunk or face. They may also extend over joints and cause flexion contractures with functional impairment. Numerous modalities including penicillin, penicillamine, anti-malarial drugs, cyclosporin A, interferon-γ, and topical or systemic glucocorticosteroids have been employed; but in general, there is no effective curative or symptomatic therapy for localized scleroderma.

In this regard, it is of particular interest that sclerosis of skin lesions appears to result from an increased synthesis of type-I and type-III collagen (3,31,32). Evidence has been provided that a major cause for this excessive collagen deposition is a malfunction of dermal fibroblasts, in particular adecreased collagenase I expression (33). It is possible to increase synthesis of collagenase I in cultured human dermal fibroblasts by in vitro exposure to UVA-1 radiation

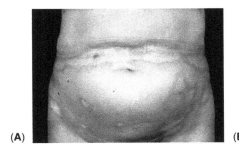
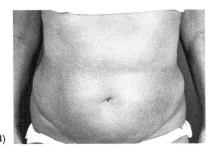

(A)   **(B)**

FIGURE 3   Sclerotic plaques in the abdominal region of a patient with localized scleroderma before (**A**) and after (**B**) UVA-1 phototherapy (30 × 130 J/cm² UVA-1).

(34,35). In these studies, UVA-1 radiation-induced collagenase production was associated with a dose-dependent upregulation of collagenase I mRNA expression, and maximal induction was achieved in vitro by UVA-1 radiation doses, which are equivalent to those used in high-dose UVA-1 phototherapy of atopic dermatitis or urticaria pigmentosa patients. It has, therefore, been hypothesized that UVA-1 radiation, by virtue of its capacity to increase collagenase I expression, may have beneficial effects for patients with localized scleroderma (36,37). This hypothesis has been tested in an open study, in which 10 patients with histologically proven localized scleroderma were exposed 30 times to 130 J/cm² of UVA-1 radiation (37) (Fig. 3). In all patients, UVA-1 therapy softened sclerotic plaques, and complete clearance was observed in 4 out of 10 patients. In addition, 20 MHz sonography revealed that UVA-1 therapy significantly reduced thickness and increased elasticity of plaques (Fig. 4). These changes were not due to spontaneous remission of skin lesions in these patients because they could only be observed in UVA-1-irradiated, but not in unirradiated, control plaques of the same patients. It has also been suggested that similar therapeutic effects can be achieved by exposing patients with localized scleroderma to low doses (20 J/cm²) of UVA-1 radiation (38,39). Direct comparison of low- versus high-dose UVA-1 phototherapy, however, revealed that high-dose UVA-1 therapy was superior to low-dose UVA-1 therapy for all parameters assessed (clinical evaluation, thickness of plaques, and cutaneous elastometry) (37). Patients were followed up for a total of three months after cessation of therapy. Termination of UVA-1 therapy was not associated with a loss of the beneficial effects achieved in any of these patients. Accordingly, in six out of seven patients, skin thickness values obtained at the end of the follow-up period were identical to those measured immediately after the last high-dose UVA-1 irradiation. In one patient, a partial relapse of skin symptoms was observed, but skin thickness after the three-month follow-up period was still significantly below values obtained before phototherapy was started. In none of the patients, further improvement of skin symptoms was observed after UVA-1 therapy was stopped.

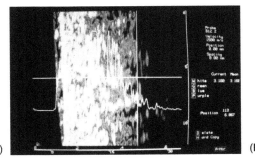
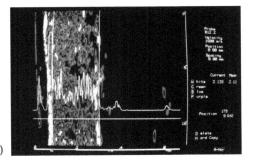

(A)   **(B)**

FIGURE 4   Sonography (20 MHz) of a sclerotic plaque of a patient with localized scleroderma before (**A**) and after (**B**) UVA-1 phototherapy (30 × 130 J/cm² UVA-1).

The precise mechanism(s) by which UVA-1 therapy may act in localized scleroderma are currently unknown. The rationale for employing a high-dose UVA-1 radiation regimen for this indication was based on previous in vitro observations that UVA-1 irradiation induced collagenase I expression in cultured human dermal fibroblasts in a dose-dependent manner (34,36). This concept is strongly supported by recent studies, in which sequential biopsies before and after high-dose UVA-1 therapy were obtained from sclerotic skin lesions of patients with localized scleroderma. UVA-1 radiation-induced clinical improvement and reduction of skin thickness were found to be associated with about a 20-fold upregulation of collagenase I mRNA expression in irradiated sclerotic plaques (47). Taken together, these studies strongly indicate that UVA-1 phototherapy is effective for localized scleroderma. Effectiveness is UVA-1 dose-dependent and associated with induction of collagenase I expression.

In addition to localized scleroderma, UVA-1 phototherapy has also been reported to be of benefit for patients with systemic sclerosis. Morita et al. (40) exposed lesional skin on the forearms of five patients with systemic sclerosis to single doses of $60 \, J/cm^2$ UVA-1. In all patients, UVA-1 phototherapy treated skin lesions were markedly softened after 10 to 30 exposures. Clinical improvement was associated with an increase in joint passive range of motion values, skin temperature, and cutaneous elasticity.

Histological evaluation of skin specimens obtained, before and after therapy, revealed loosening of collagen bundles and the appearance of small collagen fibers. A half-side comparison in one patient revealed that improvement of these parameters was only observed in UVA-1-treated, but not in unirradiated control skin (40). This study further supports the concept that UVA-1 phototherapy is a valuable treatment option for patients suffering from scleroderma. The fact that, currently no other treatment options with proven efficacy for the management of diseases associated with skin sclerosis are available, should further stimulate the interest in UVA-1 phototherapy.

It should be noted that in addition to UVA-1 therapy, systemic as well as topical PUVA therapy have been reported to be of benefit for patients with localized scleroderma and systemic sclerosis (41,42). Future studies will therefore have to compare UVA-1 versus PUVA therapy for both therapeutic efficacy and unwanted side effects. At least in the in vitro situation, PUVA treatment, but not UVA-1 irradiation, induced terminal differentiation of cultured human fibroblasts, indicating that PUVA therapy may be associated with a greater risk for photoaging. In addition, clinical improvement in patients with systemic sclerosis required an average of 50 PUVA treatments given over a period of four to five months (16). In contrast, UVA-1 phototherapy required a total of 30 irradiations to achieve maximal therapeutic effects (24). Since UVA-1, in contrast to PUVA therapy, was given on a daily basis, the total treatment time was reduced to between 1 to 1.5 months, and UVA-1 phototherapy thus yielded beneficial effects much faster than PUVA.

UVA-1 for HIV-Positive Patients

The safety of UVB or PUVA in the treatment of patients with skin disorders remains controversial. On the one hand, clinical studies have not shown dramatic adverse effects on immune status or plasma viral load. On the other hand, laboratory studies have clearly demonstrated that UVB or PUVA can activate HIV in cultured cells and in vivo in transgenic animals. The debate has been further stimulated by recent studies, in which HIV-1 (gag) expression was analyzed in a semiquantitative manner in human skin using a PCR-based assay. It was observed that UVB administered in vivo in suberythemogenic doses can activate the virus in lesional skin and nonlesional skin of seropositive patients with psoriasis or eosinophilic folliculitis. Previous in vitro studies have demonstrated that the only wavelength range within the UV that does not activate the HIV promoter is UVA-1 (43). Since psoriasis is currently being regarded as a T-cell-mediated skin disease and since UVA-1 phototherapy has proven to be highly effective for the treatment of T-cell-mediated inflammatory responses in human skin, it was obvious to assess whether UVA-1 phototherapy can be used for the treatment of psoriasis in HIV+ individuals. In an open, uncontrolled trial, HIV+ patients ($n = 3$) showed a beneficial response to UVA-1 phototherapy, which was given on a daily base as a high-dose regimen (44) (Fig. 5).

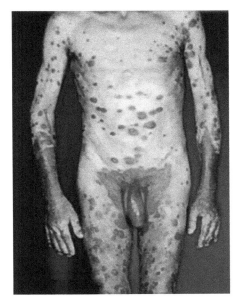 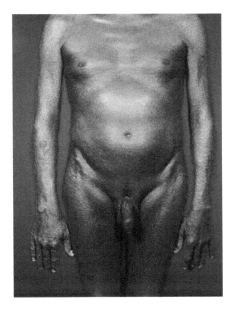

FIGURE 5 HIV + patient with psoriasis before (**A**) and after (**B**) UVA-1 phototherapy (20×130 J/cm^2).

Prior to initiation of whole-body UVA-1 phototherapy, the safety of UVA-1 phototherapy in HIV+ patients was assessed. For this purpose, paired lesional and nonlesional skin specimens were obtained from all patients after a single exposure to UVB (150 mJ/cm^2), UVA-1 (130 J/cm^2), or sham irradiation. By employing the quantitative PCR-based HIV assay, it was observed that UVB-treated skin showed a 6- to 15-fold increase in HIV count compared to unirradiated skin. By contrast, there were no differences in the HIV count of UVA-1 treated versus unirradiated skin. Moreover, complete clearance of psoriasis was observed in these patients after 20 to 30 UVA-1 irradiations. Importantly, there were also no increments in the skin viral counts of HIV+ patients with psoriasis after UVA-1 phototherapy (up to 41 total-body UVA-1 radiation exposures). These studies indicate that (*i*) UVA-1 is an effective treatment for psoriasis in HIV+ patients and (*ii*) that UVA-1, unlike UVB, does not activate HIV in human skin. At least from the perspective of safety, UVA-1 phototherapy, therefore, seems to represent the phototherapy of choice in HIV+ patients.

Miscellaneous Indications for UVA-1

In an open pilot study, 12 patients with an acute exacerbation of their chronic vesicular dyshidrotic hand eczema were subjected to a local UVA-1 phototherapy (18). Palms and backs of hands were exposed to 15 UVA-1 irradiations with a dose of 40 J/cm^2 per day over a period of three weeks. After one week of treatment, all but one patient reported a marked relief of itch. After the three-week treatment period, significant clinical improvement was noted in 10 out of 12 patients. This report is consistent with the observed therapeutic efficacy of UVA-1 phototherapy for atopic dermatitis and other T-cell-mediated skin diseases (45,7). Local UVA-1 phototherapy may thus prove to be an effective therapeutic option in the management of patients with chronic vesicular hand eczema.

A recent case report indicates that UVA-1 phototherapy is of benefit for patients with keloids and hypertrophic scars (46). A 37-year-old man (skin type IV) with a 17-year history of a stable chest keloid secondary to severe acne was treated 22 times with single exposures of 130 J/cm^2 UVA-1. Only two-thirds of the keloid were treated, whereas the remaining served as the unirradiated control. Already, after three weeks, and even more so after six weeks, of UVA-1 phototherapy, marked softening and flattening of the irradiated, but not the unirradiated parts of the keloid were noted. Histological evaluation revealed the reappearance of normal-looking collagen and elastic fibers in this keloid after phototherapy. These very preliminary but exciting results indicate that UVA-1 phototherapy could be of great help to patients with large scars such as burn scars for whom surgical remodeling or intralesional corticosteroid injection can be difficult.

Combined UVA-1 radiation and acitretin therapy has been reported as a treatment option in one patient with pityriasis rubra pilaris (47). From this case report, the relative contribution of UVA-1 and acitretin to the therapeutic response remains unclear.

It has been suggested that daily low-dose UVA-1 irradiation is beneficial to patients with lupus erythematosus. In support of this concept has been the publication of an open study of 10 patients with systemic lupus erythematosus who were treated with single doses of $6\,J/cm^2$ UVA-1 for various durations (15 days–8 months) (48). There was a decrease in clinical indices of disease activity as well as in titers of anti-SSA or antinuclear antibodies. This study has recently been confirmed in an 18-week, two-phase study (49). During the initial six-week prospective, double blind, placebo-controlled phase, 26 female patients were divided into two groups. Group A patients were exposed to $6\,J/cm^2$ UVA-1 and group B patients for an equal amount of time to visible light. Each group was subsequently crossed over for three weeks. This was followed by a second phase of 12 weeks, in which patients and physicians were unblinded and patients were treated with progressively decreasing levels of UVA-1 radiation. In patients from group A, disease activity was significantly decreased after three weeks of UVA-1 therapy but relapsed to baseline levels after three weeks of visible light treatment. In contrast, group B patients showed no significant response to the initial three weeks of visible light treatment or to the following three weeks of UVA-1 therapy. In both groups, however, significant improvement of clinical symptoms was detected after six weeks of UVA-1 phototherapy, which was given under uncontrolled conditions in phase two. These single center studies, however, have not yet been confirmed by other groups. Also, treatment of a UV-sensitive autoimmune disease such as lupus erythematosus with UVA-1 phototherapy may not be without risk, in particular, when UVA-1 is used at higher doses for SCLE patients who might develop a systemic form due to phototherapy (50).

SIDE EFFECTS OF UVA-1 AND VISIBLE LIGHT THERAPY

UVA-1 phototherapy may not be performed in patients with UVA-sensitive photodermatoses or photosensitive atopic dermatitis. It is necessary to exclude these diseases prior to initiation of phototherapy. This can easily be accomplished by photoprovocation testing. Except for eczema herpeticatum, no acute side effects have been observed in any patient treated with UVA-1. No other side effects have been observed, although its potential carcinogenic risk is a concern. Exposure of hairless albino Skh-hr1 mice to high doses of UVA-1 radiation has been shown to induce squamous cell carcinoma (51). The actual contribution of UVA-1 radiation to the development of malignant melanoma in humans is under debate and at this point cannot be excluded (52). These theoretical concerns are mainly relevant for atopic dermatitis patients who usually are at a younger age. Until more is known about UVA-1 phototherapy, its use in patients with atopic dermatitis should be limited to periods of acute exacerbation, and one treatment cycle should not exceed 10 to 15 exposures once or twice a year. As a general rule, children should not be treated with UVA-1 phototherapy except for severe cases of scleroderma where other treatment options do not exist (13). For other indications such as CTCL, urticaria pigmentosa, and connective tissue diseases, the benefits achieved by UVA-1 phototherapy probably outweigh its potential long-term risks.

No side effects have been reported with UV-free phototherapy, and in general, it can be assumed that UV-free phototherapy, in contrast to UV phototherapy, does not cause skin cancer and thus may be considered safe to be used in children, young adults, and in combination with immunosuppressive drugs.

PERSPECTIVES

UVA-1 phototherapy has almost always been used as a monotherapy in order to unambiguously prove its efficacy. Combination regimens integrating UVA-1 phototherapy are, however, of obvious clinical interest and practical benefit because they should allow for the maximization of therapeutic efficacy and safety at the same time. Combinations of interest include the use of UVA-1 together with topical steroids or novel immunosuppressants for atopic dermatitis or UVA-1 with systemic retinoids or interferon-α for CTCL.

Analysis of the mechanism of action of UVA-1 phototherapy has led to a rapid expansion of its indication spectrum. It is anticipated that this development will continue within the near future. In this regard, it has been of particular interest to learn that the generation of singlet oxygen by UVA-1 radiation represents a central photobiological mechanism required for the achievement of therapeutic effects (7). It is thus conceivable to assume that strategies directed at the amplification of singlet-oxygen-mediated effects as well as the development of alternative modes for singlet oxygen generation in human skin such as UV-free phototherapy will prove to be superior to UVA-1 phototherapy, as it is currently being employed. All these efforts will eventually contribute to the further development of UVA-1 and visible light phototherapy as one of the driving forces of modern photomedicine.

REFERENCES

1. Mutzhas MF, Hölzle E, Hofmann C, et al. A new apparatus with high radiation energy between 320–460 nm: physical description and dermatological applications.J Invest Dermatol 1981; 76:42–47.
2. Krutmann J, Schöpf E. High-dose UVA1 therapy: a novel and highly effective approach for the treatment of patients with acute exacerbation of atopic dermatitis. Acta Derm Venereol (Stockh) 1992; 176:120–122.
3. LeRoy EC. Increased collagen synthesis by scleroderma skin fibroblasts in vitro. J Clin Invest 1979; 54:880–889.
4. Jekler J, Larkö O. Combined UV-A–UV-B versus UVB phototherapy for atopic dermatitis. J Am Acad Dermatol 1990; 22:49–53.
5. Krutmann J. Phototherapy for atopic dermatitis. Dermatol Ther 1996; 1:24–31.
6. Godar DE. UVA 1 radiation mediates singlet-oxygen and superoxide-anion production which trigger two different final apoptotic pathways: the S and P site of mitochondria. J Invest Dermatol 1999; 112:3–12.
7. Morita A, Werfel T, Stege H, et al. Evidence that singlet oxygen-induced human T helper cell apoptosis is the basic mechanism of ultraviolet-A radiation phototherapy. J Exp Med 1997; 186:1763–1768.
8. Grewe M, Gyufko K, Schöpf E, et al. Lesional expression of interferon-γ in atopic eczema. Lancet 1994; 343:25–26.
9. Grewe M, Bruijnzeel-Koomen CAFM, Schöpf E, et al. A role for Th1 and Th2 cells in the immunopathogenesis of atopic dermatitis. Immunol Today 1998; 19:359–361.
10. Plettenberg H, Stege H, Megahed M, et al. Ultraviolet A1 (340–400 nm) phototherapy for cutaneous T-cell lymphoma. J Am Acad Dermatol 1999; 41:47–50.
11. Krutmann J, Czech W, Diepgen T, et al. High-dose UVA-1 therapy in the treatment of patients with atopic dermatitis. J Am Acad Dermatol 1992; 26:225–230.
12. Costa C, Rillet A, Nicolet M, Saurat JH. Scoring atopic dermatitis: the simpler the better. Acta Derm Venereol (Stockh) 1989; 69:41–47.
13. Czech W, Krutmann J, Schöpf E, et al. Serum eosinophil cationic protein is a sensitive measure for disease activity in atopic dermatitis. Br J Dermatol 1992; 126:351–355.
14. Kobyletzki G, Pieck C, Hoffmann K, et al. Medium-dose UVA1 cold-light phototherapy in the treatment of severe atopic dermatitis. J Am Acad Dermatol 1999; 41:931–937.
15. Kolde G, Frosch PJ, Czarnetzki BM. Response of cutaneous mast cells to PUVA in patients with urticaria pigmentosa: histophotometric, ultrastructural, and biochemical investigations. J Invest Dermatol 1984; 83:175–178.
16. Meffert H, Sönnichsen N, Herzog M, et al. UVA-1 cold light therapy of severe atopic dermatitis. Dermatol Monatsschr 1992; 78:291–296.
17. Krutmann J, Diepgen T, Luger TA, et al. High-dose UVA1 therapy for atopic dermatitis: results of a multicenter trial. J Am Acad Dermatol 1998; 38:589–593.
18. Schmidt T, Abeck D, Boeck K, et al. UVA1 irradiation is effective in treatment of chronic vesicular dyshidrotic hand eczema. Acta Derm Venereol (Stockh) 1998; 78:318–319.
19. Krutmann J, Medve-Koenigs K, Ruzicka, et al. UV-free phototherapy of atopic hand and foot eczema. Photodermatol Photoimmunol Photomed 2005; 21:59–61.
20. Kowalzick L, Kleinhenz A, Weichenthal M, et al. Low dose versus medium dose UVA-1 treatment in severe atopic dermatitis. Acta Derm Venereol (Stockh) 1995; 75:43–45.
21. Krutmann J. Therapeutic photomedicine: phototherapy. In: Freedberg IM, Eisen AZ, Wolff K, Austen KF, Goldsmith LA, Katz SI, Fitzpatrick TB, eds. Fitzpatrick's Dermatology in General Medicine. 5th ed. New York: McGraw-Hill, 1999:2870–2879.

22. Zane C, Leali C, Airo P, et al. High-dose UVA1 therapy of large plaques and nodular lesions of cutaneous T-cell lymphoma. J Am Acad Dermatol 2001; 44:629–633.
23. Plettenberg H, Stege H, Mang R, et al. A comparison of Ultraviolet A-1 and PUVA therapy for early stages of cutaneous T-cell lymphoma. Photodermatol Photoimmunol Photomed 2001; 17:149–155.
24. Yamauchi R, Morita A, Yasuda Y, et al. Different susceptibility of malignant versus nonmalignant human T cells toward ultraviolet A-1 radiation-induced apoptosis. J Invest Dermatol 2004; 122(2):477–483.
25. Grabbe J, Welker P, Humke S, et al. High-dose UVA1 therapy, but not UVA/UVB therapy, decreases IgE binding cells in lesional skin of patients with atopic eczema. J Invest Dermatol 1996; 107:419–423.
26. Stege H, Schöpf E, Ruzicka T, et al. High-dose-UVA1 for urticaria pigmentosa. Lancet 1996; 347:64.
27. Stege H, Budde M, Kürten V, et al. Induction of apoptosis in skin-infiltrating mast cells by high-dose ultraviolet A-1 radiation phototherapy in patients with urticaria pigmentosa. J Invest Dermatol 1999; 112:561.
28. Christophers E, Hönigsmann H, Wolff K, et al. PUVA treatment of urticaria pigmentosa. Br J Dermatol 1978; 98:701–702.
29. Granerus G, Roupa G, Swanbeck G. Decreased urinary histamine levels after successful PUVA treatment of urticaria pigmentosa. J Invest Dermatol 1981; 76:1–3.
30. Rosenwasser TA, Eisen AZ. Scleroderma. In: Fitzpatrick TB, Eisen AZ, Wolff K, Freedberg IM, Austen KF, eds. Dermatology in General Medicine. 4th ed. New York: McGraw-Hill, 1993:2156–2167.
31. Fleischmajer R. Localized and systemic scleroderma. In: Lapiere CM, Krieg T, eds. Connective Tissue Diseases of the Skin. New York: Dekker, 1993:295–313.
32. Rodnan GP, Lipinski I, Luksick J. Skin collagen content in progressive systemic sclerosis (scleroderma) and localized scleroderma. Arthritis Rheum 1979; 22:130–140.
33. Takeda K, Hahamochi A, Ueki H, et al. Decreased collagenase expression in cultured systemic sclerosis fibroblasts. J Invest Dermatol 1994; 103:359–363.
34. Petersen MJ, Nasen C, Craig S. Ultraviolet A irradiation stimulates collagenase production in cultured human fibroblasts. J Invest Dermatol 1992; 99:440–442.
35. Scharffetter K, Wlaschek M, Hogg A, et al. UVA irradiation induces collagenase in human dermal fibroblasts in vitro and in vivo. Arch Dermatol Res 1991; 283:506–511.
36. Kerscher M, Dirschka T, Volkenandt M. Treatment of localized scleroderma by UVA1 phototherapy. Lancet 1995; 346:1166.
37. Stege H, Humke S, Berneburg M, et al. High-dose ultraviolet A1 radiation therapy of localized scleroderma. J Am Acad Dermatol 1996; 36:938–943.
38. Gruss C, Strucker M, Kobyletzki G, et al. Low dose UVA1 phototherapy in disabling pansclerotic morphea. Br J Dermatol 1997; 136:293–294.
39. Kerscher M, Volkenandt M, Gruss C, et al. Low-dose UVA1 phototherapy for treatment of localized scleroderma. J Am Acad Dermatol 1998; 38:21–26.
40. Morita A, Kobayashi K, Isomura I, et al. Ultraviolet A-1 (340–400 nm) phototherapy for systemic sclerosis. J Am Acad Dermatol 2000; 43:670–674.
41. Morita A, Sakakibara S, Sakakibara N, et al. Successful treatment of systemic sclerosis with topical PUVA. J Rheumatol 1995; 22:2361–2365.
42. Scharfetter-Kochanek K, Goldermann R, et al. PUVA therapy in disabling pansclerotic morphea of children. Br J Dermatol 1995; 132:830–831.
43. Zmudzka BZ, Olvey KM, Lee W, et al. Reassessment of the differential effects of ultraviolet and ionizing radiation on HIV promoter: the use of cell survival as the basis for comparisons. Photochem Photobiol 1994; 59:643–649.
44. Breur-McHam J, Simpson E, Dougherty I, et al. Activation of HIV in human skin by ultraviolet B radiation and its inhibition by NF-κB blocking agents. Photochem Photobiol 2001; 74:805–810.
45. Krutmann J. UVA1 induced immunomodulation. In: Krutmann J, Elmets CA, eds. Photoimmunology. Oxford: Blackwell Science, 1995:246–256.
46. Asawananda P, Khoo LS, Fitzpatrick TB, et al. UV-A1 for keloid. Arch Dermatol 1999; 135:348–349.
47. Herbst RA, Vogelbruich M, Ehnis A, et al. Combined ultraviolet A1 radiation and acitretin therapy as a treatment option for pityriasis rubra pilaris. Br J Dermatol 2000; 142:574–575.
48. McGrath H Jr. Ultraviolet-A1 irradiation decreases clinical disease activity and autoantibodies in patients with systemic lupus erythematosus. Clin Exp Rheumatol 1994; 12:129–135.
49. McGrath Jr H, Martinez-Osuna P, Lee FA. Ultraviolet A-1 (340–400 nm) irradiation in systemic lupus erythematosus. Lupus 1996; 5:269–274.
50. Soennichsen N, Meffert H, Kunzelmann V. UV-A-1 Therapie bei subakut-kutanem Lupus erythematodes. Hautarzt 1993; 44:723–725.
51. Sterenborg HJ, van der Leun JC. Tumorigenesis by a long wavelength UV-A source. Photochem Photobiol 1990; 51:325–330.
52. Setlow RB, Grist E, Thompson K, et al. Wavelengths effective in induction of malignant melanoma. Proc Natl Acad Sci USA 1993; 90:6666–6670.

24 | Psoralen Photochemotherapy

Warwick L. Morison
Department of Dermatology, Johns Hopkins University, Baltimore, Maryland, U.S.A.

Herbert Hönigsmann
Department of Dermatology, Medical University of Vienna, Vienna, Austria

- The acronym PUVA refers to the combined use of photoactive psoralens and UVA radiation.

- The most widely used form of PUVA therapy consists of oral administration of methoxsalen and exposure to UVA fluorescent bulbs.

- The goal of PUVA therapy is to clear skin disease, but the treatment has two constraints: the risk of erythema from being too aggressive and the risk of developing too much pigmentation from being too conservative.

- PUVA therapy is an effective treatment for many inflammatory and neoplastic skin diseases.

- The commonest disease treated with PUVA therapy is psoriasis and it is effective in >90% of patients with psoriasis vulgaris.

- Excessive exposure to PUVA therapy causes photoaging of the skin and is associated with an increased risk of developing nonmelanoma skin cancer and possibly melanoma.

- Topical PUVA therapy is an alternative approach to treatment and avoids systemic exposure to psoralens.

INTRODUCTION

P soralens are a group of phototoxic compounds that can interact with various components of cells and then absorb photons to produce photochemical reactions that alter the function of cellular constituents. The acronym PUVA refers to the combined use of psoralens (P) and long-wave ultraviolet radiation (UVA). A combination of drug and radiation results in a therapeutic effect after repeated controlled phototoxic reactions. Psoralens may be administered orally or be applied topically to the skin; the initial discussion will be restricted to oral PUVA therapy and topical therapy will be addressed later in the chapter.

PSORALENS
Background and History

Psoralens belong to the furocoumarin group of compounds and the parent compound, psoralen, and many of its derivatives are naturally occurring compounds found in a large number of plants. The medicinal properties of psoralens have been known for centuries and their use in the treatment of vitiligo was recorded as long ago as 1550 BC (1). Three psoralens are used in PUVA therapy (Fig. 1). Methoxsalen or 8-methoxypsoralen is obtained from the seeds of a plant called *Ammi majus* and it is the most widely used psoralen and the only one available in the United States. Bergapten or 5-methoxypsoralen and trioxsalen or 4,5′,8-trimethylpsoralen are available in Europe and elsewhere.

Pharmacology
Absorption

Psoralens are poorly soluble in water and this is a limiting factor in their absorption from the gastrointestinal tract. There is a lot of interindividual variation in the absorption of the drug in terms of both the amount absorbed and the rate of absorption (2). Peak blood levels vary a great deal and timing also varies. Therefore, it is important to treat patients at a consistent time after ingestion. There is also some intra-individual variation in the absorption of psoralens and this is mainly due to what the patient has eaten and the time of day.

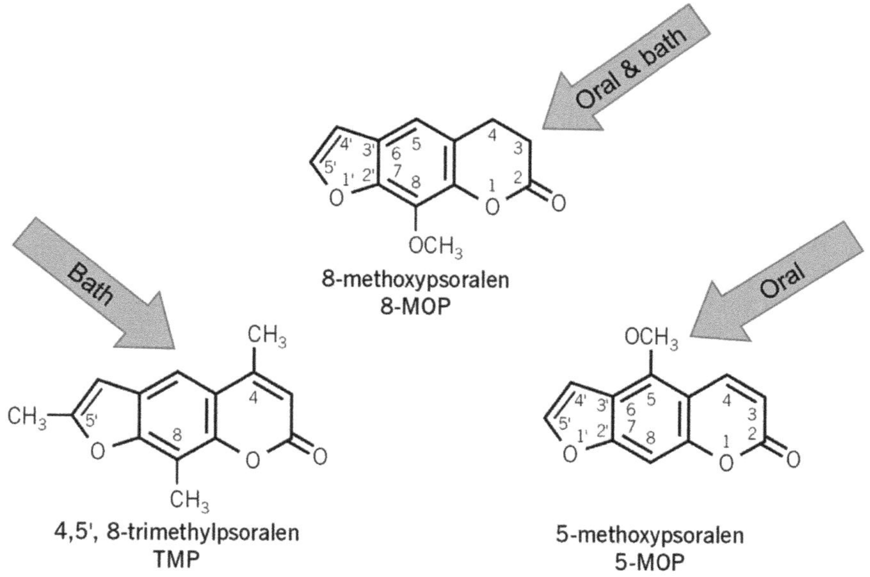

FIGURE 1   Psoralens used in therapy.

First-Pass Effect

Psoralens are subject to a significant but saturable first-pass effect in the liver (3). This means that a proportion of any dose is metabolized by the liver after absorption and never reaches the skin. However, since this effect can be saturated, as the dose is raised, the proportion of active compound reaching the skin rises.

Concentration in Skin

The concentration level that is of importance is the level at the target site in the skin since it is there that an interaction with UVA radiation will yield therapeutic benefit. Direct measurement of the phototoxic response of skin is the only means available for assessing the cutaneous content of psoralens.

Metabolism and Excretion

After oral administration, psoralens are distributed to all organs of the body, but in the absence of photochemical binding, excretion is rapid. The compounds are metabolized in the liver by cytochrome P-450 enzymes and drugs activating these enzymes accelerate metabolism of psoralens (4).

Photobiology

Determinations of action spectra in vivo have shown that psoralen photosensitization occurs with wavelengths >320 nm. Early studies in guinea pigs and humans indicated that the action spectrum for delayed erythema with psoralens was between 340 and 380 nm and this led to the use of UVA bulbs with a peak emission at those wavelengths; these are the bulbs still used in therapy. More recent studies suggest that maximal photosensitization occurs at the shorter wavelengths of 320 to 340 nm, but the precise action spectrum has not been defined (5).

UVA RADIATION

Psoralens are mainly used in combination with broadband sources of UVA radiation. The most commonly used source is fluorescent light bulbs, typically labeled PUVA lamps, having a maximum emission at 352 nm and some emission in both UVB and visible light. Metal halide lamps with suitable filters have also been used as a source of UVA radiation for activating psoralens. Their main advantage is a high irradiance so that treatment times are short.

Several sources of UVA radiation are not suitable for activating psoralens. The sun is a very convenient source of UVA radiation but it is not a safe radiation source for use with psoralens because the therapeutic dose is close to the phototoxic dose. A high content of UVB in sunlight might contribute to this problem. Black-light bulbs are also in general unsafe because the emission spectrum is quite different from that of PUVA bulbs in most cases. Tanning lamps are also unsuitable as a source of UVA radiation because they usually emit a significant amount of UVB radiation and this will add to the unpredictability in psoralen activation.

CUTANEOUS RESPONSES
Erythema

PUVA-induced erythema follows a different time course than that of UVB-induced erythema. PUVA-induced erythema usually appears after 36 to 48 hours but in some patients may be delayed until 72 hours. The peak of the erythema response is also delayed and may not be reached until 96 to 120 hours after exposure and an erythema can persist for up to two or even three weeks (6). Pruritus is a marked feature of PUVA-induced erythemas and often occurs as a deep burning itch, feeling like insects crawling under the skin, and this can persist for weeks or even months. This response is probably due to a direct phototoxic injury of cutaneous nerves.

Pruritus

PUVA itch may occur as a symptom of phototoxicity in the absence of erythema and this typically begins on the outer aspect of the arms and thighs, the buttocks, and in women on the breasts.

Pigmentation

PUVA produces pigmentation in all patients with functioning melanocytes. Pigmentation after oral administration of psoralen and exposure to UVA radiation is usually darker and lasts longer than the tan associated with a comparable UVB-induced erythema. Pigmentation following topical application of psoralens and exposure to UVA radiation can last for months. Pigmentation combined with hyperplasia of the epidermis and thickening of the stratum corneum is effective in raising the threshold for erythema from subsequent exposure to UV radiation with or without psoralens.

CELLULAR RESPONSES

Photoactive psoralens intercalate between the bases of DNA in the absence of radiation. Absorption of photons by psoralens results in photochemical binding to a pyrimidine molecule to give a monofunctional adduct. With some compounds, including methoxsalen, trimethylpsoralen, and 5-methoxypsoralen, a second photon can be absorbed resulting in a cross-link to a pyrimidine molecule on the sister strand of DNA. Such cross-links are also called bifunctional adducts (7). Psoralens also react with RNA, protein, and cell membranes, but the importance of these reactions is unknown.

TREATMENT
Psoralen Dosing

Both 5-methoxypsoralen and 8-methoxypsoralen are available as crystals in a capsule and as a liquid in a soft gelatin capsule. The liquid formulation is preferred as it gives better and more consistent absorption (8). The dose of 5-methoxypsoralen used is typically 1.2 mg/kg and that of 8-methoxypsoralen is 0.4 to 0.6 mg/kg. The higher dose of 5-methoxypsoralen is necessary to compensate for lower absorption (9). These compounds can be administered one or two hours prior to exposure to UVA radiation but the time must be kept constant in any given patient.

Determination of Sensitivity to PUVA Therapy

Two methods are used for determination of the initial dose of UVA radiation, skin typing, and measurement of the minimal phototoxic dose (MPD). Phototesting to determine the MPD is a superior approach in terms of requiring fewer treatments to clear disease but the total cumulative dose and the frequency of erythema are higher with this technique (10).

Skin Typing

The patient is asked about their response to a 30-minute noontime exposure to sunlight at the beginning of summer to determine skin types I through IV, whereas skin types V and VI are decided on the basis of examination of the skin, skin type V being brown individuals and skin type VI being black individuals. Suitable starting doses of UVA radiation and dose increments for a twice weekly or three times a week treatment schedule are given in Table 1.

Determination of the MPD

Dose ranges of UVA radiation for determining the MPD are given in Table 2. The phototest is usually read at 72 hours and the starting dose of UVA radiation is 50% to 70% of the MPD and the UVA radiation dose is increased weekly by 30% as tolerated (11).

TABLE 1 Dose of UVA Radiation Determined by Skin Types

Skin type	UVA radiation dose (J/cm^2)	
	Initial	Increments
I	1.5	0.5
II	2.5	0.5
III	3.5	0.5–1.0
IV	4.5	1.0
V	5.5	1.0
VI	6.5	1.0–1.5

TABLE 2 Exposure Doses for MPD Test

With oral PUVA (J/cm^2)						
Skin types I–IV						
UVA dose (8-MOP)	0.5	1	2	3	4	5
UVA dose (5-MOP)	1	2	4	6	8	10
With bath PUVA (J/cm^2)						
Skin types I and II						
UVA dose (8-MOP)	0.25	0.5	1	1.5	2	2.5
Skin types III and IV						
UVA dose (8-MOP)	0.5	1	2	3	4	5

Abbreviation: MPD, minimal phototoxic dose.

Treatment Schedules

Various treatment schedules have been used in PUVA therapy. A schedule using twice weekly or three treatments a week appears to be equally efficacious. Treatments spaced at least 48 hours apart can determine whether erythema is developing from the previous treatment, and the dose of UVA radiation is increased for each treatment provided no erythema is present. A four times a week schedule is used in some centers with treatment on Monday, Tuesday, Thursday, and Friday. The dose of UVA radiation is increased on Monday and Thursday. For all schedules, if faint erythema is present, the dose of UVA radiation should be held constant, but if widespread definite or tender erythema is present, treatment is stopped until it has faded. Localized erythema, such as on the breasts or buttocks, can be managed by shielding with clothing while treatment is continued.

MAINTENANCE THERAPY

One of the main advantages of PUVA therapy is that it is possible to maintain patients in a relatively clear state using infrequent treatment, once their disease is controlled (12). The last clearance dose of UVA radiation is held constant as the maintenance dose. There is no fixed schedule of treatment for maintenance because individual responses are very variable and the schedule outlined in Table 3 should only be used as a guide. If the patient has had four months of monthly treatment without any significant recurrence, treatment can probably be stopped. However, in our own left–right comparison study with psoriatics, short-term PUVA maintenance treatment over two months did not increase the length of remission (13).

TABLE 3 Maintenance Schedule for PUVA Therapy

Four treatments at weekly intervals (Q.W)
Then four treatments every other week (Q.2W)
Then four treatments every third week (Q.3W)
Then four treatments at monthly intervals (Q.M)

TABLE 4 Protection During PUVA Therapy

During radiation
  Eyes shielded by UVA-opaque goggles
  Male genitalia covered with a jockstrap
  Face protected
After ingestion of psoralen
  Eyes protected by UVA-opaque glasses
  Skin protected by clothing and sunscreens and avoidance of outdoor activities
Nontreatment days
  Exposure to sunlight minimized
  UV-blocking sunglasses worn

PRECAUTIONS

Attention must be focussed in two directions. First, psoralens enter all cells in the body and not just those affected by the disease process. Second, there is a large amount of UVA radiation in sunlight that can activate psoralens from the time of ingestion of the drug until it is excreted. The eye is the most important consideration. Psoralens enter the eye and UVA radiation is absorbed by the lens, so cataracts are a risk after repeated phototoxic insults. Clinical evaluation of patients who neglected careful eye protection has shown no increase in lens opacities (14). Obviously, there is no risk with topical or bath PUVA. Requirements for protection during PUVA therapy are outlined in Table 4.

CONTRAINDICATIONS TO PUVA THERAPY

Table 5 lists the absolute and relative contraindications to therapy (15).

Short-Term Side Effects

The short-term problems with PUVA therapy are outlined in Table 6 (16). Most of these are minor and can be easily overcome so that few patients cease treatment because of adverse effects. Gastrointestinal disturbances, such as anorexia and nausea, and central nervous system (CNS) disturbances, such as dizziness and insomnia, are the most common side effects and are probably related to a high blood level of psoralen. Taking psoralen with food, splitting the dose so that half is taken 90 minutes before treatment and the other half is taken one hour before treatment or reducing the dose by 10 mg overcomes these problems in most patients. With 5-MOP, these symptoms are much rarer. Symptomatic erythema is the most troubling short-term problem of PUVA therapy and it occurs in around 10% of patients during the clearance phase of treatment. There is no specific treatment for PUVA-induced erythema and supportive measures such as cool baths, liberal use of moisturizing creams,

TABLE 5 Contraindications to PUVA Therapy

Absolute
  Xeroderma pigmentosum
  Albinism
  Lactation
  Lupus erythematosus with a history of photosensitivity or
  a positive Ro antibody test
Relative
  History or family history of melanoma
  Past history of nonmelanoma skin cancer
  Extensive solar damage
  Uremia and severe hepatic failure
  Pemphigus and pemphigoid
  Immunosuppression
  Pregnancy
  Young age

TABLE 6 Short-Term Side Effects

Due to methoxsalen
    Gastrointestinal effects
    CNS symptoms
    Bronchoconstriction
    Drug fever
    Exanthema
Phototoxicity
    Erythema
    Pruritus
    Subacute phototoxicity
    Photo-onycholysis
    Koebner Phenomenon
    Friction blisters
    Phytophotodermatitis
    Ankle edema
Nonphototoxic reactions
    Cardiovascular stress
    Hypertrichosis
    Herpes simplex

Abbreviation: CNS, central nervous system.

aspirin, and antipruritics offer some relief. Unfortunately, some patients develop a new rash as a side effect of treatment and the causes are listed in Table 7.

Long-Term Side Effects

Large prospective studies in the United States and Europe combined with smaller studies from other areas have provided more than 25 years of follow-up data on the adverse effects of PUVA therapy. Photoaging of the skin occurs with long-term treatment and is most marked with skin types I and II, whereas little or no change is seen in skin types V and VI. Non-melanoma skin cancer, mainly squamous cell carcinomas, has also been seen in patients receiving large doses of treatment and again there is a strong correlation with skin type, with the lower skin types being more susceptible (17–19). A small increase in basal cell carcinomas has been observed with lesions mainly occurring on the trunk (20). An increased incidence of melanoma began to appear in one multicenter study 15 years after the start of treatment and the incidence increased steadily in that study (21). This has not been observed in other studies but the duration and completeness of follow-up in those studies may be inadequate.

    The potential ocular risk of PUVA therapy is cataracts and there are anecdotal reports of several patients who developed cataracts following a course of PUVA therapy, but this has not been revealed as a problem in a large prospective study (14).

DISEASES RESPONSIVE TO PUVA THERAPY
Psoriasis

Most forms of psoriasis are responsive to PUVA therapy with improvement after 6 to 10 treatments and clearance occurring in 20 to 30 treatments in about 90% of patients (12,22,23). The

TABLE 7 Rashes Complicating Treatment

Polymorphous light eruption
Lupus erythematosus
Transient acantholytic disease
Bullous pemphigoid
Guttate psoriasis
Sebborrheic dermatitis
Porokeratosis
Actinic lichen planus
Chronic actinic dermatitis

most common indication for PUVA therapy is disabling psoriasis unresponsive to topical therapy but there is no clear-cut definition of disability so it must be determined on a case-by-case basis. In addition, generalized pustular psoriasis (24), palmoplantar pusulosis (25), and erythrodermic psoriasis (26) have been reported to respond to PUVA therapy alone.

Combination therapy is often indicated in patients with severe inflammatory psoriasis, erythrodermic, and generalized pustular psoriasis, in patients with thick plaques, or in those with high skin types. Commonly used second agents are acitretin (27), methotrexate (28), and broadband UVB (29). All these agents appear to improve the clearance rate and decrease the duration of therapy.

Vitiligo

Vitiligo was the first indication for PUVA therapy, although it is less used now since narrow-band UVB phototherapy has been demonstrated as an effective alternative for repigmentation of this condition. Patients are treated as skin type I individuals with the aim of maintaining minimal, light pink, phototoxicity in patches of vitiligo. It requires 100 to 200 exposures to produce maximal repigmentation and about 70% of patients respond (30,31). Treatments are given two or three times weekly. Combination therapy using topical corticosteroids or topical calcipotriene may enhance the response to PUVA therapy (32).

Mycosis Fungoides

Mycosis fungoides in the most common of the cutaneous T-cell lymphomas, a group of disorders that arise from malignant CD4+ helper T-cells and localize within the skin and associated lymph nodes. The early phases of this disease, the so-called patch and plaque phases, respond well to PUVA therapy with clearance rates of 70% to 90% (33). A high relapse rate when short-term maintenance treatment alone is used may indicate a need for long-term maintenance therapy in this condition; this approach has not been carefully evaluated (34). According to the Swedish National Central Bureau of Statistics, it seems probable that PUVA may be the main reason for a significant decrease in the death rate for mycosis fungoides, which has dropped more than 50% since the introduction of PUVA (35). The addition of systemic retinoids or combination with interferons may be beneficial but this requires more controlled investigations (36,37).

Eczema

Most forms of eczema are responsive to PUVA therapy including atopic eczema (38) and hand eczema (39). Clearance usually requires 30 to 50 treatments and maintenance is required for several months.

Photodermatoses

Polymorphous light eruption is essentially prevented by PUVA therapy. A schedule of three weekly exposures for three to four weeks is usually sufficient to prevent the rash and regular sun exposure is required to keep up protection for the whole summer season (40). Solar urticaria is also responsive to PUVA therapy with treatment of this condition requiring careful dosimetry so as not to precipitate widespread urticaria (41). Chronic actinic dermatitis can also be suppressed by PUVA therapy and this usually requires suppression with systemic corticosteroids in the early phase of treatment (42).

Other Dermatoses

In addition to the diseases of the skin that have already been discussed, there are at least 30 other diseases reported to respond to PUVA therapy. Many of these conditions are rare, and experience is limited to case reports but some have been studied in controlled or open trials (Table 8).

TABLE 8 Other Dermatoses Responsive to PUVA Therapy

Alopecia areata (43,44)
Amyloidosis (45)
Darier's disease (46)
Dermatitis herpetiformis (47)
Eosinophilic cellulitis (48)
Eosinophilic fasciitis (49)
Eosinophilic pustular folliculitis (50)
Erythema multiforme (51)
Flegel's disease (52)
GVH disease (53,54)
Granuloma annulare (55,56)
Granuloma faciale (57)
Histiocytosis X (58)
Ichthyosis linearis circumflexa (59)
Keratosis lichenoides chronica (60)
Lichen planus (61,62)
Lymphomatoid papulosis (63)
Mastocytosis (64,65)
Necrobiosis lipoidica (66)
Papulerythroderma (67)
Pigmented purpuric dermatoses (68,69)
Pityriasis lichenoides (70)
Pruritus—polycythemia vera (71)
Sclerosing skin diseases
   Morphea (72,73)
   Systemic sclerosis (74)
   Lichen sclerosis et atrophicus (75)
   Scleredema (76,77)
   Scleromyxedema (78,79)
Subacute prurigo (80)
Subcorneal pustular dermatosis (81)
Transient acantholytic dermatosis (82,83)
Vasculitis (84)

TOPICAL PUVA THERAPY

Direct application of psoralens to the skin combined with subsequent exposure to UVA radiation is widely used as a treatment, particularly in Europe (85). The psoralen is usually applied as a dilute solution in a bath or in a small container for local treatment of the hands and feet, the so-called soak PUVA therapy. Methoxsalen is the preferred psoralen in most centers because it gives a brief duration of photosensitivity, with all photosensitivity cleared within four hours. Trimethylpsoralen has been used in Scandinavia but has the disadvantage of causing prolonged photosensitivity that can last up to 48 hours.

Bath PUVA

The patient bathes in a dilute methoxsalen solution at 37°C immersed up to the neck for 15 minutes, then dries, and is given immediate exposure to UVA radiation. Various concentrations of methoxsalen have been used ranging from 0.5 up to 3 mg/L. The initial dose of UVA radiation is usually determined by measuring the MPD, although skin typing has also been used as a guide for treatment. Phototoxicity is the main adverse effect reported in studies and its frequency depends on the aggressiveness of the treatment protocol. Gastrointestinal disturbances and CNS symptoms are not seen with this form of PUVA therapy. Because of the very low serum levels that occur with topical PUVA therapy, the potential risk of cataracts should be nonexistent. There is no long-term safety data available for topical methoxsalen PUVA therapy, but based on studies in Swedish and Finnish patients, bath PUVA with TMP (86) and 8-MOP (87) appeared to have no relevant risk of carcinogenesis. Perhaps related to lower cumulative UVA doses, these data on the long-term safety of bath PUVA are encouraging but no premature conclusions should be drawn.

Other Forms of Therapy

Soak PUVA therapy uses a basin containing about 5 L of water and is useful for treating hand and foot diseases. Methoxsalen in a cream or gel has been used for local treatments and the kinetics of photosensitivity are similar to bath PUVA.

REFERENCES

1. Pathak MA, Fitzpatrick TB. The evolution of photochemotherapy with psoralens and UVA (PUVA): 2000 BC to 1992 AD. J Photochem Photobiol B: Biol 1992; 14:3–22.
2. Herfst MJ, De Wolff FA. Intraindividual and interindividual variability in 8-methoxypsoralen kinetics and effect in psoriatic patients. Clin Pharmacol Ther 1983; 34:117–125.
3. Brikl R, Schmid J, Koss FW. Pharmacokinetics and pharmacodynamics of psoralens after oral administration: considerations and conclusions. Natl Cancer Inst Monogr 1984; 66:63–67.
4. Tantcheva-Poór I, Servera-Llaneras M, Scharffetter-Kochanek K, et al. Liver cytochrome P450 CYP1A2 is markedly inhibited by systemic but not by bath PUVA in dermatological patients. Br J Dermatol 2001; 144:1127–1132.
5. Cripps DJ, Lowe NJ, Lerner AB. Action spectra of topical psoralens: a re-evaluation. Br J Dermatol 1982; 107:77–82.
6. Ibbotson SH, Farr PM. The time-course of psoralen ultraviolet A (PUVA) erythema. J Invest Dermatol 1999; 113:346–349.
7. Dall'Acqua F. Furocoumarin photochemistry and its main biological implications. In: Hönigsmann H, Stingl G, eds. Current Problems in Dermatology. Vol. 15. Therapeutic Photomedicine. Basel: Karger, 1986:137–163.
8. Hönigsmann H, Jaschke E, Nitsche V, et al. Serum levels of 8-methoxypsoralen in two different drug preparations. Correlation with photosensitivity and UVA dose requirements for photochemotherapy. J Invest Dermatol 1982; 79:233–236.
9. Stolk LML, Westerhof W, Corman RH, et al. Serum and urine concentrations of 5-methoxypsoralen after oral administration. Br J Dermatol 1981; 105:415–420.
10. Collins P, Wainwright NJ, Amorim I, et al. 8-MOP PUVA for psoriasis: a comparison of a minimal phototoxic dose-based regimen with a skin-type approach. Br J Dermatol 1996; 135:248–254.
11. Wolff K, Gschnait F, Hönigsmann H, et al. Phototesting and dosimetry for photochemotherapy. Br J Dermatol 1977; 96:1–10.
12. Melski JW, Tanenbaum L, Fitzpatrick TB, et al. Oral methoxsalen photochemotherapy for the treatment of psoriasis: a cooperative clinical trial. J Invest Dermatol 1977; 68:328–335.
13. Tanew A, Radakovic-Fijans, Seeber A, et al. PUVA maintenance treatment for psoriasis. J Invest Dermatol 2001; 117(3):816.
14. Stern RS, Parrish JA, Fitzpatrick TB. Ocular findings in patients treated with PUVA. J Invest Dermatol 1985; 85:269–273.
15. American Academy of Dermatology Committee on Guidelines of Care. Guidelines of care for psoriasis. J Am Acad Dermatol 1994; 31:643–648.
16. Morison WL. Phototherapy and Phototherapy of Skin Disease. 3rd ed. Boca Raton, FL: Taylor & Francis Group, 2005.
17. Stern RS, Lunder EJ. Risk of squamous cell carcinoma and methoxsalen (psoralen) and UV-A radiation (PUVA). Arch Dermatol 1998; 134:1582–1585.
18. Stern RS, Thibodeau LA, Kleinerman RA, et al. Risk of cutaneous carcinoma in patients treated with oral methoxsalen photochemotherapy for psoriasis. N Eng J Med 1979; 300:809–813.
19. Henseler T, Christophers E, Hönigsmann H, et al. Skin tumors in the European PUVA study. J Am Acad Dermatol 1987; 16:108–116.
20. Katz KA, Marcil I, Stern RS. Incidence and risk factors associated with a second squamous cell carcinoma or basal cell carcinoma in psoralen + ultraviolet A light-treated psoriasis patients. J Invest Dermatol 2002; 118:1038–1043.
21. Stern RS, Nichols KT, Väkevä LH. Malignant melanoma in patients treated for psoriasis with methoxsalen (psoralen) and ultraviolet A radiation (PUVA). N Engl J Med 1997; 336:1041–1045.
22. Parrish JA, Fitzpatrick TV, Tanenbaum L, et al. Photochemotherapy of psoriasis with oral methoxsalen and long wave ultraviolet light. N Engl J Med 1974; 291:1207–1211.
23. Hönigsman H, Fitzpatrick TB, Pathak MA, et al. Oral photochemotherapy with psoralens and UVA (PUVA): principles and practice. In: Fitzpatrick TB, Eisen AZ, Wolkk F, et al., eds. Dermatology in General Medicine. 4th ed. New York: McGraw-Hill, 1993:1728–1754.
24. Hönigsmann H, Gschnait F, Konrad K, et al. Photochemotherapy for pustular psoriasis (von Zumbusch). Br J Dermatol 1977; 97:119–126.
25. Murray D, Corbett MF, Warin AP. A controlled trial of photochemotherapy for persistent palmoplantar pustulosis. Br J Dermatol 1980; 102:659–665.
26. Vukas A. Photochemotherapy in treatment of psoriatic variants. Dermatologica 1977; 155:355–361.

27. Tanew A, Guggenbichler A, Hönigsmann H, et al. Photochemotherapy for severe psoriasis without or in combination with acitretin: a randomized, double-blind comparison study. J Am Acad Dermatol 1991; 25:682–684.
28. Morison WL, Momtaz K, Parrish JA, et al. Combined methotrexate-PUVA therapy in the treatment of psoriasis. J Am Acad Dermatol 1982; 6(1):46–51.
29. Momtaz-T K, Parrish JA. Combination of psoralens and ultraviolet A and ultraviolet B in the treatment of psoriasis vulgaris: a bilateral comparison study. J Am Acad Dermatol 1984; 10:481–486.
30. Pathak MA, Mosher DB, Parrish JA, et al. Relative effectiveness of three psoralens & sunlight in repigmentation of 365 vitiligo patients (abstract). J Invest Dermatol 1980; 74:252.
31. Grimes PE, Minus HR, Chakrabarti SG, et al. Determination of optimal topical photochemotherapy for vitiligo. J Am Acad Dermatol 1982; 7:771–778.
32. Ermis O, Alpsoy E, Cetin L, et al. Is the efficacy of psoralen plus ultraviolet A therapy for vitiligo enhanced by concurrent topical calcipotriol? A placebo-controlled double-blind study. Br J Dermatol 2001; 145:472–475.
33. Gilchrest BA, Parrish JA, Tanenbaum LT, et al. Oral methoxsalen photochemotherapy of mycosis fungoides. Cancer 1976; 38:683–689.
34. Hönigsmann H, Brenner W, Rauschmeier W, et al. Photochemotherapy for cutaneous T cell lymphoma. J Am Acad Dermatol 1984; 10:238–245.
35. Swanbeck G, Roupe G, Sandström MH. Indications of a considerable decrease in the death rate in mycosis fungoides by PUVA treatment. Acta Derm Venereol 1994; 74:465–466.
36. Mostow EN, Neckel SL, Oberhelman L, et al. Complete remissions in psoralen and UV-A (PUVA)-refractory mycosis fungoides-type cutaneous T-cell lymphoma with combined interferon Alfa and PUVA. Arch Dermatol 1993; 129:747–752.
37. Stadler R, Otte HG, Luger T, et al. Prospective randomized multicenter clinical trial on the use of interferon $\propto$ 2a plus acitretin versus interferon $\propto$ 2a plus PUVA in patients with cutaneous T-cell lymphoma stages I and II. Blood 1998; 10:3578–3581.
38. Morison WL, Parrish JA, Fitzpatrick TB. Oral psoralen photochemotherapy of atopic eczema. Br J Dermatol 1978; 98:25–30.
39. Tegner E, Thelin I. PUVA treatment of chronic eczematous dermatitis of the palms and soles. Acta Derm Venereol (Stockh) 1985; 65:451–453.
40. Ortel B, Tanew A, Wolff K, et al. Polymorphous light eruption: action spectrum and photoprotection. J Am Acad Dermatol 1986; 14:748–753.
41. Parrish JA, Jaenicke KF, Morison WL, et al. Solar urticaria: treatment with PUVA and mediator inhibitors. Br J Dermatol 1982; 106:575–580.
42. Yokel BK, Hood AF, Morison WL. Management of chronic photosensitive eczema. Arch Dermatol 1990; 126:1283–1285.
43. Claudy AL, Gagnaire D. Photochemotherapy for alopecia areata. Acta Dermatol Venereol (Stockh) 1979; 60:171–172.
44. Healy E, Rogers S. PUVA treatment for alopecia areata—does it work? A retrospective review of 102 cases. Br J Dermatol 1993; 129:42–44.
45. Jin AGT, Por A, Wee LKS, et al. Comparative study of phototherapy (UVB) vs. photochemotherapy (PUVA) vs. topical steroids in the treatment of primary cutaneous lichen amyloidosis. Photodermatol Phtoimmunol Photomed 2001; 17:42–43.
46. Sönnichsen VN, Brenke A, Diezel W. Dyskeratosis follicularis vegetans (Morbus Darier) therapie mit dem aromaitschen retinoid RO 10-9359 (Tigason®) in kombination mit systemischer photochemotherapie (ReUVA). Dermatol Monatsschr 1982; 168:520–522.
47. Kalimo K, Lammintausta K, Viander M. PUVA treatment of dermatitis herpetiformis. Photodermatol 1986; 3:54–55.
48. Diridl E, Hönigsmann H, Tanew A. Wells' syndrome responsive to PUVA therapy. Br J Dermatol 1997; 137:479–481.
49. Schiener R, Behrens-Williams SC, Gottlöber P, et al. Eosinophilic fasciitis treated with psoralen-ultraviolet A bath photochemotherapy. Br J Dermatol 2000; 142:804–807.
50. Buchness MR, Lim HW, Hatcher LA, et al. Eosinophilic pustular folliculitis in the acquired immunodeficiency syndrome. N Eng J Med 1988; 318:1183–1186.
51. Morison WL, Anhalt GJ. Therapy with oral psoralen plus UV-A for erythema multiforme. Arch Dermatol 1997; 133:1465–1466.
52. Cooper SM, George S. Flegel's disease treated with psoralen ultraviolet A. Br J Dermatol 2000; 142:340–342.
53. Vole-Platzer B, Hönigsmann H, Hinterberger W, et al. Photochemotherapy improves chronic cutaneous graft-versus-host disease. J Am Acad Dermatol 1990; 23:220–228.
54. Wolff D, Anders V, Corio R, et al. Oral PUVA and topical steroids for treatment of oral manifestations of chronic graft-vs-host disease. Photodermatol Photoimmunol Photomed 2004; 20:184–190.
55. Hindson TC, Spiro JG, Cochrane H. PUVA therapy of diffuse granuloma annulare. Clin Exp Dermatol 1988; 13:26–27.

56. Kerker BJ, Huang CP, Morison WL. Photochemotherapy of generalized granuloma annulare. Arch Dermatol 1990; 126:359–361.

57. Hudson LD. Granuloma faciale: treatment with topical psoralen and UVA. J Am Acad Dermatol 1983; 8:559.

58. Iwatsuki K, Tsugiki M, Yoshizawa N, et al. The effect of phototherapies on cutaneous lesions of histiocytosis X in the elderly. Cancer 1986; 57:1931–1936.

59. Manabe M, Yoshiike T, Negi M. Successful therapy of ichthyosis linearis circumflexa with PUVA. J Am Acad Dermatol 1983; 8:905–906.

60. Lang PG. Keratosis lichenoides chronica. Arch Dermatol 1981; 117:105–108.

61. Gonzalez E, Momtaz TK, Freedman S. Bilateral comparison of generalized lichen planus treated with psoralens and ultraviolet A. J Am Acad Dermatol 1984; 10:958–961.

62. Lundquist G, Forsgren H, Gajecki M, et al. Photochemotherapy of oral lichen planus. Oral Surg Oral Med Oral Pathol Oral Radio Endod 1995; 79:554–558.

63. Volkenandt M, Kerscher M, Sander C, et al. PUVA-bath photochemotherapy resulting in rapid clearance of lymphomatoid papulosis in a child. Arch Dermatol 1995; 131:1094.

64. Briffa DV, Eady RAJ, James MP, et al. Photochemotherapy (PUVA) in the treatment of urticaria pigmentosa. Br J Dermatol 1983; 109:67–75.

65. Mackey S, Pride HB, Tyler WB. Diffuse cutaneous mastocytosis. Arch Dermatol 1996; 132:1429–1430.

66. Ling TC, Thomson KF, Goulden V, et al. PUVA therapy in necrobiosis lipoidica diabeticorum. J Am Acad Dermatol 2002; 46:319–320.

67. Mutluer S, Yerebakan O, Alpsoy E, et al. Treatment of papuloerythroderma of Ofuji with re-PUVA: a case report and review of the therapy. J Eur Acad Dermatol Venereol 2004; 18:480–483.

68. Krizsa J, Hunyadi J, Dobozy A. PUVA treatment of pigmented purpuric lichenoid dermatitis (Gougerot-Blum). J Am Acad Dermatol 1992; 27:778–780.

69. Ling TC, Goulden V, Goodfield MJD. PUVA therapy in lichen aureus. J Am Acad Dermatol 2001; 45:145–146.

70. Boelen RE, Faber WR, Lambers JCCA, et al. Long-term follow-up of photochemotherapy in pityriasis lichenoides. Acta Derm Venereol (Stockh) 1982; 62:442–444.

71. Morison WL, Nesbitt JA. Oral psoralen photochemotherapy (PUVA) for pruritus associated with polycythemia vera and myelofibrosis. Am J Heratol 1993; 42:409–410.

72. Morison WL. Psoralen UVA therapy for linear and generalized morphea. J Am Acad Dermatol 1997; 37:657–658.

73. Todd DJ, Askari A, Ektaish F. PUVA therapy for disabling pansclerotic morphoea of children. Br J Dermatol 1998; 138:201–202.

74. Hofer A, Soyer HP. Oral psoralen-UV-A for systemic scleroderma. Arch Dermatol 1999; 136:603–604.

75. Reichrath J, Reinhold J, Tilgen W. Treatment of genito-anal lesions in inflammatory skin diseases with PUVA cream photochemotherapy: an open pilot study in 12 patients. Dermatology 2002; 205(3):245–248.

76. Grundmann-Kollman M, Ochsendorf F, Zollner TM, et al. Cream PUVA therapy for sclerodema adultorum. Br J Dermatol 2000; 142:1058–1059.

77. Hager CM, Sobhi HA, Hunzelmann N, et al. Bath-PUVA therapy in three patients with scleredema adultorum. J Am Acad Dermatol 1998; 38:240–242.

78. Adachi Y, Iba S, Horio T. Successful treatment of lichen myxoedematosus with PUVA photoche- motherapy. Photodermatol Photoimmunol Photomed 2000; 16:229–231.

79. Farr PM, Ive FA. PUVA treatment of scleromyxedema. Br J Dermatol 1984; 110:347–350.

80. Clark AR, Pa C, Jorizzo JL, et al. Papular dermatitis (subacute prurigo "itchy red bump" disease): pilot study of phototherapy. J Am Acad Dermatol 1998; 38:929–933.

81. Todd DJ, Bingham EA, Walsh M, et al. Subcorneal pustular dermatosis and IgA paraproteinaemia: response to both etretinate and PUVA. Br J Dermatol 1991; 125:387–389.

82. Lüftl M, Degitz K, Plewig G, et al. Bath psoralen-UV-A therapy for persistent Grover disease. Arch Dermatol 1999; 135:606–607.

83. Paul BS, Arndt KA. Response of transient acantholytic dermatosis to photochemotherapy. Arch Dermatol 1984; 120:121–122.

84. Choi HJ, Hann SK. Livedo reticularis and livedoid vasculitis responding to PUVA therapy. J Am Acad Dermatol 1999; 40:204–207.

85. Halpern SM, Anstey AV, Dawe RS, et al. Guidelines for topical PUVA: a report of a workshop of the British Photodermatology Group. Br J Dermatol 2000; 142:22–31.

86. Hannuksela-Svahn A, Sigurgeirsson B, Pukkala E, et al. Trioxsalen bath PUVA did not increase the risk of squamous cell skin carcinoma and cutaneous malignant melanoma in a joint analysis of 944 Swedish and Finnish patients with psoriasis. Br J Dermatol 1999; 141:497–501.

87. Hannuksela-Svahn A, Pukkala E, Koulu L, et al. Cancer incidence among Finnish psoriasis patients treated with 8-methoxypsoralen bath PUVA. J Am Acad Dermatol 1999; 40:694–696.

25 | Extracorporeal Photochemotherapy (Photopheresis)

Robert Knobler
*Division of Special and Environmental Dermatology, Department of Dermatology,
Medical University of Vienna, Vienna, Austria, and Department of Dermatology, College of Physicians and
Surgeons, Columbia University, New York, New York, U.S.A.*

Peter W. Heald
*Department of Dermatology, West Haven VA Medical Center, Yale University School of Medicine,
New Haven, Connecticut, U.S.A.*

- Efficacy of treating CTCL with skin directed therapies such as PUVA lead to the refinement of this therapeutic approach, where the target cells responsible for the disease pathology are directly treated. In ECP, extracorporeal PUVA therapy of the peripheral blood mononuclear cells (lymphocyte enriched, red cell depleted buffy coat) is performed.

- Photopheresis is approved by the Food and Drug Administration for the palliative treatment of refractory erythrodermic CTCL (Sézary's syndrome); however, the results in plaque and tumor stage disease are not impressive. Photopheresis has engendered numerous therapeutic trials with a wide range of other applications, particularly, acute and chronic GVHD, which has become the second most common application, and solid organ transplant rejection.

- Photopheresis for the treatment of systemic scleroderma and other autoimmune diseases and bullous dermatoses, although reportedly successful in several studies, is still under investigation. The efficacy of this treatment for these diseases, except for systemic scleroderma, has not been established by controlled clinical trials.

- Since its introduction, ECP has been shown to have only limited side effects, most of which are associated with volume changes during treatment, rarely anticoagulation toxicity such as bleeding or hypersensitivity reactions (Table 2).

- Recent progress in the understanding of the mechanisms of action, including possible induction of regulatory T-cells, may provide future developments that can be tested in future clinical trials and new indications within and outside dermatology.

INTRODUCTION

M
any of the therapeutic effects of irradiating diseased skin arise from the unique susceptibility of the pathogenic leukocytes in the skin to ultraviolet therapy when compared to
normal resident cells. Hence, in the management of cutaneous T-cell lymphoma (CTCL),
Psoralen plus UVA (PUVA) has repeatedly demonstrated its efficacy (see chap. 24). Patients
with the mycosis fungoides type of CTCL have malignant lymphocytes infiltrating the epidermis and dermis. When those are the only lesions present, PUVA is an appropriate therapy. The
disease can progress by several mechanisms to spread beyond this epidermal-dermal unit.
When malignant lymphocytes accumulate in the blood and diffusely infiltrate the skin, patients
become erythrodermic (Fig 1). Thus, PUVA therapy of the peripheral blood became a concept
in the early 1980s. The major physical problem with irradiating circulating lymphocytes
is that they are surrounded with erythrocytes containing hemoglobin, providing multiple
interruptions to the delivery of UVA to the lymphocyte. Another obvious problem is that
not all lymphocytes can be exposed, most are in tissue, and even if they were in circulation,
the entire peripheral compartment cannot be removed. To effect a session of extracorporeal
photochemotherapy or photophoresis ECP, the peripheral blood would need to be pheresed,
returning removed erythrocytes to the patient. This creates a buffy coat, enriched for lymphocytes,
with a hematocrit of between 2% and 4%. This population of collected cells, some 10% of the circulating pool, can be dosed with 8-methoxypsoralen (MOP) and perfused through a UVA emitting
light source. In the initial clinical trial, it was decided to perform consecutive days of therapy to
expose at least 20% of the circulating lymphocytes. The intervals between treatments would determine the size of the clinical trial, and intervals of four weeks were selected. As will be discussed in
the applications, efficacy and safety were noted and this two half-day-per-month schedule was
adopted. Since those initial developments, some of the patents on photophoresis have expired,
and there are now derivations developing that accentuate one or more aspects in the overall
process, to develop a wider range of phototherapy products than what was initially offered.

Photophoresis has engendered numerous therapeutic trials, a wide range of applications
(Table 1), immunologic insights, and concepts for future development that are presented in this

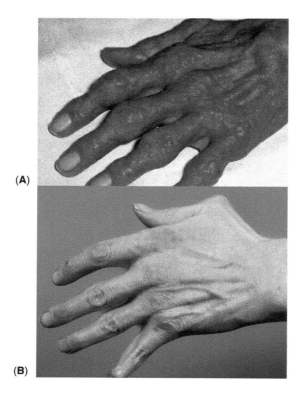

(A)

(B)

FIGURE 1 Erythrodermic cutaneous T-cell lymphoma (**A**) with diffuse involvement of the hands prior to photophoresis, and (**B**) in remission (patient remained in complete remission for over 12 years).

chapter. The therapeutic applications are presented to portray the scope of the therapy. This is followed by an attempt to project where this photoimmunotherapy will develop based on current research.

APPLICATIONS OF PHOTOPHERESIS IN DISEASE
Cutaneous T-Cell Lymphoma

As mentioned, the current photopheresis regimens still reflect the schedules in the initial multi-center clinical trial (1). In that initial study, the erythrodermic form of CTCL was noted to be the variant most responsive to photopheresis. Based on the success of this schedule, most CTCL patients undergo the two-day every four-week regimen.

The results of the initial clinical trials and follow-up studies showed that, as a monother-apy, photopheresis (Fig. 2) can induce a remission in approximately one-fourth of the patients treated (Figs. 1,3) (2). One-half of the patients with erythrodermic CTCL had a significant partial response and the remaining one-fourth had no response or progressive disease. This same proportion of responses was observed in the smaller series of CTCL (3–5). From these clinical experiences, several other common features were found. The response to photopheresis is gradual; a periodic assessment of tumor burden measures should be conducted every four to eight weeks with a time to response of typically 12 to 16 weeks into therapy. Peripheral blood studies would include flow cytometry, following the lymphocyte population that expresses CD4, but not CD7 (CD4+/CD7−). Along with a skin score, this is an objective parameter in the management of erythrodermic CTCL patients (6). In the absence of this investigation, one could also follow CD4:CD8 ratios as a measure of tumor burden in the peripheral blood (7). Dose responsiveness of photopheresis has not been striking, but in one report, a patient was treated using an every two-week regimen at the initiation of therapy. The CTCL patient in that report had hyperleukocytic disease and after the leukemia improved, the patient was put on a four-week cycle (8). Several other centers have since adopted this accelerated delivery schedule at the initiation of therapy. After 12 to 16 weeks, a trend in the patient's clinical status should be evident. If there are signs of improvement, the therapy should be continued to maximize the therapeutic response. Complete clearing may occur after six to eight months of gradual improvement. Patients with incomplete responses at three to six months are usually considered for adjunctive therapy.

Adjunctive therapy with photopheresis is as vast as the therapeutic armamentarium for this disease in general. However, the major principle guiding the use of adjunctive therapy is that the disease at this point is immunosuppressive in itself (7), so that therapies that avoid immuno-suppression or even stimulate the immune system are preferred. There are agents used in conjunction with photopheresis from all three categories of CTCL therapy: (*i*) skin-directed

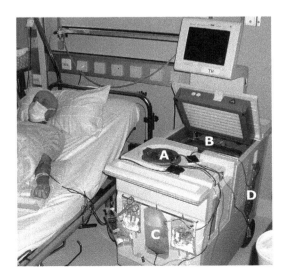

FIGURE 2 A patient being treated with photopheresis. The recumbent position or in bed (as illustrated) is maintained for at least three hours. The device opened to display the various components: A. Centrifuge, B. Irradiation Chamber, C. Pheresed erythrocytes to be returned, and D. Photoinactivated lymphocytes to be reinfused.

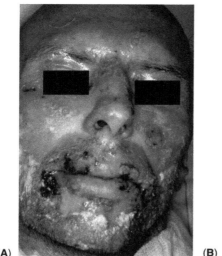 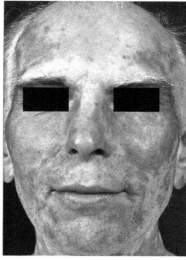

(A)   **(B)**

FIGURE 3 Response of facial features of Sézary syndrome (**A**) before (with vegetating herpes simplex), and (**B**) after photopheresis (pre-existing vitiligo became evident).

therapy, (*ii*) biologic response modifiers, and (*iii*) low-dose chemotherapy. In patients with significant tumor burden, a reduction of that tumor burden with a skin-directed treatment can work synergistically with photopheresis. Debulking of CTCL can reliably be performed with radiotherapy (total skin electron beam therapy). In one series, patients treated with photopheresis and total skin electron beam had improved survival, when compared with similarly staged patients at the same institution treated with total skin electron beam therapy alone (9). More recently, however, the failing immunity in erythrodermic CTCL patients has become the target of adjunctive therapy. This began with alfa-interferon (IFN-α).

In a review of a decade of using IFN-α with photopheresis, a greater response rate was noted than with historic controls (10,11). Once the oral retinoid bexarotene was found to have unique activity against CTCL, combinations of this with photopheresis have been reported. The most intriguing results have now been reported with the combination of IFN-α, oral bexarotene, and photopheresis (12). This multimodality regimen is useful in that it can minimize toxicity of the injected and oral agents by using low doses. Enough complete remissions have been induced with this regimen to prompt discussion regarding the approach to managing photopheresis patients (13). Typically, patients are started on monotherapy and if responding, adjuncts are added to achieve a complete response. An alternative approach would be to commence with the best chance of a response, with all the three therapies, and taper off if a complete response has been achieved.

The failing immunity of advancing CTCL is the major reason why traditional high-dose chemotherapy has been unsuccessful in treating CTCL, because it is too toxic. However, low-dose chemotherapy has been employed with beneficial results. There are two oral agents that

TABLE 1 Indications for Photopheresis

Good evidence available	
Erythrodermic CTCL	Chronic graft-versus-host disease
Acute graft-versus-host disease	Organ transplant rejection
Experimental and investigational	
Scleroderma	Nephrogenic fibrosing dermopathy
Bullous dermatoses	Lichen planus
Crohn's disease	Multiple sclerosis

Abbreviation: CTCL, cutaneous T-cell lymphoma.

TABLE 2 Side Effects of Photopheresis

Volume loading with saline: exacerbation of congestive heart failure
Anticoagulation toxicity: bleeding, hypersensitivity
Venipuncture pain and prolonged recumbency

have theoretical and anecdotal benefits for photopheresis patients (14,15). Photochemotherapy induces DNA damage and requires rescue from pathways that are inhibitable by methotrexate and enzymes that are inhibited by etoposide. Each of these agents has an impact in the oral low-dose therapy of CTCL. Oral corticosteroids can be palliative in CTCL patients, but their immunosuppressive effects have been shown to negate the therapeutic effects of photopheresis in an experimental model (16).

In summary, photopheresis can be used as monotherapy in patients with erythrodermic CTCL, or as part of a multiagent regimen for CTCL patients with refractory disease or multiple tumors. The goal of therapy should be to achieve palliation and, less frequently, remission. After achieving the therapy goal, photopheresis is gradually tapered. The taper schedule used in the majority of the initial study patients was to add a seven-day interval every three cycles of therapy. Once patients achieved eight-week intervals, and their skin remained clear for a period of six months, they were taken off therapy. Patients with an unacceptable response or progressive disease while receiving photopheresis should have their next line of therapy introduced before discontinuing treatment completely. Therapeutic effects of photopheresis are sometimes not appreciated until they are unmasked by a disease flare with the cessation of therapy.

Once photopheresis became an available modality for CTCL treatment, dermatologists began exploring the therapeutic effects in other difficult to treat dermatoses. The majority of these have been with autoimmune diseases. After therapeutic effects were noted and defined, photopheresis was then utilized in the undeniably autoimmune disease of graft-versus-host disease (GVHD) in allogeneic bone marrow and stem cell transplants. GVHD has become the second most common application.

Graft-vs.-Host Disease

GVHD is a frequent complication of allogeneic bone marrow transplantation (BMT) and peripheral blood stem cell transplantation. GVHD is mediated by donor T-cells, reactive against the recipient's major, and minor histocompatibility antigens. Photopheresis is capable of eliciting an immunoregulatory response against such pathogenic T-cells in a mouse model system (17). There has been a growing clinical experience in the use of photopheresis as treatment of acute and chronic GVHD (18–26).

The largest single center group of patients with chronic GVHD treated with photopheresis involved 15 patients (19). In this study, patients had extensive chronic GVHD, representing a spectrum from lichenoid to sclerodermoid forms. They received photopheresis every two weeks for the first three months, and monthly thereafter. Out of the 15 patients, 12 (80%) obtained complete clearing of their cutaneous involvement. Of note, 11 of 11 patients with oral mucosal involvement and 7 of 10 patients with liver involvement demonstrated complete resolution of their extracutaneous involvement. Patients received photopheresis for 7 to 31 months, during which time corticosteroid therapy could be discontinued after a median of 80 days. In an independent study, 11 patients with chronic GVHD were treated with photopheresis twice monthly for four months, then once monthly thereafter. Although nearly all patients initially demonstrated an improvement in skin and mucosal involvement by a blinded observer scoring at the fourth month, the effects on visceral manifestations were less impressive. For example, elevated liver enzymes improved in one of six patients but worsened in three patients receiving photopheresis (20). In another report, four of five patients with chronic GVHD (two of which had extensive cutaneous involvement) demonstrated improvement with photopheresis, and three patients achieved complete remission. These complete responders were able to eventually discontinue all treatment modalities (20). Although these reports and others are very encouraging, a large ongoing trial will more clearly delineate the role of photopheresis in the treatment of chronic GVHD (21–26).

Experience with photopheresis in the treatment of acute GVHD is equally promising, but more limited than for chronic GVHD. As part of the study mentioned above, six patients with histologic grade II to IV acute GVHD were treated with photopheresis twice monthly (18). All were unresponsive to immunosuppressive therapy with combination of cyclosporine and methylprednisolone. Overall, four of the six patients obtained complete resolution of disease after only two to three months, at which time photopheresis was halted. Of note, prednisone was tapered off completely in the first two to four weeks of photopheresis, whereas low-dose cyclosporine was continued as a maintenance modality. Prospective multicenter studies under way should in the near future help delineate the significance of photopheresis in the treatment of acute GVHD.

In a novel approach to using photopheresis in the management of GVHD, photopheresis was reported to prevent the development of GVHD. The therapeutic regimen utilized the combination of photopheresis, pentostatin, and radiotherapy in a series of 55 patients, where only 9% developed greater than grade II GVHD (26).

Given the problems with the toxicity of the current standard of care therapy for GVHD (i.e., various immunosuppressive medications) and the increasing incidence of GVHD as a result of an expanding use of allogeneic BMT and peripheral blood stem cell transplantation, photopheresis has grown in its use for GVHD. This is now the second largest group of patients treated with photopheresis, behind CTCL.

Scleroderma

Scleroderma has been considered as a disorder of T-cells, a notion heavily reinforced by its occurrence in the setting of allogeneic bone marrow or stem cell transplantation. The early phase of scleroderma is characterized by an inflammatory infiltrate and edema within the dermis. It is hypothesized that activated helper T-cells within the infiltrate help stimulate the production of collagen synthesis and subsequent fibrosis. The degree to which fibrosis is reversible in patients with scleroderma is unknown. One would anticipate that any successful modality for scleroderma would demonstrate its greatest therapeutic effect in patients with relatively recent disease onset. For that reason, the initial clinical trial of photopheresis for scleroderma focused on patients diagnosed within two years of starting therapy. The randomized, parallel-group, single-blinded, multicenter clinical trial involved 79 patients and its goal was to demonstrate safety and efficacy of photopheresis in the treatment of scleroderma (27). Patients who had worsening of cutaneous involvement of at least 30% during the preceding six months were randomized to receive photopheresis or oral D-penicillamine (maximum dose of 750 mg daily) for six months. Exclusion criteria included significant renal disease (serum creatinine >3 mg/dL) or pulmonary involvement (carbon monoxide diffusing capacity less than 50% of normal). Clinical examiners, blinded to the treatment-type delivered, recorded a skin score based on skin thickness, percentage surface area involved, oral aperture diameter, and the capacity for hand closure. A significant improvement in skin score occurred in 68% (21 of 31) of patients receiving photopheresis and 32% (8 of 25) of patients on D-penicillamine, whereas significant worsening was observed in 10% (three patients) receiving photopheresis and 32% (eight patients) receiving D-penicillamine. The difference between the two groups was statistically significant ($P = 0.02$). Furthermore, adverse reactions in the photopheresis study group were minimal, and all patients in the photopheresis group completed the study. This is in contrast to the D-penicillamine group; 24% of these patients had to permanently discontinue the treatment directly, because of adverse effects of this medication.

There were nine subjects in an open trial of scleroderma treated with photopheresis for 6 to 21 months. These patients demonstrated significant improvement in their skin, musculoskeletal system, functional index, and symptoms including Raynaud's phenomenon, dyspnea, fatigue, dysphagia, and arthralgias (28). Again, patients in this study were relatively early in their disease onset, with a history of scleroderma findings for only six months to four years. However, there are two separate open trials of eight patients (29) and seven patients (30), where subjects showed little response or worsening despite treatment with photopheresis.

Average disease duration in both trials was longer than in the randomized multicenter trial discussed before. Furthermore, patients were not excluded on the basis of severe internal organ involvement. In a recent randomized, double-blinded, placebo-controlled trial with 64 patients, the efficacy of photopheresis on skin and joint involvement was also reported (31).

A scleroderma variant, eosinophilic fasciitis, has been treated with photopheresis. There have been reports of response in this autoimmune fibrotic disorder that can also occur in the setting of GVHD. In a pilot study of eosinophilic fasciitis, two of three patients showed softening of indurated skin as determined by a computerized measurement of skin elasticity (32).

Autoimmune Bullous Diseases

Autoimmune bullous diseases (pemphigus vulgaris, pemphigus foliaceus, and epidermolysis bullosa acquisita) represent disorders of humoral immunity with the elaboration of circulating antibodies against distinctive structural proteins in the skin. In patients with pemphigus vulgaris, production of autoantibodies against the desmoglein-3 protein component of keratinocyte desmosomes leads to blister and erosion formation of cutaneous and mucosal surfaces. Although the majority of patients are adequately controlled with the use of various immunosuppressive medications (i.e., high-dose corticosteroids, azathioprine, cyclosporin, or cyclophosphamide), long-term treatment with these medications often results in significant adverse effects. Thus, mortality remains around 5% to 15%, largely because of complications from these drugs. Because photopheresis has a few adverse effects profile, it is a potential treatment for pemphigus patients failing systemic drug therapy that is often immunosuppressing and toxic.

The initial report of photopheresis efficacy involved four patients (ages 61–78 years) with extensive and refractory pemphigus vulgaris, despite large doses of immunosuppressive medications (33). Patients continued to receive prednisone alone or with azathioprine. All four patients showed clinical improvement and a drop in antidesmosomal antibody titers, despite tapering of immunosuppressive medications. After 36 to 48 months, three of the four patients demonstrated a complete remission (no clinical evidence of active disease and undetectable antidesmosomal antibody titers), which lasted an average 19.3 months (range 7–36 months). Relapses in the three patients responded to reinitiation of photopheresis after three to four monthly cycles. Similar beneficial results of photopheresis for pemphigus vulgaris have been reported in individual case reports. One involved a 31 year old man with a four-year history of severe disease (34), and a woman, 37 years of age, with a five-year history of severe pemphigus vulgaris (35). More recently, reported a beneficial effect of photopheresis in the treatment of severe pemphigus foliaceus (36).

These case reports suggest that photopheresis may be a promising and relatively safe treatment for the selective cases of pemphigus vulgaris. A randomized, controlled study would be helpful to define its role.

Another notoriously difficult to treat bullous disease is epidermolysis bullosa acquisita (EBA). In this disorder of antitype VII collagen antibodies, patients develop blisters and, in addition, marked skin fragility. In an initial study of three adult patients with refractory EBA, photopheresis treatment demonstrated objective improvements in blistering, whereas two of three patients had significant subjective improvement in skin fragility (37). Certainly further studies are necessary before photopheresis proves to be an effective treatment option for aggressive forms of EBA.

Systemic Lupus Erythematosus

Disordered T-cell immunity has notoriously been associated with systemic lupus erythematosus (SLE). Abnormal circulating B-cells and T-cells result in autoantibody production against various nuclear and cytoplasmic antigens. The disease is usually controlled to some degree with standard therapies, including antimalarials, corticosteroids, and other immunosuppressive agents. A murine model of lupus has been modulated by infusions of

8-methoxypsoralen/UVA-light treated lymphocytes (38). This led to the concept of a clinical trial in lupus patients. The initial investigators proceeded cautiously with concern that photodamaged DNA would be infused into patients with anti-DNA antibodies.

The initial study of photopheresis in the treatment of SLE consisted of 10 patients who met the American College of Rheumatology criteria for SLE (39). Study patients had their disease adequately controlled with low-dose prednisone, chloroquine, azathioprine, or cyclophosphamide; however, all patients had disease flares with multiple drug tapering attempts. Strict inclusion criteria resulted in a study population with mild-to-moderate systemic involvement. Patients were treated on two consecutive days every month for six months, then every two months for another six months. In the eight patients who completed the study, disease activity decreased as measured by the SLE Activity Index Scoring System (40). The SIS score, based on a combination of clinical and laboratory findings, dropped from a median seven (range 4–9) down to one (range 0–5). In all patients except one, the dosages of corticosteroids and immunosuppressive medications were reduced during this time. A marked resolution of cutaneous lesions was observed in six patients after four to six months of photopheresis. Laboratory abnormalities showed no difference from baseline values (39).

Oral Lichen Planus

The striking clinical similarities of lichen planus and GVHD continue into their respective therapies. Photopheresis has been investigated in patients with lichen planus suffering from one of the most symptomatic presentations: erosive oral lichen planus. In a study of seven patients resistant to multiple medications, all patients demonstrated complete remission of disease activity after a mean of 12 cycles (41).

PHOTOBIOLOGY OF PHOTOPHERESIS

Given the variety of immunomodulated diseases in dermatology, it would not be surprising to see the repertoire of therapeutic applications increase over the next few years. Perhaps, these clinical extensions will proceed from some of the parallel investigations being made in ex-vivo studies of photoinactivated lymphocytes infusions. To date, no single mechanism is consistent with the observations made, clinically or at the bench.

Investigators observed that CTCL patient's peripheral lymphocytes that are isolated by the photopheresis unit, after exposure to UVA in the presence of 8-MOP, undergo a programmed cellular death (apoptosis) (42,43). Thus, an alternative, nonimmunologic theory as to the efficacy of photopheresis for CTCL is that repeated treatments eventually result in the exposure of nearly all peripheral tumor cells to the induction of apoptosis. The explanation may be limited by the asymptotic nature of such an exposure curve and by the fact that many of the tumor cells are not in the peripheral circulation at any given time, although they may repeatedly migrate in and out of the skin. Nonetheless, apoptotic malignant T-cells may be actively phagocytized by antigen presenting cells (APC), which may facilitate the presentation of relevant tumor antigens necessary to generate clone-specific, antitumor immunity.

Photopheresis has been shown to induce large numbers of peripheral blood monocytes to express markers of dermal dendritic cells (DC) (44). These cells have the capacity to actively ingest 8-MOP/UVA-induced apoptotic T-cells, including malignant or autoreactive T-cells that may be present in the circulation, which further stimulates DC activation and maturation. Hence, photopheresis has been conjectured to result in the production and reinfusion of putative T-cell-loaded APC capable of stimulating immunity against the pathogenic T-cells. Importantly, especially in consideration of the mechanism of inhibition of autoreactivity, it is also possible that under certain immune states, photopheresis may induce the production of sufficient numbers of (e.g., immature) DC that may provide tolerogenic signals (45).

Recent experimental data suggest that infusion of autologous haptenated cells in which apoptosis was induced by 8-MOP/UVA induces immunologic tolerance. The nature of this tolerance is primarily due to regulatory T-cells, because transfer in an animal model conferred similar protection. The demonstration of the induction of regulatory T-cells may explain why, in humans, ECP exerts a beneficial effect in a wide variety of diseases, which would be amenable to such activity. The generation of age-specific regulatory T-cells may explain why generalized immunosuppression has not been noted with ECP (46).

The insight into the mechanism of photopheresis has provided several therapeutic developments that can be tested in future clinical trials. The conjecture that APC play a critical role in photopheresis-induced activation of CD8+ T-cells leads to the conjectured use of cytokines (e.g., GM-CSF) to activate APCs. Injections prior to a session of photopheresis would appear to be the most timely, but post therapy may also be an important time of administration. Not many dimensions of the photopheresis session can be manipulated (both the volume of blood removed and the patient's willingness to sit for long periods of time have limits); however, the time that the lymphocytes are out of the body may also be increased in an attempt to enhance efficacy (47). Future trials involving these and other adaptations of photopheresis are anticipated.

REFERENCES

1. Edelson R, Berger C, Gasparro F, et al. Treatment of cutaneous T-cell lymphoma by extracorporeal photochemotherapy. Preliminary results. N Engl J Med 1987; 316(6):297–303.
2. Heald P, Rook A, Perez M, et al. Treatment of erythrodermic cutaneous T-cell lymphoma with extracorporeal photochemotherapy. J Am Acad Dermatol 1992; 27(3):427–433.
3. Zic J, Arzubiaga C, Salhany KE, et al. Extracorporeal photopheresis for the treatment of cutaneous T-cell lymphoma. J Am Acad Dermatol 1992; 27(5):729–736.
4. Armus S, Keyes B, Cahill C, et al. Photopheresis for the treatment of cutaneous T-cell lymphoma. J Am Acad Dermatol 1990; 23(5):898–902.
5. Bisaccia E, Gonzalez J, Palangio M, et al. Extracorporeal photochemotherapy alone or with adjuvant therapy in the treatment of cutaneous T-cell lymphoma: A 9-year retrospective study at a single institution. J Am Acad Dermatol 2000; 43(2):263–271.
6. Stevens SR, Baron ED, Masten S, et al. Circulating CD4+ CD7 lymphocyte burden and rapidity of response: predictors of outcome in the treatment of Sézary syndrome and erythrodermic mycosis fungoides with extracorporeal photopheresis. Arch Dermatol 2002; 138(10):1347–1350.
7. Heald P, Yan SL, Latkowski J, Edelson R. Profound deficiency in normal circulating T-cells in erythrodermic cutaneous T-cell lymphoma. Arch Dermatol 1994; 130(2):198–203.
8. Bowen GM, Steens SR, Dubin HV, et al. Diagnosis of Sézary syndrome in a patient with generalized pruritus based on early molecular study and flow cytometry. J Am Acad Dermatol 1995; 33(4):678–680.
9. Wilson LD, Licata AL, Braverman IM, et al. Systemic chemotherapy and extracorporeal photochemotherapy and T3 and T4 cutaneous T-cell lymphoma patients who have achieved a complete response to total skin electron beam therapy. Int J Rad Oncol 1995; 32(4):987–995.
10. Rook A, Prystowsky M, Cassin M, et al. Combined therapy for Sézary syndrome with extracorporeal photochemotherapy and low dose interferon alfa therapy. Arch Dermatol 1991; 127(10):1535–1540.
11. Gottlieb SL, Wolfe JT, Fox F, et al. Treatment of cutaneous T-cell lymphoma with extracorporeal photopheresis monotherapy and in combination with recombinant interferon alfa: a 10-year experience at a single institution. J Am Acad Dermatol 1996; 35(6):946–957.
12. Shapiro M, Rook AH, Lehrer MS, et al. Novel multimodality biologic response modifier therapy, including bexarotene and long-wave ultraviolet A for a patient with refractory stage IVa. J Am Acad Dermatol 2002; 47(6):956–961.
13. Knobler R, Jantschitsch C. Extracorporeal photoimmunotherapy in cutaneous T-cell lymphoma. Tranfus Apheresis Sci 2003; 28:81–89.
14. Zackheim HS, Epstein EH. Low dose methotrexate for Sézary syndrome. J Am Acad Dermatol 1989; 21(4):757–762.
15. Molin L, Thomsen K, Volden G, et al. Epipodophyllotoxin (VP-16-23) in mycosis fungoides: a report for the Scandinavian mycosis fungoides group. Acta Derm Venereol 1979; 59(1):84–90.
16. Perez MI, Edelson RL, LaRoche L, et al. Inhibition of anti-skin allograft immunity by infusions with syngeneic photoinactivated effector lymphocytes. J Invest Dermatol 1989; 92(5):669–674.
17. Girardi M, Heald P, Tigelaar RE. Specific suppression of lupus-like graft-versus-host disease using extracorporeal photochemical attenuation of effector lymphocytes. J Invest Dermatol 1995; 104(2):177–182.
18. Greinix HT, Volc-Platzer B, Rabitsch W, et al. Successful use of extracorporeal photochemotherapy in the treatment of severe acute and chronic graft-versus-host disease. Blood 1998; 92(9):3098–3104.
19. Child FJ, Ratnavel R, Watkins P, et al. Extracorporeal photopheresis (ECP) in the treatment of chronic graft-versus-host disease (GVHD). Bone Marrow Transplant 1999; 23(9):881–887.

20. Besnier D, Chabannes D, Mahè B, et al. Treatment of graft-versus-host disease by extracorporeal photochemotherapy. Transplantation 1997; 64(1):49–54.
21. Owsianowski M, Gollnick H, Siegert W, et al. Successful treatment of chronic graft-versus-host disease with extracorporeal photopheresis. Bone Marrow Transplant 1994; 14(5):845–848.
22. Dall'Amico R, Rossetti F, Zulian F, et al. Photopheresis in paediatric patients with drug-resistant chronic graft-versus-host disease. Br J Haematol 1997; 97(4):848–854.
23. Rossetti F, Zulian F, Dall'Amico R, et al. Extracorporeal photochemotherapy as single therapy for extensive, cutaneous, chronic graft-versus-host disease. Transplantation 1995; 59(1):49–51.
24. Konstantinow A, Balda B-R, Starz H, et al. Chronic graft-versus-host disease: successful treatment with extracorporeal photochemotherapy: a follow-up. Br J Dermatol 1996; 135(6):1003–1017.
25. Richter H, Stege H, Ruzicka T, et al. Extracorporeal photopheresis in the treatment of acute graft-versus-host disease. J Am Acad Dermatol 1997; 36(5 Pt 1):787–789.
26. Miller KB, Roberts TF, Chan G, et al. A novel reduced intensity regimen for allogeneic hematopoietic stem cell transplantation associated with a reduced incidence of graft-versus-host disease. Bone Marrow Transplant 2004; 33(9):881–999.
27. Rook AH, Freundlich B, Jegasothy BV, et al. Treatment of systemic sclerosis with extracorporeal photochemotherapy. Results of a multicenter trial. Arch Dermatol 1992; 128(3):337–346.
28. Di Spaltro FX, Cottrill C, Cahill C, et al. Extracorporeal photochemotherapy in progressive systemic sclerosis. Int J Dermatol 1993; 32(6):417–421.
29. Zachariae H, Bjerring P, Heickendorff L, et al. Photopheresis in systemic sclerosis: clinical and serological studies using markers of collagen metabolism. Acta Derm Venereol 1993; 73(5):356–361.
30. Cribier B, Faradji T, Le Coz C, et al. Extracorporeal photochemotherapy in systemic sclerosis and severe morphea. Dermatology 1995; 191(1):25–31.
31. Knobler RM, French LE, Kim Y, et al. A randomized, double-blind, placebo-controlled trial of photopheresis in systemic sclerosis. J Am Acad Dermatol 2006; 54(5):793–796.
32. Romano C, Rubegni P, De Aloe G, et al. Extracorporeal photochemotherapy in the treatment of eosinophilic fasciitis. J Eur Acad Dermatol Venereol 2003; 17(1):10–13.
33. Rook AH, Jegasothy BV, Heald P, et al. Extracorporeal photochemotherapy for drug-resistant pemphigus vulgaris. Ann Intern Med 1990; 112(4):303–305.
34. Liang G, Nahass G, Kerdel FA. Pemphigus vulgaris treated with photopheresis. J Am Acad Dermatol 1992; 26(5 Pt 1):779–780.
35. Gollnick HP, Owsianowski M, Taube KM, et al. Unresponsive severe generalized pemphigus vulgaris successfully controlled by extracorporeal photopheresis. J Am Acad Dermatol 1993; 28(1):122–124.
36. Azana JM, de Misa RF, Harto A, et al. Severe pemphigus foliaceus treated with extracorporeal photochemotherapy. Arch Dermatol 1997; 133(3):287–289.
37. Miller J, Stricklin GP, Fine JD, et al. Remission of severe epidermolysis bullosa acquisita induced by extracorporeal photochemotherapy. Br J Dermatol 1995; 133(3):467–471.
38. Berger CL, Perez M, Laroche L, et al. Inhibition of autoimmune disease in a murine model of systemic lupus erythematosus induced by exposure to syngeneic photoinactivated lymphocytes. J Invest Dermatol 1990; 94(1):52–57.
39. Knobler RM, Graninger W, Lindmaier A, et al. Extracorporeal photochemotherapy for the treatment of systemic lupus erythematosus. A pilot study. Arthritis Rheum 1992; 35(3):319–324.
40. Brunner HI, Feldman BM, Bombardier C, et al. Sensitivity of the systemic lupus erythematosus disease activity index, British isles lupus assessment group index, and Systemic Lupus Activity Measure in the evaluation of clinical change in childhood-onset systemic lupus erythematosus. Arthritis Rheum 1999; 42(7):1354–1360.
41. Bécherel PA, Bussel A, Chosidow O, et al. Extracorporeal photochemotherapy for chronic erosive lichen planus. Lancet 1998; 351(9105):805.
42. Yoo E, Rook A, Elenitsas R, et al. Apoptosis induction by ultraviolet light A and photochemotherapy in cutaneous T-cell lymphoma: relevance to mechanism of therapeutic action. J Invest Dermatol 1996; 107(2):235–242.
43. Miracco C, Rubegni P, DeAloe G, et al. Extracorporeal photochemotherapy induces apoptosis of infiltrating lymphoid cells in patients with mycosis fungoides in early stages. A quantitative histological study. Br J Dermatol 1997; 137(4):549–557.
44. Berger CL, Xu AL, Hanlon D, et al. Induction of human tumor-loaded dendritic cells. Int J Cancer 2001; 91(4):438–447.
45. Lamioni A, Parisi F, Isacchi G, et al. The immunological effects of extracorporeal photopheresis unraveled: induction of tolerogenic dendritic cells in vitro and regulatory T cells in vivo. Transplantation 2005; 79(7):846–850.
46. Maeda A, Schwarz A, Kernebeck K, et al. Intravenous infusion of syngeneic apoptotic cells by photopheresis induces antigen-specific regulatory T cells. J Immunol 2005; 174(10):5968–5976.
47. Girardi M, Schechner J, Glusac E, et al. Transimmunization and the evolution of extracorporeal photochemotherapy. Transfus Apheresis Sci 2002; 26(3):181–190.

26 | Photodynamic Therapy

Sally H. Ibbotson
*Department of Dermatology, Ninewells Hospital and Medical School,
University of Dundee, Dundee, Scotland, U.K.*

Rolf-Markus Szeimies
Department of Dermatology, Regensburg University Hospital, Regensburg, Germany

- The efficacy of 5-aminolevulinic acid/methyl aminolevulinate PDT in the treatment of nonmelanoma skin cancer, particularly actinic keratoses, Bowen's disease, and superficial basal cell carcinomas, has been sufficiently documented and justifies that PDT is to be considered among the standard therapeutic procedures for these diseases.

- The proven advantages of PDT include the simultaneous treatment of multiple tumors, subclinical and large lesions, relatively short healing times, good patient tolerance, and excellent cosmesis.

- The potential tumor control in immunocompromised patients (i.e., transplant recipients) is very promising.

- Cost-effectiveness analysis indicates that with relatively low costs for permanent equipment, topical PDT is probably no more expensive than conventional therapy when its lower side-effect profile is considered.

- PDT may also find a place in the treatment of patients with inflammatory dermatoses.

- Nevertheless, the limitations of PDT, including its topical variant, have to be kept in mind. Crucial parameters are the depth of penetration of both sensitizer and light into the skin. Moreover, for the treatment of skin cancers with metastatic potential, patients need to be selected carefully, and histologic diagnosis and determination of tumor thickness are a prerequisite.

INTRODUCTION AND HISTORICAL ASPECTS

The first attempt to use the amplifying effect of light in the presence of a chemical substance was undertaken by Oscar Raab, a medical student at the Department of Pharmacology at the University of Munich, Germany. The Head of Department, Hermann von Tappeiner was looking for new antimalarials and Raab's task was to study the influence of acridine orange and its derivatives on infusoria and other protozoa. Raab discovered that the cell-killing effects of the drug were potentiated by the presence of light. In 1904, von Tappeiner coined the term "photodynamic reaction."

This new therapeutic approach was then applied to patients. Together with Albert Jesionek, a young assistant professor at the Department of Dermatology, University of Munich, von Tappeiner started the first experiments in man in February 1903. Their first paper of three was published in 1903 and dealt with the photodynamic treatment of cancerous, syphilitic, and tuberculous skin conditions.

In 1902, Georges Dreyer in Copenhagen examined the effect of light on bacteria. Besides bacteria and animal skin, he also sensitized living human skin to demonstrate the phototoxic effect.

In 1903, Dreyer started his first experiments in patients with lupus vulgaris by intra- and subcutaneous injection of a sterile erythrosine solution and illumination after four to eight hours. Within 24 hours, a severe phlegmonous reaction resulted which resolved leaving prominent scar formation. The patients suffered from severe pain during irradiation and Dreyer therefore, terminated his experiments.

In contrast, von Tappeiner and Jesionek reported on good results using topical application of eosin or other dyes. In 1905, they extended their trial on patients with superficial skin cancer and observed efficacy with repetitive photodynamic therapy (PDT) using topically applied 0.1% to 5% eosin dye (Fig. 1) (1).

Today, it is known that PDT requires the simultaneous presence of a photosensitizer, light, and oxygen inside the diseased tissue. The photosensitizer accumulates in the target cells and absorbs light of a certain wavelength. The energy is transferred to oxygen and highly reactive oxygen species, mainly singlet oxygen, are generated. Following an appropriate light dose, the reactive oxygen species (ROS) directly lead to cell and tissue damage by inducing necrosis and apoptosis or indirectly stimulate inflammatory cell mediators (Fig. 2).

In recent years, PDT has gained worldwide popularity as an experimental therapy for a variety of human cancers. To date porphyrins, chlorine derivatives, or phthalocyanines have been studied for primary or adjuvant cancer therapy (2). However, for dermatological

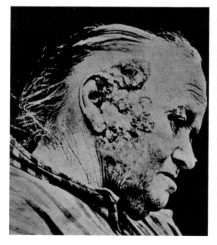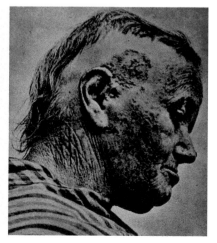

FIGURE 1 (*Left*): Seventy-year-old countrywoman with multiple skin cancers. The lesions were painted consecutively with eosin dye plus intratumoral injection of eosin and were then exposed to sunlight or light from a carbon arc lamp for six to eight hours a day. (*Right*): Reduction of tumors two months later.

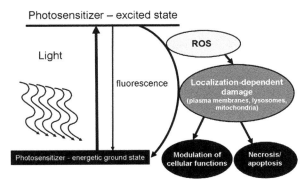

FIGURE 2 Upon illumination, a photosensitizer molecule transformed to the excited state is able to reach ground state by either release of photons (fluorescence) or by induction of reactive oxygen species, mainly singlet oxygen (reaction type-II). Depending on the subcellular localization of the photosensitizer, site-specific damage occurs, thus leading to necrosis/apoptosis or modulation of cellular functions. *Abbreviation*: ROS, reactive oxygen species.

purposes, only hematoporphyrin derivatives (HPDs) such as porfimer sodium (Photofrin®), benzoporphyrin derivative (Visudyne®), or porphyrin-inducing precursors such as 5-aminolevulinic acid (ALA, Levulan® Kerastick) or methyl aminolevulinate (MAL, Metvix®/Metvixia®) are of practical use. As systemic photosensitizing drugs induce prolonged phototoxicity (3), topical photosensitizers are preferred for use in dermatology. There is a growing interest in the use of topical PDT not only for nonmelanoma skin cancer (NMSC), but also for other skin tumors such as lymphoma as well as for non-oncological indications such as psoriasis, localized scleroderma, acne, or skin rejuvenation (4–6).

MECHANISM OF ACTION

During illumination, the photosensitizer absorbs light, a process followed by conversion to an energetically higher status, the "singlet-status." After a short half-life period (approximately 10^{-9} seconds), the activated photosensitizer returns to the ground state after emission of fluorescence and/or internal conversion. Alternatively, the activated photosensitizer changes from the singlet state into the more stable triplet state with a longer half-life period (10^{-3} seconds) (a process referred to as "intersystem crossing"). In the type-I photo-oxidative reaction, there is a direct hydrogen- and electron transfer from the triplet state of the photosensitizer to a substrate. This reaction results in the generation of radicals of the substrate. These radicals are able to react directly with molecular oxygen and form peroxides, hydroxy-radicals, and superoxide anions. This type-I reaction is strongly concentration-dependent. Direct damage to the cells by this reaction can occur, especially when the photosensitizer is bound to easily oxidizable molecules. In the type-II photo-oxidative reaction, electrons or energy are directly transferred to molecular oxygen in the ground state (triplet) and singlet oxygen is formed. The highly reactive state of singlet oxygen results in very effective oxidation of biological substrates. Both reaction types can compete in parallel, as substrate and molecular oxygen compete for the photosensitizer in the triplet state. What kind of reaction preferably happens depends on the photosensitizer used, its subcellular localization, and the substrate, and oxygen supply around the activated photosensitizer. Indirect experiments in vitro indicate that singlet oxygen is the main mediator of PDT-induced biological effects (2,7).

Depending on the amount and localization in the target tissue, ROS, in particular singlet oxygen, either modify cellular functions or induce cell death by necrosis or apoptosis (Fig. 2).

PHOTOSENSITIZERS FOR PHOTODYNAMIC THERAPY

Topically applied dyes such as eosin red or erythrosine were the first "photosensitizers" used to treat conditions such as pityriasis versicolor, psoriasis, molluscum contagiosum, syphilis, lupus vulgaris, or skin cancer (1). The tumor localizing effects of porphyrins have been studied since 1908. The late 1970s witnessed a renaissance of PDT, as Thomas Dougherty used HPD for the treatment of skin cancer (1,2). The main problem in the use of HPD is the prolonged skin photosensitization that lasts for several weeks (8). Topical application of these drugs is not possible since the rather large HPD molecules (tetrapyrrol rings) do not penetrate the skin. Therefore, the introduction of porphyrin precursors such as ALA by Kennedy and coworkers in 1990 or MAL was a significant milestone in the development of PDT in dermatology. These small molecules easily penetrate the epidermis due to their low molecular weight (2,7). Currently in Europe, MAL is approved under the name of Metvix® for the treatment of basal cell carcinoma (BCC), actinic keratoses (AK) and Bowen's disease (BD) in combination with red light. In the United States, Metvixia® was approved for treating AKs in 2004, whereas 5-ALA hydrochloride (Levulan® Kerastick) was approved for photodynamic treatment of AKs in combination with blue light in 1999 (3). The ALA-based photosensitizers are not photoactive by themselves, but show a preferential intracellular accumulation inside rapidly proliferating dysplastic and neoplastic cells (and to a lesser extent, normal skin). These substances are then metabolized in the heme biosynthesis pathway to protoporphyrin IX (PpIX), a potent photosensitizing porphyrin, in a milieu of depleted iron and ferrochelatase, the rate limiting cofactor, and enzyme in the formation of heme (Fig. 3). If no surface illumination is given, the photoactive porphyrins are metabolized to the photodynamically inactive heme within the next 24 to 48 hours (2,7).

Since proliferating, relatively iron-deficient tumor cells of epithelial origin are remarkably sensitized by ALA or MAL, tissue damage is mostly restricted to the sensitized cells, thus almost sparing the surrounding tissue, especially cells of mesenchymal origin like fibroblasts,

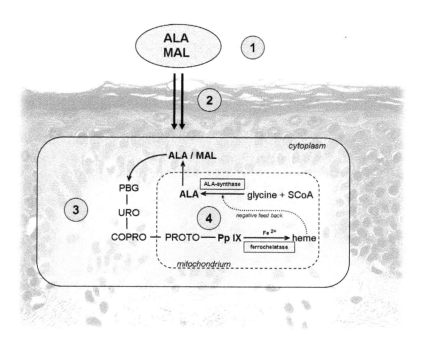

FIGURE 3 Upon topical application (*1*) of the small molecules aminolevulinic acid (ALA) or its methyl ester (methyl aminolevulinate, MAL) on the targeted tissue, there is an enhanced penetration through abnormal stratum corneum overlying epithelial skin tumors (*2*). Due to the need for heme proteins in rapidly proliferating cells, uptake of ALA and MAL into altered keratinocytes is augmented. Since the rate-limiting step of heme biosynthesis is bypassed then, fast synthesis of tetrapyrolic porphyrins occur (*3*), thus resulting in accumulation of protoporphyrin IX (PpIX), the actual photosensitizer (*4*). The relative lack of ferric ions within tumor cells and the lower activity of the enzyme ferrochelatase, further increases the amount of PpIX compared to the surrounding tissue thus leading to a high ratio [up to 10 (8)]. *Abbreviations*: COPRO, coproporphyrinogen III; PBG, porphobilinogen; PROTO, protoporphyrinogen IX; SCoA, succinyl coenzyme A; URO, uroporphyrinogen III.

resulting in excellent cosmesis (9). Aside from two case reports which were possibly coincidental, there are no reports of carcinogenic potential of ALA/MAL-PDT (9). In fact, patients with erythropoietic protoporphyria, who have a chronic excess of PpIX, are not at increased risk of developing skin cancers. Moreover, a recent study showed that long-term topical application of ALA and subsequent irradiation with blue light in a hairless mouse model did not induce skin tumors (10). In a similar experimental setting, Stender et al. showed a delay of photoinduced carcinogenesis in mice following repetitive treatments with ALA-PDT (11).

Although topically applicable photosensitizers are most commonly used in dermatology, recent investigations have shown that the prolonged photosensitivity after systemic application of photosensitizers can be alleviated by chemical modification. *Meso*-tetrahydroxyphenylchlorine or verteporfin have recently been studied with good success for BD and BCC with significantly lower side effects than those reported for the first-generation photosensitizers like HPD (12,13).

LIGHT SOURCES

Historically, PDT has been performed using laser sources, although these are expensive and require a considerable amount of technical support. More recently, diode lasers, which are compact, easy to use semiconductor devices, have facilitated the use of lasers for PDT and these can be used in systemic PDT with endoscopic light delivery via fiber optic (14).

When using ALA or MAL, PpIX accumulates and can be activated by a range of wavelengths in the Soret band. However, with respect to PDT treatment of skin, tissue penetration in the blue light part of the spectrum is poor (1–2 mm), whereas red light can penetrate up to approximately 6 mm in depth (9,15). On this basis, although the efficiency of blue light activation of PpIX is greater than that of red light, light delivery for PDT of skin is a compromise and generally red light sources are chosen for their depth of penetration. ALA with blue light irradiation is the approved form of PDT in the United States for the treatment of AK (16).

For topical PDT, there is no evidence that laser irradiation is superior to the noncoherent and much cheaper light sources. Broad spectrum, filtered sources have been successfully used to treat superficial NMSC, dysplasia, and other nonmalignant skin diseases. Typically, filtered xenon arc sources or tungsten filament quartz halogen sources have been used with emission ranges between 600 and 700 nm. Other commercially available metal halide sources, such as the Waldmann PDT 1200L, are also widely used and are convenient if requiring treatment of large areas up to 20 cm in diameter. For the treatment of superficial NMSC, there is evidence that laser and nonlaser light sources are of equivalent efficacy (17,18).

More recently, light emitting diode (LED) arrays have increasingly been used for PDT (19). These have relatively narrow emission spectra with greater photosensitizer activation efficiency and, therefore, lower dose requirements. These sources are much less expensive than conventional sources and have facilitated the availability of PDT. Preliminary work indicates that these LED sources may be more efficient than broader emission noncoherent sources, although the validation of their use in terms of outcomes and patient tolerance of treatment has yet to be substantiated (20). In general, irradiances of less than 150 mW/cm^2 are used to avoid hyperthermia, and indeed, the lower the irradiance, the less pain appears to occur with treatment and outcomes may be improved (17,21).

The efficiency of different light sources for PDT can be considered in the concept of the total effective fluence, which indicates that green light is more effective than red to a depth of 2 mm, whereas red light provides more uniform radiation at greater tissue depth and is more widely applicable for the treatment of lesions at or below 2 mm (22).

A wide variety of light sources, irradiances, and doses has been used in PDT (37–540 J/cm^2), which makes comparison between studies difficult (Table 1). It is essential that regular calibration of light sources is carried out by PDT clinic staff as a lack of uniformity in irradiance may otherwise go undetected (19).

Fractionation of light delivery may improve the PDT effect by allowing tissue reoxygenation, although the importance of this phenomenon in cutaneous PDT is not clear

TABLE 1   Examples of Commercial Light Sources Used for Topical Photodynamic Therapy

Type of source	Trade name	Peak/range of emission (nm)	Skin surface irradiance (mW/cm²)
Semiconductor diode laser	Diomed®	630	120
Metal halide	Waldmann PDT 1200L	580–740	70–90
Tungsten filament	Curelight®	560–710	<150
LED	Aktilite 16®	632 ± 19 full width at half maximum	Approximately 77
LED	Aktilite 128®	632 ± 19 full width at half maximum	Approximately 65
LED	Omnilux®	633 ± 15	Approximately 80
Xenon arc	Phototherapeutics®	630 ± 15	<130
Sodium (phosphor coated)	Medeikonos®	590–670	100

Abbreviations: LED, light emitting diode; PDT, photodynamic therapy.

(23). It is interesting that with the development of films for ALA delivery and the potential use of LEDs, chemiluminescence and polymers for light delivery, ambulatory home delivery of PDT may be feasible and this requires further study (24–27).

PHOTODYNAMIC THERAPY AND ITS ADVERSE EFFECTS

Patients with histologically-confirmed BD, superficial BCC ≤2 mm in histological thickness, and non-hyperkeratotic AK, particularly on face and scalp, are appropriately treated by topical PDT. Nodular BCC may be treated by PDT if the lesion or patient is not suitable for surgery. Nodular, morphoeic, or heavily pigmented BCCs should not routinely be treated by PDT, and if treatment is performed, adequate surface curettage should be undertaken first. Lesions on the lower legs and multiple lesions are particularly suited to PDT (9).

Assessment of the site and maximum diameter of the lesion is necessary and photographic documentation may be helpful. Application of petrolatum or debriding agents to the lesion(s) for a few days prior to treatment may loosen surface crust or hyperkeratosis and, if heavy crusting is present, surface preparation with either a spatula or curette without local anesthetic is commonly practiced, although there is no evidence that this improves treatment outcomes. The photosensitizer pro-drug, generally ALA, 20% w/v in an oil in water base (Crawford's Pharmaceuticals, U.K.; Photonamic, Germany, or alternative commercial or in-house preparations) or MAL 160 mg/g (Galderma, France) is applied to the lesion under occlusion with a 5 mm rim of surrounding normal tissue for three hours (MAL), four hours (ALA for BD or AK), or six hours (ALA for BCC). A test area may be advisable if a large field is to be treated. If the lesion is on a sunlight-exposed site, such as head and neck, an additional light-opaque dressing is required to protect the treatment site prior to irradiation. This can all be performed on an outpatient basis and the patient will then return for irradiation later that day (28).

After the incubation period, ALA/MAL is removed and the lesion examined using Wood's light illumination or a fluorescence-imaging device to determine the sensitivity and specificity of PpIX fluorescence. On the basis of naked eye and Wood's light examination the irradiation field is mapped out to include a 5 mm rim of clinically normal appearing tissue and the maximum diameter of the field documented. Irradiation is performed with one of several possible light sources, as discussed (Table 1). Generally, doses of 37 to 75 J/cm² are used with LED sources and 75 to 150 J/cm² for noncoherent, broadband, or laser sources. Lower doses have been used for nonmalignant disease (29).

The majority of patients will find irradiation during topical PDT uncomfortable and will describe a burning, painful sensation, usually maximal in the first few minutes of treatment. The mechanisms of PDT-induced pain and pain relief are poorly understood (9,30). However, talking to patients to put them at ease, use of a cooling fan, xylocaine spray, and a device such as the Cynosure®/Zimmer cold air blower, which delivers a jet of chilled air to the skin surface may be helpful. At least 20% of patients will report topical PDT as being significantly painful (17). Ametop® and EMLA are not significantly effective when compared with placebo for PDT pain relief and injectable local anesthetic does not necessarily abolish discomfort (30–32). MAL may be less painful than ALA-PDT, although this has not been formally studied in patients (33).

During irradiation, erythema, edema, urticaria, and exudation can occur (34). These changes are maximal during and immediately after irradiation and usually subside within 24 to 48 hours of treatment, although inflammation and crusting will occur over one to two weeks. Persistent erythema and hypo- or hyper-pigmentation may occur at the treatment site for a few weeks after treatment, but usually resolve leaving no more than an extremely faint scar and excellent cosmetic outcome (35). Infection, ulceration, and hair loss and increase are also rarely reported. Generalized photosensitivity has not been reported as most ALA/MAL-induced PpIX is cleared within 24 hours (36). PDT in vitro can induce DNA damage and there are two reported cases of melanoma and squamous cell carcinoma arising at sites of previous PDT treatments in humans (37,38). However, these cases may well have been unrelated to PDT itself and there is no evidence of a significant risk of carcinogenicity in humans (9).

There is evidence that two PDT treatments are more effective than one, although it is unclear when the second treatment should be performed, and this may vary from one week to 8 to 12 weeks (18,39–41). Review after PDT by medical staff is advised and will generally be performed three to six months after the last treatment, when treatment outcome and remaining adverse events such as erythema, pigmentation, scarring, or milia will be recorded. If persistent disease remains, treatment can be repeated and there is no evidence of cumulative damage from PDT, although in our own center, if lesions do not clear within four treatments, alternative therapeutic approaches are taken. There is evidence that late recurrences beyond one to two years after PDT may occur and, therefore, long-term follow-up is theoretically advised (18).

All aspects of the PDT procedure can be performed by fully trained nursing staff or technicians and this may be appropriate depending on local expertise and staff availability. However, the assessment of lesion responses by medical staff is strongly advised, as it may sometimes be difficult to distinguish whether persistent erythema is representative of residual disease or merely the result of treatment.

DYPLASIA/NONMELANOMA SKIN CANCER

Regarding oncologic indications, AK, nodular or superficial BCC and BD are approved indications for MAL and ALA/MAL PDT is recommended by evidence-based guidelines in Britain (9). However, for therapy of single lesions several efficient alternative treatments are available, for example, cryotherapy or surgery, whereas for therapy of multiple lesions PDT is among the first choice, in particular for AK of the scalp and face or in cases of basal cell nevus syndrome (2). An international consensus for guidelines on the use of PDT for NMSC has been established (42).

Actinic Keratoses

The efficacy of ALA-PDT has been observed so far in six open studies of 323 AK situated on the face and scalp in Caucasian populations (Fig. 4). Clearance rates ranged from 71% to 100% after a single treatment (9,43). For illumination purposes, either blue light (417 nm) or red (635 nm) have been used (43,44).

In a European, multicenter, randomized prospective study, MAL-PDT was compared to cryosurgery in the treatment of AK. A total of 193 patients (95%) with 699 lesions completed the trial. Patients received either a single treatment with MAL-PDT (repeated after one week in 8% of cases) or a double freeze-thaw course of liquid nitrogen cryosurgery. MAL was applied for three hours after slight lesion preparation, followed by illumination with broad-spectrum red light (75 J/cm^2). A follow-up visit was performed three months after treatment. The efficacy

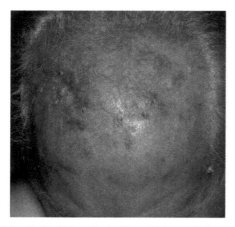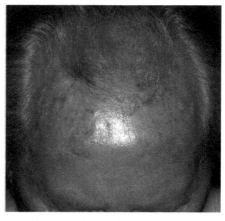

FIGURE 4   (*Left*): Male patient with multiple actinic keratoses on his face and scalp. Single treatment session with 5-aminolevulinic acid-photodynamic therapy (PDT) (20% w/o cream, incubation for four hours, illumination with the Waldmann PDT 1200L; 150 mW/cm^2; 120 J/cm^2). (*Right*): Clinical outcome after two months with significant improvement, a second PDT-treatment was scheduled for the same day.

for MAL-PDT (single application) was 69% versus 75% for cryosurgery, the difference being of no statistical significance. Thin lesions on the scalp had the highest response rates (80% and 82% for PDT and cryosurgery, respectively). Cosmetic outcome, as judged by the investigator, was superior for MAL-PDT (96% vs. 81%) (40).

In accordance with this trial, another was conducted in Australia. Here MAL-PDT was used as a dual cycle, with two treatment sessions, one week apart. PDT was compared to a single course of cryosurgery or placebo in 204 patients. Lesion response was assessed after three months. A significantly higher complete remission rate (91%) with MAL-PDT was observed compared with 68% remission with cryosurgery and 30% with placebo. The cosmetic result was rated excellent in 81% of MAL-PDT patients compared with 51% treated with cryotherapy (41).

A multicenter, randomized, double blind, placebo-controlled study with two MAL-PDT cycles was performed in 80 patients with AK in the United States. PDT treatment parameters were similar to the aforementioned trials. Assessment after three months revealed a complete lesion response rate of 89% for MAL-PDT versus 38% for placebo. An excellent or good cosmetic outcome was reported in more than 90% of MAL-treated patients (45) MAL PDT has also been shown to be effectice for AK in transplant recipients in a randomzied, double-blind placebo controlled study (46).

Also for ALA-PDT in the treatment of AK a randomized, placebo-controlled, uneven-parallel-group study was published recently. In 243 patients, clinical response, based on lesion clearance, was assessed at weeks 8 and 12. Patients were randomized to receive either vehicle or ALA (Levulan® Kerastick), followed within 14 to 18 hours by illumination with visible blue light (BLU-U®, DUSA, low pressure fluorescent lamps). Complete response rates for ALA-PDT patients with ≥75% of the treated lesions clearing at weeks 8 and 12 were 77% and 89%, respectively. In the placebo group, clearing rates were 18% and 13%. The 12-week clearing rates included 30% of patients who received a second ALA-PDT course. Moderate to severe discomfort during illumination was reported by at least 90% of patients; however, only 3% of patients required discontinuation of therapy (44).

For the purpose of lowering the amount of side effects of ALA-PDT, shorter incubation periods (one, two, and three hours), in conjunction with pretreatment with 40% urea in order to enhance ALA penetration and the use of topical 3% lidocaine hydrochloride to decrease discomfort were also evaluated. One and five months after therapy in 18 patients with at least four non-hypertrophic AK, a reduction of lesions up to 90% in the target area was observed. No difference was seen between the three incubation periods nor did pretreatment with urea or lidocaine have an influence on the therapeutic outcome (6).

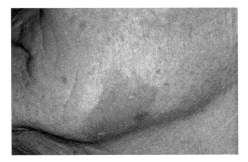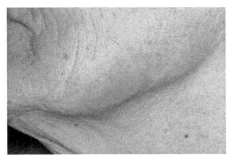

FIGURE 5 (*Left*): Bowen's disease on the lower right cheek in this 72-year-old woman. Two cycles of methyl aminolevulinate-photodynamic therapy (repetitive treatment after one week; three hours incubation; illumination with the Aktilite light emitting diode; 37 J/cm^2). (*Right*): Situation after two months. Complete clinical remission, slight erythema, no scar formation.

Bowen's Disease and Initial Squamous Cell Carcinoma

There have been several reports on the use of systemic PDT in BD (13), but these reports now have been superseded by topical therapies with higher tolerability. Topical PDT using 20% ALA has been extensively assessed in BD with more than 14 open and three randomized comparison studies (9,46). Cure rates reported so far are the best for all epithelial cancers or precursors (up to 100%). In a study by Salim et al., ALA-PDT was compared to topical 5-fluorouracil (5-FU). In this bicenter, randomized, phase-III trial, 40 patients with one to three lesions of histologically proven BD received either PDT or 5-FU. ALA 20% in an o/w-emulsion was applied four hours prior to illumination with an incoherent red light source (Paterson lamp, Photo therapeutics, U.K.; 50–90 mW/cm^2, 100 J/cm^2). Treatment with 5-FU was once daily in week one and then twice daily during weeks two to four. At first follow-up at week six, both ALA-PDT and 5-FU application were repeated, if required. Twenty-nine of 33 lesions (88%) treated with PDT showed complete response, versus 67% after 5-FU (22 of 33). After one-year of follow-up, further recurrences reduced the complete clinical clearance rates to 82% and 42%, respectively (47).

MAL-PDT has recently been studied in one of the largest existing studies in the treatment of BD (Fig. 5). In a multicenter, comparative randomized controlled trial with a total of 225 patients carrying 275 lesions, MAL-PDT was compared to cryotherapy, topical 5-FU, and placebo. At 12 months, the estimated sustained lesion complete response rate was 80% for MAL-PDT, 67% for cryotherapy, and 69% for 5-FU. The cosmetic outcome was likewise superior for MAL-PDT (94% vs. 66% cryotherapy vs. 76% 5-FU) (48).

Basal Cell Carcinoma

Numerous studies concerning ALA/MAL-PDT for BCC have been conducted in recent years (3,7,49–53). The weighted average complete clearance rates, after follow-up periods varying between 3 and 36 months, were 87% in 12 studies treating 826 superficial BCCs and 53% in 208 nodular BCCs (3,9). Available compiled data from other trials have shown an average clearance of 87% for superficial BCCs and 71% for nodular BCCs (2).

In order to improve poor outcome after PDT of thicker BCC lesions, Thissen et al. treated 23 patients with 24 nodular BCCs once with ALA-PDT (incoherent red light; 100 mW/cm^2, 120 J/cm^2) three weeks after debulking of the BCCs. The former tumor areas were excised three months later and histopathologically evaluated for residual tumor. Twenty-two (92%) of the 24 nodular BCCs showed both clinical and histological complete response (50).

In a prospective phase-III trial comparing ALA-PDT with cryosurgery, Wang et al. included 88 superficial and nodular BCCs. A 20 % ALA/water-in-oil cream was applied for six hours under an occlusive dressing, followed by irradiation with a laser at 635 nm (80 mW/cm^2, 60 J/cm^2). In the cryosurgery arm, lesions were treated with liquid nitrogen in the open spray technique using two freeze-thaw cycles for 25 to 30 seconds each time.

After three months, punch biopsies were performed and revealed a recurrence rate of 25% in the PDT group and 15% in the cryosurgery group. However, the clinical recurrence rates were only 5% for ALA-PDT and 13% for cryosurgery. Besides better cosmetic outcome, healing time was also shorter in the PDT treated group (53).

Solèr and colleagues studied the long-term effects of MAL-PDT in 59 patients with 350 BCCs. Nodular tumors were curetted before PDT and MAL (160 mg/g) was applied to all tumors for 24 or 3 hours prior to irradiation with a broad-band halogen light source (50–200 J/cm^2). Patients were followed for two to four years (mean 35 months). The overall cure rate was 79%, cosmetic outcome was excellent or good in 98% of the completely responding lesions (49).

In a recent open, uncontrolled, prospective, multicenter trial, both patients with superficial and/or nodular BCC who were at risk of complications, poor cosmetic outcome, disfigurement, and/or recurrence using conventional therapy were studied. Ninety-four patients were treated with a single cycle of MAL-PDT involving two treatment sessions one week apart, and followed-up at three months, at which time nonresponders were retreated. The clinical lesion remission rate after three months was 92% for superficial BCC and 87% for nodular BCC. Histological cure rate at this time point was 85% in superficial BCC and 75% in nodular BCC. At 24 months after treatment, the overall lesion recurrence rate was 18% (51).

In another European multicenter, open, randomized trial, MAL-PDT for nodular BCC was compared with surgery. A total of 101 patients were included and received either PDT twice, seven days apart (75 J/cm^2 red light), or surgical excision. The primary end point of this trial was the clinically assessed lesion clearance at three months after treatment, besides cosmetic outcome. The cure rate after three months was similar with MAL-PDT or surgery (91% vs. 98%), the 24 months recurrence rate was 10% with MAL and 2% with surgery. The cosmetic result was rated good/excellent in 85% of the patients receiving PDT versus 33% with surgery (52).

ALA-PDT can be used also for adjuvant therapy in combination with Mohs surgery, as reported recently by Kuijpers et al. In four patients, who underwent Mohs micrographic surgery for extensive BCC, first the central infiltrating tumor part was excised. After re-epithelialization, ALA-PDT of the surrounding tumor rims (2–5 cm) bearing remaining superficial tumor parts, was performed. This led to a complete remission of the tumors with excellent clinical and cosmetical results (follow-up period up to 27 months) (54).

However, even if clinical studies support the use of PDT as an effective treatment of BCC, the relatively short follow-up of most of the studies to date have to be considered. Mandatory indications for surgical treatment are different histological subtypes such as pigmented or morphoeic BCCs or BCCs located in the area of the facial embryonic fusion clefts as well as all BCCs thicker than 3 mm if no debulking procedure is performed prior to PDT.

NONMELANOMA SKIN CANCER INDICATIONS

Despite the increasing acceptance of topical PDT for superficial NMSC and dysplasia, its use in other dermatological conditions has not been widely validated. Many benign skin conditions show specificity of photosensitizer accumulation after ALA/MAL application and this observation has led to the study of topical PDT in other non-NMSC conditions (Table 2) (4).

Recalcitrant Viral Warts and Viral Skin Diseases

After application of ALA to a pared viral wart, PpIX fluorescence can be demonstrated (55). There is a clinical need for adjunctive treatments for recalcitrant viral warts, particularly in immunosuppressed patients. However, much of the work with PDT has been done in immunocompetent subjects.

Retrospective analysis of 62 patients showed that 58% of those who completed treatment cleared with no recurrence up to 17 months follow-up, although pain was a significant adverse effect. However, of the five-immunocompromized patients only one responded (56).

The same group compared PDT with cryotherapy for recalcitrant warts (57). Randomization in comparative treatment groups was performed: white light (22 mW/cm^2) three times (W3) or

TABLE 2 Skin Conditions Other than Nonmelanoma Skin Cancer in Which Topical Photodynamic Therapy has been Applied

Most studied	Case reports/series	
Acne	Actinic cheilitis/oral leukoplakia	Lichen sclerosus
Cutaneous T-cell lymphoma	Alopecia areata[a]	Lymphadenosis benigna cutis
Psoriasis[b]	Bowenoid papulosis	Melanoma[b]
Warts	Breast metastases[b]	Molluscum contagiosum
	Chondrodermatitis nodularis helicis	Nevus sebaceous
	Condylomata acuminata	Photoaging
	Darier's disease	Porokeratosis[b]
	Epidermodysplasia verruciformis	Port wine stain[b]
	Erythroplasia of Queyrat	Sarcoidosis
	Extramammary Paget's	Scleroderma
	Goltz syndrome	Sebaceous hyperplasia
	Hailey–Hailey	Superficial mycoses/antibacterial
	Hidradenitis suppurativa[a]	Vulval intraepithelial neoplasia[a]
	Hirsutism	X-ray dermatitis
	Keratoacanthoma	
	Leg ulcers	
	Leishmaniasis	
	Lichen planus	

[a]Contradictory evidence.
[b]Poor response to photodynamic therapy.

once (W1) in 10 days; red light (17.5 mW/cm^2) three times in 10 days (R3); blue light (22 mW/cm^2) three times in 10 days (B3) or cryotherapy with a double 10-second freeze/thaw cycle, repeated up to four times over two months. The total light dose in the PDT-treated groups was 40 J/cm^2. Re-treatment was performed four to six weeks later for partial responders. Complete responders were followed-up for 12 months, with no recurrence. Re-treatment was needed in 78% of the W1 and W3, 40% of R3, and 22% of B3 groups. Significantly higher clearance rates occurred after white light than red or blue light PDT or cryotherapy: 73% (W3), 71% (W1), 42% (R3), 28% (B3), and 20% (cryotherapy), respectively. White-light PDT three times in 10 days was most effective, although pain was significant in the majority.

A definitive study in immunocompetent patients with hand and foot warts randomized to receive either ALA-PDT or placebo-PDT was performed with weekly treatment for three weeks, repeated one month later if warts persisted (55). Clearance of warts at week 18 follow-up was seen in 56% of actively treated and 43% of placebo-treated subjects. There was also a significant decrease in wart area in the active treatment group compared with placebo. The relatively low overall response rates and high placebo response rates probably indicate the effect of regular paring and keratolysis and that patients had treatment-resistant disease. Pain was significant and may be limiting, particularly in children. Others have confirmed the efficacy of ALA-PDT for viral warts (58).

To conclude, multiple treatments with ALA-PDT, combined with paring and keratolysis are more effective than placebo or cryotherapy for recalcitrant viral warts, although optimal treatment regimes need to be established in order to minimize pain. Immunosuppressed patients may respond less well and this requires further study. There is potential for the use of ALA-PDT in planar warts and others have shown that combined PDT and pulsed dye laser may be effective, although this requires substantiation (59,60).

High response rates were seen in four of seven patients with condylomata acuminata, using ALA (14 hours) and argon dye laser irradiation (630 nm, 75 or 150 mW/cm^2, 100 J/cm^2) (61). Topical ALA-PDT was effective (95% clearance) and well tolerated with low recurrence rates (5%) in patients with urethral condylomata ($n = 164$) and 66% clearance rates for vulval and vaginal condylomata ($n = 16$) have also been reported (62,63).

There may also be potential for the use of topical PDT for the treatment of epidermodysplasia verruciformis (64). PDT may also be effective for molluscum contagiosum in HIV patients ($n = 6$) (65,66). It is likely that direct virucidal action and cytotoxicity are important determinants of the effects of PDT for viral diseases (60).

Acne Vulgaris, Diseases of the Sebaceous Gland, and Bacterial/Fungal Diseases

Visible light phototherapy for acne vulgaris has been investigated (67,68). *Propionibacterium acnes* contain endogenous porphyrins and fluoresce (69). Indeed, *P. acnes* toxicity has been shown in vitro on irradiation with blue light (70,71).

Improvement in inflammatory and comedonal acne occurs after visible light phototherapy, where combined red and blue light seems to be the most effective regime and it is likely that anti-inflammatory, immunomodulatory, and endogenous PDT effects are operative (72).

The use of PDT was examined in moderate trunkal acne in an open, randomized controlled study ($n = 22$, three hours ALA and visible light irradiation; 550–700 nm; 150 J/cm^2) (73). Each subject received either one or four treatments with appropriate intra-subject controls, and significant reduction in sebum, *P. acnes* fluorescence, and sebaceous gland size occurred with clinical improvement for up to 20 weeks after four treatments. However, significant side effects of pigmentation, folliculitis, and pain were seen.

Ten patients with mild to moderate trunkal acne were randomized to receive test sites of either ALA-PDT, ALA alone, light alone, or untreated (three hours ALA, 635 nm diode laser, 25 mW/cm^2, 15 J/cm^2 weekly for three weeks). Reduction in inflammatory acne was seen with ALA-PDT, but no change in sebum excretion or *P. acnes* counts. Significant phototoxicity and pigmentation were seen, although permanent damage to sebaceous glands may be avoided with this lower irradiation regime (74). More recently, the efficacy of MAL-PDT (two treatments of three hours MAL; 37 J/cm^2 Aktilite 128) for inflammatory lesions in moderate to severe facial acne was shown in a randomized, controlled, investigator-blinded study ($n = 21$ MAL-PDT; $n = 15$ control, no treatment) (75). However, severe pain and adverse effects of erythema, pustular eruptions, and exfoliation occurred. In another blinded, prospective, randomized, placebo-controlled multicenter, MAL-PDT split-face study with 30 patients with moderate to severe acne, patients received MAL- or placebo cream for three hours, followed by illumination with red light. The treatment was repeated after two weeks. Inflammatory and non-inflammatory acne lesions were counted at baseline, 6 and 12 weeks later. MAL-PDT resulted in a statistically significant greater reduction in inflammatory lesion count than placebo at week 12 (median reduction 54% vs. 20%) However, MAL-PDT was associated with more pain than placebo-PDT (76).

Topical PDT has also been applied to hidradenitis suppurativa, where 75% to 100% clearance rates were reported in four subjects using a well-tolerated regime (77). This was remarkable as short contact ALA and blue light with very limited tissue penetration were used. In contrast, a study in four patients showed no sustained response of hidradenitis suppurativa to topical PDT using red light (78). There are also reports of efficacy of topical PDT for nevus sebaceous and sebaceous hyperplasia, which require further clarification.

The potential use of topical PDT for bacterial and fungal disease is of considerable interest. ALA-PDT has been reported to be effective for inter-digital mycoses although associated with rapid recurrence, and in vitro studies suggest possible efficacy of bioadhesive patch ALA-PDT for Trichophyton interdigitale and Candida albicans (79,80).

Psoriasis

There are reports of PDT efficacy for psoriasis as far back as 1937 (81). Selective photosensitizer-induced fluorescence in psoriatic plaque and photobleaching on irradiation occurs, although uniform fluorescence is not seen (82). Peak fluorescence occurs approximately six hours after ALA application to a psoriatic plaque (83).

An initial study in three patients showed topical PDT to be comparable in efficacy to dithranol, although subsequent studies have not been encouraging (84). Improvement in lesion severity was seen after topical PDT ($n = 14$) (85). However, in 22 subjects treated with ALA (four hours) and irradiation with a modified slide projector (400–650 nm, 25 mW/cm^2, up to 16 J/cm^2) 10 of 36 sites within psoriatic plaques cleared but all relapsed within two weeks (86). Multiple treatments [four hours ALA, slide projector irradiation (15 mW/cm^2; 8 J/cm^2) up to three times a week and a maximum of 12 treatments] resulted in clinical improvement in 8 of 10 subjects but clearance in only 4 of 19 treated sites (87). PpIX fluorescence varied within and between patients, there was variation in treatment response and treatment was painful (87,88).

A randomized, within-patient observer-blinded study ($n = 29$) using 1% ALA and 5 to 20 J/cm^2 irradiation showed a 59% improvement with PDT, although a 25% improvement was seen with keratolysis alone and, overall, responses and tolerance of treatment were poor (89). In the second study, different ALA concentrations (0.1%, 1%, 5%) were used at a light dose of 20 J/cm^2. Treatment was conducted twice a week until complete clearance or for a maximum of 12 irradiations. Again, clinical efficacy was disappointing with and unfavorable adverse event profile (90). Certainly, ALA-PDT seems to be less effective than UVB phototherapy for psoriasis and there is a concern about potential for koebnerisation (91). Thus, the role of topical ALA-PDT with current regimes is questionable.

Cutaneous T-cell Lymphoma

Patients with limited patch or plaque stage cutaneous T-cell lymphoma (CTCL) whose disease is resistant to conventional therapies present a particular therapeutic challenge. Selective accumulation of PpIX in lymphocytes after ALA application and PDT-induced cytotoxicity occurs in vitro (92–96). In two patients with plaque stage CTCL, ALA-PDT was performed on up to five occasions (four to six hours ALA, irradiation with a modified slide projector; 44 mW/cm^2; 40 J/cm^2) (97). Lesion-specific ALA-induced PpIX fluorescence was seen and clinical and histological clearance achieved. Treatment was well tolerated and clearance maintained for 14 months in one patient, with recurrence in the other at eight months. In contrast, a single PDT treatment in one patient showed clinical clearance but residual disease histologically (98). These studies support the need for multiple treatments in order to obtain histological disease resolution (97,99–102).

In a study in two patients with four lesions of CTCL, a 50% response rate occurred with a single treatment (four to six hours ALA, 630 nm laser irradiation, <110 mW/cm^2, 60 J/cm^2) and a fluorescence ratio of 5:1 for ALA-induced PpIX accumulation in tumor compared with adjacent normal tissue was seen (103). It appears that tumor stage disease is not as responsive, although clearance can be achieved with multiple treatments (100,101).

The optimal treatment parameters for topical PDT in CTCL are unclear, and ALA applications at 10 and 20% and up to 24 hours and irradiation doses of up to 380 J/cm^2 have been used (99,102). Higher intensity irradiation may spare the epidermis and specifically target the dermal lymphocytic infiltrate, although this requires substantiation. PDT can also be used in combination with other therapies such as radiotherapy and may be used as a debulking procedure for more infiltrative disease (104,105). Treatment may also be of benefit for CTCL in patients with HIV and other types of cutaneous lymphoma such as anaplastic lymphoma and pagetoid reticulosis (105,106).

Encouraging Data for the Use of Topical Photodynamic Therapy in Other Skin Diseases

Topical PDT can be effective for actinic cheilitis, oral leukoplakia, and verrucous hyperplasia, with complete response rates in the majority of patients ($n = 3–12$) (107–110). The rationale for use in these diseases is similar to that in AK. There have also been encouraging outcomes for keratoacanthoma ($n = 4$) treated by topical PDT (111). Topical PDT has been used for erythroplasia of Queyrat ($n = 4$) and was shown to be effective for limited stage disease and MAL-PDT may also be effective (112,113). Extramammary Paget's disease is difficult to treat and often multiple treatment modalities are required with high recurrence rates after surgery. However, PDT may be of benefit and can be combined with other therapies (114–117). Interestingly, low dose multiple PDT treatments may be effective for chronic nonmalignant inflammatory diseases. For example, 100% response rates and prolonged remission were achieved in cutaneous scleroderma.

Conditions that Require Additional Investigation

Subjective improvement of vulval lichen sclerosus was reported in two studies, although without documented objective improvement. Topical PDT has also been used to treat

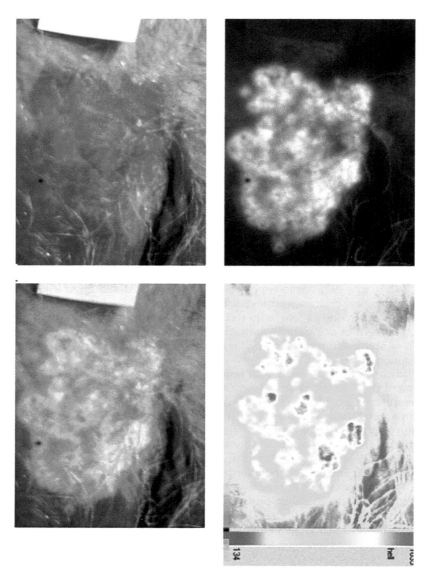

FIGURE 6 Fluorescence diagnosis of a superficial basal cell carcinoma at the mons pubis. (*Upper left*): Clinical image after topical application of a 16% methyl aminolevulinate-cream for three hours. (*Upper right*): Sharp demarcation of the lesion under excitation with CCD-Camera system (Dyaderm professional, Biocam, Germany) (b/w-fluorescence). (*Lower left*): Real-time fusion image of both the upper left and upper right image (overlay technique). (*Lower right*): False color-coded image of the original fluorescence image (*upper right*).

hirsutism, and interestingly, 50 to 100% response rates were achieved using 100 to 200 J/cm² irradiations after ALA application. In a quite different condition, lesions of cutaneous leishmaniasis have been reported to be effectively treated by either ALA- or MAL-PDT. Six patients with Darier's disease also responded with sustained responses to topical ALA-PDT. However, for each of the above examples, perhaps besides leishmaniasis, these preliminary observations require more robust study before PDT should definitively be considered.

Other conditions that require further substantiation but for which there are isolated reports of topical PDT efficacy are lichen planus, Hailey–Hailey disease, cutaneous sarcoidosis, chondrodermatitis nodularis helicis, Bowenoid papulosis, lymphadenosis benigna cutis, X-ray dermatitis, and Goltz syndrome.

Contradictory Evidence Relating to the Use of Photodynamic Therapy

Single treatment topical ALA-PDT was shown to be ineffective for vulval intraepithelial neoplasia. However, complete response rates of between 33 and 52% have been reported with multiple treatments ($n = 9-25$) and PDT may be as effective as surgery or laser treatment (118–120). Multi-focal high-grade disease, the presence of HPV, lack of cell-mediated immunity, hyperpigmentation, and hyperkeratosis are all predictors of poor response to PDT (118,121). Future use of bioadhesive patch delivery of ALA may also facilitate PDT at this difficult body site (26).

There have also been contradictory reports of the use of topical PDT for alopecia areata with an initial report in two patients showing regrowth of hair up to four months after topical PDT using hematoporphyrin and UVA. More recently, ALA-PDT was shown to be completely ineffective for alopecia areata even with multiple treatments ($n = 6$) (122).

Poor Response to Photodynamic Therapy

Not all conditions investigated have responded to topical PDT. These include porokeratosis, cutaneous breast metastases, malignant melanoma, and port wine stains.

In summary, topical PDT may be useful for the treatment of recalcitrant viral warts and acne vulgaris, and early studies in CTCL are encouraging. The potential in psoriasis and other diseases requires further investigation, and controlled, comparative studies are required in larger numbers of patients. Furthermore, most of the studies performed to date have used ALA and it will be of interest to determine whether ALA esters may be of benefit in some of these conditions.

FLUORESCENCE DIAGNOSIS

The tissue selectivity of the porphyrin induction after topical application of ALA or MAL can also be exploited for diagnostic purposes. The porphyrin-containing tissue can be illuminated with blue light at the Soret band, thus inducing the emission of pink fluorescent light (Fig. 2), which then enables the delineation of the tumor due to the high ratio of the porphyrin content in the tumor versus the surrounding tissue (123,124).

This procedure is called fluorescence detection (FD), although misleadingly the term "photodynamic diagnosis" is often used. FD can enable the dermatologist to perform either a guided biopsy or a controlled and complete resection of the tumor, sparing unaffected tissue. By combination of this procedure with a digital CCD camera system, together with digital imaging, the contrast of the acquired fluorescence images can be enhanced significantly (Fig. 6). This allows determination of a threshold, which can be utilized either for a directed biopsy or for pre- and intra-operative planning when Mohs' surgery is scheduled (125). In addition, FD may be a helpful tool to demonstrate the efficacy of PDT. However, at present the routine employment of such systems is still being assessed in prospective trials.

REFERENCES

1. Szeimies RM, Dräger J, Abels C, et al. History of photodynamic therapy in dermatology. In: Calzavara-Pinton PG, Szeimies RM, Ortel B, eds. Photodynamic Therapy and Fluorescence Diagnosis in Dermatology. Amsterdam: Elsevier, 2001:3–16.
2. Zeitouni NC, Oseroff AR, Shieh S. Photodynamic therapy for nonmelanoma skin cancers. Mol Immunol 2003; 39:1133–1136.
3. Marmur ES, Schmults CD, Goldberg DJ. A review of laser and photodynamic therapy for the treatment of nonmelanoma skin cancer. Dermatol Surg 2004; 30:264–271.
4. Ibbotson SH. Topical 5-aminolaevulinic acid photodynamic therapy for the treatment of skin conditions other than non-melanoma skin cancer. Br J Dermatol 2002; 146:178–188.
5. Karrer S, Abels C, Landthaler M, et al. Topical photodynamic therapy for localized scleroderma. Acta Derm Venereol 2000; 80:26–27.
6. Touma D, Yaar M, Whitehead S, et al. Short incubation δ-ALA photodynamic therapy for treatment of actinic keratoses and facial photodamage. Arch Dermatol 2004; 140:33–40.

7. Szeimies RM, Karrer S, Abels C, et al. Photodynamic therapy in dermatology. In: Krutmann J, Hönigsmann H, Elmets CA, et al., eds. Dermatological Phototherapy and Photodiagnostic Methods. Berlin: Springer, 2001:209–247.

8. Schweitzer VG. Photofrin-mediated photodynamic therapy for treatment of aggressive head and neck nonmelanomatous skin tumors in elderly patients. Laryngoscope 2001; 111:1091–1098.

9. Morton CA, Brown SB, Collins S, et al. Guidelines for topical phototherapy therapy: report of a workshop of the British Photodermatology Group. Br J Dermatol 2002; 146:552–567.

10. Liu Y, Viau G, Bissonnette R. Multiple large-surface photodynamic therapy sessions with topical or systemic aminolevulinic acid and blue light in UV-exposed hairless mice. J Cutan Med Surg 2004; 8:131–139.

11. Stender IM, Bech-Thomsen N, Poulsen T, et al. Photodynamic therapy with topical delta-aminolevulinic acid delays UV photocarcinogenesis in hairless mice. Photochem Photobiol 1997; 66:493–496.

12. Baas P, Saarnak AE, Oppelaar H, et al. Photodynamic therapy with meso-tetrahydroxyphenylchlorin for basal cell carcinoma: a phase I/II study. Br J Dermatol 2001; 145:75–78.

13. Lui H, Hobbs L, Tope WD, et al. Photodynamic therapy of multiple nonmelanoma skin cancers with verteporfin and red light-emitting diodes. Two-year results evaluating tumor response and cosmetic outcomes. Arch Dermatol 2004; 140:41–46.

14. Brancaleon L, Moseley H. Lasers and non-laser light sources for photodynamic therapy. Lasers Med Sci 2002; 17:173–186.

15. Henderson BW, Dougherty TJ. How does photodynamic therapy work? Photochem Photobiol 1992; 55:145–157.

16. Ormrod D, Jarvis B. Topical aminolevulinic acid HCl photodynamic therapy. Am J Clin Dermatol 2000; 1:133–139.

17. Clark C, Bryden A, Dawe RS, et al. Topical 5-aminolaevulinc acid photodynamic therapy for cutaneous lesions: outcome and comparison of light sources. Photodermatol Photoimmunol Photomed 2003; 19:134–141.

18. Moseley H, Ibbotson S, Woods J, et al. Clinical and research applications of photodynamic therapy in dermatology: Experience of the Scottish PDT Centre. Lasers Surg Med 2006; 38:403–416.

19. Moseley H. Light distribution and calibration of commercial PDT LED arrays. Photochem Photobiol Sci 2005; 4:911–914.

20. Juzeniene A, Juzenas P, Ma LW, et al. Effectiveness of different light sources for 5-aminolevulinic acid photodynamic therapy. Lasers Med Sci 2004; 19:139–149.

21. Ericson MB, Sandberg C, Stenquist B, et al. Photodynamic therapy of actinic keratosis at varying fluence rates: assessment of photobleaching, pain and primary clinical outcome. Br J Dermatol 2004; 151:1204–1212.

22. Moseley H. Total effective fluence: a useful concept in photodynamic therapy. Lasers Med Sci 1996; 11:139–143.

23. Robinson DJ, de Bruijn HS, Star WM, et al. Dose and timing of the first light fraction in two-fold illumination schemes for topical ALA-mediated photodynamic therapy of hairless mouse skin. Photochem Photobiol 2003; 77:319–323.

24. Lieb S, Szeimies RM, Lee G. Self-adhesive thin films for topical delivery of 5-aminolevulinic acid. Eur J Pharm Biopharm 2002; 53:99–106.

25. Zelickson B, Counters J, Coles C, et al. Light patch: preliminary report of a novel form of blue light delivery for the treatment of actinic keratosis. Dermatol Surg 2005; 31:375–378.

26. McCarron PA, Donnelly RF, Zawislak A, et al. Evaluation of a water-soluble bioadhesive patch for photodynamic therapy of vulval lesions. Int J Pharm 2005; 293:11–23.

27. Moseley H, Allen JW, Ibbotson S, et al. Ambulatory photodynamic therapy: a new concept in delivering photodynamic therapy. Br J Dermatol 2006; 154:747–750.

28. Ibbotson SH. How to treat a superficial basal cell carcinoma with topical photodynamic therapy in Dundee. Photodiagn Photodyn Ther 2006; 3:128–131.

29. Szeimies RM, Landthaler M, Karrer S. Non-oncologic indications for ALA-PDT. J Derm Treat 2002; 13(suppl 1):S13–S18.

30. Grapengiesser S, Gudmundsson F, Larko O, et al. Pain caused by photodynamic therapy of skin cancer. Clin Exp Dermatol 2002; 27:493–497.

31. Holmes MV, Dawe RS, Ferguson J, et al. A randomized, double-blind, placebo-controlled study of the efficacy of tetracaine gel (Ametop®) for pain relief during topical photodynamic therapy. Br J Dermatol 2004; 150:337–340.

32. Langan SM, Collins P. Randomized, double-blind, placebo-controlled prospective study of the efficacy of topical anaesthesia with a eutetic mixture of lignocaine 2.5% and prilocaine 2.5% for topical 5-aminolaevulinic acid-photodynamic therapy for extensive scalp actinic keratoses. Br J Dermatol 2006; 154:146–149.

33. Wiegell SR, Stender I-M, Na R, et al. Pain associated with photodynamic therapy using 5-aminolevulinic acid or 5-aminolevulinic acid methylester on tape-stripped normal skin. Arch Dermatol 2003; 139:1173–1177.

34. Clark C, Dawe RS, Moseley H, et al. The characteristics of erythema induced by topical 5-aminolaevulinic acid photodynamic therapy. Photodermatol Photoimmunol Photomed 2004; 20:105–107.
35. Monfrecola G, Procaccini EM, D'Onofrio D, et al. Hyperpigmentation induced by topical 5-aminolaevulinic acid plus visible light. J Photochem Photobiol B-Biol 2002; 68:147–155.
36. Rhodes LE, Tsoukas MM, Anderson RR, et al. Iontophoretic delivery of ALA provides a quantitative model for ALA pharmacokinetics and PpIX phototoxicity in human skin. J Invest Dermatol 1997; 108:87–91.
37. Wolf P, Fink-Puches R, Reimann-Weber A, et al. Development of malignant melanoma after repeated topical photodynamic therapy with 5-aminolevulinic acid at the exposed site. Dermatology 1997; 194:53–54.
38. Varma S, Holt PJA, Anstey AV. Erythroplasia of Queyrat treated by topical aminolaevulinic acid photodynamic therapy: a cautionary tale. Br J Dermatol 2000; 142:825–826.
39. Haller JC, Cairnduff F, Slack G, et al. Routine double treatments of superficial basal cell carcinomas using aminolaevulinic acid-based photodynamic therapy. Br J Dermatol 2000; 143:1270–1274.
40. Szeimies RM, Karrer S, Radakovic-Fijan S, et al. Photodynamic therapy using topical methyl 5-aminolevulinate compared with cryotherapy for actinic keratosis: a prospective, randomized study. J Am Acad Dermatol 2002; 47:258–262.
41. Freeman M, Vinciullo C, Francis D, et al. A comparison of photodynamic therapy using topical methyl aminolevulinate (Metvix®) with single cycle cryotherapy in patients with actinic keratosis: a prospective, randomized study. J Derm Treat 2003; 14:99–106.
42. Braathen LR, Szeimies RM, Basset-Seguin N, et al. Guidelines on the use of photodynamic therapy (PDT) for non-melanoma skin cancer—an international consensus. J Am Acad Dermatol. In press.
43. Sidoroff A. Actinic keratosis. In: Calzavara-Pinton PG, Szeimies RM, Ortel B, eds. Photodynamic Therapy and Fluorescence Diagnosis in Dermatology. Amsterdam: Elsevier, 2001:199–216.
44. Piacquadio DJ, Chen DM, Farber HF, et al. Photodynamic therapy with aminolevulinic acid topical solution and visible blue light in the treatment of multiple actinic keratoses of the face and scalp: investigator-blinded, phase 3, multicenter trials. Arch Dermatol 2004; 140:41–46.
45. Pariser DM, Lowe NJ, Stewart DM, et al. Photodynamic therapy with topical methyl aminolevulinate for actinic keratosis: results of a prospective randomized multicenter trial. J Am Acad Dermatol 2003; 48:227–232.
46. Dragieva G, Hafner J, Dummer R, et al. Topical photodynamic therapy in the treatment of actinic keratoses and Bowen's disease in transplant recipients. Transplantation 2004; 77:115–121.
47. Salim A, Leman JA, McColl JH, et al. Randomized comparison of photodynamic therapy with topical 5-fluorouracil in Bowen's disease. Br J Dermatol 2003; 148:539–543.
48. Morton CA, Horn M, Leman J, et al. Comparison of topical methyl aminolevulinate photodynamic therapy with cryotherapy or fluorouracil for treatment of squamous cell carcinoma in situ. Arch Dermatol 2006; 142:729–735.
49. Solèr AM, Warloe T, Berner A, et al. A follow-up study of recurrence and cosmesis in completely responding superficial and nodular basal cell carcinomas treated with methyl 5-aminolevulinate-based photodynamic therapy alone and with prior curettage. Br J Dermatol 2001; 145: 467–471.
50. Thissen MR, Schroeter CA, Neumann HA. Photodynamic therapy with delta-aminolaevulinic acid for nodular basal cell carcinomas using a prior debulking technique. Br J Dermatol 2000; 142:338–339.
51. Horn M, Wolf P, Wulf HC, et al. Topical methyl aminolaevulinate photodynamic therapy in patients with basal cell carcinoma prone to complications and poor cosmetic outcome with conventional treatment. Br J Dermatol 2003; 149:1242–1249.
52. Rhodes LE, de Rie M, Enstrom Y, et al. Photodynamic therapy using topical methyl aminolevulinate vs surgery for nodular basal cell carcinoma: results of a multicenter randomized prospective trial. Arch Dermatol 2004; 140:17–23.
53. Wang I, Bendsoe N, Klinteberg CA, et al. Photodynamic therapy vs. cryosurgery of basal cell carcinomas: results of a phase III clinical trial. Br J Dermatol 2001; 144:832–840.
54. Kuijpers DI, Smeets NW, Krekels GA, et al. Photodynamic therapy as adjuvant treatment of extensive basal cell carcinoma treated with Mohs micrographic surgery. Dermatol Surg 2004; 30:794–798.
55. Stender IM, Na R, Fogh H, et al. Photodynamic therapy with 5-aminolaevulinic acid or placebo for recalcitrant foot and hand warts: randomised double-blind trial. Lancet 2000; 355:963–966.
56. Stender IM, Wulf CH. Photodynamic therapy of recalcitrant warts with 5-aminolevulinic: a retrospective analysis. Acta Dermato-Venereol 1999; 79:400–401.
57. Stender IM, Lock-Anderson J, Wulf HC. Recalcitrant hand and foot warts successfully treated with photodynamic therapy with topical 5-aminolaevulinic acid: a pilot study. Clin Exp Dermatol 1999; 24:154–159.
58. Schroeter CA, Pleuins J, van Nispen tot Pannerden C, et al. Photodynamic therapy: new treatment for therapy-resistant plantar warts. Dermatol Surg 2005; 31:71–75.

59. Mizuki D, Kaneko T, Hanada K. Successful treatment of topical photodynamic therapy using 5-aminolevulinic acid for plane warts. Br J Dermatol 2003; 149:1087–1088.

60. Smucler R, Jatsova E. Comparative study of aminolevulinic acid photodynamic therapy plus pulsed dye laser versus pulsed dye laser alone in treatment of viral warts. Photomed Laser Surg 2005; 23:202–205.

61. Frank RG, Bos JD, Meulen FW, et al. Photodynamic therapy for condylomata acuminata with local application of 5-aminolevulinic acid. Genitourin Med 1996; 72:70–71.

62. Fehr MK, Hornung R, Degen A, et al. Photodynamic therapy of vulvar and vaginal condyloma and intraepithelial neoplasia using topically applied 5-aminolevulinic acid. Lasers Surg Med 2002; 30:273–279.

63. Wang XL, Wang HW, Wang HS, et al. Topical 5-aminolaevulinic acid-photodynamic therapy for the treatment of urethral condylomata acuminata. Br J Dermatol 2004; 151:880–885.

64. Karrer S, Szeimies RM, Abels C, et al. Epidermodysplasia verruciformis treated using topical 5-aminolaevulinic acid photodynamic therapy. Br J Dermatol 1999; 140:935–938.

65. Moiin A. Photodynamic therapy for molluscum contagiosum infection in HIV-coinfected patients: review of 6 patients. J Drugs Dermatol 2003; 2:637–639.

66. Gold MH, Boring MM, Bridges TM, et al. The successful use of ALA-PDT in the treatment of recalcitrant molluscum contagiosum. J Drugs Dermatol 2004; 3:187–190.

67. Cunliffe WJ, Goulden V. Phototherapy and acne vulgaris. Br J Dermatol 2000; 142:855–856.

68. Morton CA, Scholefield RD, Whitehurst C, et al. An open study to determine the efficacy of blue light in the treatment of mild to moderate acne. J Dermatol Treat 2005; 16:219–223.

69. Lee WLS, Shalita AR, Poh-Fitzpatrick MB. Comparative studies of porphyrin production in Propionibacterium acnes and Propionibacterium granulosum. J Bacteriol 1978; 133:811–815.

70. Kjeldstad B, Johnsson A. An action spectrum for blue and near ultraviolet inactivation of Propionibacterium acnes: with emphasis on a possible porphyrin photosensitization. Photochem Photobiol 1986; 43:67–70.

71. Arakane K, Ryu A, Hayashi C, et al. Singlet oxygen (1 delta g) generation from coproporphyrin in Propionibacterium acnes on irradiation. Biochem Biophys Res Commun 1996; 223:578–582.

72. Papageorgiou P, Katsambas A, Chu A. Phototherapy with blue (415 nm) and red (660 nm) light in the treatment of acne vulgaris. Br J Dermatol 2000; 142:973–978.

73. Hongcharu W, Taylor CR, Chang Y, et al. Topical ALA-photodynamic therapy for the treatment of acne vulgaris. J Invest Dermatol 2000; 115:183–192.

74. Pollock B, Turner D, Stringer MR, et al. Topical aminolaevulinic acid-photodynamic therapy for the treatment of acne vulgaris: a study of clinical efficacy and mechanism of action. Br J Dermatol 2004; 151:616–622.

75. Wiegell SR, Wulf HC. Photodynamic therapy of acne vulgaris using methyl aminolaevulinate: a blinded, randomized, controlled trial. Br J Dermatol 2006; 154:969–976.

76. Hörfelt C, Funk J, Frohm-Nilsson M, et al. Topical methyl aminolaevulinate photodynamic therapy for treatment of facial acne vulgaris: results of a randomized, controlled study. Br J Dermatol 2006; 155:608–613.

77. Gold M, Bridges TM, Bradshaw VL, et al. ALA-PDT and blue light therapy for hidradenitis suppurativa. J Drugs Dermatol 2004; 3(1 suppl):S32–S35.

78. Strauss RM, Pollock B, Stables GI, et al. Photodynamic therapy using aminolaevulinic acid does not lead to clinical improvement in hidradenitis suppurativa. Br J Dermatol 2005; 152:803–804.

79. Calzavara-Pinton PG, Venturini M, Capezzera R, et al. Photodynamic therapy of interdigital mycoses of the feet with topical application of 5-aminolevulinic acid. Photodermatol Photoimmunol Photomed 2004; 20:144–147.

80. Donnelly RF, McCarron PA, Lightowler JM, et al. Bioadhesive patch-based delivery of 5-aminolevulinic acid to the nail for photodynamic therapy of onychomycosis. J Controlled Release 2005; 103:381–392.

81. Silver H. Psoriasis vulgaris treated with hematoporphyrin. Arch Dermatol Syphilol 1937; 36:1118–1119.

82. Boehncke WH, König K, Kaufmann R, et al. Photodynamic therapy in psoriasis: suppression of cytokine production in vitro and recording of fluorescence modification during treatment in vivo. Arch Dermatol Res 1994; 286:300–303.

83. Fritsch C, Lehmann P, Stahl W, et al. Optimum porphyrin accumulation in epithelial skin tumours and psoriatic lesions after topical application of delta-aminolaevulinic acid. Br J Cancer 1999; 79:1603–1608.

84. Boehncke WH, Sterry W, Kaufmann R. Treatment of psoriasis by topical photodynamic therapy with polychromatic light. Lancet 1994; 343:801.

85. Weinstein GD, McCullough JL, Jeffes EW, et al. Photodynamic therapy (PDT) of psoriasis with topical delta aminolevulinic acid (ALA): a pilot dose-ranging study. Photodermatol Photoimmunol Photomed 1994; 10:92.

86. Collins P, Robinson DJ, Stringer MR, et al. The variable response of plaque psoriasis after a single treatment with topical 5-aminolaevulinic acid photodynamic therapy. Br J Dermatol 1997; 137:743–749.

87. Robinson DJ, Collins P, Stringer MR, et al. Improved response of plaque psoriasis after multiple treatments with topical 5-aminolaevulinic acid photodynamic therapy. Acta Derm Venereol 1999; 79:451–455.

88. Stringer MR, Collins P, Robinson DJ, et al. The accumulation of protoporphyrin IX in plaque psoriasis after topical application of 5-aminolevulinic acid indicates a potential for superficial photodynamic therapy. J Invest Dermatol 1996; 107:76–81.

89. Radakovic-Fijan S, Blecha-Thathammer U, Schleyer V, et al. Topical aminolaevulinic acid-based photodynamic therapy as a treatment option for psoriasis? Results of a randomized, observed-blinded study. Br J Dermatol 2005; 152:279–283.

90. Schleyer V, Radakovic-Fijan S, Karrer S, et al. Disappointing results and low tolerability of photodynamic therapy with topical 5-aminolaevulinic acid in psoriasis. A randomized, double-blind phase I/II study. J Eur Acad Dermatol 2006; 20:823–828.

91. Beattie PE, Dawe RS, Ferguson J, et al. Lack of efficacy and tolerability of topical PDT for psoriasis in comparison with narrowband UVB phototherapy. Clin Exp Dermatol 2004; 29:560–562.

92. Malik Z, Ehrenberg B, Faraggi A. Inactivation of erythrocytic, lymphocytic and myelocytic leukemic cells by photoexcitation of endogenous porphyrins. J Photochem Photobiol B Biol 1989; 4:195–205.

93. Boehncke WH, König K, Rück A, et al. In vitro and in vivo effects of photodynamic therapy in cutaneous T-cell lymphoma. Acta Dermato-Venereol 1994; 74:201–205.

94. Rittenhouse-Diakun K, van Leengoed H, Morgan J, et al. The role of transferrin receptor (CD71) in photodynamic therapy of activated and malignant lymphocytes using the heme precursor delta-aminolevulinic acid (ALA). Photochem Photobiol 1995; 61:523–528.

95. Boehncke WH, Rück A, Naumann J, et al. Comparison of sensitivity towards photodynamic therapy of cutaneous resident and infiltrating cell types in vitro. Lasers Surg Med 1996; 19:451–457.

96. Grebenova D, Cajthamlova H, Bartosova J, et al. Selective destruction of leukaemic cells by photo-activation of 5-aminolaevulinic acid-induced protoporphyrin IX. J Photochem Photobiol B Biol 1998; 47:74–81.

97. Wolf P, Fink-Puches R, Cerroni L, et al. Photodynamic therapy for mycosis fungoides after topical photosensitisation with 5-aminolevulinic acid. J Am Acad Dermatol 1994; 31:678–680.

98. Ammann R, Hunziker T. Photodynamic therapy for mycosis fungoides after topical photosensitisation with 5-aminolevulinic acid. J Am Acad Dermatol 1995; 33:541.

99. Orenstein A, Halik J, Tamir J, et al. Photodynamic therapy of cutaneous lymphoma using 5-aminolevulinic acid topical application. Dermatologic Surg 2000; 26:765–769.

100. Edstrom DW, Porwit A, Ros AM. Photodynamic therapy with topical 5-aminolevulinic acid for mycosis fungoides: clinical and histological response. Acta Dermato-Venereol 2001; 81:184–188.

101. Markham T, Sheahan K, Collins P. Topical 5-aminolevulinic acid photodynamic therapy for tumour-stage mycosis fungoides. Br J Dermatol 2001; 144:1262–1263.

102. Leman JA, Dick DC, Morton CA. Topical 5-ALA photodynamic therapy for the treatment of cutaneous T-cell lymphoma. Clin Exp Dermatol 2002; 27:516–518.

103. Svanberg K, Andersson T, Killander D, et al. Photodynamic therapy of non-melanoma malignant tumours of the skin using topical delta-aminolevulinic acid sensitisation and laser irradiation. Br J Dermatol 1994; 130:743–751.

104. Coors EA, von den Driesch P. Topical photodynamic therapy for patients with therapy-resistant lesions of cutaneous T-cell lymphoma. J Am Acad Dermatol 2004; 50:363–367.

105. Umegaki N, Moritsugu R, Katoh S, et al. Photodynamic therapy may be useful in debulking cutaneous lymphoma prior to radiotherapy. Clin Exp Dermatol 2004; 29:42–45.

106. Berroeta L, Lewis-Jones MS, Evans AT, et al. Woringer-Kolopp (localised pagetoid reticulosis) treated with topical photodynamic therapy (PDT). Clin Exp Dermatol 2005; 31:1–2.

107. Stender IM, Wulf HC. Photodynamic therapy with 5-aminolaevulinic acid in the treatment of actinic cheilitis. Br J Dermatol 1996; 135:454–456.

108. Hauschild A, Lischner S, Lange-Asschenfeldt B, et al. Treatment of actinic cheilitis using photodynamic therapy with methylaminolevulinate: report of three cases. Dermatol Surg 2005; 31:1344–1348.

109. Sieron A, Adamek M, Kawczyk-Krupka A, et al. Photodynamic therapy (PDT) using topically applied delta-aminolevulinic acid (ALA) for the treatment of oral leukoplakia. J Oral Pathol Med 2003; 32:330–336.

110. Chen HM, Chen CT, Yang H, et al. Successful treatment of oral verrucous hyperplasia with topical 5-aminolevulinic acid-mediated photodynamic therapy. Oral Oncol 2004; 40:630–637.

111. Calzavara-Pinton PG. Repetitive photodynamic therapy with topical delta-aminolaevulinic acid as an appropriate approach to the routine treatment of superficial non-melanoma skin tumours. Photochem Photobiol B Biol 1995; 29:53–57.

112. Stables GI, Stringer MR, Robinson DJ, et al. Erythroplasia of Queyrat treated by topical aminolaevulinic acid photodynamic therapy. Br J Dermatol 1999; 140:514–517.

113. Lee MR, Ryman W. Erythroplasia of Queyrat treated with topical methyl aminolevulinate photodynamic therapy. Australas J Dermatol 2005; 46:196–198.

114. Henta T, Itoh Y, Kobayashi M, et al. Photodynamic therapy for inoperable vulval Paget's disease using delta-aminolaevulinic acid: successful management of a large skin lesion. Br J Dermatol 1999; 141:347–349.

115. Zollo JD, Zeitouni NC. The Roswell Park Cancer Institute experience with extramammary Paget's disease. Br J Dermatol 2000; 142:59–65.

116. Shieh S, Dee AS, Cheney RT, et al. Photodynamic therapy for the treatment of extramammary Paget's disease. Br J Dermatol 2002; 146:1000–1005.

117. Madan V, Loncaster J, Allan D, et al. Extramammary Paget's disease treated with topical and systemic photodynamic therapy. Photodiagn Photodyn Ther 2005; 2:309–311.

118. Martin Hirsch PL, Whitehurst C, Buckley CH, et al. Photodynamic treatment for lower genital tract intraepithelial neoplasia. Lancet 1998; 351:1403.

119. Hillemanns P, Untch M, Dannecker C, et al. Photodynamic therapy of vulvar intraepithelial neoplasia using 5-aminolevulinic acid. Int J Cancer 2000; 85:649–653.

120. Fehr MK, Hornung R, Schwarz VA, et al. Photodynamic therapy of vulvar intraepithelial neoplasia III using topically applied 5-aminolevlinic acid. Gynecol Oncol 2001; 80:62–66.

121. Abel-Hady E-S, Martin-Hirsch P, Duggan-Keen M, et al. Immunological and viral factors associated with the response of vulval intraepithelial neoplasia to photodynamic therapy. Cancer Res 2001; 61:192–196.

122. Bissonnette R, Shapiro J, Zeng H, et al. Topical photodynamic with 5-aminolaevulinic acid does not induce hair regrowth inpatients with extensive alopecia areata. Br J Dermatol 2000; 143:1032–1035.

123. Ackermann G, Abels C, Bäumler W, et al. Simulations on the selectivity of 5-aminolevulinic acid-induced fluorescence in vivo. J Photochem Photobiol B: Biol 1998; 47:121–128.

124. Ericson MB, Sandberg C, Gudmundson F, et al. Fluorescence contrast and threshold limit: implications for photodynamic diagnosis of basal cell carcinoma. J Photochem Photobiol B: Biol 2003; 69:121–127.

125. Bäumler W, Abels C, Szeimies RM. Fluorescence diagnosis and photodynamic therapy in dermatology. Med Laser Appl 2003; 18:47–56.

27 | The Principles and Medical Applications of Lasers and Intense-Pulsed Light in Dermatology

Iltefat Hamzavi
Department of Dermatology, Henry Ford Hospital, Detroit, and Hamzavi Dermatology, Port Huron, Michigan, U.S.A.

Harvey Lui
Department of Dermatology and Skin Science, Vancouver Coastal Health Research Institute, University of British Columbia, Vancouver, British Columbia, Canada

- In order to exert their effect, lasers and IPL must get photons of radiation into the skin/chromophore and then an absorption event must happen.

- Tissue optics dictate how light gets to a particular structure and most often thermal effects dictate the clinical result.

- There are different physical qualities of lasers and IPL, but both devices can work for certain conditions.

- Q-switched lasers are best at removing tattoos with minimal scarring but require many treatments and do not always clear tattoos.

- Laser hair removal can also be used for noncosmetic indications such as dissecting cellultis.

- UV lasers and targeted phototherapy target diseased skin while sparing uninvolved skin.

- Lasers and IPL with or without PDT may have a role in acne but it is too early to say if they are better than medical therapy.

- Laser-activated PDT can be less painful for actinic keratosis than noncoherent light activation but long-term efficacy has not been defined yet.

aser and light sources offer a potential benefit to many dermatology patients, but the rate of advance within the field can confuse even the experienced laser user without a proper understanding of the principles, which lie behind their use. This chapter highlights some of the most important advances in the medical use of lasers by relating how these advances pertain to basic optical principles. Regardless of the device or dermatologic indication, specific biophysical laws govern how all light affects the skin. This chapter will go on to cover the medical uses of laser while deferring most of the cosmetic uses for photodamage and ethnic skin to other chapter of this book. The distinction between cosmetic and medical can be arbitrary and is often made by third party payers, but for the purposes of this chapter noncarcinogenic UV-induced effects on the skin and hair removal are considered cosmetic while other indications will fall within either the medical laser section or the ethnic laser section.

The key to developing and refining any type of light-based therapy is understanding how to efficiently and effectively deliver this energy to cutaneous structures in a highly targeted fashion so as to limit collateral light-induced trauma or to modify certain immune-based tissue responses. While the term "light" is sometimes restricted to electromagnetic radiation that is visible to the human eye (i.e., 400–700 nm), in this chapter, the entire region from ultraviolet to infrared will be referred to as either light or radiation. Treating the skin with light can be considered in two stages: (*i*) understanding how to selectively deliver photons to specific structural targets in the skin, that is, tissue optics; and (*ii*) understanding the biological processes that occur after a skin target absorbs light photons, that is, photobiological reactions. The overwhelming majority of refinements to phototherapeutic devices such as lasers and intense-pulsed light (IPL) exploit either one or both of these two aspects, and the advances highlighted in the article will be discussed using this mechanistic perspective.

UNDERSTANDING TISSUE OPTICS AND PHOTOBIOLOGICAL REACTIONS

A detailed explanation of tissue optics and photobiological reactions is covered in the section on radiation sources (chap. 3), but certain basic biophysical principles warrant a brief summary. The interaction of radiation with tissue is governed by three basic processes that can occur when a photon of light reaches the skin: reflection, scattering, and absorption (Fig. 1). Radiation that is *reflected* from the skin and perceived by the human visual system provides the means for diagnosing skin disease, but reflected radiation does not itself result in any direct therapeutic effect. In the absence of an absorption event (see below), the forward propagation of radiation deeper within the skin is influenced by the degree to which its direction of travel has been *scattered* by tissue structures. Tissue scattering of ultraviolet, visible, and near-infrared light is wavelength-dependent, and in general longer wavelength radiation penetrates the skin more deeply because longer wavelengths tend to scatter less in the skin. Thus, targets that are deeper in the skin require the use of devices that can deliver longer wavelength radiation.

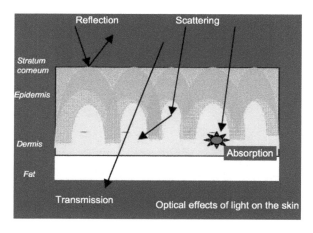

FIGURE 1   The various optical effects of photons on the skin.

Absorption is an important biophysical event that involves the transfer of energy from radiation to tissue. The structure which absorbs energy is referred to as a chromophore. Absorption is strictly defined as when a molecule, which makes up the chromophore, absorbs electromagnetic energy with a characteristic efficiency given by the molecules extinction coefficient in a wavelength-dependent manner (1). Without photon absorption, energy will not be taken up by the skin and no biological or therapeutic effect will occur. The absorption of photons by specific molecules within the skin also influences light penetration, since any photon that is absorbed is no longer capable of propagating through the skin, as that particular photon no longer exists (2). Like scattering, absorption is wavelength-dependent, but in a somewhat more complicated manner since it depends on the absorption profile or "spectrum" of the chromophore. With the possible exception of the UVB wavelength excimer laser, the specific chromophores for most light-based therapies are precisely known, which include hemoglobin, melanin, water, exogenous dyes (i.e., tattoo pigment), and photosensitizing drugs (i.e., psoralens and PDT photosensitizers). These chromophores absorb light over a broad spectrum of wavelengths as shown in Figures 2A and B (3,4).

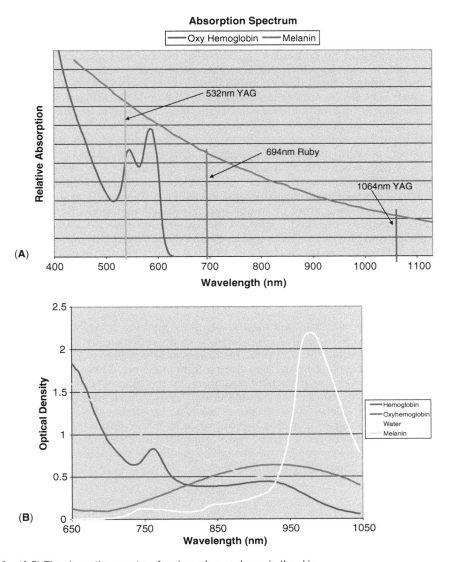

FIGURE 2 (**A,B**) The absorption spectra of various chromophores in the skin.

In summary, both scattering and absorption will determine the depth to which light will penetrate the skin, but only absorption can lead to photobiological and phototherapeutic effects. All phototherapeutic applications must, by definition be mediated by chromophores present in the skin. Thus, in order for a given photon to have a clinical effect it must actually reach the target structure within the skin and then be absorbed by a specific chromophore within that target. Whether or not these events occur and the degree to which they occur is dependent on the wavelength of light used, the structures of the skin which affect reflection/scattering, and the concentration and location of chromophores.

Once the photon is absorbed by the chromophore, the source's radiation energy is transferred to the skin to either (*i*) generate heat, or (*ii*) drive photochemical reactions. The former scenario encompasses the mechanism behind the majority of lasers and IPLs in dermatology, all of which, in essence involve the selective and irreversible alteration of tissue using heat (2). In contrast, ultraviolet phototherapy using lasers or IPL and laser-assisted/IPL-assisted Photodynamic therapy (PDT) do not primarily involve the use of light to generate heat, but rather rely on photon absorption to energize photochemistry. In the case of ultraviolet therapy, it is now generally accepted that the therapeutically useful photochemical reactions culminate in cutaneous immunosuppression although the exact sequence of reactions is less clear. In laser-/IPL-assisted PDT, the first two photochemical reactions are very clearly defined. The energy of the excited chromophore is first transferred to molecular oxygen to form singlet oxygen which then reacts with a diverse range of biomolecules (2). The ever-expanding indications for PDT partly mirrors the multiple ways by which singlet oxygen generated by light can affect the skin.

In clinical parlance, there is often an undue preoccupation with the technical specifications for a given light device rather than a well grounded understanding of the desired underlying photobiological and phototherapeutic endpoints. The reality is that for any clinical indication a multiplicity of possible photonic devices are often available. This simply reflects the fact that from the point of view of the tissue and its chromophores, the exact source of the photons (e.g., laser vs. intense-pulsed light vs. light emitting diode vs. fluorescent lamp) matters far less than whether the photons are of the appropriate wavelength and delivered to the target in sufficient quantity to cause irreversible tissue changes to particular structures without collateral damage to surrounding skin. As with any therapeutic modality, the ultimate arbiters for the bewildering array of competing light-based therapies and devices are well-designed and rigorously executed controlled clinical studies which must be evaluated with photobiological principles in mind. Clinical trials information must be coupled to the operators comfort level with regards to the devices ease of use for the particular indication for which the patient seeks treatment.

USING LASERS AND INTENSE-PULSED LIGHT TO HEAT THE SKIN

Since most lasers in dermatology are used to precisely heat the skin, the advances for these applications are related to increasing the selectivity of these devices by fine-tuning the wavelength, spot size, and pulse duration (i.e., the time over which the laser energy is delivered) (5,6), and simultaneously cooling the skin during light exposure. These variables are used to selectively thermally damage particular structures in the skin. These modifications have increased the safety and efficacy for photothermal lasers/IPL in dermatology, particularly for targeting larger or deeper skin structures such as larger blood vessels, melanosomes, porphyrins, and hair follicles. Another driving force in the evolution of lasers and IPL has been the need to minimize "down-time" from postprocedure purpura to elaborate wound care protocols. More information on the cosmetic uses of IPL and laser can be found in the cosmetic laser chapter (chap. 29) within this book.

Intense-Pulsed Light

IPL sources are now very popular in medicine and have been heavily marketed to the public as well as dermatologists, other physicians, and nonmedical practitioners. IPL devices are not lasers, but like most cutaneous lasers, produce their desired effect by generating heat. The core technology is relatively simple and involves the use of polychromatic broadband flashlamps equipped with optical filters that allow preselected visible to infrared wavebands (500–1200 nm) to reach the skin (7). Since multiple wavelengths are delivered, several different chromophores including hemoglobin, melanin, and perhaps, even water can be targeted with the same light exposure. In practical terms, multiple IPL treatment sessions are often required, and due to the complexity of selecting the appropriate wavelength cut-off filter, fluence, and pulse duration there is a risk for developing side effects secondary to nonspecific thermal damage. These side effects include crusting, pigmentary changes, hair loss, and paradoxical increases in hair growth (8). Another potential area of concern with IPL relates in part to the multiplicity of repeat treatments that are often advocated for both the initial treatment and subsequent maintenance sessions. Lastly, the ergonomics of IPL make visualizing the skin while firing a laser difficult when compared to laser technology (9). However, IPL is one of the better treatment options to simultaneously treat pigment and telangiectasias. The versatility and effective marketing of these devices is a driving force behind their popularity. In addition, there is a much lower acquisition and maintenance cost along with their multiple uses which have made them an often used technology (9).

CLINCIAL INDICATIONS
Getting the Red Out

The principle for treating vascular lesions such as port wine stains with yellow 577/585/595 nm light was originally based on hemoglobin's absorption spectrum, red to infrared light appears to better target blood vessels that are situated more deeply (Fig. 3) (Table 1). In addition, vascular laser pulse durations have been extended from the sub-microsecond to millisecond domain for two reasons. A longer duration of exposure will heat a greater tissue volume, which is necessary for larger caliber vessels. Second, longer pulses will conduct heat more gradually within blood vessels resulting in a lesser tendency to immediate purpura which, although temporary, patients find very disfiguring. The long-pulsed neodymium:YAG and later-model pulsed-dye lasers both expand the range of blood vessels that can be treated by incorporating these parameter changes. The longer penetration of the long-pulsed 1064 nm neodymium:YAG laser facilitates its use for leg veins including blue veins up to 3 mm in diameter. The depth of penetration of these wavelengths are enhanced using wider spot sizes which increase forward scattering which minimizes superficial thermal injury (10,11). Not unexpectedly, these lasers are often less effective for finer red telangiectasias presumably due to a mismatch between the vessel's thermal relaxation time and the laser's pulsewidth. The deeper penetration of the recently developed 595 nm, long pulse (up to 40 ms) dye laser allows the operator to obtain clearance for some port wine stains that is equivalent to the original 585 nm, 450 µs pulsed dye laser results with fewer side effects such as prolonged purpura and crusting (12). IPL can also be used to treat erythema with a minimal amount of purpura but requires more treatment and has the disadvantage of limiting the operators visualization of vessels until after they are treated (9). A more detailed explanation of vascular laser treatments can be found in the cosmetic laser chapter of this book (chap. 29).

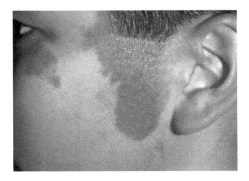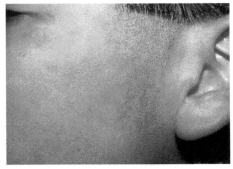

FIGURE 3   A port wine stain treated with a pulsed-dye laser (*left*: before treatment; *right*: after eight treatments).

TABLE 1 A Selected List of Lasers and Intense-Pulsed Light with Wavelength, Pulse Duration, and Clinical Indications

Type of laser	Wavelength (nm)	Target	Pulse duration/comments
Continuous wave			
CO_2	10,600	Water	Less than 1.6–2.8 ms which is the estimated thermal relaxation time of the skin
Ablative laser			
Pulsed CO_2	10,600	Water	<2 ms, but varies
Erbium	2940	Water	Automatically adjusts in most models
Fractional lasers			
Microablative laser	1550,1540,1440	Water in dermis	Creates microthermal injury zones using light arrays
Pulsed lasers for vascular, hair, collagen, and sebaceous glands thermolysis; longer pulse duration and intermediate peak power			
Flashlamp-pumped pulsed dye	585	Blood vessel (30–100 μm)	450 μs
Long-pulsed dye	595	1.5–40 ms	Blood vessels (>1 mm)
KTP (potassium titanyl phosphate)	532	1–100 ms	Blood vessels up to 1 mm
Nonablative infrared lasers			Used for acne and photoaging
Nd:YAG	1320	Water in Collagen	Precools epidermis to limit thermal effect to dermis
Diode	1450	Water in collagen and sebaceous gland	Precools epidermis to limit thermal effect to dermis
Glass Erbium	1540	Water in dermis	10–100 ms
Pulsed lasers/light sources for pigmented lesions at very high peak powers and very short pulse durations			
Q-switched ruby	694	25 ns	Melanin, black, blue, green tattoos
Q-switched alexandrite	755	50–100 ns	Melanin, black, blue, green tattoos
Q-switched Nd:YAG	1064	5-15 nsec	Melanin, black tattoos
Q-switched Nd:YAG	532 (freq-doubled)	5–15 ns	Melanin, red, orange, yellow tattoos
IPL (not Q-switched)	590–1200	Variable (ms)	Works on pigmented and vascular lesions
Hair-removal devices			
694 ruby	694	3–100 ms	Most w/ cooling device
755 nm alexandrite	755	2–40 ms	Most w/ cooling device
800 nm diode lasers	800	5–250 ms	Most w/ cooling device
1064 nm long pulsed	1064	1–350 ms	Most w/ cooling device
IPL	590–1200	Variable (ms)	Some w/ cooling device

Abbreviation: IPL, intense-pulsed light.

Getting the Melanin Out

Lasers and IPL can be used to selectively remove melanin in a variety of conditions with variable success and safety. The selectivity can be obtained by appropriate selection of the wavelength, pulse duration, spot size, and recognition of biological endpoints. There are a variety of wavelengths in the visible range which are absorbed by melanin as indicated in Figures 2A and B, but the over-riding principle of this therapy is to target the melanin in the pathological skin without destroying the normal skin. Selectivity is obtained by appropriate selection of wavelength, pulsed duration, spot size, and cooling the targeted areas. Q-switched lasers and IPL treatments are very helpful in pigmented lesions such as nevus of Ota, tattoo removal, and lentigines. Nevus of Ota and tattoos are best treated with high-peak power devices with very short pulse durations. Q-switched lasers are the best options for these conditions but lead to some crusting post-treatment with the potential side effects of hypopigmentation. In addition, they require multiple treatments. Q-switched lasers are effective devices but they do suffer from an inadequate response in some patients along with postinflammatory hyperpigmentation in Asians, in particular (9). IPL has the benefit of minimal crusting but requires multiple treatments. The response of melasma to light treatment has been less than satisfactory and this particular disorder of pigmentation must be approached differently. This is covered in more detail in the cosmetic sections and the section on treatment of ethnic skin diseases.

Tattoos

Lasers have been used to remove tattoos for more than 25 years. Initially, the CO_2 laser in continuous mode was used but resulted in significant irreversible textural changes and dyspigmentation. Other wavelengths that were specific to particular tattoo colors were added that resulted in scarring as well. However, in the 1990s, lasers were designed based on experimental data from the 1960s and 1980s, which suggested that shorter pulsed durations in the nanosecond domain of high-peak power could more specifically target smaller structures with less collateral damage. Since that time, Q-switched lasers have become the preferred modality of tattoo removal (5,13) (Fig. 4). These devices should be used by an experienced operator who is aware of their limitations. These include the following key points: (*i*) the color of the tattoo should match the wavelength used to ablate it (Table 1); (*ii*) larger spot sizes are preferred due to the deeper depth of penetration; (*iii*) the laser should have a pulse duration in the nanosecond domain; and (*iv*) skin-colored tattoos should be treated with care, since they may develop a paradoxical hyperpigmentation (14). Even if everything is optimal, laser tattoo removal requires multiple treatments, cannot treat certain inks and may cause some hypopigmentation. However, the textural changes are much improved as compared with other types of removal using heat or surgery (14). The skin-colored tattoos are best left alone, but if treatment is desired then very careful pulsed CO_2 laser can be performed with effective removal of the tattoo (15).

Cooling the Skin to Protect the Epidermis and Superficial Dermis

Although the judicious selection of wavelength, spot size, pulse duration, and fluence allows lasers and IPL sources to generate heat at specific targets within the skin, collateral heat

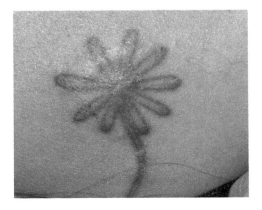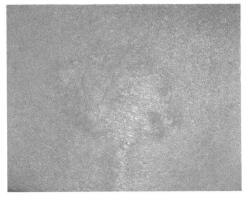

FIGURE 4   Tattoo removal with a 755 nm Q-switched laser (*Left*: before treatment; *Right*: after four treatments).

damage can still be sustained by surrounding structures, particularly the epidermis which contains melanin, a broad spectrum chromophore. Unwanted epidermal thermal damage becomes even more problematic when treating darker skin types or when using higher fluences as may be the case when treating deeper targets such as hair follicles. Cooling the skin surface during laser exposures serves to protect the epidermis and superficial dermis from unintended photothermal effects. Skin-cooling techniques include chilled probes held in contact with the skin, timed cryogen sprays directed to the skin surface, and forced cold air fans directed at the treatment site. All forms of cooling aim to prevent the superficial layers of the skin from reaching the threshold temperature for thermal damage during laser exposure, and they all differ in terms of reliability and the cost of consumables such as cyrogen. An additional benefit of skin cooling beyond the reduction of superficial crusting and dyschromia is intraoperative pain relief (16).

Treating Hair Disorders with Light

The use of lasers and IPL systems for hair removal has expanded tremendously over the decade. This has mostly been used for cosmetic indications, which are covered in other chapters of this work. In addition, Table 1 lists some of the laser hair-removal options presently available. The benefits of this technology are expanding into medical arenas such as the treatment of inflammatory scalp disorders such as pseudofolliculitis barbae, dissecting cellulites, and scarring alopecias (Fig. 5). Since many of these conditions involve an immune response to the hair, treatments that target the hair often improve the condition. Given the fact that these diseases target people of color, the longer wavelength, long-pulsed lasers have added new treatment options for these diseases. Treatment for pseudofollicultis has been documented in a randomized clinical trials (17), whereas treatment for the other conditions has not. All these conditions can often be quite disabling. There are reports of prolonged remissions of these conditions with long-pulse Nd:YAG lasers (18).

Lasers for Warts

Lasers used for the treatment of *Verrucae vulgaris* is controversial. The treatment is often nonspecific and can generate a plume of infectious smoke which must be evacuated by a filter (19). However, the treatment can be effective for recalcitrant verruca that have not responded to the traditional treatments (20). It is the author's experience that the pulsed-dye laser can be an effective treatment for multiple verruca located on the hands, but several treatments are required and the settings have to be adjusted to induce significant purpura of the affected lesions and surrounding skin. The pulsed dye is less effective for *Verruca plantaris*. These may respond to the CO_2 laser, but scarring complications are not uncommon. However, the ability to simultaneously

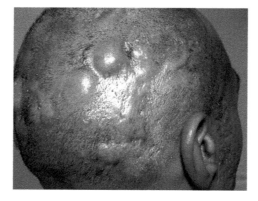 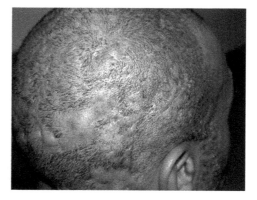

FIGURE 5 An example of dissecting cellulitis treated with Nd:YAG laser (*left*: before treatment; *right*: after six treatments).

destroy tissue while maintaining hemostasis can be very helpful and the CO_2 can compare favorably to other treatments for the treatment of recalcitrant verruca.

UV Lasers as Immunomodulators

Recent advances in ultraviolet phototherapy include a better mechanistic understanding of its biological effects, more rational dosimetry approaches, and the deployment of several novel UV sources. Although this book has a separate section on phototherapy, a quick review here will explain the rationale behind laser and targeted phototherapy systems. The basic science for UV phototherapy is characterized best for psoriasis where the induction of T-cell apoptosis has been demonstrated for broad (21) and narrowband UVB (22). Narrowband UVB phototherapy also seems to affect keratinocyte apoptosis as well (23). Multiple other cutaneous immunological reactions also occur with UV, but the T cell-depleting effects are likely pivotal for clearing inflammatory dermatoses and cutaneous T cell lymphoma. These cytolytic effects on activated immune cells may also explain why UV therapy can be considered a remittive form of psoriasis treatment. The fundamental shift in concept of UV phototherapy as a means of inducing localized cutaneous immunosuppression has provided a far more logical rationale for its general efficacy in a broad range of dermatoses.

In conventional UV phototherapy, both diseased and normal skin are simultaneously exposed to light. While the primary goal of treating inflammatory dermatoses such as psoriasis is to clear skin lesions using light, our current approach to UV dosimetry is limited by the need to avoid burning the unaffected skin. Very high-dose UV exposures—as high as several multiples of the baseline minimal erythema (UVB) (24) or phototoxic (PUVA) (25) dose—can indeed clear psoriasis fairly efficiently, but using such fluences on a "whole body" basis at the outset of therapy will cause severe burning of unaffected skin.

Novel UV Light Sources

Unlike selective photothermolysis with lasers, which is critically dependent on the rate and number (i.e., irradiance and fluence, respectively) of photons delivered to the skin, the effects of UV phototherapy are primarily determined by the total number of photons that reach the skin which result in apoptosis and other immunosuppressive effects (23,26). Thus, depending on the specific light source, psoriasis can be cleared with UV light exposures ranging from several minutes (conventional fluorescent or incandescent lamps) to fractions of a second (lasers and IPL). UV lasers and IPL sources aim to clear psoriasis more efficiently than conventional broadband UVB in three ways. First, these sources emit relatively longer wavelength UVB, or UVB, UVA, and visible light; second, they can be targeted to expose only the affected areas while sparing normal skin thereby allowing much higher fluences to be safely used; and finally, they operate at much higher irradiances so that exposure times are much shorter than with fluorescent lamps. There are now at least three commercial devices that can provide targeted phototherapy: the 308 nm excimer laser, broadband IPL, and the broadband mercury lamp with dual UVB and UVA output. There are several published controlled clinical studies to show that psoriasis responds to the excimer laser and other targeted phototherapy systems (24,27,28). The disadvantages to targeted phototherapy are the higher cost and the relatively time-consuming aspect of covering broad plaques on the body with a series of relatively small spot size exposures. Parenthetically, non-UV lasers have been successfully used for psoriasis (29), but these techniques have not been widely adapted in dermatology, presumably because of practical limitations.

In addition to psoriasis, UV wavelength lasers have been shown to be effective in vitiligo as well. They do appear to repigment skin faster than conventional UV light sources, but they still have the issue of not being able to completely repigment most patient on most locations of the skin (30).

Laser-/Intense-Pulsed Light-activated Photodynamic Therapy

Following its approval by the Food and Drug Administration (FDA) in 1999 for treating actinic keratoses, PDT was initially slow to catch on in dermatology, and this was largely due to the low reimbursement for dermatologic PDT in the United States by third party payers. The concept of PDT is a century old, and its dependence on oxygen-related photochemistry has been well known for most of that time. In clinical practice, the treatment involves the administration of a photosensitizer followed by exposing the skin to light. The drug-activating photons can come from lasers or noncoherent light sources. The photosensitizer, incubation period, and wavelength used to activate the photosensitizer allow the nonthermal selective destruction of neoplastic keratinocytes, sebaceous glands, and hair follicles to be fine-tuned. Indications for PDT can include oncological uses and destruction of appendegeal structures.

The efficacy of topical PDT using 20% aminolevulinic acid (ALA) and a blue light has been documented in the treatment of actinic keratosis (31). However, the procedure as approved by the FDA is painful and requires two visits on separate days. A few studies where the incubation period was reduced to a few hours and a pulsed-dye laser or IPL used to activate the photodynamic reactions reduced the pain and overall patient treatment time (32). In addition, there are reports of using lasers/IPL and ALA to treat photodamaged skin (33).

Lasers and Intense-Pulsed Light for Acne

Acne is a potential area of dermatology that lasers may impact. There are few studies comparing light-based devices to standard topical or oral medications, but there are several split-faced no treatment/treatment-controlled studies showing a benefit (34,35). There have been several reports suggesting that lasers may be helpful in the treatment of acne (34). There also have been reports to the contrary stating that the lasers do not offer a treatment benefit (36). Long pulsed-dye lasers may offer a benefit, but the optimal settings and the desired biological endpoint have not been determined. There are reports that the 1450 nm laser which targets water in the sebaceous gland is effective for up to 12 months (35). There is also absorption of this wavelength by water in the epidermis, but the use of cryogen cooling prevents the epidermis from suffering significant thermal damage while the sebaceous gland is heated (37).

The use of PDT to ablate appendegeal structures is an area of active investigation. There has been one case study on the use of topical 20% ALA to treat truncal acne with good results. However, significant postinflammatory hyperpigmentation and pain were reported (38). Recently, this technique has been modified by decreasing the incubation period and activating the photosensitizer by a laser or IPL. This has been shown to be less painful and may induce a clinical remission of moderate acne (39). However, the long-term ability of PDT to induce a clinical remission of acne cannot be confirmed at this time. To date, no controlled trials have been published.

CONCLUSION

It is no longer possible to practice dermatology without drawing on the healing power of lasers and light. As compared to drugs, light therapy is in general vastly more versatile with an equal or better safety profile. The range of indications for using light in dermatology cuts across all areas including chronic inflammatory dermatoses, pigmentary disorders, cancer, infections, and cosmetic applications. Physicians can remain current in their understanding of current and evolving modalities by mastering the basic biophysical principles outlined in this chapter. Once these concepts are understood all the advances in lasers and IPL can be kept in perspective. Physicians can then apply the most appropriate technology to the care of their patients while informing patients and themselves about the potential limitations and pitfalls of over-marketed but inadequately proven strategies.

ACKNOWLEDGMENT

The authors gratefully acknowledge Michael Owen, BS, Graduate Student, Wayne State University for formatting the images in this chapter.

REFERENCES

1. Stamatas GN, Zmudzka BZ, Kollias N, Beer JZ. Non-invasive measurements of skin pigmentation in situ. Pigment Cell Res 2004; 17(6):618–626.
2. Hamzavi I, Lui H. Using light in dermatology: an update on lasers, ultraviolet phototherapy, and photodynamic therapy. Dermatol Clin 2005; 23(2):199–207.
3. Dover JS, Arndt KA, Geronemus RG, Alora MB. Cutaneous and Aesthetic Laser Surgery. 2nd ed. Stamford: Appleton and Lang, 2000.
4. Attas M, Hewko M, Payette J, Posthumus T, Sowa M, Mantsch H. Visualization of cutaneous hemoglobin oxygenation and skin hydration using near-infrared spectroscopic imaging. Skin Res Technol 2001; 7(4):238–245.
5. Anderson RR, Parrish JA. Selective photothermolysis: precise microsurgery by selective absorption of pulsed radiation. Science 1983; 220(4596):524–527.
6. Nouri K, Chen H, Saghari S, Ricotti CA, Jr. Comparing 18- versus 12-mm spot size in hair removal using a gentlease 755-nm alexandrite laser. Dermatol Surg 2004; 30(4 Pt 1):494–497.
7. Raulin C, Greve B, Grema H. IPL technology: a review. Lasers Surg Med 2003; 32(2):78–87.
8. Moreno-Arias GA, Castelo-Branco C, Ferrando J. Side-effects after IPL photodepilation. Dermatol Surg 2002; 28(12):1131–1134.
9. Ross EV. Laser versus intense pulsed light: competing technologies in dermatology. Lasers Surg Med 2006; 38(4):261–272.
10. Sadick NS, Prieto VG, Shea CR, Nicholson J, McCaffrey T. Clinical and pathophysiologic correlates of 1064-nm Nd:Yag laser treatment of reticular veins and venulectasias. Arch Dermatol 2001; 137(5):613–617.
11. Omura NE, Dover JS, Arndt KA, Kauvar AN. Treatment of reticular leg veins with a 1064 nm long-pulsed Nd:YAG laser. J Am Acad Dermatol 2003; 48(1):76–81.
12. Greve B, Raulin C. Prospective study of port wine stain treatment with dye laser: comparison of two wavelengths (585 nm vs. 595 nm) and two pulse durations (0.5 milliseconds vs. 20 milliseconds). Lasers Surg Med 2004; 34(2):168–173.
13. Goldman L, Wilson RG, Hornby P, Meyer RG. Radiation from a Q-switched ruby laser. Effect of repeated impacts of power output of 10 megawatts on a tattoo of man. J Invest Dermatol 1965; 44:69–71.
14. Bernstein EF. Laser treatment of tattoos. Clin Dermatol 2006; 24(1):43–55.
15. Hamzavi I, Lui H. Surgical pearl: removing skin-colored cosmetic tattoos with carbon dioxide resurfacing lasers. J Am Acad Dermatol 2002; 46(5):764–765.
16. Tunnell JW, Chang DW, Johnston C, et al. Effects of cryogen spray cooling and high radiant exposures on selective vascular injury during laser irradiation of human skin. Arch Dermatol 2003; 139(6):743–750.
17. Ross EV, Cooke LM, Overstreet KA, Buttolph GD, Blair MA. Treatment of pseudofolliculitis barbae in very dark skin with a long pulse Nd:YAG laser. J Natl Med Assoc 2002; 94(10):888–893.
18. Krasner B, Hamzavi F, Murakawa G, Hamzavi I. Dissecting cellulitis treated with the long pulsed Nd:YAG laser. Dermatol Surg 2006; 32(8):1039–1044.
19. Garden JM, O'Banion MK, Bakus AD, Olson C. Viral disease transmitted by laser-generated plume (aerosol). Arch Dermatol 2002; 138(10):1303–1307.
20. Kopera D. *Verrucae vulgares*: flashlamp-pumped pulsed dye laser treatment in 134 patients. Int J Dermatol 2003; 42(11):905–908.
21. Krueger JG, Wolfe JT, Nabeya RT, et al. Successful ultraviolet B treatment of psoriasis is accompanied by a reversal of keratinocyte pathology and by selective depletion of intraepidermal T cells. J Exp Med 1995; 182(6):2057–2068.
22. Ozawa M, Ferenczi K, Kikuchi T, et al. 312-nanometer ultraviolet B light (narrow-band UVB) induces apoptosis of T cells within psoriatic lesions. J Exp Med 1999; 189(4):711–718.
23. Aufiero BM, Talwar H, Young C, et al. Narrow-band UVB induces apoptosis in human keratinocytes. J Photochem Photobiol B 2006; 82(2):132–139.
24. Trehan M, Taylor CR. High-dose 308-nm excimer laser for the treatment of psoriasis. J Am Acad Dermatol 2002; 46(5):732–737.
25. Taylor CR, Kwangsukstith C, Wimberly J, Kollias N, Anderson RR. Turbo-PUVA: dihydroxyacetone-enhanced photochemotherapy for psoriasis: a pilot study. Arch Dermatol 1999; 135(5):540–544.
26. Bianchi B, Campolmi P, Mavilia L, Danesi A, Rossi R, Cappugi P. Monochromatic excimer light (308 nm): an immunohistochemical study of cutaneous T cells and apoptosis-related molecules in psoriasis. J Eur Acad Dermatol Venereol 2003; 17(4):408–413.
27. Dierickx C. Optimalization of treatment of psoriasis with B clear system(abstract). Lasers Surg Med 2003; 32(suppl 15):37.
28. Asawanonda P, Chingchai A, Torranin P. Targeted UV-B phototherapy for plaque-type psoriasis. Arch Dermatol 2005; 141(12):1542–1546.
29. Zelickson BD, Mehregan DA, Wendelschfer-Crabb G, et al. Clinical and histologic evaluation of psoriatic plaques treated with a flashlamp pulsed dye laser. J Am Acad Dermatol 1996; 35(1):64–68.
30. Hong SB, Park HH, Lee MH. Short-term effects of 308-nm xenon-chloride excimer laser and narrow-band ultraviolet B in the treatment of vitiligo: a comparative study. J Korean Med Sci 2005; 20(2):273–278.

31. Jeffes EW, McCullough JL, Weinstein GD, Kaplan R, Glazer SD, Taylor JR. Photodynamic therapy of actinic keratoses with topical aminolevulinic acid hydrochloride and fluorescent blue light. J Am Acad Dermatol 2001; 45(1):96–104.

32. Alexiades-Armenakas MR, Geronemus RG. Laser-mediated photodynamic therapy of actinic keratoses. Arch Dermatol 2003; 139(10):1313–1320.

33. Avram DK, Goldman MP. Effectiveness and safety of ALA-IPL in treating actinic keratoses and photodamage. J Drugs Dermatol 2004; 3(suppl 1):S36–S39.

34. Seaton ED, Charakida A, Mouser PE, Grace I, Clement RM, Chu AC. Pulsed-dye laser treatment for inflammatory acne vulgaris: randomised controlled trial. Lancet 2003; 362(9393):1347–1352.

35. Jih MH, Friedman PM, Goldberg LH, Robles M, Glaich AS, Kimyai-Asadi A. The 1450-nm diode laser for facial inflammatory acne vulgaris: dose-response and 12-month follow-up study. J Am Acad Dermatol 2006; 55(1):80–87.

36. Orringer JS, Kang S, Hamilton T, et al. Treatment of acne vulgaris with a pulsed dye laser: a randomized controlled trial. JAMA 2004; 291(23):2834–2839.

37. Paithankar DY, Ross EV, Saleh BA, Blair MA, Graham BS. Acne treatment with a 1450 nm wavelength laser and cryogen spray cooling. Lasers Surg Med 2002; 31(2):106–114.

38. Hongcharu W, Taylor CR, Chang Y, Aghassi D, Suthamjariya K, Anderson RR. Topical ALA-photodynamic therapy for the treatment of acne vulgaris. J Invest Dermatol 2000; 115(2):183–192.

39. Goldman MP, Boyce SM. A single-center study of aminolevulinic acid and 417 nm photodynamic therapy in the treatment of moderate to severe acne vulgaris. J Drugs Dermatol 2003; 2(4):393–396.

Lasers and Energy Sources for Skin Rejuvenation and Epilation

Robert A. Weiss
Department of Dermatology, Johns Hopkins University School of Medicine, Baltimore, and Maryland Laser Skin & Vein Institute, Hunt Valley, Maryland, U.S.A.

Michael Landthaler
Department of Dermatology, University Clinic Regensburg, Regensburg, Germany

- Type I photorejuvenation includes treatment of vascular and pigmentary changes associated with photoaging, including lentigines, telangiectasias, dull skin tone, diffuse redness, and rosacea.

- Type II photorejuvenation includes treatment of structural changes in collagen and connective tissue, resulting in improvement in pore size, elastosis, and rhytides.

- Visible light sources and lasers have more influence on type I photorejuvenation treating telangiectatic and melanocytic components of photoaging. These sources can be subdivided into coherent, single wavelength, broadband (flash lamps) or narrowband, such as light emitting diode.

- Infrared wavelengths with primarily water absorption are used to create thermal dermal and collagen injury to effect type II photorejuvenation. The most commonly employed devices are 1320 nm, 1450 nm, and 1540 nm lasers.

- Fractional or microthermal resurfacing refers to small, localized regions of significant thermal injury (coagulation columns) surrounded by circumscribed areas of untreated skin. As a result of direct micro-columnar thermal coagulation of tissue, microrejuvenation techniques stimulate direct replacement of photoaged dermal collagen, resulting in improved skin texture and reduction of fine-to-moderate rhytids.

- Clinical tissue tightening following radiofrequency treatment is thought to result from heat-induced immediate collagen contraction, subsequent collagen remodeling, and neocollagenesis of the dermis and subcutis.

- Multiple lasers and intense pulse light can be used for epilation; most patients will achieve 90% hair reduction. However, regrowth may occur in 6 to 12 months.

PHOTOREJUVENATION
INTRODUCTION

Photorejuvenation is the process whereby light or other energy sources are utilized to reverse the process of photo- or sun-induced aging or environmental damage to the skin. Nonablative photorejuvenation accomplishes this without disturbance of the overlying epidermis. Nonablative typically refers to controlled wounding by thermal means inducing photothermolysis of targeted structures. In addition, there is a relatively new modality of nonwounding/nonthermal, termed photomodulation. The newest treatment for cosmetic improvement is fractional resurfacing, which describes discrete micro-thermal zones of injury, 100 to 250 μ wide and 300 to 700 μ deep with a zone of surrounding unaffected skin. The goal of photorejuvenation with these devices is a reorganization in dermal structural elements and an increase in dermal volume with minimal stimulation of epidermal turnover or injury.

Dermal remodeling without epidermal injury evolved further from initial observations with the use of the pulsed dye laser (PDL) for treatment of surface telangiectasia, but with a secondary effect of skin textural smoothing (1). Subsequently, the development of the 1320 nm, 1450 nm, and 1540 nm infrared lasers with some form of epidermal protection whether cryogen spray, contact cooling, or forced air cooling allowed deeper collagen remodeling with targeted depths of 300 to 500 μ for treatment of deeper scars and rhytids. Complete cosmetic enhancement of the skin must also evolve to include reversal of some of the visible changes that occur from photoaging, not entirely relating to structural changes. Reduction of superficial dyspigmentation (both dermal and epidermal), reduction of dermal telangiectasias, and the appearance of an overall smoother texture and tone became essential elements. As a result, two types of photorejuvenation have been described (2). Type I deals with the elements of vascular and pigmentary changes associated with photoaging, lentigines, telangiectasias, dull skin tone, diffuse redness, and rosacea. Type II involves the structural changes in collagen and connective tissue and can be associated with improvement in pore size, elastosis, and rhytides. Type I and II skin rejuvenation represent photothermal nonablative therapies, as traditionally described.

CLASSIFICATION AND USE OF LASERS/LIGHT SOURCES
FOR PHOTOREJUVENATION

Table 1 outlines the main classifications of laser, light, and other energy sources utilized for cosmetic improvement of the skin. All such classifications are arbitrary, as many devices are capable of delivering multiple wavelengths or energy forms. The first category is visible light lasers or light sources, which have more absorption by hemoglobin and melanin. These visible light sources and lasers have more influence on the telangiectatic and melanocytic components of photoaging. These sources can be subdivided into coherent, single wavelength, broadband (flash lamps) or narrowband, such as light emitting diode (LED). Intense pulsed light (IPL) is a broadband light source with filters used to limit the lower end of the emitted spectrum.

The next category is infrared with absorption predominantly by water. Infrared wavelengths with primarily water absorption are used to create thermal dermal and collagen injury. The most commonly employed devices are 1320 nm, 1450 nm, and 1540 nm lasers, although narrowband infrared LED devices and other filtered light sources and possibly ultrasound may be available in the future. A variant of this is fractional resurfacing. This method can be thought of as microthermal, namely, small zones of thermal injury, tens to hundreds of microns wide are placed into the dermis in a pixel-like fashion. The epidermis is not ablated in these pinpoint thermal columns due to laser design and the use of rigorous skin cooling. There are presently three devices; two use a 1550 nm wavelength and one uses a 1440 nm wavelength to create small microthermal zones of thermal injury about 100 to 300 μ in diameter. It is speculated that this pixel-like microthermal dermal heating will result in skin contraction, dermal collagen remodeling, and thickening and replacement of elastotic collagen. Hence, a cosmetic improvement in the rhytid portion of photoaging.

TABLE 1 Classification of Lasers, Light, and Energy Sources

Visible laser light sources
Frequency doubled Nd:YAG, KTP (green 532 nm)
Pulsed dye (yellow 585–595 nm)
Long pulse versus short PDL
Visible nonlaser light sources
Intense pulsed light—broadband filtered light of various origins
Visible infrared
LED—narrowband
UV, visible, infrared
Infrared lasers (target pigment, hemoglobin and water)
Q-switched and millisecond domain Nd:YAG 1064 nm
Infrared lasers (target water only)
1320 nm Nd:YAG laser
1450 nm diode laser
1540 nm erbium glass laser
Microablative infrared lasers (target water)
1440 nm microarray
1540 nm microarray
1550 nm scanned
Radio-frequency, microwave, and ultrasound

Abbreviations: KTP, potassium-titanyl-phosphate; LED, light emitting diode; Nd:YAG, neodymium : yttrium-aluminum-garnet; PDL, pulsed dye laser.

When selecting an energy source for cosmetic improvement, it is critical to understand the physics behind the wavelength or energy source and thoroughly understand the method of delivery and histologic changes. Having knowledge of the output of a device, with understanding whether the target is hemoglobin, melanin or water (or all three) with spot size and method of delivery, the physician may be better able to choose the correct system for the correct application. For example, photorejuvenation of pigmented lesions would not be possible with a unit emitting 1450 nm for which the target is water and not melanin. This knowledge is also vital for the clinician to minimize possible adverse clinical events in darker ethnic skin types. Visible light, more strongly absorbed by melanin, must therefore be used with greater caution in darker skin. An algorithm for approaches to specific cosmetic conditions is outlined in Table 2.

Visible Light Lasers

Frequency Doubled Nd:YAG, KTP (Green 532 nm)

This has been effectively used for the pigment and telangiectatic component of photoaging for many years and has become an accepted modality for comprehensive photorejuvenation (3). It can be enhanced by the simultaneous use of 1064 nm Nd:YAG laser. The use of this device for many years was very technique-dependent, as the 532 nm light could only be delivered via a relatively small spot size of 4 to 5 mm. The newest version of this device (Gemini, Laserscope, San Jose, California, U.S.A.) allows implementation of a 10 mm spot size of 532 nm green so that a rapid technique to treat a cheek in one to three passes can be employed with reproducible results. In a bilateral comparison of IPL versus large spot 532 nm, the large spot 532 nm was actually a little bit faster than the IPL and delivered slightly better results on pigmentation (4). This is predicted by the higher absorption of 532 nm by melanin over wavelengths cut off at 560 nm with the IPL device. It is now thought that the large spot size 532 nm is an additional to the armamentarium of cosmetic rejuvenation. It compares favorably to some of the broadband devices that deliver energy in large spot sizes so that the entire face can be treated quickly (Fig. 1).

Pulsed Dye (Yellow 585–595 nm) (Pulsed Dye Laser)

The first nonablative wavelength cleared by the FDA for periocular wrinkling for both the 585 and 595 nm wavelengths, this laser has become popular for several components of photoaging

TABLE 2 Algorithm by Photoaging Problem for Nonablative Skin Photorejuvenation

Telangiectasias
  IPL
  PDL LP
  Nd:YAG LP 532 nm

Diffuse redness (nonvisible telangiectasia)
  IPL
  LED photomodulation

Mottled pigmentation
  IPL
  Nd:YAG LP 532 nm
  LED photomodulation

Mild rhytides
  LED photomodulation
  IPL
  PDL
  Nonablative infrared lasers
  Microthermal infrared lasers

Moderate rhytides
  Infrared
  Microthermal infrared lasers

Deeper rhytids
  Infrared wavelengths beyond main hemoglobin and melanin absorption
    1320 nm, 1450 nm, and 1540 nm
  Radiofrequency (more effective for skin tightening)
  Radiofrequency plus additional energy source

Abbreviations: IPL, intense pulse light; LED, light emitting diode; LP, long pulse; PDL, pulsed dye laser.

with newer longer pulse durations. By avoiding the purpura of the original 0.45 msec pulse durations, pulse durations from 6 to 40 msec and/or low fluences of 2 to 3 J/cm^2 are being utilized for the thermal remodeling effects on the dermis at lower energies. The utility of this wavelength is that higher energies provide excellent reduction of telangiectasias (Fig. 2).

Light Sources
Intense Pulsed Light
One of the most controversial light-based technologies initially, IPL was first introduced as a radically new concept with not being a coherent laser wavelength in 1994, and cleared by the FDA in late 1995 as the Photoderm^{TM} (Lumenis, Santa Clara, California, U.S.A.). IPL is a noncoherent filtered flash lamp IPL source. It was initially launched and promoted as a

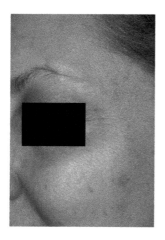
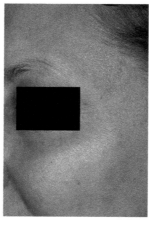

FIGURE 1 Photorejuvenation with the Gemini (Laserscope, San Jose, CA) 10 mm spot 532 nm laser. This 42-year-old patient was treated with two passes of 10 mm spot size, 532 nm green. At one month there is textural improvement as well as reduction in telangiectasias and pigmentation.

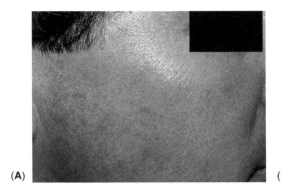 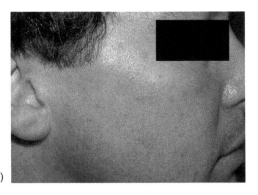

(A) **(B)**

FIGURE 2 Use of extended pulsed dye laser for photorejuvenation. This 39-year-old patient was treated with the extended pulsed dye laser (V-Star, Cynosure, Westford, Massachusetts, U.S.A.). The patient complained of flushing episodes and facial telangiectasia (**A**). The patient was treated with stacked pulsing, three pulses per stack, of 595 nm, 10 mm spot, 7 J/cm^2 and use of forced air cooling. This is the appearance at one month after one treatment with a 75% reduction of telangiectasia (**B**). The patient's facial flushing intensity and frequency was reduced.

radical improvement over existing methods for elimination of leg telangiectasias with reduction in the risks of purpura common to PDLs of the time. It was quickly adapted to facial vessels, which is presently the number one application of IPL. Present day IPL indications have expanded to include nonablative facial rejuvenation, facial telangiectasias, pigmentation, poikiloderma of Civatte, and treatment of scars (5).

In a study of IPL for poikiloderma, 135 patients randomly selected with typical changes of poikiloderma of Civatte on the neck and/or upper chest were treated with one to five treatments using IPL (6). Results indicated clearance of more than 75% of telangiectasias and hyperpigmentation. The incidence of side effects was 5%, including pigment changes. In many cases, improved skin texture was noted both by physician and patient. The authors concluded that IPL was an effective mode of therapy for poikiloderma of Civatte. Cutoff filters utilized in these treatments included primarily 550 to 570 nm. Median number of treatments to achieve results was three. The significance of this study was to demonstrate that cosmetic improvement with these devices was not confined to the face but could be used for necks, chests, back, and so on.

Bitter (7) reported facial rejuvenation in 49 patients using similar parameters and cut-off filters, with 550 to 570 nm cut-off filters and double pulsing of 2.4 to 4.7 pulses with varying inter-pulse intervals. Subjects were treated with a series of four or more full-face treatments at three-week intervals with fluences varying from 30 to 50 J/cm^2. Subject evaluation and skin biopsies were used to assess treatment results. The results reported were that all aspects of photodamage, including telangiectasia, irregular pigmentation, wrinkling, skin coarseness, and pore size, showed visible improvement in more than 90% of subjects with minimal downtime and no scarring. Eighty-eight percent of subjects were satisfied with the overall results of their treatments. Side effects of edema mild blistering and transient pigmentation changes were observed in a small percentage of patients. Collagen synthesis was noted in the biopsy sample.

The longevity of improvement with light-based devices has always been questioned. A recent study demonstrated that a five-year follow-up of 80 randomly selected patients with skin types I–IV who were treated by IPL during 1996 and 1997 showed that at five years following initial treatment, skin textural improvement was noted in 83% of the subjects (8). Photos and patient self-assessment were also graded for telangiectasia severity and dyspigmentation. For those patients practicing rigorous UV-blocking methods, telangiectasias were improved in 82% of subjects, whereas pigmentation remained improved in 79% over the five year period (Fig. 3).

Photomodulation and Low Energy Light Emitting Diodes

The LEDs are narrowband emitters of a broad range of electromagnetic radiation ranging from UV-visible to IR. The LEDs themselves are typically assembled on small chips or equipped with

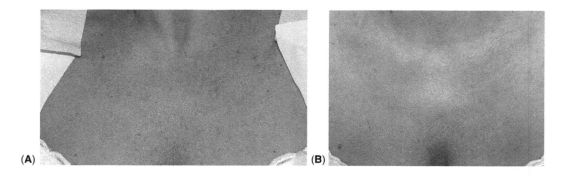

FIGURE 3 Use of intense pulsed light (IPL) for photorejuvenation of the chest. The IPL is well suited for rejuvenation of large surface areas due to the large crystal size, which often ranges to several cm². This 52-year-old patient presented with extensive photodamage of the face, chest, and neck. The images are before and after one treatment at one month. The settings on the Quantum IPL (Lumenis, Santa Clara, California, U.S.A.) device were Program one with a slight modification. The 560-nm filter with a setting of 2.4 msec, 10 msec delay, and 4 msec pulse shows a dramatic reduction in pigmentation and improvement of surface texture.

tiny lenses and assembled into small lamps (typically up to 3–5 mm in diameter, but 10 mm and larger lamps are available). These LEDs typically emit low intensity of light in the milliwatt domain. However, the LEDs may be assembled into larger arrays or panels, and higher energy intensities may also be generated, although the life of the LED is typically shortened. The LEDs are extremely versatile and durable, exhibiting good resistance to temperature, dirt, vibration, and other environmental insults with a typical lamp life of up to 100,000 hours. Also, they do not require expensive or dangerous high voltage power supplies or complex optics, and thus alignment issues and maintenance tend to be very minimal. This therapy is painless, and large LED panel arrays can be assembled so that the entire face may be treated in a few minutes or less.

Typically, LEDs emit light in a ±10 to 20 nm band around the dominant emitted wavelength. We use 590 nm yellow most commonly in a 250 msec pulse duration. (Gentlewaves™, LightBioScience, Virginia Beach, Virginia, U.S.A.). The output of these LEDs is 90% 590 nm light, far greater than a yellow LED in a laptop computer. For this scenario, packages of specifically pulsed photons are absorbed by the "antenna molecules" in mitochondria, thus activating the electron transport system that amplifies the cell signals, eventually resulting in increased production of the cell's normal products. For fibroblasts in culture this translates into production of extracellular matrix proteins, such as collagen and elastin, but without being mediated via thermal injury. Laboratory in vitro testing suggests that a greater net increase in total collagen may be created using nonthermal LED photomodulation than with thermal injury techniques. Initial studies of over 90 patients treated with the Gentlewaves™ LED device showed up to 90% improvement in some aspect of cosmetic appearance of wrinkles or skin tone or textural smoothness (9).

A multi-center clinical trial was also conducted on 90 photoaged females (10). One week after the last treatment, the global improvement in appearance of skin in periorbital region was 62%. Upper lip improvement was 36%. Other observations in periorbital area included reduction of 27% in skin roughness, 30% in elastosis, 14% in pore size, and 25% in redness. Histopathology and immunohistopathology showed increase in several key extracellular matrix proteins associated with clinical improvement in wrinkles. Data up to one-year post-treatment in these same subjects indicate that improvement peaked at four to six months, but that without further treatments of photomodulation, the results decline from 6 to 12 months. On the basis of this study, the FDA cleared the Gentlewaves™ (LightBioScience, Virginia Beach, Virginia, U.S.A.) LED photomodulation device for improvement of periocular rhytids. The patients underwent a series of eight treatments over a four-week interval, and then maintenance treatment was performed once a month. It was also found that the use of LED

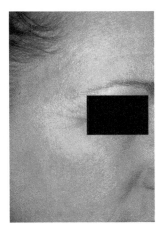 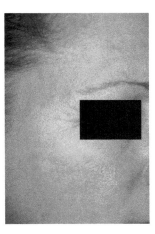

FIGURE 4 Gentlewaves™ light emitting diode photomodulation (LightBioScience, Virginia Beach, Virginia, U.S.A.) for mild photoaging. A 38-year-old patient presents with mild photoaging changes, including mild periocular rhytids and slight dyspigmentation (**A**). The after image was taken at four months following eight treatments given over four weeks. Each treatment was delivered as 100 pulses of 250 msec each, at an extremely low fluence of 0.1 J/cm² (**B**). Treatments are easily tolerated since no heat is involved. This device is cleared by the FDA for improvement of periocular rhytids. This treatment regimen used alone is best for mild or early onset photoaging. Strict sun protection measures must be enforced for patients to benefit from photomodulation.

photomodulation after other photorejuvenation procedures, such as IPL or fractional resurfacing, improves results of textural smoothing and more rapidly reduces the thermal effects of erythema and edema (Fig. 4) (11).

Infrared Lasers (Melanin, Hemoglobin, and Water Absorbing)
Short Pulse Q-switched Nd:YAG (1064 nm)
Although 1064 nm is typically used in the millisecond domain, it has been on the market for over a decade as Q-switched laser for tattoos and pigmented lesions. Owing to the deep penetration of 1064 nm and the safety with very small amounts of heat generated in the nanosecond pulse domain, the Q-switched nanosecond domain 1064 nm laser was actually one of the first lasers used for nonablative skin rejuvenation. Used at a fluence of 5.5 J/cm² at around 40 nsec pulse duration, Q-switched 1064 nm was employed in an attempt to smooth the skin of 11 patients (12). This initial group demonstrated pinpoint bleeding at this fluence, thus making this more of an epidermal ablative treatment rather than a nonablative one. Rhytid improvement was scored at about 25% by relatively nonobjective means, but fluences utilized were low at 2.5 J/cm² and so the goals of a nonablative were achieved.

Infrared Lasers (Water Absorbing Only)
1320 nm Nd:YAG
The 1320 nm wavelength is thought to accomplish collagen production by scattering thermal energy throughout the laser-irradiated dermis after nonspecific absorption by dermal water. Typical pulse durations are 30 to 50 msec with fluence ranging from 15 to 30 J/cm². Once slight thermal damage of collagen has been induced, the same mechanisms are triggered for collagen regeneration as for other collagen damaging lasers. The 1320 nm wavelength has an advantage in that inherent scatter allows penetration to at least 500 μ with some estimates of up to 2 mm into the dermis (13). Theoretically, this wavelength has the deepest penetration into the dermis, since water absorption is the least of the available water-only targeted infrared lasers. This penetration is unimpeded by absorption by hemoglobin or melanin, which occurs at lower wavelengths. Deeper heating than 200 to 300 μ may be detrimental to collagen synthesis as reported with the erbium glass laser (14). A study in a mouse model has shown that 60 days after two treatments with 1320 nm laser, formation of collagen type I and III was observed (15).

In the latest iteration of the 1320 nm delivery system (CoolTouch3, CoolTouch Corp., Roseville, California, U.S.A.), the epidermis is thermally protected from injury with a 20 to 30 msec cryogen spray delivered 10 msec pre-, mid pulse and 10 msec postlaser pulse. Typical parameters are 16 to 19 J/cm², fixed 50 msec pulse duration, 10 msec precooling, 5 to 10 msec mid-cooling, and 10 msec postcooling. The goal of this system, similar to other nonablative systems, is improvement of rhytids without the creation of a visible epidermal wound. In a study with 1320 nm without coordinated epidermal cooling, 10 patients received laser treatments of their peri-ocular rhytids and postauricular skin (16). Postauricular skin biopsies from before treatment and three months post-treatment showed a small post-treatment increase in the amount of dermal collagen in three patients. Without epidermal cooling, complications included hyperpigmentation in three patients and pitted scarring in three patients. More recently, Nelson (17), using the dynamic cryogen cooling technique before the laser pulse, showed that one or more passes of a 1320 nm Nd:YAG laser on photoaged skin led to improved facial rhytids at two months after treatment. Mild edema and erythema appeared in the treated skin immediately after treatment, which disappeared within hours.

A recent histologic study was reported on the preauricular cheek of 10 patients who were biopsied following one to three laser passes of dynamically cooled millisecond domain Nd:YAG 1320 nm laser (18). Biopsies were performed at one hour and at three days following a single treatment. The number of passes was varied from one to three and T_{max} (peak temperature measured by integrated radiometer) during treatment was targeted for 45 to 48°C. At one hour post-treatment, epidermal spongiosis and edema of the basal cell layer were present in all the specimens treated with three passes. At three days, the three pass samples also showed micro-thrombosis, widened vessels, sclerosis of the vessel-walls, and infiltration of neurophilic granulocytes. The clinical findings in our experience with the 1320 nm wavelength are improvement in rhytids, more effectively on nondynamic lines as well as significant improvement in acne scarring. This defines the meaning of "non-ablative subsurface resurfacing," which involves dermal heating over 1000 μ into the dermis (Fig. 5).

1450 nm Diode
This mid-infrared wavelength is thought to penetrate the skin to a maximum of 500 μm. It is sold as a low power diode system with pulsed cryogen cooling delivered in small pulses throughout the typical delivery cycle of 250 msec (Smoothbeam, Candela, Wayland,

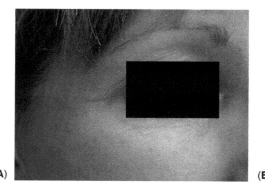 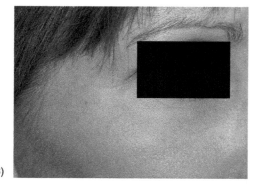

(A)   **(B)**

FIGURE 5   CoolTouch 3 (CoolTouch Corp., Roseville, California, U.S.A.) 1320 nm collagen remodeling. A 44-year-old patient presents with periocular rhytids and lower lid laxity (**A**). Three passes were performed for each treatment at a fluence of 17 J/cm² (**B**). Both the spot size and pulse duration are fixed at 10 mm and 50 msec, respectively. The parameters of cooling utilized were 20 msec precooling to a final skin temperature of 45°C after three passes. Prior treatment for 30 minutes with a topical anesthetic, such as LMX (Ferndale Labs, Ferndale, Michigan, U.S.A.), makes the treatment tolerable. Enhancement of results can be obtained with administration of botulinum toxin immediately after the first treatment.

Massachusetts, U.S.A.). Relatively long times are required to achieve dermal heating, which range up to 250 msec. Fluence typically ranges from 10 to 20 J/cm^2. Preliminary results have shown improvement in mean wrinkle score (19). Rhytid scores improved from a baseline score of 2.3 to 1.8 at six months after treatment ($P > 0.05$). Patient acceptance of the treatment was high, but most felt that there was little improvement of the treated rhytids. The device has also recently received FDA clearance for the treatment of active acne, as sebaceous activity seems to be diminished by this device. This device was found to be most useful for sebaceous hyperplasia and acne scarring on the chin. It is also effective and FDA-cleared for active acne. It shares this in common with the 1320 nm wavelength. Heating of sebaceous glands with subsequent reduced activity is thought to be the mechanism.

1540 nm Erbium Glass
The 1540 nm erbium glass laser is delivered in 10 to 100 msec pulses with fluences ranging from 20 to 30 J/cm^2, although relatively long pulses comprised of pulselets are necessary to effect dermal heating. The biggest problems for clinical treatment are the small spot size (4 mm), very long pulse length (1–2 seconds for the entire pulse train envelope), and uncontrolled contact cooling. In one study, immediate post-treatment biopsies demonstrated thermal damage in a 333 μ thick band (mean range from 311 to 644 μ deep in the dermis). Dermal fibrosis was observed two months after treatment in a 272 μ band (mean range from 148 to 420 μ) (19). In earlier experiments with less sophisticated cooling, heat effects were seen at up to 1.3 mm deep with some scarring-like effect, but this effect was considered a bit too deep for optimal results with rhytids (13). The authors felt that the optimal depth for thermal effects on rhytids was a 0.1 to 0.4 mm band of the dermis just below the epidermis. A clinical study of 10 patients demonstrated some improvement in periocular rhytids, but some changes in pigmentation; thus leading the authors to conclude that this wavelength had the potential only to be used for collagen remodeling under the right conditions (20).

Microthermal, Fractional Resurfacing or Microrejuvenation (1440–1550 nm)

As opposed to the relatively large spot sizes (4–10 mm) macropulses traditionally used with the infrared lasers described earlier, these wavelengths have most recently been applied to the concept of "microrejuvenation." Cosmetic outcomes for dermal photoaging can be improved by the creation of small, localized regions of significant thermal injury (coagulation columns) surrounded by circumscribed areas of untreated skin (Fig. 6). These methods produce significant tissue alterations that extend into the mid-dermis, a similar depth of treatment as that associated with ablative methods. However, the effects are limited to a small proportion of the tissue, surrounding each column with unaffected tissue, and thereby allowing rapid healing. This approach appears to minimize much of the inflammatory wound healing response and associated side effects of other ablative and nonablative rejuvenation methods (21).

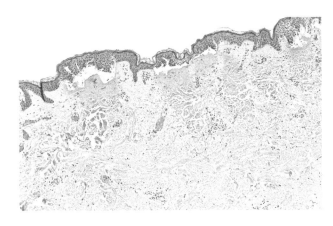

FIGURE 6 Micro-thermal zones of injury with microablative resurfacing. Zones are seen as darker zones of collagen with overlying dermal-epidermal separation with H&E staining (20×).

As a result of direct micro-columnar thermal coagulation of tissue, microrejuvenation techniques stimulate direct replacement of photoaged dermal collagen, resulting in improved skin texture and reduction of fine-to-moderate rhytids. It can also be used for scar remodeling. Most treatments have been performed one month apart for a total series of five treatments. The immediate effects are urtication (hours) and erythema (100%), which can last for up to several days (22). Other side effects include occasional patients with short-term bruising, bleeding, edema, and crusting or bronzing (22).

Fraxel™ (Reliant Technologies, Palo Alto, California, U.S.A.)

This 1550 nm device scans a linear array of "dots," which are 100 μ wide and 300 to 350 μ deep and at a density of 125 to 250 microthermal zones (MTZ) or dots/cm². The biggest downside of the scanning mode is the need for application of blue dye for optical scanning purposes. The removal of the blue dye is difficult and may be visible as a blue hue on the patient's skin for up to three days. The treatment requires multiple passes, typically eight, to insure uniformity of MTZ application, as the head of the device delivers a single row of microablative points.

Affirm™ (Cynosure, Westford, Massachusetts, U.S.A.)

This device uses a microlens array to divide a 1440 nm beam into multiple diffractive elements. The combined apex pulse (CAP™) array contains a laser-etched array of approximately 1000 diffractive elements in a 10-mm spot. These elements redistribute the laser's uniform energy into regions of high- and low-fluence treatment to tissue. Histologically, the high-fluence CAP columns are limited to approximately 300-μm in depth, constraining treatment to the zone of superficial photodamage. The treatment is performed by "stamping" this 10-mm wide microarray with a 50% overlap. Only one to two passes are required. Cooling is provided by a forced air system. Improvement is seen in wrinkles and scars with three to five treatments spaced one month apart (Fig. 7).

Lux1540 Fractional 1540 nm™ (Palomar, Burlington, Massachusetts, U.S.A.)

This hand piece for the Starlux™ platform also delivers light in an array of high precision microbeams. These microbeams create narrow, deep columns of tissue coagulation that penetrate well below the epidermis and into the dermis, while sparing the tissue surrounding the columns from damage. A sapphire water-cooled hand piece protects the epidermis from injury. Uniform microbeam delivery is more consistent and uniform than the scanned approach. The 10-mm spot size head delivers fluences up to 100 mJ/mb and creates a 100 mb/cm² array of columns for deep coagulation. The 15-mm spot size head delivers fluences

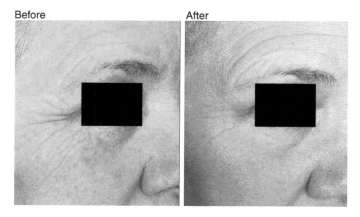

Before   After

FIGURE 7 Affirm™ (Cynosure, Westford, Massachusetts, U.S.A.) resurfacing for superficial wrinkling. Note improvement in periocular wrinkles after five treatments spaced one month apart.

up to 15 mJ/mb and creates a 320-mb/cm^2 array of narrower columns for relatively more shallow coagulation. This treatment is also performed by "stamping" this 10-mm wide microarray with a 50% overlap. Only one to two passes are required. Similar erythema for 24 to 48 hours is seen.

Radio-Frequency

Primary effects of radio frequency (RF) energy on living tissue are considered to be thermal. Clinical tissue tightening following radiofrequency treatment is thought to result from heat-induced immediate collagen contraction, subsequent collagen remodeling, and neocollagenesis of the dermis and subcutis.

The most frequently utilized device is a monopolar RF device in which the patient has a grounding pad placed on the back or flank and RF energy is delivered through a inductive capacitance membrane, which distributes RF evenly over a 1.5 cm^2 area. Patients experience heat in the region of each pulse. It is thought that the RF energy causes not only dermal heating, but heating in the fibrous septae attaching the dermis to the fascial fascia below, thus causing contraction and lifting of the skin. In a recent study, patients with facial and/or neck skin laxity were treated over several years with a monopolar radiofrequency device (Thermacool, Thermage Corp., Haywood, California, U.S.A.) (23). Treatment was delivered with one of three different tips as each became available. Mild self-limited erythema and edema were the most common treatment responses. Complications included one patient with a slight 1 cm^2 depression, which resolved without intervention at six weeks. Although depressions have been reported with the 1 cm^2 standard tip, it is believed that they were due to higher fluence, use of injectable anesthetics and/or IV sedation, and the slower cycle tip.

Finzi et al. (24) reported 25 patients (skin types I to V) with mild-to-severe facial and neck laxity receiving one treatment session with a multipass vector technique consisting of four to five passes targeted over specific skin areas. Energy levels were kept low and ranged from 62 to 91 J/cm^2 per pulse. In the Finzi study all patients experienced some immediate erythema and edema, which had completely resolved in most patients within 48 hours. No severe side effects were seen, and specifically no scarring or dyspigmentation was noted. Efficacy was high, as digital images revealed cosmetic improvement in facial and neck laxity in 96% (Fig. 8).

CONCLUSIONS

Nonablative skin rejuvenation and cosmetic appearance improvement techniques produce dermal remodeling without the obvious epidermal injury and the wound created with earlier ablative approaches (16,18,25). The popularity of these new techniques lies significantly in the lack of wound care and downtime as well as reduced costs. Experience with attempts to control dermal thermal injury more subtly than the CO$_2$ laser has led to the belief that induction of collagen and ECM is possible with less injury. This has led to the development of the infrared lasers with cryogen cooled epidermal protection and low fluence PDLs. A new theory of photomodulation proposes that cosmetic improvements in skin appearance, structure, and function may be achieved via a different nonthermal pathway without the traditional activation of the wound healing mechanism. Total nonablative rejuvenation must encompass surface, deep dermal, or structural and subcutaneous tightening for skin laxity. Reversal of some of the visible changes that occur from photoaging are not entirely relating to structural changes. These include reduction of superficial dyspigmentation (both dermal and epidermal), reduction of dermal telangiectasias, and the appearance of an overall smoother texture and tone. The visible wavelength lasers and IPL are especially useful for these aspects of photoaging. Deep dermal photoaging can be treated with fractional microthermal approaches. Tissue tightening requires the contraction of collagen-based fibrous septae connection skin with subcutaneous tissue. Ongoing studies continue to delineate the role of lasers, light, and other energy sources in the cosmetic improvement in the appearance of photoaged skin.

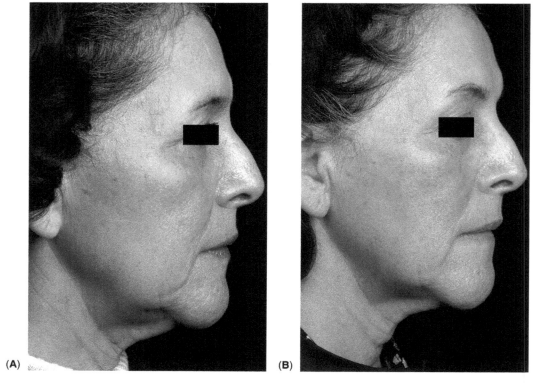

FIGURE 8   Monopolar radiofrequency (Thermacool, Thermage Corp., Haywood, California, U.S.A.) skin tightening. Two months after one treatment of 438 pulses over the cheeks, jowls, and chin, visible lifting of the malar and buccal fat pads is seen. (**A**, before; **B**, after) The mechanism is believed to be contraction of fibrous septae. Tightening continues for six months following treatment.

PHOTOEPILATION
INTRODUCTION

The density of hair on scalp, face, and body and extremities on different individuals is highly variable. There are three different types of increase in visible hair. In hypertrichosis, vellus hair is transformed into dark and thick terminal hair. Wide variations exist depending on the ethnic groups. Hypertrichosis can also be caused by medication, for example, by cyclosporin, interferons, minoxidil, and d-penicillamine. Hirsutism is defined as male pattern hair growth under the influence of testosterone; typically, upper lip, cheeks, chin, breasts, and the pubic triangle are involved. In virilism, hirsutism is accompanied by other signs of masculinization.

Three phases of hair growth can be distinguished as: (*i*) growing phase (anagen); (*ii*) transitional phase (catagen); and (*iii*) resting phase (telogen). The duration of hair cycles and the percentage of hair in these three phases vary according to body areas (Table 3) (26). For long-lasting epilation, destruction of the stem cell area of the hair bulb is necessary, that is, the bulb region and the hair papilla (27). Since hair follicles are rather superficial in the early anagen phase, that would be the ideal time for treatment.

Laser therapy may result in a synchronization of hair cycles and hair in the anagen phase change to telogen phase. Regrowing hair in the early anagen phase is then more receptible to laser therapy. Regrown hair is usually thinner compared to the original hair, a change that has been termed miniaturization.

The absorption of light energy in hair requires melanin as absorber. Phaeomelanin in blond and red hair has a different maximum of absorption compared to dark hair. Thus,

TABLE 3 Hair Cycle in Different Body Areas

Localization	Anagen (%)	Anagen (duration)	Telogen (%)	Telogen (duration)	Depth of hair follicle (mm)
Upper lip	65	16 wk	35	6 wk	1–2.5
Chin	70	1 yr	30	10 wk	1–2.5
Axilla	30	4 mo	70	3 mo	3.5–4.5
Bikini area	30	2 mo	70	3 mo	3.5–4.5
Arms	20	3 mo	80	4.5 mo	2.5–3.5
Legs	20	4 mo	80	6 mo	2.5–4.5

Source: Adapted from Ref. 26.

blond and red hair does not respond to laser therapy. Furthermore, physical parameters, such as pulse duration, fluence, and spot size, are very important for efficacy. Longer wavelengths (between 700 and 1000 nm) penetrate deeper into the dermis compared to shorter wavelengths, and are less absorbed by melanin. A large spot size is important, since depth of penetration increases with a larger spot size, and technically, the treatment is easier to perform. Theoretically, optimal pulse duration should be between the thermal relaxation time of hair follicles (40–100 msec) and the epidermis (3–10 msec); however, but in comparative studies, this concept could no be proven (28).

PULSED RUBY LASER (694 nm)

Wimmershoff et al. (29) treated 74 patients with a follow-up of up to six months. After six weeks, hair reduction of 50% to 75% could be seen, after six months this rate decreased to less than 25%. Similar results were published by other groups (30).

ALEXANDRITE LASER (755 nm)

This wavelength is less absorbed by epidermal melanin; therefore, the risk of epidermal damage is reduced. Protection of epidermis is increased by an additional cooling device. The effectiveness of the alexandrite laser for epilation has been demonstrated in many studies. In several studies, the influence of pulse duration was investigated; none showed any significant influence. Nouri et al. (31) investigated the influence of spot sizes and found better results with increasing spot size. Drosner et al. (32) investigated different fluences (5, 10, 15, and 20 J/cm^2) and did not find any statistically significant differences; the low fluences of 5 and 10 J/cm^2 were nearly as effective with less pain and less side effects.

DIODE LASERS (800/810 nm)

This wavelength penetrates deeper into the dermis and is less absorbed in the epidermis. Long pulse durations and high fluences require an epidermal cooling device. Sadick et al. (33) found a hair reduction of 75% after three and six months; the best results were seen in patients with skin type III. Better results with greater spot size has been reported.

PULSED ND:YAG LASER (1064 nm)

This wavelength, being the longest, has the highest penetration into the dermis and is less absorbed in melanin. Therefore, this laser can also be used for epilation in patients with dark skin. Since treatment is painful, cooling devices are necessary. The effectiveness of the pulsed Nd:YAG laser has been proven in many studies (34–36). Hair reduction of 30% to 60% after four to six treatments over several months has been reported. Best results were obtained with larger spot sizes and longer pulse duration.

INTENSE PULSED LIGHT SOURCES (590–1200 nm)

A cutoff filter at 600 nm and pulse duration of 15 to 20 msec are usually used for epilation (Fig. 9). Hair reduction of 36% to over 80% was reported after several treatments (37). Up to 10% of the patients showed side effects, such as pain, erythema, and hyperpigmentation.

Comparative Studies

Bjerring et al. (38) compared IPL and ruby laser and found the IPL to be more effective. Comparative studies between the pulsed diode laser and the alexandrite laser did not show any significant differences between these two lasers (39,40) (Table 4).

Side Effects

Complications are mainly due to absorption of light energy by melanin in pigmented epidermis, or caused by incorrect physical parameters. Immediately after laser or IPL therapy, perifollicular erythema and edema may occur, and in some patients, with blistering and crusting. Hypo- and hyper-pigmentations are usually transient. Reticular erythema resembling livido reticularis has been observed in patients suffering from perniosis. Scarring is rare and is mainly due to incorrect physical parameters.

Paradoxically, hair growth was observed in patients with dark skin and black hair following alexandrite laser therapy (41). This could be explained by a synchronization of the hair cycle by the stimulation of hair growth by light. Hair growth was also observed after IPL therapy of women with hirsutism who had increased hair growth in untreated neighboring areas (42).

Other reported side effects include leukotrichia, changes in melanocytic nevi located in epilated areas, and the development of lichen planus and permanent scarring alopecia following ruby laser epilation in a patient with mucosal lichen planus.

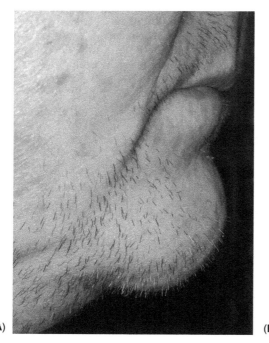 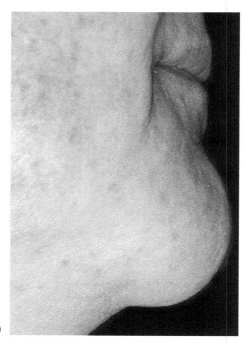

(A)   **(B)**

FIGURE 9   Hypertrichosis in a 65-year-old patient. Result of five intense pulsed light treatments.

TABLE 4 Comparative Studies

Type of laser	Patients	Parameters	Treatments	Follow-ups	Hair reduction	Reference
IPL versus ruby	31	600—950 nm, 48 × 10 mm, 5–40 msec, 18.4 J/cm^2 694 nm, 5 mm, 0.9 msec, 19.5 J/cm^2	3	6 mo	49.3% versus 21.3%	(38)
Diode versus alexandrite	20	800 nm, 9 mm, 12.5 msec, 25–40 0.9 J/cm^2 755 nm, 10 mm, 2 msec, 25 J/cm^2	3	6 mo	No significant difference	(39)
Diode versus Alexandrite	15	800–810 nm, 9 mm, 30–35 J/cm^2 755 nm, 12 mm, 3 msec, 6–40 J/cm^2	4	12 mo	84% versus 85%	(40)
Diode versus Nd:YAG	15	800 nm, 9 mm, 30–35 J/cm^2 1964 nm, 5 mm, 78–80 J/cm^2	1	9 mo	No significant difference	(43)
Nd:YAG versus alexandrite versus diode	75	1064 nm, 6–8 mm, 25–32 msec, 40–55 J/cm^2	5.5	3 mo	42.5 %	(44)
		755 nm, 8–10 mm, 10–20 msec, 15–25 J/cm^2	5.2		65.6 %	
		800 nm, 9 mm, 10–30 msec, 25–40 J/cm^2	2.6		46.8%	

Source: Adapted from Ref. 26.

CONCLUSION

For epilation, different lasers and IPLs can be used. Multiple treatments in four- to six-week intervals for face, or two to three months for back, are necessary for achieving a significant reduction of hair growth. Most patients will have 90% hair reduction; however, there will always be some sparse and thinner diameter hair growth. As regrowth of hair can be observed after 6 to 12 months, repeated treatments are necessary.

REFERENCES

1. Zelickson BD, Kilmer SL, Bernstein E, et al. Pulsed dye laser therapy for sun damaged skin. Lasers Surg Med 1999; 25(3):229–236.
2. Weiss RA, McDaniel DH, Geronemus RG. Review of nonablative photorejuvenation: reversal of the aging effects of the sun and environmental damage using laser and light sources. Semin Cutan Med Surg 2003; 22(2):93–106.
3. Lee MW. Combination visible and infrared lasers for skin rejuvenation. Semin Cutan Med Surg 2002; 21(4):288–300.
4. Butler EG, McClellan SD, Ross EV. Split treatment of photodamaged skin with KTP 532 nm laser with 10 mm handpiece versus IPL: a cheek-to-cheek comparison. Lasers Surg Med 2006; 38(2): 124–128.
5. Goldman MP, Weiss RA, Weiss MA. Intense pulsed light as a nonablative approach to photoaging. Dermatol Surg 2005; 31(9 Pt 2):1179–1187.
6. Weiss RA, Goldman MP, Weiss MA. Treatment of poikiloderma of Civatte with an intense pulsed light source. Dermatol Surg 2000; 26(9):823–827.
7. Bitter PH. Noninvasive rejuvenation of photodamaged skin using serial, full-face intense pulsed light treatments. Dermatol Surg 2000; 26(9):835–842.
8. Weiss RA, Weiss MA, Beasley KL. Rejuvenation of photoaged skin: 5 years results with intense pulsed light of the face, neck, and chest. Dermatol Surg 2002; 28(12):1115–1119.
9. Weiss RA, Weiss MA, Geronemus RG, McDaniel DH. A novel non-thermal non-ablative full panel led photomodulation device for reversal of photoaging: digital microscopic and clinical results in various skin types. J Drugs Dermatol 2004; 3(6):605–610.
10. Weiss RA, McDaniel DH, Geronemus R, Weiss MA. Clinical trial of a novel non-thermal LED array for reversal of photoaging: clinical, histologic, and surface profilometric results. Lasers Surg Med 2005; 31:1099–1205.
11. Weiss RA, Weiss MA, Beasley KL, Munavalli G. Our approach to non-ablative treatment of photo-aging. Lasers Surg Med 2005; 37(1):2–8.
12. Goldberg DJ, Whitworth J. Laser skin resurfacing with the Q-switched Nd:YAG laser. Dermatol Surg 1997; 23(10):903–906.
13. Hardaway CA, Ross EV. Nonablative laser skin remodeling. Dermatol Clin 2002; 20(1):97–111:ix.

14. Ross EV, Sajben FP, Hsia J, Barnette D, Miller CH, McKinlay JR. Nonablative skin remodeling: selective dermal heating with a mid- infrared laser and contact cooling combination. Lasers Surg Med 2000; 26(2):186–195.

15. Dang YY, Ren QS, Liu HX, Ma JB, Zhang JS. Comparison of histologic, biochemical, and mechanical properties of murine skin treated with the 1064-nm and 1320-nm Nd:YAG lasers. Exp Dermatol 2005; 14(12):876–882.

16. Menaker GM, Wrone DA, Williams RM, Moy RL. Treatment of facial rhytids with a nonablative laser: a clinical and histologic study. Dermatol Surg 1999; 25(6):440–444.

17. Nelson JS, Millner TD, Dave D, et al. Clinical study of non-ablative laser treatment of facial rhytides. Lasers Surg Med 1998; 17(suppl. 9):150. Ref type: abstract.

18. Fatemi A, Weiss MA, Weiss RA. Short-term histologic effects of nonablative resurfacing: results with a dynamically cooled millisecond-domain 1320 nm Nd:YAG Laser. Dermatol Surg 2002; 28(2):172–176.

19. Hardaway CA, Ross EV, Barnette DJ, Paithankar DY. Non-ablative cutaneous remodeling with a 1.45 micron mid-infrared diode laser: phase I. J Cosmet Laser Ther 2002 Mar; 4(1):3–8.

20. Levy JL, Besson R, Mordon S. Determination of optimal parameters for laser for nonablative remodeling with a 1.54 microm Er:glass laser: a dose-response study. Dermatol Surg 2002; 28(5):405–409.

21. Geronemus RG. Fractional photothermolysis: current and future applications. Lasers Surg Med 2006; 38(3):169–176.

22. Fisher GH, Geronemus RG. Short-term side effects of fractional photothermolysis. Dermatol Surg 2005; 31(9 Pt 2):1245–1249.

23. Burns AJ, Holden SG. Monopolar radiofrequency tissue tightening—how we do it in our practice. Lasers Surg Med 2006; 38(6):575–579.

24. Finzi E, Spangler A. Multipass vector (mpave) technique with nonablative radiofrequency to treat facial and neck laxity. Dermatol Surg 2005; 31(8 Pt 1):916–922.

25. Goldberg DJ. Nonablative resurfacing. Clin Plast Surg 2000; 27(2):287–292, xi.

26. Gottschaller C, Hohenleutner U. Laser- und lichtepilation. In: Landthaler M, Hohenleutner U, eds. Lasertherapie in der Dermatologie. 2nd edn. Heidelberg: Springer, 2006:179–192.

27. Kolinko VG, Littler CM. Mathematical modeling for the prediction and optimization of laser hair removal. Lasers Surg Med 2000; 26:164–176.

28. Stangl S, Hertenberger B, Drosner M. Does pulse duration influence efficacy of photo-epilation? Med Laser Appl 2005; 19:205–211.

29. Wimmershoff MB, Scherer K, Lorenz S, Landthaler M, Hohenleutner U. Hair removal using a 5-msec long-pulsed ruby laser. Dermatol Surg 2000; 26:205–209.

30. Polderman MC, Pavel S, le Cessie S, Grevelink JM, van Leeuwen RL. Efficacy, tolerability, and safety of a long-pulsed ruby laser system in the removal of unwanted hair. Dermatol Surg 2000; 26:240–243.

31. Nouri K, Chen H, Saghari S, Ricotti CA. Comparing 18- versus 12-mm spot size in hair removal using a GentleLase 755-nm Alexandrite laser. Dermatol Surg 2004; 30:494–497.

32. Drosner M, Stangl S, Hertenberger B, Klimek H, Pettke-Rank C. Low dose epilation by alexandrite laser: a dose response study. Med Laser Appl 2001; 16:293–298.

33. Sadick NS, Prieto VG. The use of a new diode laser for hair removal. Dermatol Surg 2003; 29: 30–34.

34. Lorenz S, Brunnberg S, Landthaler M, Hohenleutner U. Hair removal with the long-pulsed Nd:YAG laser: a prospective study with one year follow-up. Lasers Surg Med 2002; 30:127–134.

35. Tanzi EL, Alster TS. Long-pulsed 1064-nm Nd:YAG laser-assisted hair removal in all skin Types. Dermatol Surg 2004; 30: 13–17.

36. Raff K, Landthaler M, Hohenleutner U. Optimizing treatment parameters for hair removal using long-pulsed Nd:YAG-lasers. Lasers Med Sci 2004; 18:219–222.

37. El Bedewi AF. Hair removal with intense pulsed light. Lasers Med Sci 2004; 19:48–51.

38. Bjerring P, Cramers M, Egekvist H, Christiansen K, Troilius A. Hair reduction using a new intense pulsed light irradiator and a normal mode ruby laser. J Cutan Laser Ther 2000; 2:63–71.

39. Handrick C, Alster T. Comparison of long-pulsed diode and long-pulsed alexandrite lasers for hair removal: a long-term clinical and histologic study. Dermatol Surg 2001; 27:622–626.

40. Eremia S, Li C, Newman N. Laser hair removal with alexandrite versus diode laser using four treatment sessions: 1-year results. Dermatol Surg 2001; 27:925–930.

41. Alajlan A, Shapiro J, Rivers JK, MacDonald N, Wiggin J, Harvey L. Paradoxical hypertrichosis after laser epilation. J Am Acad Dermatol 2005; 53:85–88.

42. Moreno-Arias G, Castelo-Branco C, Ferrando J. Paradoxical effect after IPL photoepilation. Dermatol Surg 2002; 28:1013–1016.

43. Chan HH, Ying S-Y, Ho W-S, Wong DSY, Lam L-K. An in vivo study comparing the efficacy and complications of diode laser and long-pulsed Nd:YAG laser in hair removal in Chinese patients. Dermatol Surg 2001; 27:950–954.

44. Bouzari N, Tabatabai H, Abbasi Z, Firooz A, Dowlati Y. Laser hair removal: comparison of long-pulsed Nd:YAG, long-pulsed alexandrite, and long-pulsed diode lasers. Dermatol Surg 2004; 30:498–502.

29 | Laser Treatment on Ethnic Skin

Henry Hin Lee Chan
Division of Dermatology, Department of Medicine, University of Hong Kong, and Department of Medicine and Therapeutics, Chinese University of Hong Kong, Hong Kong, China

Brooke Jackson
Skin and Wellness Center of Chicago, Chicago, Illinois, U.S.A.

- Cutaneous manifestations of photoaging in ethnic skin differ from those in Caucasian skin, with more pigmentary changes and less wrinkling.

- Some conditions, such as nevus of Ota and dermatosis papulosa nigra, are more common in ethnic skin.

- Ethnic skin, with its higher epidermal melanin context, is more likely to develop adverse pigmentary reactions following laser surgery.

- Nonablative skin rejuvenation with low down time and minimal risk of adverse effects is particularly popular among patients with ethnic skin.

- Fractional resurfacing can be used for the treatment of acne scarring and melasma in ethnic skin.

- Effective skin cooling allows protection of the epidermis and enables laser procedures such as laser-assisted hair removal and the treatment of vascular lesions to be performed.

- Longer pulsed width further improves laser safety for laser-assisted hair removal in ethnic skin.

INTRODUCTION

Cutaneous laser surgery has been a mainstay of dermatologic therapy for more than a decade. Yet, the published literature has until recently focussed on the Caucasian patient. Based on statistics from the 2000 U.S.A. census, it is evident that the face of the patient who is seeking aesthetic services is changing to be more representative of the increasing ethnic diversity of the United States population. Besides cosmetic procedures, conditions such as nevus of Ota and dermatosis papulosa nigra are particularly common in ethnic skin. Furthermore, ethnic skin, with its higher epidermal melanin context, is more likely to develop adverse pigmentary reactions following laser surgery. As a result, it is imperative that the dermatologic laser surgeon has not only an awareness of the unique needs of those with ethnic skin, but is also well versed in the available laser technology to select an appropriate modality for the treatment of the ethnic patient.

CUTANEOUS MANIFESTATIONS OF AGING ETHNIC SKIN

Ninety five percent of the visible signs of aging are caused by sun exposure, which begins in infancy and continues throughout life (1). Other intrinsic factors such as gravity and external factors (pollution) that are unrelated to sun exposure also contribute to the cutaneous aging process. Crows feet, lipstick lines, and fine perioral and periorbital lines seen as early as the 20s in the Caucasian patient, tend not to occur in the patient with more darkly complexed skin tones. Aging in patients with darker skin manifests not only ten to twenty years later than age-matched Caucasian counterparts, but also occurs in the deeper muscular layers of the face rather than within the skin. Other cutaneous manifestations of aging ethnic skin include the development of benign cutaneous growths such as dermatosis papulosa nigra and the development of solar lentigenes.

ETHNIC SKIN: SPECIAL PRECAUTIONS

When treating skin of any type, an understanding of laser tissue interaction and laser physics is necessary (2–7). Hemoglobin, melanin, and water are the primary organic chromophores within the skin, each with specific wavelengths of peak absorption on the electromagnetic spectrum (5). The broad absorption spectrum of melanin on the electromagnetic spectrum, and the increased melanin content of ethnic skin create significant therapeutic challenges for cutaneous laser surgeons when treating patients with ethnic skin (6). The highly melanized epidermis of ethnic skin absorbs and/or interferes with the absorption of laser energy that is intended for another target, such as pigment within the hair follicle, a blood vessel, or tattoo ink within the dermis. The unique features of ethnic skin must be considered when selecting treatment parameters.

PREOPERATIVE CONSIDERATIONS

In general, ethnic patients wish to preserve and enhance their unique features, not westernize them. Their darker skin is prone to dyschromia and scarring, which are often why these patients initially seek cosmetic consultation. However, corrective procedures each carry their own risks of dyschromia and scarring, both of which should be discussed in detail preoperatively.

Patients with darker skin tones are less likely to wear photoprotection on a daily basis because such products are marketed toward the prevention of skin cancer, which many darkly completed patients feel will not affect them. Although the majority of people with darkly completed skin may never develop skin cancer, many are at increased risk of developing other systemic diseases, such as hypertension and diabetes, that require medications, which are photosensitizing. All laser patients in our practice are advised to wear daily sun protection throughout the course of treatment.

MEDICAL HISTORY

A history of treatment with isotretinoin should be obtained before the initiation of any surgical corrective procedure (8). Disorders such as sickle cell anemia, thalassemia, and glucose 6-phosphate dehydrogenase (G6PD) deficiency are more prevalent in African, American, Mediterranean, and Southeast Asian patients. A detailed medical history should be taken in an effort to determine the personal or family history of these hereditary hemolytic diseases that may affect postoperative healing. Given our mobile society, the physician should also be aware of dermatologic conditions that are endemic to certain areas of the world, such as cutaneous leishmaniasis. This parasitic infection is endemic in the Middle East, Central and South America, and Africa, and often causes cutaneous scarring for which patients may request cosmetic correction.

CULTURAL CONCERNS

The preprocedure consultation is an opportunity to not only identify and discuss therapeutic options for the patient's chief complaint, but also to understand whether the patient's expectations of the procedure, postoperative period, and outcome are realistic. To achieve a successful procedural outcome, a surgeon's understanding of cultural differences and preferences among ethnic patients is equally as important as technical proficiency in the procedures to be performed. Cultural preferences can be understood through open discussion with the patient and knowledge of the way in which cultural variations affect communication. For example, Asian cultures place great importance on physical beauty to the extent that there is a belief that prospects for personal success in life are related to one's physical traits. In general, most Asian patients have great respect for authority, which may limit communication with the physician by the patient assuming the physician will understand and do what the patient desires (9). Questioning authority is considered to be disrespectful in some cultures. The surgeon should encourage the patient to verbalize concerns and expectations. Additionally, because of strong cultural beliefs in fate and destiny, Asian patients may often have associated feelings of guilt after undergoing procedures that may alter given physical characteristics, as this act is perceived to be disrespectful to one's parents (9). These feelings of guilt may lead to postoperative withdrawal.

ABLATIVE AND NONABLATIVE SKIN REJUVENATION IN ETHNIC SKIN
The Use of a Laser/Light Source for the Treatment of Solar Lentigines, Seborrhoeic Keratosis, and Dermatosis Papulosa Nigra in Ethnic Skin

For many years, Q-switched (QS) lasers have been used to treat lentigines, and although the approach is mostly effective, postoperative postinflammatory hyperpigmentation (PIH) occurs in 10% to 20% of darker-skinned patients. Several years ago, a study compared the efficacy and complication rates in Chinese patients who were treated with QS 532 nm neodymium: yttrium-aluminum-garnet (Nd:YAG) laser to those who were treated with long-pulsed 532 nm Nd:YAG laser, and found that although the two groups had similar degrees of clearing, treatment with the QS device was associated with a greater risk of PIH (10).

The study created controversy as the authors suggested that QS lasers were not suitable for the removal of lentigines in Asians due to the photomechanical effect of these systems that can lead to a greater risk of PIH. Since then, others looking at the use of intense pulsed light (IPL) source and long-pulsed 532 nm Nd:YAG laser in the treatment of lentigines in dark-skinned patients have confirmed the observation (11,12). A recent study looking at the use of QS Alexandrite (QS Alex) laser versus IPL for the treatment of freckles and lentigines in Chinese further confirmed the risk of PIH, when QS laser is used in ethnic skin (13).

By choosing a pulse width (millisecond domain) that matches the thermal relaxation time of the epidermis (10 msec), the risk of thermal injury to the dermis is minimized (Fig. 1).

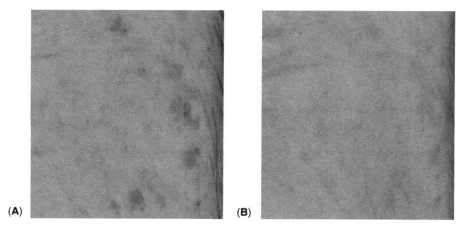

(A)   **(B)**

FIGURE 1   Lentigines under cross polarized light: (**A**) before treatment, (**B**) after second treatment with long-pulsed 532 nm neodymium: yttrium-aluminum-garnet laser with 2 mm spot size, 2 millisecond pulse duration, 12 J/cm².

Most pigment laser/light source is also absorbed to a lesser degree by hemoglobin. Therefore, besides the use of long pulsed rather than QS laser, another means of further reducing the risk of PIH is to compress and empty the dermal vessels and, in doing so, reduce the risk of dermal vascular damage (14). A recent study compared the efficacy and complications of QS ruby laser to those of long-pulsed, 595 nm pulsed dye laser (PDL) with a compression window attached for the removal of lentigines among Japanese patients. The results indicated that the group treated with the compression technique was associated with a lower risk of PIH than the group treated with QS laser, while the degree of efficacy was the same in both groups (15). Table 1 shows the suggested laser parameters and clinical endpoint to be considered for the removal of lentigines in ethnic skin.

TABLE 1   Laser/Intense Pulsed Light Source for the Treatment of Lentigines

Type of laser/IPL	Wavelength (nm)	Pulse width	Clinical endpoint	Special consideration
QS 532 nm Nd:YAG, ruby, alexandrite, laser	532,694,755	Nanosecond	Immediate whitening	Use the smallest spot size and lowest fluence to induce clinical endpoint. Useful for light color lentigines. PIH rate: 5%–50% (10,13,15) Test area especially for solar lentigo.
KTP/Nd:YAG laser	532	Millisecond	Slate gray darkening	Choose pulse width at 2 ms to match the thermal relaxation time of the epidermis, with cooling window, pulse width can be increased to 5–10 ms. Light color lentigines are not as effective.
Alexandrite	755	Millisecond	Slate gray	
Intense pulsed light	560–1200 nm	Millisecond	Erythema or darkening of the lentigines depends upon the type of IPL.	IPL with shorter pulsed width (2.5 ms) tend to have a more apparent clinical endpoint. A longer pulsed width (10–40 ms) allows greater epidermal protection, but the endpoint is more subtle and can even be delayed.

Abbreviations: IPL, intense pulsed light; KTP, potassium-titanyl-phosphate; Nd:YAG, neodymium:yttrium-aluminum-garnet; PIH, post-inflammatory hyperpigmentation; QS, Q-switching.

Another means of further reducing the risk of PIH is to use a laser/light source with a shorter wavelength (350–500 nm) and therefore confine the thermal injury to the epidermal layer (14). Interestingly, a 351 nm XeF pulsed excimer laser, one of the first used, experimentally, for the treatment of pigmented lesion when the concept of selective photothermolysis was proposed, is one such example. With the use of this laser, dermal penetration is limited (the damage is confined to 100 um within the epidermis). This lack of dermal penetr-wavelength filter is being tested at this moment for the removal of lentigines in ethnic skin. Due to the high epidermal melanin context of ethnic skin, adequate cooling is necessary to avoid epidermal injury.

Seborrhoeic keratosis and dermatosis papulosa nigra are common cutaneous manifestations of photoaging of ethnic skin. While no treatment is needed, these manifestations are often of cosmetic concern and are easily removed through a variety of means including scissor excision, electrodessication, and laser ablation. When using either the CO_2 or erbium:YAG laser, one must be careful to use a spot size that does not exceed the diameter of the lesion to minimize the risk of collateral thermal damage and PIH of the surrounding skin.

ABLATIVE AND NON-ABLATIVE SKIN REJUVENATION AND FRACTIONAL RESURFACING

Ablative skin rejuvenation is less commonly performed in ethnic skin for two reasons. First, aging in ethnic skin tends to present with more pigmentary issues rather than wrinkle, furthermore laser resurfacing in ethnic skin is associated with more adverse effects such as IPL (16). As a result, nonablative skin rejuvenation with a laser/light source is particularly popular for ethnic skin due to the lower risk of complication and limited down time (17). Nonablative skin rejuvenation involves the use of a laser/light source together with a cooling device, and in doing so improves the features of photoaging including lentigines, telangiectasia, pore size, skin texture, wrinkles, and skin laxity with minimal down time. Green and yellow laser/light sources target the epidermal pigment and papillary dermal vessels. Injury to the papillary dermal vessels not only allows effective treatment of facial telangiectasia, but also leads to the subsequent healing process and new collagen formation. Producing an effect on the microvascular supply of the sebaceous gland can reduce sebum production and improve pore size (17–20). Near-infrared and infrared lasers/light sources together with skin cooling target the water content in the dermis, and their photothermal effect, produced as a result of the laser-tissue interaction, is to cause a rise in the dermal temperature (21–24). The consequences are collagen tightening, increased fibroblastic activity, and increased collagen production. Table 2 summarizes the use of different lasers for nonablative skin rejuvenation in ethnic skin.

For non-ablative skin rejuvenation, repeated monthly treatment intervals are necessary to achieve the desired effect. More recently, combined modalities using different lasers and light sources in the same treatment session have been advocated (17,18,20). To reduce the risk of complications from such a combined approach, lower fluence is necessary.

Although the results of some studies support the use of non-ablative skin rejuvenation for the treatment of acne scarring, ablative skin resurfacing can achieve a significantly superior result and therefore remains the gold standard for the treatment of acne scarring in ethnic skin. For laser resurfacing, patients are prescribed a systemic antiviral (Famciclovir 250 mg three times daily) and a systemic antibiotic (cefuroxime 250 mg three times daily) 48 hours before laser surgery and until complete re-epithelization. To further optimize the result, a punch biopsy and subcision two weeks before surgery is recommended. A more aggressive approach (three passes of carbon dioxide laser resurfacing, followed by one pass of Erbium YAG laser) has become less popular due to the down time and potential complications that include prolonged erythema, pigmentary disturbance, and increased risk of scarring. More recently, single pass laser resurfacing has been recommended by some investigators to reduce the morbidity that is associated with this procedure (25). Postoperatively, a closed dressing is applied for 48 hours, followed by an open dressing thereafter. Daily follow up is necessary to ensure that wound infection does not occur.

TABLE 2 Laser for Nonablative Skin Rejuvenation

Type of laser	Wavelength (nm)	Pulse width	Target	Special consideration
KTP/Nd:YAG	532	Millisecond	Vessel/pigment	Better efficacy if used in combination with long pulsed 1064 nm (18)
Pulsed dye laser	585/595	Millisecond	Vessel/pigment	Mainly vessel, development of compression window allows pigment to be targeted (15) Better efficacy if combine with 1450 nm diode laser (20)
Nd:YAG	1064	Nanosecond	Water/pigment	Can be used with carbon dioxide
Nd:YAG	1064	Millisecond	Water	Better efficacy if used in combination with long-pulsed 532 nm Nd:YAG (18)
Nd:YAG	1320	Millisecond	Water	More painful than other treatments, effective for fine wrinkle and acne scarring
Diode	1450	Millisecond	Water	Postinflammatory hyperpigmentation is an issue in ethnic skin and is thought to be due to excessive cryogen injury
Erbium glass	1540	Millisecond	Water	Less painful than 1320 nm Nd:YAG and 1450 nm diode laser; the lack of clinical end point is a disadvantage

Abbreviations: KTP, potassium-titanyl-phosphate; Nd:YAG, neodymium:yttrium-aluminum-garnet.

Fractional resurfacing is a new technology that involves the use of a laser to generate microscopic spots of thermal injury that are surrounded by healthy skin tissue (26). By taking into account the discrepancy between epidermal and dermal healing properties (given the microscopic nature of the lesion, epidermal healing is completed within 24 hours, whereas dermal collagen remodeling takes 4–6 weeks), fractional resurfacing can lead to excellent clinical outcomes with minimal adverse effects. There are two main variables in fractional resurfacing: (*i*) energy expressed in minijoules, and (*ii*) density expressed as the microscopic thermal injury zone per cm^2 (MTZ). Fractional resurfacing is now approved by US Food and Drug Administration for the treatment of wrinkles, melasma, and acne scarring (Fig. 2). Multiple devices can now perform fractional resurfacing. The initial device involves the use of a scan to deliver laser injury when the device moves across the skin surface (scanning mode), and the others involve the placement of the laser handpiece on the skin surface in a stamping fashion (stamping mode). Some stamping devices are multiplatform. The advantages and disadvantages of these two different modes are summarized in Table 3.

For ethnic skin, fractional resurfacing can be particularly effective for the treatment of acne scarring, and is the main indication for its use. PIH is the main potential complication. Previous studies indicated that the risk of PIH is associated with the energy and density of

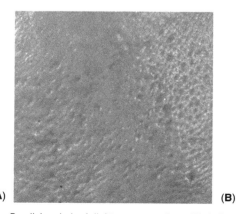
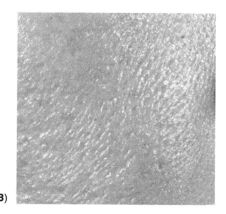

(A)   (B)

FIGURE 2 Parallel polarized light-acne scarring: (**A**) before treatment, (**B**) after 12th treatment with fractional resurfacing 20 mJ, four passes of 125 microscopic thermal injury zone per cm^2 per treatment.

TABLE 3 Advantages and Disadvantages of Fractional Device

Advantages	Disadvantages
With scanning mode	
Much published clinical data in peer review journals	Single platform
Robust and reliable	Blue dye: reduce visibility
Even distribution of MTZ	Need a separate cooling device
Faster treatment time	
With stamping mode	
Single platform with multipurposes	No published peer review data. (?Efficacy is the same as the scanning device, which particularly applies to those that are not 1540 nm in wavelength)
More space efficient	Lack of multiplatform reliability; if the device breaks down, no treatment can be performed
Cooling sapphire window	Overlapping/under treatment
Less painful	Longer treatment time

Abbreviation: MTZ, microscopic thermal injury zone per cm^2.

the laser, with density being particularly important (27,28). In one study, 7% of acne scar patients who were treated with 16 mJ, 1000 MTZ/cm^2 were found to have PIH (27). Several factors contribute to the development of PIH. Skin type and recent sun exposure are important. The degree of inflammation and the extent of derma-epidermal junction disruption are also important. To reduce the risk of PIH, several measures should be taken, including reducing the density of each treatment but increasing the total number of treatment sessions (17). The interval between treatment sessions can also be increased so that inflammation at the derma-epidermal junction can completely subside. The use of cooling is also important to reduce the risk of bulk tissue heating that occurs after repeat treatment at a short interval.

THE USE OF LASER FOR THE TREATMENT OF OTHER MELANOCYTIC LESIONS

In ethnic skin, besides pigmentary conditions that are associated with photoaging, other conditions are particularly prevalent, including melasma, Hori's macules, and nevus of Ota. Another important factor is the risk of malignant transformation. Melanoma is uncommon in ethnic skin. As a result, it is common for laser to be used for the treatment of congenital melanocytic lesions in ethnic skin.

EPIDERMAL LESIONS
Café au Lait Patch

The use of lasers in the treatment of café au lait patch has yielded variable results, and although some early studies indicated complete removal without recurrence, such findings have not always been repeated (29). A study using a Q-Switched ruby laser (QS ruby) and a frequency double QS 532 nm, Neodymium:Yttrium-Aluminum-Garnet (QS 532 nm Nd:YAG) laser found that the degree of clearance varied across lesions (30). Furthermore, categorization of the patches into histological subtypes did not help to predict the clinical outcome. One possibility is that QS lasers fail to remove the follicular melanocytic component of the café au lait patch. Based on this hypothesis, long-pulsed pigmented lasers such as normal mode ruby have been used for the removal of café au lait patch, and preliminary data has indicated a lower rate of recurrence as compared with a QS ruby laser (40% as compared to 80%) (31) (Fig. 3).

Becker's Nevus

A previous study using QS ruby laser indicated a postoperative increase in pigmentation after four weeks (32). More recently, in a study that compared the use of Erbium YAG laser to that of QS 1064 nm Nd:YAG laser, 22 patients were treated with either Erbium YAG laser or QS

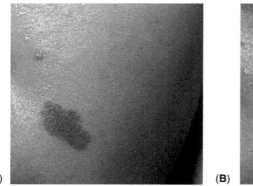
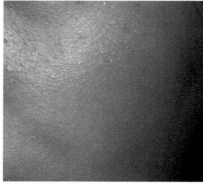

(A)   (B)

FIGURE 3   Café au lait spot. (**A**) before treatment, (**B**) two months after treatment. One treatment with long-pulsed Alexandrite 755 nm laser, 40 J/cm2, 10 mm spot size, 3 ms pulse duration.

1064 nm Nd:YAG and were followed up after two years (33). The group that was treated with Erbium YAG laser achieved a significantly better result, with complete clearance in 54% of the patients after a single treatment. For the group that was treated with QS 1064 nm Nd:YAG, multiple treatments were necessary, and only 1 out of 11 patients had significant clearing after three treatment sessions. Long-pulsed pigmented laser has also been used to remove hair and reduce pigmentation, but texture can still occur (34).

DERMAL AND MIXED LESION
Nevus of Ota and Hori's Macules

QS ruby, QS Alex, and QS 1064 nm Nd:YAG have been used for the treatment of nevus of Ota with excellent results and minimal risk of complications (16). QS ruby laser can achieve a good to excellent degree of lightening after three or more treatment sessions. The side effects were few, with transient hyperpigmentation after the first treatment being the most common (35). A study that compared the use of QS Alex and QS 1064 nm Nd:YAG lasers found that most patients better tolerated the former (36). However, QS 1064 nm Nd:YAG laser appeared to be more effective than QS Alex in the lightening of nevus of Ota after three or more treatment sessions (37). In term of complications, hypopigmentation was common, especially among those who were treated with QS ruby and those who were treated with different lasers in different treatment session (38,39). The original pigmentation could also recur in patients after complete laser-induced clearing, which is an important issue, especially for pediatric patients. The risk of recurrence is estimated to be between 0.6% and 1.2%. Nevertheless, treatment is optimal at a younger age as there is a lower number of mean treatments and a lower rate of complications (40).

Hori's macules differ from nevus of Ota because they occur in adults, are bilateral rather than unilateral, and have no mucosal involvement. Hori's macules are thought to occur due to a range of aetiological factors such as sex hormones, ultraviolet light exposure, and trauma, which lead to a dropping off of the hair follicular melanocytes to the dermis. Frequently, Hori's macules coexist with other pigmentary conditions, such as melasma and lentigines. QS ruby, QS Alex, and 1064 nm Nd:YAG lasers have been shown to be effective in the treatment of this condition (41–43). However, previous studies indicated that Hori's macules are more resistant to treatment than nevus of Ota and require shorter treatment intervals and more treatment sessions before the lesions gradually subside. Transit pigmentary disturbance is the main adverse effect, with hyperpigmentation particularly common during the first few treatment sessions. Recently, it was proposed to combine QS 532 nm Nd:YAG and QS 1064 nm Nd:YAG to obtain a greater degree of improvement (44) (Fig. 4).

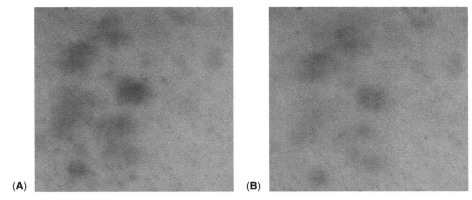

FIGURE 4 Hori's macules under cross polarized light: (**A**) before treatment, and (**B**) after fourth treatment with QS ruby 4.6, 5 J/cm², 5 mm spot size.

Melasma

The results of previous studies have discouraged the use of laser in the treatment of melasma. Over a decade ago, 510 nm PDL was found to be ineffective in the removal of melasma, and could increase pigmentation (45). The same finding was observed when melasma was treated with a QS ruby laser (46). Regardless of fluence (7.5–15 J/cm²), there was no permanent improvement and, in some cases, hyperpigmentation occurred. A more recent study indicated that IPL could lead to the manifestation of previously subtle subclinical melasma (47). Wood's light examination before any IPL treatment of ethnic skin is now recommended.

The cause for such unwanted effects is unknown, but is probably related to the pathogenesis of melasma. It has been suggested that in epidermal and mixed type melasma, which is characterized by epidermal hyperpigmentation, the pathogenesis involves an increased number of melanocytes and increased activity of melanogenic enzymes overlying dermal changes that are caused by solar radiation (48). This may explain the development of hyperpigmentation after the use of pigment laser for treatment. An increase in melanogenic enzyme activity suggests that melanocytes are hyperactive. Sublethal laser damage to these melanocytes by pigment lasers can increase the production of melanin and result in hyperpigmentation. Hence, before any laser/IPL treatment, it is important to suppress the hyperactivity of these abnormal melanocytes by the use of sunscreen and bleaching agents for at least six weeks and preferably three months (49). The prolonged use of topical treatment is necessary as it does require more than six weeks for the follicular melanocytes to be affected. Even with the prolonged application of topical treatment, there is still a risk of hyperpigmentation. A recent study in Taipei that compared 16 patients on topical treatment against 17 who received topical and IPL treatment for melasma indicated 39.8% improvement in the treatment group as compared to 11.6% in the control group (50). Despite, three months use of topical bleaching agents before recruitment into the study, two patients in the treatment group developed increases in pigmentation.

To prevent increases in pigmentation, low fluence is essential, and one should look for the mildest clinical endpoint. Slight erythema should be used for IPL. Large spot size QS 1064 nm Nd:YAG laser can also be used, and once again slight erythema is the appropriate clinical endpoint. More recently, fractional resurfacing has been used for the removal of melasma. In a small-scale study, 60% of the treated subjects were found to have a significant degree of improvement, 30% had a mild degree of improvement, and 10% had an increase in pigmentation (51). Fractional resurfacing in this study involved the formation of melanocytic epidermal necrotic debris that acted as a melanocytic shuttle and effectively removed epidermal pigmentation. Other factors that may contribute to the effectiveness of fractional resurfacing in the treatment of melasma include transit impairment of the epidermal barrier function, which allows better absorption of the topical agents, and ablative removal of abnormal hyperactive melanoctyes.

Congenital Melanocytic Nevi

The use of laser for the treatment of congenital melanocytic nevi is controversial. Advocates have proposed that by reducing the melanocytic mass of the nevi, the risk of neoplastic changes can be reduced. Opponents are skeptical because there have been cases in which the use of laser delayed the diagnosis of melanoma or contributed to an incorrect diagnosis. Furthermore, whether there are long-term complications, such as increased risk of neoplastic changes, is not known.

Whereas the use of laser for the treatment of melanocytic nevi in Caucasians is controversial, there are more justifications for doing so with dark-skinned patients (52). First, unlike in the Caucasian population, melanoma is less common among darker-skinned patients; genetic difference rather than a difference in skin type is likely to be the main reason. Indeed, among patients with skin of color, melanoma tends to be acral in nature. Furthermore, the only long-term follow up study looking at the use of laser for the treatment of congenital melanocytic nevi was from Japan, and it indicated no histological evidence of malignant changes eight years after normal ruby laser treatment for congenital nevi (53). As a result, the use of laser for the removal of melanocytic nevi can be justified in ethnic skin, provided that there is no family history of melanoma and the lesion is not acral in nature.

In terms of the treatment approach, various pigmented lasers have been used in the removal of melanocytic nevi. A study looking at the use of QS Ruby laser found that an average clearance of 76% could occur after an average of eight treatment sessions (54). However, other studies showed that depending on the depth of the nests of melanocytes, recurrence could be a problem. Normal mode ruby laser (NMRL) can be used for the treatment of melanocytic nevi based on the principle that with longer pulse durations, a greater degree of clearance is achieved when nests of cells are destroyed (55). A combined approach with a QS ruby laser followed immediately, or two weeks later, with an NMRL was used with the intention of removing the superficial pigment first with the QS ruby laser, thereby enhancing the penetration of the NMRL (56). A previous study found that although 52% of the nevi showed a visible decrease in pigment, no lesion had complete histological clearance. Subtle microscopic scarring of the underlying nevus cells was considered to be important in creating the appearance of a significant reduction in pigmentation. More recently, another study reported better clearance by first using an NMRL to remove the epidermis, immediately followed by multiple passes of a QS ruby laser (57). The removal of the epidermis allows a greater degree of penetration by the QS laser, of which multiple passes further improve the clinical efficacy (Fig. 5).

LASER-ASSISTED HAIR REMOVAL IN ETHNIC SKIN

Laser-assisted hair removal techniques have been available since the mid 1990s. The first generation of hair-removal lasers with short 2 to 5 ms pulse durations allowed for successful

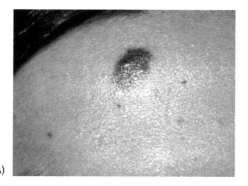 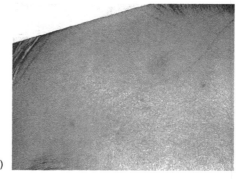

(A)   **(B)**

FIGURE 5   Congenital melanocytic nevus. (**A**) before treatment; (**B**) after sixth treatment with long-pulsed 532 mm, 6.2 J/cm², 2 mm spot size, followed immediately by Q-switching Alexandrite laser 7.5 J/cm², 2 mm spot size.

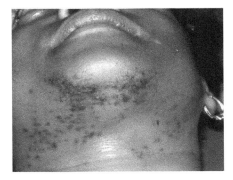 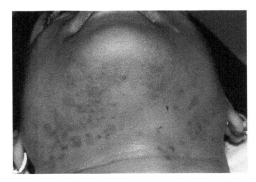

FIGURE 6 Laser hair removal using long-pulsed alexandrite, pre- (*Left*) and post- (*Right*) treatment. Effective hair removal in dark skin with some posttreatment dyschromia.

hair removal in those with fair skin and dark hair, but proved problematic in those with darker skin, resulting in blistering, dyschromia, and scarring. For effective treatment, laser energy must be transmitted unimpeded through the skin toward the intended target of melanin within the hair shaft and follicle. Darker skin (Fitzpatrick III–VI), with its increased melanin content, creates competition for the laser energy between the epidermal melanin and the targeted melanin. The selective destruction of the melanin within the hair follicle, while sparing epidermal melanin is possible through the process of thermokinetic selectivity, which is a corollary of the theory of selective photothermolysis (58,59). Smaller structures (epidermal melanocytes) dissipate heat more quickly than larger structures of the same chromophore with a greater surface to volume ratio (hair follicle). The ability of these smaller structures to dissipate heat more quickly acts as a protective mechanism. Newer generation laser hair removal devices incorporate longer pulse durations and a variety of cooling devices, thus allowing the safer treatment of dark skin.

Among all of the systems that are currently available for laser hair removal, long-pulsed Alexandrite laser, long-pulsed 800 nm diode laser (800–810 nm, 9–12 mm spot size, 30–100 msec pulse duration), and long-pulsed Nd:YAG laser (1064 nm, 10–100 msec pulse duration, 5–10 mm spot size) have fulfilled the above criteria, and may be particularly applicable to ethnic skin.

Initial studies with the long-pulsed Alexandrite laser (60,61) demonstrated effective hair removal in darker skin with pulse durations of 40 ms and fluences of 11 to 15 J/cm (Fig. 6) Although successful hair removal was achieved, post treatment dyschromia was noted in patients with very dark skin (skin type VI). Lengthening the pulsewidth to 200 ms (62) and using the long-pulsed diode laser resulted in effective hair removal and no post treatment dyschromia (Fig. 7).

Another study investigated the efficacy and complications of long-pulsed diode and long-pulsed Nd:YAG lasers in removing the hair of Chinese patients. The long-pulsed Nd:YAG laser was associated with significantly greater pain immediately after surgery and more protracted treatment time (63). Transient adverse effects were erythema and perifollicular edema, and only one patient developed hypopigmentation, at week six, which resolved by week 36. Such findings were further confirmed by Alster et al. (64), who examined twenty dark-skinned patients who were treated with long-pulsed Nd:YAG laser, which was found to be safe and effective.

A newer generation IPL sources with greater selectivity have also been shown to be effective in hair removal on ethnic skin. A recent study that looked at 28 Koreans who were treated with four sessions of IPL indicated minimal adverse effects with a clearance rate of up to 80% (65).

Laser assisted hair removal is now a successful treatment for hypertrichosis and pseudofolliculitis barbae. Despite the use of cooling devices, darker-skinned patients experience more pain with laser hair removal procedures (personal observation), are generally not able to tolerate higher fluences (58), and should be treated with conservative parameters.

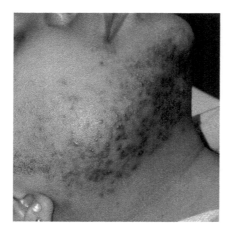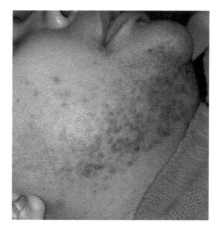

FIGURE 7 Pre- and post-treatment photos of two patients using super long-pulsed diode showing effective hair removal, no post-treatment dyschromia and resolution of pseudofolliculitis barbae. Pretreatment (*Left*), post-treatment (*Right*).

One must also be cautious while using cryogen cooling-devices in patients with darker skin tones to avoid possible hypopigmentation that is a result of the damage caused by cryogen to the melanocyte.

THE USE OF LASER FOR THE TREATMENT OF OTHER VASCULAR LESIONS

Beside facial telangiectasia, laser and IPL sources are also used for the treatment of port wine stain and proliferative hemangioma. With greater epidermal melanin context, ethnic skin is at a higher risk of adverse effects such as vesiculation and pigmentary changes after laser treatments of vascular lesions. Furthermore, with the epidermal melanin acting as a competing chromophore for hemoglobin, higher fluence or more treatment sessions are necessary to produce the desirable clinical endpoint. Before the development of skin cooling technology, studies indicated that the treatment of port wine stain in ethnic skin was associated with greater risk of transient PIH and texture changes (66,67). Adequate skin cooling allows epidermal protection, and in doing so improves safety and efficacy. Several cooling methods, including cold gel, air cooling, cryogen spray cooling (CSC), and contact cooling with a sapphire window, can be used in conjunction with vascular laser.

There is limited data on the use of air cooling with PDL for the treatment of vascular lesions in ethnic skin. Most of the published data is on CSC with pulsed dye laser (PDL-CSC) for the treatment of port wine stain. In a retrospective study, Chang and Nelson (68) found that PDL-CSC could enhance clinical efficacy, and a higher fluence could be used without an increase in complications for the treatment of port wine stain in Asian patients. Kelly et al. (69) demonstrated that PDL-CSC could be safely used at higher fluences in 20 port wine stain patients with skin types I–IV.

Another prospective study looking at 35 Chinese patients who were treated with PDL alone compared with PDL-CSC indicated that PDL-CSC was more effective, better tolerated, and had lower adverse effects than PDL alone (70) (Fig. 8). More recently, in a large-scale retrospective study, PDL-CSC was found to be effective for the treatment of a wide range of vascular lesions in 239 Korean patients (71).

Multiple intermittent cryogen spurts and laser pulses have been proposed to provide adequate epidermal protection, while permitting port wine stain photocoagulation for darker-skinned patients using heat diffusion, light distribution, and thermal damage computational models. Further clinical study using these new developments is necessary for darker-skinned patients with port wine stain (72).

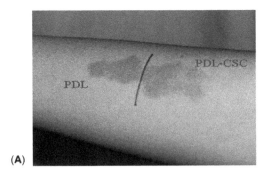
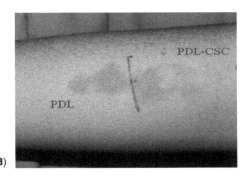

(A)   **(B)**

FIGURE 8   Thirteen-year-old Chinese female with port wine stain (PWS) of the right forearm: **(A)** before laser therapy, and **(B)** two months after fourth treatment with PDL alone and PDL-CSC using mean energy densities of 6.75 and 10.5 J/cm². *Abbreviations*: PDL, pulsed dye laser; PDL-CSC, pulsed dye laser-cryogen spray cooling.

A retrospective study that examined the results of a glass cooling chamber equipped variable pulse 532 nm Nd:YAG laser (VP 532) in the treatment of port wine stain in Chinese patients found that the VP 532 laser was only partially effective. High fluence was necessary, and even though contact cooling reduced the risk of epidermal damage, texture changes still occurred (73).

IPL sources have also been shown to be effective in the treatment of PDL resistant port wine stain. However, this method of treatment is only effective in experienced hands; complications can occur and the method should only be used as a second line therapy (74).

For proliferative hemangioma, the role of laser treatment is controversial. A previous study that looked at the use of PDL without cooling did not indicate that it had a beneficial effect (75). However, more recently, long PDL with cooling has been shown to be effective in reducing the proliferative phase of hemangioma among Japanese patients (76). Further study is necessary to confirm this finding.

CONCLUSION

When performing laser procedures in patients with ethnic skin, the challenge of effective treatment lies in one's ability to balance effective treatment with minimal risk to the patient. Untoward effects can be minimized with the use of conservative treatment parameters and lower energy settings for darker-skinned patients. Cutaneous laser surgery has been a mainstay of dermatologic therapy for more than a decade, but until recently most published studies excluded patients with ethnic skin. The changing demographics of the United States and the development of laser technologies that protect epidermal melanin from damage mean that with appropriate patient selection and proper physician training, laser surgery has become increasingly safe for darker-skinned patients.

REFERENCES

1. Matory WE. Skin care. In: Matory WE, ed. Ethnic Considerations in Facial Aesthetic Surgery. Philadelphia: Lippincott-Raven, 1998:100.
2. O'shea DC, Callen WR, Rhodes WT. Introduction to Lasers and Their Applications. Menlo Park, CA: Addison-Wesley Publishing Co, 1978.
3. Stratigos AJ, Alora MB, Uroste S, et al. Cutaneous laser surgery. Curr Probl Dermatol 1998; 10:127–174.
4. Anderson RR, parish JA. Optical properties of human skin. In: Regan JD, Parrish JA, eds. The Science of Photomedicine. New York: Plenum Press, 1982:147–194.
5. Anderson RR, Parrish JA. Selective photothermolysis: precise microsurgery by selective absorption of pulsed radiation. Science 1983; 220:524.
6. Anderson RR. Laser-Tissue Interaction. In: Goldman MP, Fitzpatrick RE, eds. Cutaneous Laser Surgery the Art and Science of Selective Photothermolysis. St Louis: Mosby, 1994.

7. Arndt KA, Noe JM, Northam DBC. Laser therapy: basic concepts and nomenclature. J AmAcad Dermatol 1981; 5:649–654.
8. Jackson BA, Junkins-Hopkins J. Super long pulsed diode laser treatment for hair removal in dark skin: clinical-pathologic correlation. 2001 oral presentation and abstract. L'Oreal Ethnic Hair and Skin Symposium.
9. McCurdy JA. Facial surgery in the asian patient. In: Matory WE, ed. Ethnic Considerations in Facial Aesthetic Surgery. Philadelphia: Lippincott-Raven, 1998:263–284.
10. Chan HH, Fung WK, Ying SY, Kono T. An in vivo trial comparing the use of different types of 532 nm Nd:YAG lasers in the treatment of facial lentigines in oriental patients. Dermatol Surg 2000; 26:743–749.
11. Rashid T, Hussain I, Haider M, Haroon TS. Laser therapy of freckles and lentigines with quasi-continuous, frequency-doubled, Nd:YAG(532 nm) laser in Fitzpatrick skin type IV: A 24 month follow up. J Cosmet Laser Ther 2002; 4:81–85.
12. Negishi K, Tezuka Y, Kudshikata N,Wakamatsu S. Photorejuvenation for Asian skin by intense pulsed light. Dermatol Surg 2001; 27:627–632.
13. Wang CC, Sue YM, Yang CH, Chen CK. A comparison of Q-switched alexandrite laser and intense pulsed light for the treatment of freckles and lentigines in Asian persons: a randomized, physician-blinded, split-face comparative trial. J Am Acad Dermatol 2006; 54:804–810.
14. Chan HH. Treatment of photoaging in asian skin. In: Rigel DS, Weiss RA, Lim HW, Dover JS, eds. Photaging. New York: Marcel Dekker, Inc, 2003:343–364. ISBN 0-8247-5450-6.
15. Kono T, Manstein D, Chan HH, Nozaki M, Anderson RR. Q-switched ruby vs. long-pulsed dye laser delivered with compression for treatment of facial lentigines in Asians. Lasers Surg Med 2006; 38:94–97.
16. Chan HH, Alam M, Kono T, Dover J. Clinical application of lasers in Asians. Dermatol Surg 2002; 28:556–563.
17. Chan HH. Recent advances in the use of lasers, light sources, and radiofrequency in Asians. Lasers Surg Med 2005; 37:179–185.
18. Lee MW. Combination visible and infrared lasers for skin rejuvenation. Semin Cutan Med Surg 2002; 21:288–300.
19. Hse TS, Zelickson B, Dover JS, et al. Multicenter study of the safety and efficacy of a 585 nm pulsed-dye laser for the nonablative treatment of facial rhytides. Dermatol Surg 2005; 31:1–9.
20. Trelles MA, Allones I, Levy JL, Calderhead RG, Moreno-Arias GA. Combined nonablative skin rejuvenation with the 595- and 1450-nm lasers. Dermatol Surg 2004; 30:1292–1298.
21. Chan HH, Lam LK, Wong DS, Kono T, Trend-Smith N. Use of 1320 nm Nd:YAG laser for wrinkle reduction and the treatment of atrophic acne scarring. Lasers Surg Med 2004; 34:98–103.
22. Tanzi EL, Williams CM, Alster TS. Treatment of facial rhytides with a nonablative 1,450 nm diode laser: a controlled clinical and histologic study. Dermatol Surg 2003; 29:124–128.
23. Goh CL, Chua SH, Ang P, Khoo L. Efficacy of smoothbeam 1,450 nm laser for treatment of acne scars in Asian skin. Lasers Surg Med 2004; S16:S76.
24. Fournier N, Dahan S, Barneon G, et al. Nonablative remodeling: a 14-month clinical ultrasound imaging and profilometric evaluation of a 1540 nm Er:Glass laser. Dermatol Surg 2002; 28:926–931.
25. Alster T, Hirsch R. Single-pass CO2 laser skin resurfacing of light and dark skin: extended experience with 52 patients. J Cosmet Laser Ther 2003; 5:39–42.
26. Manstein D, Herron GS, Sink RK, Tanner H, Anderson RR. Fractional photothermolysis: a new concept for cutaneous remodeling using microscopic patterns of thermal injury. Lasers Surg Med 2004; 34:426–438.
27. Chan HH, Shek S, Yu CY, Yeung CK, Kono T, Mainstein D. Prevalence and risk factor of post-inflammatory hyperpigmentation in Chinese patients treated with fractional resurfacing. Lasers Surg Med 2006; S18:S77.
28. Kono T, Chan HH, Manstein D, Sesova IP, Nozaki M. Comparison study of the down time and complications of fraxel laser skin rejuvenation. Lasers Surg Med 2006; S18:S20.
29. Alster TS. Complete elimination of large café au lait birthmarks by the 510 nm pulsed dye laser. Plast Reconstr Surg 1995; 96:1660–1664.
30. Grossman MC, Anderson RR, Farinelli W, Flotte TJ, Grevelink JM. Treatment of cafe au lait macules with lasers. A clinicopathologic correlation. Arch Dermatol 1995; 131:1416–1420.
31. Chan HH, Kono T. The use of lasers and intense pulsed light sources for the treatment pigmentary lesions. Skin Ther Lett 2004; 9:5–7.
32. Kopera D, Hohenleutner U, Landthaler M. Quality-switched ruby laser treatment of solar lentigines and Becker's nevus: a histopathological and immunohistochemical study. Dermatology 1997; 194:338–343.
33. Trelles MA, Allones I, Moreno-Arias GA, Velez M. Becker's naevus: a comparative study between erbium: YAG and Q-switched neodymium:YAG; clinical and histopathological findings. Br J Dermatol 2005; 152:308–313.
34. Nanni CA, Alster TS. Treatment of a Becker's nevus using a 694 nm long-pulsed ruby laser. Dermatol Surg 1998; 24:1032–1034.

35. Watanabe S, Takahashi H. Treatment of nevus of ota with the Q-switched ruby laser. N Engl J Med 1994; 331:1745–1750.

36. Chan HH, King WWK, Chan ESY, et al. An vivo trial comparing the patients' tolerability of Q-switched Alexandrite (QS Alex) and Q-switched Neodymium: Yttrium-Aluminum-Garnet (QS Nd-YAG) lasers in the treatment of nevus of ota. Laser Surg Med 1999; 24:24–28.

37. Chan HH, Ying SY, Ho WS, Kono T, King WW. An in vivo trial comparing the clinical efficacy and complications of Q-switched Alexandrite (QS Alex) and Q-switched 1064 nm Neodymium: Yttrium-Aluminum-Garnet (QS 1064 Nd-YAG) lasers in the treatment of nevus of ota. Dermatol Surg 2000; 26:919–922.

38. Chan HH, Leung RS, Ying SY, Lai CF, Kono T, Chua JK, Ho WS. A retrospective study looking at the complications of Q-switched Alexandrite (QS Alex) and Q-switched Neodymium: Yttrium-Aluminum-Garnet (QS Nd-YAG) lasers in the treatment of nevus of Ota. Dermatol Surg 2000; 26:1000–1006.

39. Kono T, Nozaki M, Chan HH, Mikashima Y. A retrospective study looking at the long-term complication of Q-switched ruby laser in the treatment of nevus of Ota. Lasers Surg Med 2001; 29:156–159.

40. Kono T, Chan HH, Ercocen AR, et al. Use of Q-switched ruby laser in the treatment of nevus of ota in different age groups. Lasers Surg Med 2003; 32:391–395.

41. Kunachak S, Leelaudomlipi P, Sirikulchayanonta V. Q-Switched ruby laser therapy of acquired bilateral nevus of ota-like macules. Dermatol Surg 1999; 25:938–941.

42. Lam AY, Wong DS, Lam LK, Ho WS, Chan HH. A retrospective study on the efficacy and complications of Q-switched. Alexandrite laser in the treatment of acquired bilateral nevus of ota-like macules. Dermatol Surg 2001; 27:937–941.

43. Polnikorn N, Tanrattanakorn S, Goldberg DJ. Treatment of Hori's nevus with the Q-switched Nd:YAG laser. Dermatol Surg 2000; 26:477–480.

44. Ee HL, Goh CL, Khoo LS, et al. Treatment of acquired bilateral nevus of ota-like macules (Hori's nevus) with a combination of the 532 nm Q-Switched Nd:YAG laser followed by the 1,064 nm Q-switched Nd:YAG is more effective: prospective study. Dermatol Surg 2006; 32:34–40.

45. Grekin RC, Shelton RM, Geisse JK, Frieden I. 510 nm pigmented lesion dye laser. Its characteristics and clinical uses. J Dermatol Surg Oncol 1993; 19:380–387.

46. Taylor CR, Anderson RR. Ineffective treatment of refractory melasma and postinflammatory hyperpigmentation by Q-switched ruby laser. J Dermatol Surg Oncol 1994; 20:592–597.

47. Kang WH, Yoon KH, Lee ES, et al. Melasma: histopathological characteristics in 56 Korean patients. Br J Dermatol 2002; 146:228–237.

48. Negishi K, Kushikata N, Tezuka Y, Takeuchi K, Miyamoto E, Wakamatsu S. Study of the incidence and nature of "very subtle epidermal melasma" in relation to intense pulsed light treatment. 2004;30:881–886; discussion 886.

49. Chan HH. The use of laser and intense pulsed light source in the treatment of melasma. Cosmet Dermatol 2007 (in press).

50. Wang CC, Hui CY, Sue YM, et al. Intense pulsed light for the treatment of refractory melasma in Asian patients. Dermatol Surg 2004; 30:1196–1200.

51. Rokhsar CK, Fitzpatrick RE. The treatment of melasma with fractional photothermolysis: a pilot study. Dermatol Surg 2005; 31:1645–1650.

52. Imayama S, Ueda S. Long- and short-term histological observations of congenital nevi treated with the normal mode ruby laser. Arch Dermatol 1999; 135:1211–1218.

53. Chan HH. Laser treatment of nevomelanocytic nevi—can results from an Asian study be applicable to the white population? Arch Dermatol 2002; 138:535.

54. Waldorf HA, Kauvar ANB, Geronemus RG. Treatment of small and medium congenital nevi with the Q-switched ruby laser. Arch Dermatol 1996; 132:301–304.

55. Vibhagool C, Randolph Byers H, Grevelink JM. Treatment of small nevomelanocytic nevi with a Q-switched ruby laser. J Am Acad Dermatol 1997; 36:738–741.

56. Duke D, Randolph Byers H, Sober AJ, Anderson RR, Grevelink JM. Treatment of benign and atypical nevi with the normal mode ruby laser and the Q-switched ruby laser. Arch Dermatol 1999; 135:290–296.

57. Kono T, Nozaki M, Chan HH, Sasaki K, Kwon SC. Combined use of a normal mode ruby laser and a Q-switched ruby laser in the treatment of congenital melanocytic nevi. Brit J Plast Surg 2001; 54:640–642.

58. Fuchs M. Thermokinetic selectivity—a new highly effective method for permanent hair removal: experience with the LPIR Alexandrite laser. Derm Prakt Dermatologie 1997; 5:1.

59. Anderson RR. Laser-Tissue interaction. In: Goldman MP, Fitzpatrick RE, eds. Cutaneous Laser Surgery the Art and Science of Selective Photothermolysis. St Louis: Mosby, 1994.

60. Jackson BA, Junkins-Hopkins JM. Effect of Pulsewidth Variation on laser Hair removal in African-American Skin. 1999 oral presentation ASDS meeting Miami, FL.

61. Jackson BA. Lasers in Ethnic skin. 1999 AAD Annual meeting focus session, New Orleans, LA.

62. Jackson BA, Junkins-Hopkins J. Super long pulsed diode laser treatment for hair removal in dark skin: clinical-pathologic correlation. 2001 Oral presentation and abstract. L'Oreal Ethnic Hair and Skin Symposium.

63. Chan HH, Ying SY, Ho WS, Wong DS, Lam LK. An in vivo study comparing the efficacy and complications of Diode laser and long-pulsed Neodymium: Yttrium-Aluminum-Garnet (Nd:YAG) laser in hair removal among Chinese patients. Dermatol Surg 2001; 27:950–954.

64. Alster TS, Bryan H, Williams CM. Long-pulsed Nd:YAG laser-assisted hair removal in pigmented skin. Arch Dermatol 2001; 137:885–889.

65. Lee JH, Huh CH, Yoon HJ, Cho KH, Chung JH. Photoepilation results of axillary hair in dark-skinned patients by IPL: a comparison between different wavelength and pulse width. Dermatol Surg 2006; 32:234–241.

66. Goh CL. Treatment response of port wine stains with the flashlamp-pulsed dye laser in the national skin centre: a report of 36 patients. Ann Acad Med Singapore 1996; 25:536–540.

67. Sommer S, Sheehan-Dare RA. Pulsed dye laser treatment of port-wine stains in pigmented skin. J Am Acad Dermatol 2000; 42:667–671.

68. Chang CJ, Nelson JS. Cryogen spray cooling and higher fluence pulsed dye laser treatment improve port wine stain clearance while minimizing epidermal damage. Dermatol Surg 1999; 25:767–772.

69. Kelly KM, Nanda VS, Nelson JS. Treatment of port-wine stain birthmarks using the 1.5-msec pulsed dye laser at high fluences in conjunction with cryogen spray cooling. Dermatol Surg 2002; 28:309–313.

70. Chiu CH, Chan HH, Ho WS, Yeung CK, Nelson JS. Prospective study of pulsed dye laser in conjunction with cryogen spray cooling for treatment of port wine stains in Chinese patients. Dermatol Surg 2003; 29:909–915.

71. Woo SH, Ahn HH, Kim SN, Kye YC. Treatment of vascular skin lesions with the variable-pulse 595 nm pulsed dye laser. Dermatol Surg 2006; 32:41–48.

72. Aguilar G, Diaz SH, Lavernia EJ, Nelson JS. Cryogen spray cooling efficiency: improvement of port wine stain laser therapy through multiple-intermittent cryogen spurts and laser pulses. Lasers Surg Med. 2002; 31:27–35.

73. Chan HH, Chan E, Kono T, Ying SY, Ho WS. The use of variable pulse width frequency doubled Nd:YAG 532 nm laser in the treatment of port-wine stain in Chinese patients. Dermatol Surg 2000; 26:657–661.

74. Ho WS, Ying SY, Chan PC, Chan HH. Treatment of port-wine stains with intense pulsed light: a prospective study. Dermatol Surg 2004; 30:887–890.

75. Batta K, Goodyear HM, Moss C, et al. Randomised controlled study of early pulsed dye laser treatment of uncomplicated childhood haemangiomas: results of a 1-year analysis. Lancet 2002; 360:521–527.

76. Kono T, Sakurai H, Groff WF, et al. Comparison study of a traditional pulsed dye laser versus a long-pulsed dye laser in the treatment of early childhood hemangiomas. Lasers Surg Med 2006; 38:112–115.

Appendix A | Phototesting

Peter M. Farr
Department of Dermatology, Royal Victoria Infirmary, Newcastle upon Tyne, England, U.K.

Robert S. Dawe
Department of Dermatology, Ninewells Hospital and Medical School, Dundee University, Dundee, Scotland, U.K.

INTRODUCTION

Phototesting is exposure of the skin to ultraviolet (UV) or visible radiation followed by the observation, recording, and evaluation of irradiated skin responses at appropriate times thereafter. In general, there are two broad phototesting categories.

1. Phototesting for therapeutic purposes. Here the minimal erythema or phototoxic dose (MED or MPD) is measured to enable choice of an appropriate UV dose with which to start a phototherapy or psoralen photochemotherapy (PUVA) course.
2. Phototesting for diagnostic purposes in patients with suspected photosensitivity. Here, measurement of the MED is again undertaken, and in appropriate clinical situations, provocation testing as well.

Phototesting can also be used to monitor changes in a condition, for example, phototesting at intervals to determine whether or not chronic actinic dermatitis (CAD) has resolved, or before and after antihistamine medication to help assess its efficacy in solar urticaria.

MEASURING THE MINIMAL ERYTHEMA DOSE PRIOR TO NARROWBAND OR BROADBAND UVB PHOTOTHERAPY

Here, it is essential that the lamp type used for phototesting is the same as that to be used for the treatment course. Closely apposed areas of skin are exposed to increasing UV doses, which given the positively skewed distribution of MED values in the normal population (see subsequently), should follow a geometric series. In general, increments of 40% (equivalent to doubling alternate doses, for example, 2.5, 3.5, 5.0, 7.1, 10, 14, 20, 28, and so on), provide an accurate enough indication of a patient's erythemal sensitivity. The exact range of doses will be determined by the predominant skin type of the population under test, with the aim in each individual of achieving a range of responses from no erythema to just above the MED. The skin site for testing may vary according to the method used, but the back is frequently chosen because the trunk is usually the most sensitive site and the back is often practically easier to test than the abdomen (1).

Two methods are available for achieving a series of doses on the skin.

1. A UV-opaque template with several apertures able to be covered or uncovered in turn is applied to the skin and different doses achieved for each uncovered site by adjusting the exposure time (Fig. 1). A special bank of fluorescent lamps may be used, or with appropriate body protection, the actual phototherapy unit to be employed for treatment. This method has the advantage that the irradiation geometry will be similar to that used for phototherapy, and dosimetry will be relatively simple. However, it is time-consuming and requires multiple interventions by trained staff.
2. A template is applied to the skin with apertures containing variably perforated metal grills that differentially attenuate the radiation (Fig. 2A) (2). A single exposure from a fluorescent

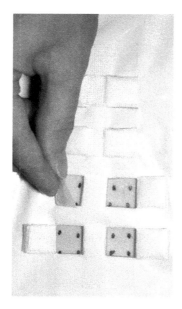
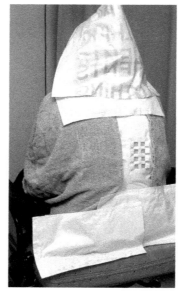
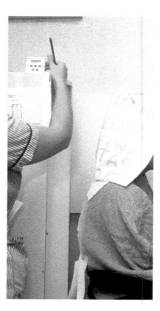

FIGURE 1 Measurement of the minimal erythema dose prior to a phototherapy course using a UV-opaque template with apertures covered in turn to achieve a series of doses. The patient's skin is protected, and a bank of fluorescent UV lamps is used to expose the test sites. *Source*: Photographs courtesy of Dr. S.H. Ibbotson.

lamp mounted closely above the template then results in a graded series of doses. This method has the advantage that testing can be performed rapidly—a dose series may be obtained with a single exposure of typically five minutes—but the irradiation geometry is unlike that to be used during the phototherapy and dosimetry can be problematic. An instrument based on these principles containing a compact fluorescent lamp is commercially available (Fig. 2B).

Whatever method is used, the exposed sites are observed at a specified time after irradiation, usually 24 hours for convenience (although UVB erythema peaks before this) (3), and the smallest dose to achieve "just perceptible erythema" is taken as the MED. It will be apparent that the MED is not an exact measurement, as the actual value can lie anywhere between the dose at which erythema is first observed and just above the dose below that in the exposure series.

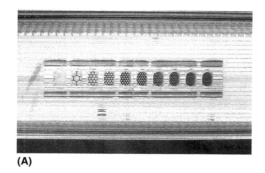
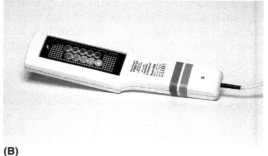

(A)   **(B)**

FIGURE 2 **(A)** A phototesting template with perforated metal grills to attenuate the radiation, allowing a series of doses to be achieved with a single exposure. **(B)** A commercially available device for minimal erythema dose measurement incorporating the attenuating template. *Source*: Figure 2A adapted from Ref. 2.

MEASURING THE MINIMAL PHOTOTOXIC DOSE PRIOR TO PSORALEN PHOTOCHEMOTHERAPY

This is performed in a similar fashion to MED testing. The appropriate psoralen dose is administered before irradiation by the appropriate route (oral or topical), and the test irradiation undertaken with the same UV source (usually broad-band UVA), as to be used for treatment. Peak PUVA erythema occurs later than after UVB or UVA alone, such that PUVA readings are usually made at 72 or 96 hours. As with MED testing, MPD assessment helps determine an appropriate UV starting dose, but also ensures before oral PUVA that sufficient drug reaches the skin to cause a reaction, given that individual variations in bioavailability, and drug and dietary interactions, may occur. If there is no response, repeat testing may be undertaken after a higher oral psoralen dose.

MEASURING THE MINIMAL ERYTHEMA DOSE WHEN INVESTIGATING PATIENTS WITH SUSPECTED PHOTOSENSITIVITY

Here, in addition to measuring the UVB MED, it is necessary also to measure the MED within the UVA and, sometimes, visible wavebands. However, UVA fluorescent lamps are not of sufficiently high irradiance to allow MED measurements except in severe photosensitivity, such that an irradiation monochromator is generally used instead.

IRRADIATION MONOCHROMATOR

An irradiation monochromator is a versatile instrument allowing small areas of skin to be exposed to specific wavelengths of radiation. It is particularly used to measure MEDs in patients under investigation for suspected abnormal photosensitivity (Table 1). It is also ideal for lesion induction in patients with solar urticaria, but not generally in other disorders, particularly polymorphic light eruption (PLE), where a larger irradiation field is required.

An irradiation monochromator typically contains a xenon arc lamp UV source providing continuous emission from the UVC (100–280 nm) into the visible region. A diffraction grating, less commonly a prism, then disperses this into its component wavelengths. Finally, a selection of specific wavelengths is shone on to the patient's skin, either by direct contact with the instrument's exit aperture, or more conveniently through a flexible liquid-filled light guide (4).

Although the term monochromator implies that a single wavelength is delivered, the spectral distribution of the emitted radiation is generally triangular in shape, with its width (or bandwidth) being varied by adjusting the size of the slits through which it passes to and from the diffraction grating. The bandwidth is typically quoted after the central wavelength, for example: 350 nm (bandwidth 30 nm or ± 15 nm), and is conventionally defined as the full width of the emission at half-maximum intensity (Fig. 3). The smaller the bandwidth, the more accurately a specific observed effect may be attributed to a specific wavelength. However, as the output irradiance, and thus the irradiation time to achieve a given dose, is highly dependent on the bandwidth, a compromise is necessary depending on the time available for testing and the specific wavelength(s) under investigation. For the UVB wavelengths, to which the skin is highly erythemally sensitive, a narrow bandwidth may be used, for example, 5 nm, whereas in the UVA region, where the skin is much less erythemally-sensitive, a bandwidth of 30 nm may be required. With such a large bandwidth, a filter is commonly used to cut off shorter wavelengths, which would otherwise contribute to the erythemal response.

The MED is measured with a monochromator by exposing adjacent areas of skin to incremental doses of radiation in turn, using a geometric dose series as described previously. Dose increments of 40% are again generally accurate enough for diagnostic purposes. Smaller dose increments (10% or 20%) might theoretically be used to improve precision, but judging whether erythema is present or not under such circumstances is often difficult, and variations in skin sensitivity, even over a defined area such as the back, also make this approach

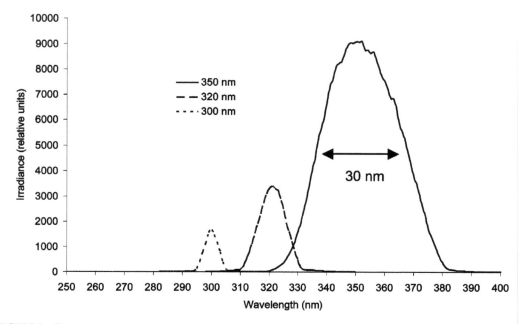

FIGURE 3 The spectral emission of an irradiation monochromator set at central wavelengths (bandwidths) of 300 (5) nm, 320 (10) nm, and 350 (30) nm. The bandwidth (full width of the emission at half-maximum intensity) is shown at 350 nm. *Source*: Spectra courtesy of Dr. J.J. Lloyd.

questionable. The results are examined at appropriate time intervals after exposure, and the lowest dose to cause just perceptible erythema is recorded, along with any abnormal morphological responses. In solar urticaria (whether idiopathic, drug-induced or associated with porphyria), wealing typically occurs within 30 minutes of irradiation. However, in porphyria, a response of erythema alone may be seen, typically maximal at around seven hours after irradiation. Additional observational time-points may be required for a few conditions, such as some drug-induced photosensitivity, xeroderma pigmentosum (XP), and psoralen-sensitized skin.

The selection of wavelengths used to investigate patients with suspected photosensitivity has not yet been standardized between specialist centers (5). As normal ranges are highly dependent upon wavelength, bandwidth, and other technical factors, they too will be specific to a particular investigating center. In the normal population, MEDs have a positively skewed, log-normal distribution (6,7), and it is therefore preferable to quote average MED values as the

TABLE 1 Summary of Photosensitivity Disorders and Phototesting Abnormalities

Diagnosis	Results of MED testing	Results of provocation testing
Polymorphic light eruption and actinic prurigo	Usually normal. Around 15% of patients may have low MEDs	Positive papular response in around 80% of patients
Solar urticaria	Normal if able to be tested	Urticarial response
Chronic actinic dermatitis	Abnormally low UVB and UVA MEDs with abnormal response to visible light in some patients	MED responses often palpable with spongiotic eczematous change on biopsy
Drug-induced photosensitivity	May be abnormal, particularly in UVA waveband	
XP	May be abnormal, particularly in UVB. In classical (not variant) XP, maximal reaction may be delayed until 72 hours	

Abbreviations: MED, minimal erythema dose; XP, xeroderma pigmentosum.

TABLE 2 Wavebands and Normal Ranges Used for Routine Irradiation Monochromator Phototesting in The Newcastle Photobiology Unit

Waveband (bandwidth) (nm)	Filter	Typical irradiance (mW/cm^2)	Normal range for MED	Dose range used
300 (5)	None	5	14–80 mJ/cm^2	2.5, 3.5, 5, 7.1, 10, 14, 20, 28, 40, and 56
320 (10)	WG305	20	1–4 J/cm^2	0.5, 0.7, 1, 1.4, and 2
350 (30)	WG320	180	14–80 J/cm^2	2.5, 3.5, 5, 7.1, 10, 14, and 20
400 (30)	WG320	190	>40 J/cm^2	20 and 40

Note: The choice of wavebands and doses varies according to the suspected diagnosis. A typical MED investigation with the wavebands shown will be completed within 30 minutes. The normal ranges are derived from unpublished data and previous publications.
Abbreviation: MED, minimal erythema dose.
Source: Adapted from Refs. 4, 7.

median, or geometric mean, rather than the arithmetic mean. Details of the routine testing methodology used in the Newcastle photobiology unit, together with the relevant normal ranges, are shown in Table 2 and Figure 3.

PROVOCATION TESTING

Provocation testing, used principally to confirm a diagnosis, involves the sometimes repeated irradiation of skin to induce a response similar to that seen following sunlight exposure (Table 1). The UV source and exposure protocol depend upon the suspected clinical diagnosis, as described subsequently.

POLYMORPHIC LIGHT ERUPTION AND ACTINIC PRURIGO

An irradiation field of several square centimetres is required, not achievable with an irradiation monochromator. Suitable UV sources include the following.

1. A solar simulator. This is a xenon arc lamp filtered to provide an emission spectrum similar to that of natural sunlight.
2. A bank of fluorescent lamps. When configured as a cylindrical array, a high irradiance may be achieved to allow provocation testing on the arm with either narrowband (NB)-UVB or broadband UVA (8).

Provocation testing may be performed on any convenient body site, frequently the arm or back. However, irradiation of recently sun-exposed or tanned skin may produce false negative results. The doses used will be limited by the possibility of normal delayed erythema for sources emitting significant UVB (such as the solar simulator and NB-UVB lamps), or by the time available for testing with UVA fluorescent lamps. Repeated exposures are generally given every 24 hours until a positive response is obtained, or the test is evaluated as negative. Positive results may be obtained in around 81% to 90% of PLE patients (8,9), although such a high success rate may perhaps be achievable only in patients with severe disease. Testing with both NB-UVB and broadband UVA increases the chances of a successful outcome (8). The percentage of patients testing positive increases from 18% after one exposure to 69% after two exposures and 81% after three (8). Positive results generally consist of small erythematous papules scattered throughout the irradiation field (Fig. 4), but other responses, such as large edematous papules or vesicles, are also possible.

SOLAR URTICARIA

The action spectrum for solar urticaria may be narrow and confined to a specific waveband within the UVB, UVA, or visible regions, or more commonly encompass a wide range of wavelengths. The monochromator is ideally suited for provocation testing in this condition, as only

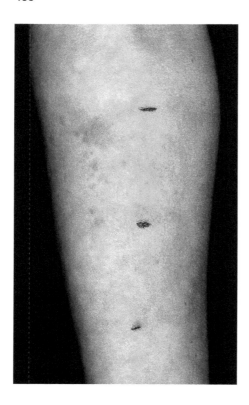

FIGURE 4 Papular lesions induced on the forearm of a patient with polymorphic light eruption after exposure to NB-UVB.

small irradiation fields are needed but testing is required at several wavelengths, including within the visible region. A typical investigation might entail a series of single exposures at 300, 320, and 350 nm, and then every 50 nm up to 500 nm (blue light) or 550 nm (green light). At 300 and 320 nm, the doses used will be limited by the need to avoid excessive delayed normal erythema, whereas at longer wavelengths, where such erythema is unlikely, a maximum of about 20 J/cm^2 may be appropriate. Irradiation sites should be observed for 10 to 15 minutes, by which time any weal and flare responses will generally be maximal (Fig. 5). An approximate action spectrum can be deduced from this initial series of tests, and a decision then made whether minimal urticarial dose testing is also needed. If so, this can be undertaken by again using a geometric dose series and examining the skin 10 to 15 minutes later to determine the smallest dose needed just to induce wealing. Typically, at doses slightly below the minimal urticarial dose, erythema alone is seen without weal or flare, and this may be termed the minimal reaction dose. Finally, if patients are taking antihistamines at the time of testing, any weal and flare responses may be inhibited, but erythema localized to the irradiation field usually still occurs (10).

CHRONIC ACTINIC DERMATITIS

Phototesting with a monochromator is very appropriate in suspected CAD as it not only determines the presence and severity of any abnormal photosensitivity but also allows definition of the responsible UV and visible wavebands. There are generally delayed responses, typically both clinically and histologically eczematous, often following extremely low irradiation doses at wavelengths nearly always including the UVB (Fig. 6). Where no monochromator is available, however, the simpler and cheaper solar simulator (see above), with filters to allow visible as well as UV testing, can instead provide sufficient information to make a probable diagnosis of CAD. Also, in the absence of a solar simulator, MED testing with UVB and UVA phototherapy units, with a slide projector as a visible light source, is an alternative

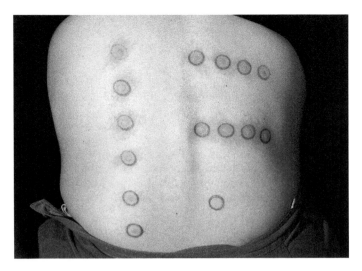

FIGURE 5 Investigating a patient with idiopathic solar urticaria. From the top of the back down, single exposures were given at 300, 320, 350, 400, 450, 500, and 550 nm (bottom of back) to define the approximate action spectrum (from 300 to 500 nm in this case). A series of reducing doses was then given at 300 nm and 350 nm in an attempt to define the minimal urticarial dose.

approach. If such a slide projector is used, a few local normal subjects should be tested first to determine suitable exposure times to avoid excessive skin heating, which may itself flare eczema and lead to an incorrect CAD diagnosis. Finally, in resource-poor settings, the sun can be used as a test irradiation source, both unfiltered and filtered with window glass, to expose small areas of unaffected skin to the solar spectrum with and without UVB. However, sunlight is unpredictably variable, making dose estimations difficult, while any associated heat might again flare the rash, possibly leading to an incorrect diagnosis of CAD.

DRUG-INDUCED PHOTOSENSITIVITY

Drug-induced photosensitivity reaction patterns include sunburn-like phototoxicity, an UV-induced dermatitis response, a porphyria cutanea tarda-like response, lichenoid reactions, urticarial, and pigmentary abnormalities. For most forms of such photosensitivity, the irradiation monochromator is again the most useful investigative tool. If abnormally low delayed MEDs are seen, particularly in the UVA waveband (7), this supports drug photosensitivity, but repeated testing is needed after the drug is stopped to confirm the

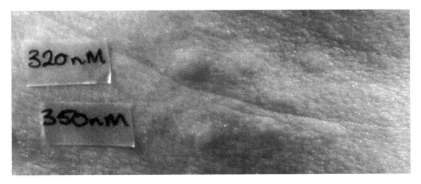

FIGURE 6 Minimal erythema dose testing at two wavelengths in a patient with chronic actinic dermatitis. A palpable response has been obtained, which would show spongiotic eczema on biopsy.

diagnosis. However, patients must sometimes be off the drug (particularly quinine or bendro-flumethiazide) for at least six months before the phototests return to normal.

OTHER DISORDERS

Similar provocation testing methods to those for PLE can induce the early lesions of hydroa vacciniforme (11).

Abnormal phototest reactions may also be found in many patients with cutaneous porphyria. Typically, early urticarial reactions and low MEDs, usually lower at seven hours than 24, occur on visible light testing, such as at 400 and 430 nm. The porphyrias are definitively diagnosed biochemically, but phototesting can sometimes help educate patients about the role of daylight in inducing their rash, for instance, if marked urticarial responses occur in erythropoietic protoporphyria, and can also help assess the responsiveness of the disorder to therapies.

Finally, in some patients with lupus erythematosus (LE), repeated exposures to broad-band UVA, UVB or both can induce abnormal reactions with histological changes in keeping with LE (12).

REFERENCES

1. Waterston K, Naysmith L, Rees JL. Physiological variation in the erythemal response to ultraviolet radiation and photoadaptation. J Invest Dermatol 2004; 123(5):958–964.
2. Gordon PM, Saunders PJ, Diffey BL, et al. Phototesting prior to narrowband (TL-01) ultraviolet B phototherapy. Br J Dermatol 1998; 139(5):811–814.
3. Man I, Dawe RS, Ferguson J, et al. An intraindividual study of the characteristics of erythema induced by bath and oral methoxsalen photochemotherapy and narrowband ultraviolet B. Photochem Photobiol 2003; 78(1):55–60.
4. Diffey BL, Farr PM, Ive FA. The establishment and clinical value of a dermatological photobiology service in a district general hospital. Br J Dermatol 1984; 110(2):187–194.
5. Bilsland D, Diffey BL, Farr PM, et al. Diagnostic phototesting in the United Kingdom. Br J Dermatol 1992; 127(3):297–299.
6. Mackenzie LA. The analysis of the ultraviolet radiation doses required to produce erythemal responses in normal skin. Br J Dermatol 1983; 108(1):1–9.
7. Diffey BL, Farr PM. The normal range in diagnostic phototesting. Br J Dermatol 1989; 120(4):517–524.
8. Das S, Lloyd JJ, Walshaw D, et al. Provocation testing in polymorphic light eruption using fluorescent ultraviolet (UV) A and UVB lamps. Br J Dermatol 2004; 151(5):1066–1070.
9. Hölzle E, Plewig G, Hofmann C, et al. Polymorphous light eruption. Experimental reproduction of skin lesions. J Am Acad Dermatol 1982; 7(1)111–125.
10. Cox NH, Higgins EM, Farr PM. Terfenadine inhibits itch and wheal, but not abnormal erythema, in physical urticarias. J Am Acad Dermatol 1989; 21:586–587.
11. Sunohara A, Mizuno N, Sakai M, et al. Action spectrum for UV erythema and reproduction of the skin lesions in hydroa vacciniforme. Photodermatol 1988; 5(3):139–145.
12. Lehmann P, Hölzle E, Kind P, et al. Experimental reproduction of skin lesions in lupus erythematosus by UVA and UVB radiation. J Am Acad Dermatol 1990; 22(2):181–187.

Appendix B | Photopatch Testing

Percy Lehmann
*Klinik für Dermatologie, Allergologie und Umweltmedizin,
HELIOS-Klinikum Wuppertal, Universitätsklinikum der
Universität Witten-Herdecke, Wuppertal, Germany*

Frank C. Victor and David E. Cohen
*Ronald O. Perelman Department of Dermatology, New York
University School of Medicine, New York, New York, U.S.A.*

INTRODUCTION

Thorough evaluation of any photosensitive patient can be difficult, there often being a legion of possible diagnoses. Where photoallergic contact dermatitis is suspected, however, the photopatch test (PPT) is the most important diagnostic procedure, potentially enabling correct diagnosis through identifying the responsible allergen or allergens. PPTs should be performed in all patients with eczema of predominantly the sun-exposed skin, in chronic actinic dermatitis, and as appropriate in other photosensitive disorders of uncertain diagnosis.

Although the investigation of photopatch testing was first described as early as 1939 by Epstein (1), the methodology used was not at all standardized until the early 1980s (2). Even since then, however, it has continued to vary between dermatological centers and countries with regard to every procedural aspect, namely the selection of test substances, their concentrations, the allergen vehicles, the time schedule for allergen application, the spectral distribution of the irradiation sources, the irradiation doses, and the reading schedules for test reactions (2).

In comprehensive multicenter studies in Scandinavia and later Germany, Austria, and Switzerland (3–8) and in several other single center studies (9–12), however, continuing efforts have been made to standardize PPT technique. The information gathered from these has led to a greatly increased knowledge of the procedure, including, in particular, the variations and limitations in interpretation of its results. However, despite such efforts towards standardization, PPT methodology still varies considerably between countries and centers.

WHO IN A CENTER SHOULD UNDERTAKE PHOTOPATCHTES?

For any given center, PPTs may be conducted by either dermatologists or nondermatologist photobiologists. This itself has influenced PPT methodology, particularly with regard to how and when allergens are irradiated. In 2001, a survey of 40 known PPT centers in Europe yielded 34 replies, most (13) with separate photo-irradiation and contact allergy services. In those with separate services, the patches were applied in the contact unit and the irradiations performed by photobiology staff. Readings were also undertaken by the photobiology staff in 14 of these 21 centers, with contact staff performing them in seven. In the 13 centers with combined units, the readings were always performed by the contact specialists.

TEST SUBSTANCES

A standard photoallergen tray should include all the local environmental agents known to be photosensitizers. Such trays normally differ between centers, reflecting the geographic location of the unit and the population being tested. Ideally, the tray should be regularly updated with the addition of new potential photosensitizers within the population at risk and removal of

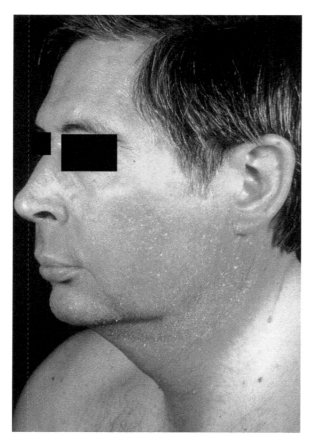

FIGURE 1 Photoallergic contact dermatitis. Dermatitis affecting predominantly exposed sites.

older products no longer used. This information is best acquired from both published reports incriminating new photoallergens and also large retrospective PPT studies, data from the latter clearly demonstrating how photoallergens change in relevance over time. Thus, in a multicenter study by Thune et al. (8), 1993 patients with a history and clinical features suggestive of photosensitivity were photopatch tested between 1980 and 1985. Photoallergic contact dermatitis was diagnosed in 10.9%, the fragrance, musk ambrette, being the most common photosensitizer responsible for 20% of positive reactions, with *para*-aminobenzoic acid the second most

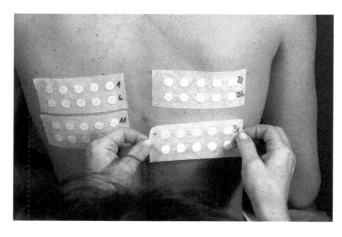

FIGURE 2 Photopatch test substances applied in duplicate on the back.

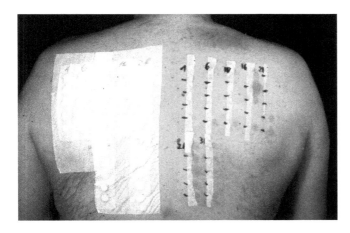

FIGURE 3 Positive photopatch test reaction (*Right side*) to ultraviolet filters. Negative test reaction at the unirradiated site (*Left*).

common and responsible for 16%. Darvay et al. (13) also conducted a retrospective analysis of 2715 patients tested between 1983 and 1998, finding that of the 2.3% of patients with photoallergic contact dermatitis, only 11% were sensitive to musk ambrette but 65% to ultraviolet (UV) sunscreen filters, most commonly benzophenone-3. This decrease in musk ambrette prevalence as a photosensitizer was the result of its removal from most world markets, whereas the UV filter increase reflected their rapidly growing use.

In the United States, between 1985 and 1990, DeLeo et al. (11) photopatch tested 187 patients with photosensitivity. Eleven percent were diagnosed with photoallergic contact dermatitis, most commonly from oxybenzone, with musk ambrette second. In another United States study, Fotiades et al. (14) tested 138 patients between 1986 and 1993, diagnosing photoallergic contact dermatitis in 12%. UV filters were again most commonly incriminated, responsible for 57% of cases, with fragrances responsible for 18%. These studies clearly illustrate how photoallergen prevalence can change over just a few years, reflecting their frequency of use in the population. The most common photosensitizers documented in retrospective PPT studies conducted between 1980 and 2002 are listed in Table 1. Such fluxes in photosensitizer prevalence reinforce the need for continuous re-evaluation of PPT allergen series.

Currently, organic sunscreens are the most common photoallergens in most populations tested and should be included in all trays. In countries where topical nonsteroidal

TABLE 1 Most Common Photosensitizers in Retrospective Studies of Photopatch Testing (1980–2002)

Location	Number of patients	Study period	% (+)	Top allergens
Scandinavia (8)	1993	1980–1985	11	Musk ambrette, *para*-aminobenzoic acid, promethazine, chlorpromazine
Minnesota (15)	70	1980–1985	20	Chlorpromazine, musk ambrette, promethazine
New York (11)	187	1985–1990	11	Sunscreen agents, antibacterials, fragrances
Austria, Germany, Switzerland (7)	1129	1985–1990	3.8	Tiaprofenic acid, fentichlor, carprofen, 4-isopropyl-dibenzoylmethane
New York (14)	138	1986–1993	12	Sunscreens, fragrances, antimicrobials
Rotterdam (9)	44	1989–1994	9	Chlorpromazine, promethazine, musk ambrette
Austria, Germany, Switzerland (7)	1261	1991–1997	8.1	Fenticlor, carprofen, chlorpromazine, 2-hydroxy-4-methoxybenzophenone
Australia (16)	81	1991–1999	39.5	Oxybenzone, benzophenone-4
France (17)	2067	1991–2001	41	Sesquiterpene lactone, ketoprofen, benzophenone, dibenzoylmethane
India (18)	50	1994–1999	20	Musk ambrette, chlorpromazine, promethazine, Balsam of Peru
Rotterdam (9)	55	1995–1999	27	Eusolex 8020, avobenzone, benzophenone-3
U.K., Europe (19)	1155	2000–2002	4	Oxybenzone

anti-inflammatory agents are routinely available, these agents should also be tested. It further seems reasonable that historic photosensitizers such as tetrachlorosalicylanilide might still be tested, as they may remain rare etiologic agents in chronic actinic dermatitis. A similar phenomenon is now commonly recognized in this disorder with airborne agents such as sesquiterpene lactone from Compositae plants (20), though this is more usually just a contact allergen. In addition to the standard photoallergens, relevant other agents should also be tested if there is an indication for this, such as, for example, chlorpromazine or in farmers olaquindox. The inclusion of plant and pesticide allergens has also been recommended (21). Thus, a modern photoallergen tray should integrate all photosensitizers relevant to the population being tested, with additional trays for special cases as suggested by the history. A comprehensive photoallergen series with recommended supplements is listed in Table 2.

Ultraviolet Dose

Although our knowledge of wavelength dependency for photoallergen activation is incomplete, the UVA (315–400 nm) radiation band is regularly used for photopatch testing, largely because most photoallergens for which information is available do react to this waveband. However, the irradiation doses used vary between centers, generally ranging between 5 and 15 J/cm^2, with 5 J/cm^2 being usual in Scandinavia, England, and Australia and 10 J/cm^2 in the United States. In patients with a known photosensitivity disorder such as chronic actinic dermatitis, however, a lower dose is often necessary to avoid flaring the underlying disease, some centers in fact performing minimal erythema dose (MED) testing beforehand and using 50% of the MED-A as the test dose (22).

METHODOLOGY

Despite the efforts toward standardization, PPT methodology varies between institutions. In all centers, however, duplicate sets of test materials should be applied in a similar array to both sides of the patient's back, starting 3 cm lateral to the vertebrae so as to avoid the paravertebral groove. MED testing may also be performed if necessary at this time. At 24 or 48 hours after application, one set of test agents should be uncovered, revealing the allergen-exposed sites for irradiation by a reliably calibrated and metered broad-spectrum UVA source. The duplicate allergen set on the contralateral back should remain fully covered and UV-protected throughout. Initial and follow-up PPT readings are then performed at specified times afterwards as discussed below. Details of PPT methodology as performed at the New York University Skin and Cancer Unit are depicted in Table 3.

There has been little consideration of exactly when allergens should be irradiated after their application, apart from in one retrospective review of 74 patients tested with three identical photoallergen sets, one irradiated at 24 hours, one at 48, and one nonirradiated as a control (23). There were 49 positive results in 15 patients, 34 consistent with photoallergy. Thirteen of these 34 were positive in both irradiated sets, five only in the set irradiated at 24 hours and 16 only in that at 48 hours. The authors therefore concluded that irradiation 48 hours after application might be more sensitive, given the greater number of positive results only in that set. Nevertheless, further studies are needed to confirm this, as well as to investigate the bioavailability of allergens at various application and irradiation times.

INTERPRETATION

Times at which PPT readings should be performed as well as the interpretation of results also vary between centers. A first reading should however be performed at either 24 or 48 hours after irradiation, with a second generally at 72 or 96 hours. The European consensus group has also agreed, in contrast with some previous recommendations in the literature (24), that readings should be recorded according to the International Contact Dermatitis Research Group scoring system (Table 4). Thus, they should include pre-irradiation, immediate post-irradiation, and 48-hour post-irradiation assessments. Further readings are also recommended

TABLE 2 Comprehensive Photoallergen Series

1	Octinoxate
2	Sulisobenzone (BZP-4) 10%
3	Thiourea (thiocarbamide) 0.1%
4	Dichlorophene 1%
5	Triclosan 2%
6	Hexachlorophene 1%
7	Chlorhexidine diacetate 0.5%
8	Sandalwood oil 2%
9	Musk ambrette 1%
10	Oxybenzone (BZP-3) 10%
11	Fenticlor (thiobis-chlorophenol) 1%
12	*Para*-aminobenzoic acid 10%
13	Octisalate
14	Tribromosalicylanilide 1%
15	Menthylanthranilate 5%
16	Sesquiterpene lactone mix 0.1%
17	Lichen acid mix 0.3%
18	Ketoprofen 5%
19	2-Hydroxy-methoxy-methyl-benzophenone 10%
20	Bithionol (thiobis-dichlorophenol) 1%
21	Octyldimethyl *para*-aminobezoic acid 10%
22	Phenylbenzimidazole sulphonic acid 10%
23	Homosalate 5%
24	Butyl methoxydibenzoylmethane 5%
25	Octyl methoxycinnamate 10%
26	4-Methylbenzylidene camphor 10%
27	Isoamyl *p*-methoxycinnamate 10%
28	Naproxen 5% in petrolatum
29	Ibuprofen 5% in petrolatum
30	Diclofenac 1% in petrolatum
31	Ketoprofen 2.5% in petrolatum
32	Tetrachlorosalicylanilide
33	Bromosalicylchloranilide
34	Buclosamide
35	Chlorpromazine
36	Chamomilla romana
37	Diallyldisulfide
38	Arnica montana
39	Taraxacum officinale
40	Achillea millefolium
41	Propolis
42	*Chrysanthemum cinerariaefolium*
43	Sesquiterpene lactone mix
44	A-methylene-Y-butyrolactone
45	Tanacetum vulgara
46	Alantolactone
47	Lichen acid mix
48	Captan
49	Zineb
50	Captafol
51	Maneb
52	Folpet
53	Pyrethrum
54	Benomyl
55	Ziram

Note: North American Contact Dermatitis Group Photoallergen Series (1–24). New York University Skin and Cancer Unit Supplemental Series (36–55).

TABLE 3   Methodology of Photopatch Testing as Performed at New York University Skin and Cancer Unit

Day 1	Perform MED testing. Apply duplicate sets of photoallergens on left and right back
Day 2	Read MEDs. Irradiate one set of allergens with UVA (10 mJ/cm^2 or 50% of MED-A, whichever is less), covering the other with an opaque material
Day 3	Remove nonirradiated patches and perform first reading of reactions to both sets of photoallergens (irradiated and nonirradiated sites)
Day 5	Perform second reading of reactions to both sets of photoallergens

Abbreviation: MED, minimal erythema dose.

TABLE 4   International Contact Dermatitis Research Group Scoring System

±	Doubtful reaction (faint erythema only)
+	Weak positive reaction (erythema, infiltration, possibly papules)
++	Strong positive reaction (erythema, infiltration, papules, vesicles)
+++	Extreme positive reaction (intense erythema, infiltration, coalescing vesicles or bulla
IR	Irritant reaction
NT	Not tested

at 72 and 96 hours to detect reaction patterns such as crescendo, decrescendo, combined or plateau, suggesting allergic, nonallergic, or combined mechanisms, respectively. This full assessment of such variations can be particularly important and sometimes specific for a photosensitizer (25), especially agents with phototoxic and photoallergic potential (26).

The interpretation of PPTs as used in most United States centers is outlined in Table 5. If there is no reaction at either the irradiated or the nonirradiated sites, this is interpreted as an absence of contact or photocontact allergy. If there is a positive reaction only at the irradiated site, this is interpreted as just photocontact allergy. If there is an equally positive reaction at both sites, this is considered as just contact allergy. Finally, if there are positive reactions at both sites but more marked at the irradiated site, a diagnosis of combined contact and photo-contact allergy is made. There is variation among centers in regard to this last interpretation; however, both the United States Mayo Clinic and Scandinavian groups regard a positive reaction at both sites as representative only of contact allergy, even if one reaction is more positive than the other. However, there has been no formal validation of this. Although it would seem logical that a reaction of greater intensity at an irradiated site compared with a non-irradiated one would establish combined contact and photocontact allergy, the converse argument is also possible. Thus, concordance studies in the evaluation of patch test results have shown that positive reactions are not always reproducible in intensity. Rietschel et al. (27), for example, evaluated 48 patients with known positive response to epoxy resin, nickel, and ethylenediamine by both the Finn Chamber and True Test methods, and found equal intensities 67% of the time, but clear differences on 27% of occasions. It therefore seems that reactions of different intensities to the same allergen in the same patient are possible through testing procedure limitations and perhaps also site-specific immunological variations. Repeat PPTs in any given patient would clearly always be necessary to try and assess the true situation.

TABLE 5   Interpretation of Photopatch Tests

	Reading	
Diagnosis	Irradiated site	Nonirradiated site
No sensitivity	−	−
Photocontact allergy	+	−
Contact allergy	+	+
Photocontact allergy and contact allergy[a]	++	+

[a]The Mayo Clinic and Scandinavian groups do not recognize a diagnosis of combined photoallergy and contact allergy. This outcome would be read as contact allergy only.

Nevertheless, it is essential that PPT interpretation guidelines should always remain consistent within a given center.

RELEVANCE

Subsequent to the evaluation of PPT reactions, an interpretation of their relevance to the patient is also essential. A system developed for the similar assessment of positive patch test reactions (COADEX) (28) may also be used for PPTs as follows:

- Current relevance (the patient has had allergen exposure during the current episode of dermatitis and improved when exposure ceased)
- Cross-reaction (the patient has had exposure to a cross-reacting allergen)
- Old or past relevance (the patient has had a past dermatitis from allergen exposure)
- Actively sensitized (the patient has presented with a late sensitization reaction from allergen exposure during testing)
- Do not know (the patient has had allergen exposure but it is not clear if this is current or old)
- EXposed (the patient has a history of allergen exposure but no dermatitis or no history of exposure but a definite positive allergic patch test).

[*C*, current; *O*, old; *A*, actively sensitized; *D*, do not know; *EX*, exposed (COADEX)].

CONCLUSION

Photopatch testing remains the gold standard for the detection of chemical substances responsible for the onset and perpetuation of dermatitis on photo-exposed skin. It is also the only established method potentially able to distinguish between contact and photocontact allergy. Although some variability exists worldwide regarding the methodology of such testing, these differences may be clinically minimized through a careful study of the at-risk population and its allergen exposure and the consistent execution of established PPT protocols.

REFERENCES

1. Epstein S. Photoallergy and primary photosensitivity to sulphanilamide. J Invest Dermatol 1939; 2:43–51.
2. Hölzle E, Plewig G, Hoffmann C, Braun-Falco O. Photpatchtesting: results of a survey on test procedures and experimental findings. Z Hautkr 1985; 151:361–365.
3. Hölzle E, Neumann J, Hausen B, et al. Photopatch testing: the 5-year experience of the German, Austrian, and Swiss Photopatch Test Group. J Am Acad Dermatol 1991; 25:59–68.
4. Jansen CT, Wennersten G, Rystedt I, Thune P, Brodthagen H. The Scandinavian standard photopatch test procedure. Contact Dermatitis 1982; 8:155–158.
5. Neumann NJ, Hölzle E, Plewig G, et al. Photopatch testing: the 12-year experience of the German, Austrian, and Swiss photopatch test group. J Am Acad Dermatol 2000; 42:183–192.
6. Neumann NJ, Fritsch C, Lehmann P. Photodiagnostic test methods. 1: stepwise light exposure and the photopatch test. Hautarzt 2000; 51:113–125.
7. Neumann NJ, Lehmann P. The photopatch test procedure of the German, Austrian and Swiss photopatch test group. Photodermatol Photoimmunol Photomed 2003; 19:8–10.
8. Thune P, Jansen C, Wennersten G, Rystedt I, Brodthagen H, McFadden N. The Scandinavian multicenter photopatch study 1980–1985: final report. Photodematol 1988; 6:261–269.
9. Bakkum RSLA, Heule F. Results of photopatch testing in Rotterdam during a 10-year period. Br J Dermatol 2002; 146:275–279.
10. Berne B, Ros AM. 7-years experience of photopatch testing with sunscreen allergens in Sweden. Contact Dermatitis 1998; 38:61–64.
11. DeLeo VA, Suarez SM, Maso MJ. Photoallergic contact dermatitis: results of photopatch testing in New York; 1985–1990. Arch Dermatol 1992; 128:1513–1518.
12. Schauder S, Ippen H. Contact and photocontact sensitity to sunscreens: review of a 15-year experience of the literature. Contact Dermatitis 1997; 37:221–232.
13. Darvay A, White IR, Rycroft RJG, Jones AB, Hawk JLM, McFadden JP. Photoallergic contact dermatitis is uncommon. Br J Dermatol 2001; 145(4):597–601.
14. Fotiades J, Soter NA, Lim HW. Results of evaluation of 203 patients for photosensitivity in a 7.3-year period. J Am Acad Dermatol 1995; 33:597–602.

15. Menz J, Muller SA, Connolly SM. Photopatch testing: a six-year experience. J Am Acad Dermatol 1988; 18:1044–1047.
16. Lee PA, Freeman S. Photosensitivity: the 9-year experience at a Sydney contact dermatitis clinic. Australas J Dermatol 2002; 43:289–292.
17. Leonard F, Adamski H, Bonnevalle A, et al. The prospective multicenter study on standard photo-patch tests by the French Society of Photodermatology from 1991–2001. Ann Dermatol Venereol 2005; 132(4):313–320.
18. Kanchan PA, Shenoi SD, Balachandran C. Five years' experience of photopatch testing in 50 patients. Indian J Dermatol Venereol Leprol 2002; 68:86–87.
19. Bryden AM, Ibbotson SH, Ferguson J. Photopatch testing: results of the U.K. multicentre photopatch study. Br J Dermatol 2003; 149(suppl 64):3.
20. Lim HW, Cohen D, Soter NA. Chronic actinic dermatitis: results of patch and photopatch tests with *Compositae*, fragrances, and pesticides. J Am Acad Dermatol 1998; 38:108–111.
21. Mark KA, Brancaccio RR, Soter NA, Cohen DE. Allergic contact and photoallergic contact dermatitis to plant and pesticide allergens. Arch Dermatol 1999; 135(1):67–70.
22. Przybilla B, Hölzle E, Enders F, Gollhausen R, Ring J. Photopatch testing with different ultraviolet A sources can yield discrepant test results. Photodermatol Photoimmunol Photomed 1991; 8:57–61.
23. Batchelor RJ, Wilkinson SM. Photopatch testing—a restrospective review using the 1 day and 2 day irradiation protocols. Contact Dermatitis 2006; 54:75–78.
24. Bruynzeel DP, Ferguson J, Andersen K, et al. Photopatch testing: a consensus methodology for Europe. J Eur Acad Dermatol Venereol 2004; 18:679–682.
25. Neumann NJ, Hölzle E, Lehmann P, Benedikter S, Tapernoux B, Plewig G. Pattern analysis of photopatch test reactions. Photodermatol Photoimmunol Photomed 1994; 10:65–73.
26. Neumann NJ, Hölzle E, Lehmann P. Guidelines for phototoxic and photoallergic reactions. J Dtsch Dermatol Ges 2004; 2:710–716.
27. Rietschel RL, Marks JG, Adams RM, et al. Preliminary studies of the TRUE Test patch test system in the United States. J Am Acad Dermatol 1989; 21:841–843.
28. Bourke J, Coulson I, English J. Guidelines for care of contact dermatitis. Br J Dermatol 2001; 145:877–885.

Appendix C

Guidelines for Setting Up a Phototherapy Referral Center or an Office-Based Phototherapy Unit

Michael Zanolli
Division of Dermatology, Vanderbilt University Medical Center, Vanderbilt University, Nashville, Tennessee, U.S.A.

Roy Palmer
Photobiology Unit, St. John's Institute of Dermatology, St. Thomas' Hospital, London, England, U.K.

INTRODUCTION

Phototherapy for psoriasis and other photoresponsive dermatoses remains an essential therapeutic tool for a dermatologist. Specialized facilities with the full range of irradiation options serve as a major resource for the region or city they serve. In general, such a phototherapy referral center is located in a densely populated urban area to serve a large referring physician and patient base, and should preferably also be the location for photodiagnostic procedures to help evaluate difficult photodermatoses. In a less-populated local community or rural region, the needs and basic services clearly differ from those of such a major referral center. Although a small office- or clinic-based phototherapy unit will be limited in equipment and staffing, the majority of patients likely to undergo the treatment will have psoriasis and need only simple whole-body UVB treatment as either broadband (BB) or narrowband (NB) UVB. These patients are better served locally rather than needing to travel to a major center, where specialized treatments such as bath psoralen plus ultraviolet A (PUVA) or UVA-1 therapy will also be available at a site designed to accommodate a high volume of patients.

Much is justifiably made of the sophisticated equipment and physical facilities necessary for the high quality patient evaluations and treatment offered at such centers. The experience of the authors however also recognizes the invaluable contributions of their staff, also a major contribution in office-based units. The dermatologist can certainly evaluate and set forth an appropriate course of action but unless there are trained personnel to execute and monitor the treatments, the results will often not be optimal or even effective. Careful consideration must therefore be given to dedicated staffing when planning a center and also when considering adding an ultraviolet (UV) unit in the office.

The guidelines set forth here concerning the two main type of treatment settings mentioned above are intentionally concise and discuss only the essential points needed.

PHOTOTHERAPY REFERRAL CENTER (TABLE 1)
Space

Within the hospital, a phototherapy unit benefits greatly from being close to the dermatology outpatient center, to ensure close cooperation between the two units. This phototherapy center needs its own reception and waiting area, in addition to individual patient phototherapy rooms or cubicles, a bath or shower facility, a storage area, and a patient lounge.

When determining the number of treatment rooms or cubicles required, it should be remembered that a minimum patient treatment slot is about 15 minutes. Therefore, given that a typical unit is open for about eight hours per day, and that some patients may wish for or need twice weekly therapy (Tuesday and Thursday) and others three times weekly

TABLE 1 Requirements for a University Center Treating Approximately 75 Patients Per Week with Phototherapy

Space	80 m²
Equipment	1 UVA whole-body unit
	1 Medium dose UVA-1 unit (optional)
	1 NBUVB whole-body unit
	1 BBUVB whole-body unit
	1 combined NBUVB/UVA whole-body unit
	1 Canopy unit
	1 Bath
	1 Hand-foot unit or localized delivery unit
	1 Shower
	Waiting room
	Reception area
	Storage room
Staff	2 Full-time nursing staff
	1 Administrative staff (receptionist)

Abbreviations: BBUVB, broadband ultraviolet B; NBUVB, narrowband ultraviolet B.

(Monday, Wednesday, and Friday), the theoretical maximum number of patients able to be treated each week in one room or cubicle is 64. In reality, however, taking account of logistical factors, it will be less than this. Some phototherapy cabinets offer a choice of two types of lamp giving increased flexibility, but each exposure then takes longer because of the decreased irradiance from the smaller numbers of each lamp type. The special electrical supply required needs to be installed in collaboration with a competent electrician and, in many cases, will be of relatively high voltage such as, for example, 415 V. Dedicated air flow, both intake and outlet, and cooling systems are essential within the treatment rooms or cubicles to maintain a comfortable temperature and efficient functioning of the lamps, since major heat output is a by-product of all irradiation units. This is an even more critical consideration if a UVA-1 unit is installed, whether for high or medium dose irradiation.

Most stand-up commercial irradiation cabinets measure approximately 1.4 × 1.4 m, and a similarly sized adjoining area is required for the patient to undress. Curtains suspended from the ceiling, or room walls and doors, are essential to provide patient privacy in the undressing area. Hand and foot units on the other hand measure approximately 0.7 × 0.7 m and do not necessarily require such a large adjoining area or any partitioning. Localized UVB delivery is also now available from units on desktops or on carts, to enable transport from room to room.

The waiting area is important because it may often be where patients spend most of their time: magazines, music, and educational posters should be made available as appropriate. A floor of nondark color so as to conceal any psoriatic scale is preferable. A shower for patients who perspire significantly during treatment and to wash off topical therapies is also essential. Finally, storage areas are necessary for spare lamps, towels, gowns, pillowcases, emollients, sunscreens, and cleaning supplies.

Staff

A receptionist, phototherapy technician, who may often be a nurse, and a lead nurse are the core staffing. Either special training at courses designed for phototherapy technicians or a set of procedures to be taught by the lead nurse is essential to achieve the level of care required of a phototherapy center, especially since nursing school curricula do not provide adequate course work for this.

Flexibility within the working week is another important point for consideration. In most instances, phototherapy is optimally delivered two or three times weekly, and many patients therefore prefer the convenience of attending slightly outside normal working hours, so a center offering appointments between 8 am and 7 pm on at least two days a week is much appreciated. It should also be remembered that many other patients prefer their treatments at peak hours, such that multiple treatments will be needed simultaneously, and staffing arrangements should take note of this. Further, it is not unusual for patients to arrive early or late, or to have taken their psoralen medication at the wrong time, or to have additional requirements such as requests for advice concerning topical therapies, and flexibility to cope with these variations is also essential. Procedure manuals should provide full guidelines concerning all these matters.

Equipments
Stand-Up Whole-Body Units
For most patients affected by generalized eruptions, these are most appropriate. Such units should always be open at the top to allow heat release and give patients a less claustrophobic impression.

Hand and Foot Units
Hand and foot units are very useful, both for supplemental treatment to palms and soles for patients having whole-body therapy, and also for the dedicated therapy of those only affected on the hands and feet. Palms and soles respond very poorly to BB and usually also NBUVB therapy, and PUVA units are therefore preferable for this therapy.

Canopy Units
These consist of flat or nearly flat panels of lamps for the treatment of localized areas. They are also useful for minimal erythema dose (MED) and minimal phototoxic dose (MPD) testing prior to whole-body phototherapy, provided that the lamps are the same as those in the whole-body units and that the lamp calibrations are in close agreement. They are useful too for UVA delivery during diagnostic photopatch testing and also for provocation testing in abnormal photosensitivity.

Localized Delivery
The excimer laser is a self-contained unit not requiring a separate cooling supply, which may be used to target localized psoriatic lesions. More recent compact BB and NBUVB delivery systems are also available, and these may also be conveniently placed on a desktop or else on a cart for easy transport from room to room.

Fluorescent Lamps
Broadband UVB
Two of the commonest of these are the Waldmann UV6 and Waldmann UV21 lamps, the latter identical also to the Philips TL-12. The output of all is predominantly within the UVB range, but the UV21 and TL-12 tubes emit a greater proportion of wavelengths below 290 nm, more erythemogenic, and also ineffective against psoriasis (1), such that the UV6 is theoretically preferable for BBUVB phototherapy.

Narrowband UVB (TL-01)
These Philips lamps have a very narrow emission spectrum, emitting predominantly within the range of 311 to 312.

PUVA
There are several UVA lamps marketed for PUVA therapy, all with similar emission spectra and all appropriate for such use.

Ultraviolet A-1
There is a major distinction between the equipment necessary to deliver high dose and medium dose UVA-1 phototherapy. Only very specialist referral centers will wish to provide the major weight bearing and demanding cooling requirements necessary for high dose systems. However, medium dose units are similar in size and specification to routine PUVA units, apart from their much longer treatment times and greater heat generation.

All the above lamps also emit at least some visible light, such that it is clear when they are switched on. In addition, they should have Perspex screens or Teflon sleeves to protect patients from falling against and breaking them, although still allowing adequate UV transmission. They will also prevent injury if a lamp implodes, which is very rarely possible.

Procedures
Dosimetry
In the past, some centers have used treatment times as the only monitored variable. This is extremely undesirable, however. A knowledge of the actual dose administered through accurate dosimetry being essential for safe phototherapy. There are two options to achieve this:

1. Automatic dosimetry (radiometry). In this situation, the operator enters the *dose* to be administered, and a built-in dosimeter measures the accumulating radiation during exposure before terminating the session, when the desired dose has been achieved. This is convenient, but for safety any such unit should sound an immediate alarm if the measured irradiance suddenly decreases, suggesting that the patient's body may suddenly have blocked the detector. The detector should also be cleaned regularly to remove any dirt obscuring it. Internal dosimeters require regular checks for accuracy, for example, every six months, as described next.
2. Intermittent dosimetry (radiometry). In this case, the output of the unit is regularly measured, for example, every four weeks. This measured output is then used to calculate the exposure time required according to time = dose/irradiance, such that for each treatment the operator enters the *time* to be administered.

Calibration of dosimeters has been found to vary considerably between centers, NBUVB output measurements varying by a factor of at least 2.7 between units in the United Kingdom (2). A detailed description of dosimetry and calibration procedures is provided elsewhere (3), but in brief, preferably under the supervision of a medical physicist or the cabinet manufacturer's engineer, the irradiance within a stand-up unit may be checked accurately with a radiometer on a tripod ("indirect method"), or else by a member of staff in protective clothing standing within the unit holding the dosimeter ("direct method"). This latter method produces a reading more accurately representing "real-life" patient irradiance, and is typically 20% less, depending on the cabinet design, than the former. If this variation is always taken into account through the use of the appropriate "shielding factor" to correct up to the true dose, the indirect method is acceptable. Shielding factors for some cabinets have been published (4), but should be checked at least annually for each cabinet to allow for possible changes in the unit's optical properties. Dosimeters themselves also require validation, preferably annually, by a recognized physics laboratory. Finally, within any center, all these procedures for dosimetry should be rigorously standardized.

Records should also be kept by each unit detailing the dates of lamp replacement, numbers of hours of lamp use, and dosimeter calibration dates with the measured irradiances at those times.

Because changes in lamp temperature during operation influence their output, manufacturers' advice on lamp warming prior to the therapy should always be followed if a lamp has been allowed to cool, and especially at the start of a working day.

Lamp Changes
By 12 hours of use, lamp outputs will have always reduced by approximately 10%, by 2000 hours by more than 50%, and by 3000 hours they will have ceased to function entirely. There are two approaches to dealing with this:

1. Replacing all lamps at 1000 to 2000 hours. This has the disadvantages of being costly and resulting in abrupt output changes requiring fresh calibration.
2. Waiting until approximately three or four lamps within a unit have ceased to operate and replacing only those. If the unit dosimeter is not built in, it will have to be recalibrated at

this time. Treatment times will be longer with this approach but output changes with new lamps will be less marked.

Therapy Guidelines

The administration of phototherapy requires many choices, examples including the following. Will the center employ starting doses based on skin type, or MED and MPD testing? If the former, will localized test doses be administered beforehand to exclude pathological photo-sensitivity? If the latter, what anatomical site will be used to test the MED or MPD, and what will be the timing of the MPD reading (72 or 96 hours)? What doses will be used to assess the MED and MPD? For bath PUVA, what concentration of psoralen will be used in the bath water? Will there be a maximum dose for therapy?

Unfortunately, for many such issues the evidence base is weak. However, some off-the--shelf guidance is available, as in "Phototherapy Treatment Protocols" (5) and "Evidence-Based Phototherapy Guidelines" (6).

Recording Treatments

Computerized methods for recording patient exposure data have been developed but are infre-quently used, paper records still being usual. Whatever method is used, however, it is essential to record the following at each patient visit: date of visit, patient side effects after last session, increment in dose since previous visit, exposure dose at this visit, cumulative dose, additional or reduced therapy to particular anatomical sites, and exposure time if an external dosimeter is used.

In most major phototherapy centers, patient phototherapy records are kept separately from the main hospital notes. It is therefore highly beneficial if the number of phototherapy ses-sions, cumulative dose, side effects, and efficacy of therapy are made available to the dermatol-ogist by the phototherapy unit for patient consultations.

Safety Guidelines

In most settings, local rules for UV installations apply. These details, for example, that eye protection for staff and patients is mandatory, and that eyewear should be checked regularly for UV transmission. For staff working close to cabinets, it is also important that the environ-mental UV level be checked when open-topped cabinets are switched on; U.K. regulations state that UVA exposure should not exceed 1 mW/cm^2. This is facilitated if the ceiling is not reflective, and high curtains surround the cabinets.

Forms

Arrangements should be made prior to therapy for patients to receive information about their therapy in the form of a handout (describing, for example, the importance of using emollients, correct posture in the cabinet, proper use of eye protection, and so on) and sign a consent form. Arrangements to review the patient every 6 to 10 sessions should be made. For children, phototherapy units may be very daunting, and time should be spent explaining to them how the machine works and how it helps their skin. Regular audit of activity is also important to ensure continuing effective and safe phototherapy.

Ancillary Equipment

In addition to the equipment above, many other miscellaneous items are essential, particularly goggles, visors, glasses, pillowcases, gowns, sunscreens, stopwatches, and a hand-held dosimeter to ensure there is no UV transmission through patients' spectacles.

OFFICE-BASED PHOTOTHERAPY UNIT
Space

The estimate of one treatment every 15 minutes holds true for both office and hospital clinic-based phototherapy units. The room used for the phototherapy does not have to be any larger than a normal clinic examination room and should be an integral part of the design of the clinic also accommodating patients, administrative staff, nurses, and dermatologists. Storage space for eye protection, gowns, and other immediate necessities for treatment can be kept in this same room.

The modifications to an existing examination room needed to transform it into a phototherapy room are: special electrical requirements dependent on manufacturers' regulations and local requirements, probable modifications to the air intake and outflow systems to permit increased heat disposal, and privacy curtains for patient dressing and undressing.

Staff

There should not be any need for added personnel in the office or hospital clinic while a new phototherapy service is being initiated, just a slight adjustment to the normal clinic flow to enable a nurse to act also as a phototherapy technician. However, as the number of photo-therapy treatments moves above 15 treatments a day, the unit will come to need more space and staffing.

Equipment
Whole-Body Unit

The single most useful phototherapy unit is an upright whole-body cabinet, whereas the most useful and safest therapeutic waveband for the widest variety of problems seen in the private office or hospital clinic is NBUVB. A question the clinician must also address is whether or not there is a need for PUVA to treat cutaneous T cell lymphoma (CTCL) in the clinic. If not, because CTCL patients are referred to a major phototherapy center, an NBUVB unit will provide treatment for most patients requiring UV therapy, although severe psoriatics may sometimes do better with PUVA. In addition, there are also creditable reports of efficacy for stages 1A and 1B CTCL with NBUVB.

Combination units offering both NBUVB and UVA lamps are an option for units wishing to provide both NBUVB and PUVA. However, this approach will lengthen the time needed for both treatments, since the numbers of lamps in the unit providing each will be smaller.

Another consideration is to make available a localized delivery system for UVB offering a small spot size. These units are now more readily available and obviate the need for a laser device. They might also be used for localized treatment of the hands and feet, so avoiding the need for a separate hand and foot fluorescent unit.

Procedures
Dosimetry

Dosimetry is just as important for the single unit in the office as for a large treatment center. Internal dosimetry is more convenient in most cases since patients will not be switching cabinets during a treatment course, as often happens in a large center. Even so, periodic cali-bration of the internal sensor should be undertaken as described above for major referral centers to ensure accurate UV dose calculation, particularly as patients moving to another city will need to take a correct dose record with them for future treatment.

Lamp Changes

This is the major expense of the unit after the initial cabinet purchase cost. Lamp life depends on the number of hours of use. Two approaches for changing lamps have been previously suggested for major referral centers. In an office or clinic with only one unit, however, it is easier to change all the lamps at one time, either after 2000 hours of operation or once the irradiance of a unit appreciably diminishes. This decreases the need for lamp storage and also prevents uneven distribution of light within the cabinet.

Protocols are available for both MED-based treatments and treatment courses based on the Fitzpatrick skin type of the individual. Attending nursing staffs need a set protocol to enable them to advance patient therapy, without constant review by the attending physician. Measurement of the MED is not a complicated procedure even in an office-based treatment setting, and gives valuable information such as a basis for the treatment starting dose and also whether there may be abnormal patient photosensitivity.

Defined protocols as stated above are available in at least two manuals, namely "Phototherapy Treatment Protocols" (5), and "Evidence-Based Phototherapy Guidelines" (6).

Recording Treatments

It is essential that the following information be recorded each time a patient visits the unit: date of visit, side effects after last session, increment in dose since previous visit, exposure dose at this visit, cumulative dose, additional or reduced therapy to particular anatomical sites, and exposure time if an external dosimeter is used. Examples of such daily treatment records are again available in the referenced treatment protocol and treatment guidelines manuals previously mentioned (5,6).

Safety Guidelines

In most settings, the development of specific local rules for UV installations is essential. These will detail, for example, that eye protection for staff and patients is mandatory and that eyewear must be checked regularly for efficacy of UV protection. Close to cabinets, it is important that the environmental UV level be checked when open-topped cabinets are switched on; U.K. regulations, for example, state that UVA exposure should not exceed 1 mW/cm^2. This is easier to achieve if the ceiling is not reflective, and high curtains surround the cabinets.

Forms

Arrangements should be made prior to therapy for patients to sign a consent form, receive a handout containing information about their therapy (describing, for example, the importance of using emollients, correct posture in the cabinet, proper use of eye protection, and so on). Arrangements for the attending physician to review the patient every 6 to 10 sessions should also be made. For children, phototherapy units may be very daunting, and time should therefore be spent explaining to them how the machine works and how it helps their skin. Regular audit of activity is also important to ensure continuing effective and safe phototherapy.

REFERENCES

1. Ibbotson SH, Bilsland D, Cox NH. An update and guidance on narrowband ultraviolet B phototherapy: a British Photodermatology Group Workshop Report. Br J Dermatol 2004; 151(2):283–297.
2. Lloyd JJ. Variation in calibration of hand-held ultraviolet (UV) meters for psoralen plus UVA and narrow-band UVB phototherapy. Br J Dermatol 2004; 150(6):1162—1166.
3. Taylor DK, Anstey AV, Coleman AJ, et al. Guidelines for dosimetry and calibration in ultraviolet radiation therapy: a report of a British Photodermatology Group workshop. Br J Dermatol 2002; 146(5):755–763.
4. Moseley H. Scottish UV dosimetry guidelines, "ScUViDo". Photodermatol Photoimmunol Photomed 2001; 17(5):230–233.
5. Zanolli MD, Feldman SR, eds. Phototherapy Treatment Protocols for Psoriasis and Other Phototherapy Responsive Dermatoses. 2nd ed. London: Taylor and Francis, 2005.
6. Palmer RA, Garibaldinos T, Hawk JLM. Evidence-Based Phototherapy Guidelines. Available from: Dr Roy Palmer, Photobiology Unit, Second Floor, St. John's Institute of Dermatology, St. Thomas' Hospital, London, U.K.

FURTHER READING

Coleman AJ. A Template of Local Rules for Operation of a Phototherapy Unit.

Available from: Dr AJ Coleman, UV Calibration Unit, Medical Physics Department, St. Thomas' Hospital, London, U.K.

Morison WL. Phototherapy and Photochemotherapy of Skin Disease. 3rd ed. Taylor and Francis, 2005.

Taylor CR, Ortel B. Basic guidelines on the establishment of a UVB/PUVA treatment centre. Appendix C. In: Hawk JLM, ed. Photodermatology. London: Arnold, 1999.

Appendix D
Guidelines for Setting Up a Laser Center

Macrene R. Alexiades-Armenakas
Department of Dermatology, Yale University School of Medicine, New Haven, Connecticut, U.S.A.

Jeffrey S. Dover
Department of Dermatology, Yale University School of Medicine, New Haven, Connecticut, and Dartmouth Medical School, Hanover, New Hampshire, U.S.A.

INTRODUCTION

In setting up a laser center, the major considerations include the selection of lasers for the practice and laser safety guidelines. The major categories of laser and light treatment, including treatment of vascular and pigmented lesions, hair removal, tattoo removal, wrinkle reduction, and skin rejuvenation, should ideally be offered in a comprehensive unit. At least one device should be selected in each category and strict laser safety guidelines and staff training should be implemented. Laser use standards must be maintained among laser practices to ensure proper protection to office staff and patients.

LASER SELECTION

Tables 1–4 list the most commonly employed laser systems in each main category of treatment. A thorough examination of each group should be considered along with the patient population in one's practice. For example, if one is commonly treating facial erythema and telangiectasia, more than one laser from the vascular category might be selected. If one's practice treats a significant proportion of dark-skinned patients, lasers that are safest in this patient group should be selected from each category. In most cases, at least one laser or other light source should be selected from each category.

LASER SAFETY

The other crucial step in setting up a laser center is to implement guidelines for laser safety. The American National Standards Institute (ANSI) is a private, nonprofit organization, which provides voluntary standardization and assessment of laser practices. Its pertinent standards regarding laser safety include ZI36.3-2005, the Safe Use of Lasers in Health Care Facilities, Z136.1-2000, the Safe Use of Lasers, and Z136.5-2000, the Safe Use of Lasers in Educational Institutions (1–3). Among these, ANSI ZI36.3 is the general standard for laser centers to follow (1). The key points to these standards include the appointment of a laser safety officer (LSO) and control measures for prevention of accidents or injury.

The LSO serves as the liaison between regulatory agencies and the center. The officer's responsibilities include monitoring and reporting hazards, enforcing compliance with control measures, providing policies and procedures in writing, evaluating and approving protective gear, implementing safety training and education, arranging maintenance and service of laser equipment, supervising daily operations, and reviewing and updating standards, regulations, and legal requirements. It is generally agreed that an individual be appointed as an LSO and assume these important responsibilities at the outset of setting up the center (4).

The second main components to the ANSI standards are control measures to protect patients and staff from both direct and nonbeam laser hazards (1,4). Such control measures include engineering controls, which comprise the built-in safety features of the laser

TABLE 1   Vascular Lasers

Laser options	Wavelengths (nm)	Indications
Pulsed dye	585, 590, 595, and 600	Port-wine stains, rosacea, facial telangiectasia, hemangiomas, cherry angiomas, spider leg telangiectasia, keloids, striae, and verrucae
Variable pulsed green	532	Facial telangiectasia, rosacea, spider leg telangiectasia, venous malformations, and cherry angiomas
Long-pulsed alexandrite	755	Spider leg telangiectasia and nodular port-wine stains
Diode	800–810	Spider leg venulectasia and telangiectasia, reticular blue veins
Long-pulsed Nd:YAG	1064	Spider leg venulectasia and telangiectasia, reticular blue veins, facial telangiectasia, and nodular port-wine stains
Intense pulsed light	400–1200	Rosacea, facial telangiectasia, and spider leg telangiectasia

systems. These include the key lock, emission indicators, and aperture covers or shutters. Administrative control measures include the LSO and their responsibilities, education and training programs for all staff, and a system in place for reporting hazards. Procedural control measures involve the steps taken prior to and during every laser operation, such as limiting treatment room access to laser-trained personnel, preparation of a nonflammable operative site, placement of proper protective eyewear, plume evacuation, and assisting the physician (5). Finally, protective equipment control measures encompass the provision of labeled protective eyewear, window barriers, room signage, fire extinguishers, facemasks, plume evacuators, nonflammable drapes, and anodized instruments. These control measures serve to address the hazards unique to laser operation.

The ANSI standards provide a credible basis for laser safety guidelines within a laser center. The U.S. Occupational Safety and Health Administration (OSHA) cites the ANSI standards. The OSHA also has guidelines for laser safety and hazard assessment (STD 01-05-001 (1991) (6). In addition, once these laser safety standards have been put in place, accreditation confirming that the center is in conformity with such standards may be attained (7). The ANSI provides accreditation services, as does the Joint Commission for Accreditation of Healthcare Organizations (JCAHO) and the Accreditation Association for Ambulatory Health Care (AAAHC). While accreditation is costly and time-consuming, making it unrealistic for most small laser centers, it is the highest standard towards which facilities may strive to achieve.

DOCUMENTATION
Consent Forms

In starting a laser practice, it is imperative to review all the potential complications of each type of laser system and prepare written documentation for patient consent forms. The most common complications are included in the consenting process. It is very helpful to have a separate consent form for every group of lasers and light sources. Having a single general consent to cover all laser, light-based and surgical procedures is not considered the highest

TABLE 2   Lasers for Pigmented Lesions and Tattoos

Laser type	Wavelength (nm)	Target skin structure	Tattoo color
Q-switched lasers			
Q-switched Nd:YAG	532	Lentigines, ephelids, and CALM	Yellow, orange, red, and purple
Q-switched ruby	694	Lentigines, nevi, and CALM	Green, blue, and black
Q-switched alexandrite	755	Lentigines, nevi, and CALM	Green, blue, and black
Q-switched Nd:YAG	1064	Nevi and CALM	Blue and black
Long-pulsed lasers			
Diode	800	Lentigines and Nevi	NA
Nd:YAG (1064 nm)	1064	Nevi	NA
Intense pulsed light	500–1200	Lentigines	NA

Abbreviations: CALM, café au lait macule; NA, not applicable; Nd:YAG, neodymium:yttrium-aluminum-garnet.

TABLE 3 Lasers for Hair Removal

Laser type	Wavelength (nm)	Skin type
Long-pulsed lasers		
Alexandrite	755	I–III
Diode	800	I–VI
Nd:YAG	1064	I–VI
Intense pulsed light	510–1200	I–III

standard of care. However, one consent form can be created to cover a group of laser procedures. An example of a general laser consent form is shown in Figure 1.

Operative Report

The type of laser used, wavelength, fluence, spot size, pulse duration, and areas treated need to be documented in reproducible fashion. Many laser centers employ standard forms for the physician, an example of which is shown in Figure 2.

Postoperative Instructions

The postoperative period following laser treatment contains unique sequelae, which require their own instruction sheet. Considerations during post-laser recovery include the avoidance of sun exposure, possibility of blistering, crusting or dyspigmentation, and specific wound care. An example of a postlaser instruction sheet is shown in Figure 3.

PRACTICAL CONSIDERATIONS FOR THE PHYSICIAN

When first starting laser surgery, it is imperative to be very familiar with the parameters of each laser system and the potential complications. It is often helpful for the beginner to attach parameter guidelines to each laser, which can be used as a reference during treatment. Beginner

TABLE 4 Lasers for Wrinkle Reduction and Skin Rejuvenation

Laser	Advantages	Disadvantages
Nonablative		
Vascular lasers (LP 532 nm, PDL 585 nm and 595 nm)	Excellent safety, no recovery time, and improvement in telangiectasia	Minimal efficacy, multiple treatments necessary
Near-infrared lasers (1320 nm, 1450 nm, and 1540 nm)	Excellent safety, no recovery time, higher efficacy for rhytides, and acne scars	Modest efficacy, painful, multiple treatments necessary
Intense pulsed light	Moderate safety, no recovery time, and improvement in telangiectasia and pigment	Minimum-to-modest efficacy, multiple treatments necessary
Radiofrequency	Excellent safety, no recovery time, and efficacy for laxity	Moderate efficacy, multiple treatments necessary
Fractional		
1320 nm Er:Glass	Higher efficacy than nonablative for rhytides, some recovery time	Two- to three-day recovery time, multiple treatments necessary but fewer than nonablative with higher efficacy
1.5 U Er:Glass	Higher efficacy than nonablative for rhytides, some recovery time	Two- to three-day recovery time, multiple treatments necessary but fewer than nonablative with higher efficacy
Ablative		
Carbon dioxide 10,600 nm	Excellent efficacy for rhytides and photodamage	Two-week recovery time, higher risk profile
Erbium 2940 nm	Excellent efficacy for rhytides and photodamage	Two-week recovery time or less depending on extent of treatment, higher risk profile

Abbreviations: LP, long-pulsed; PDL, pulsed dye laser.

I hereby authorize Dr. _____ and his/her associates/assistants to perform upon the named patient or me the following surgical/medical/laser procedure(s), invasive test(s), and/or treatment(s) for my condition which has been explained to me: Procedure(s)/Test(s)/Treatment(s): _____
Diagnosis/Condition(s): _____

1. Nature, Purpose, Risks and Benefits of Procedure(s)/Test(s)/Treatment(s)
   The nature and purpose of the procedure(s), test(s), and/or treatment(s) have been explained to me. The expected benefits and possible complications or risks have also been explained. I understand that there is no guarantee of a specific result or cure, and that discomforts, risks and complications may arise. The possible alternatives to proposed treatment, including no treatment, have been explained to me. I have been given the opportunity to ask questions and all of my questions have been answered fully and to my satisfaction.
2. Possibility of Additional Unplanned Procedure(s)/Test(s)/Treatment(s)
   I understand that during the course of the procedure/test/treatment, unforeseen conditions may require that different and/or additional procedures/tests/treatments be performed. I therefore consent to the above-named physician and assistants to perform such additional procedures/tests/treatments, as they consider necessary.
3. Risks and Complications
   - I understand that surgical procedures, incisions, and laser procedures may result in scars, hyperpigmentation (darkening of skin), hypopigmentation (lightening of skin), or localized hair loss in hair-bearing areas that are treated. I confirm that the areas to be treated have been delineated in advance of the procedure with my approval. I understand that scars, hyperpigmentation, and hypopigmentation may be amenable to additional procedures or treatments in the future in order for them to be improved.
   - I understand that laser procedures may result in a burn. I have informed my physician of any recent tanning or prior history of laser procedures.
   - I understand that other common side effects or complications from surgical procedures/tests/and/or treatments include bleeding and infection. I understand that the risk of bleeding either during or after the procedure is increased when taking certain medications or supplements, and I have informed my doctor as to which medications and supplements I am taking. The risk of infection is increased in individuals with certain medical problems, and I have informed my doctor as to my medical conditions.
   - I understand that uncommonly allergic reactions may occur, which may manifest as a red bump at the site of injection, incision, procedure, test or treatment; theoretically, an extreme, severe form of allergy may result in anaphylaxis, which manifests as itching, skin swellings, difficulty breathing, and exceedingly rarely, even death. I have informed my physician of any allergies that I am known to have.
   - Other risks include blood clot formation in a superficial (thrombophlebitis) or deep (deep venous thrombosis) vessel; bruising, swelling or tenderness at the treated areas; or delayed wound healing, which may require additional procedures/tests/treatments. Such risks are increased in smokers, and if I am a smoker, understand that I should discontinue smoking for at least two weeks following the procedure, test, or treatment.
   - Unusual risks include superficial nerve damage at the treated sites, which may result in prolonged pain, disturbed sensation, or impaired movement at the treated areas.
4. Laser Hair Removal Information
   I understand that laser hair removal results in most cases in gradual thinning of hairs, with the potential for long-term hair loss. I understand that in some cases the hair may regrow completely, and that multiple treatments are necessary. A rare complication is the darkening of hairs in treated areas; I understand that should this occur, further treatments with laser are advised.
5. Laser Tattoo Removal and Cosmetic Tattoo Information
   I understand that tattoos that are red, flesh-toned, white, or brown in color may permanently darken following laser treatment. I have informed my doctor of any cosmetic tattoos I may have. I understand that tattoo removal requires multiple treatments, that removal may result in lightening or discoloration of the skin, and that complete removal may not be achieved.
6. Post-Treatment Instructions
   I understand the post-operative instructions given to me.
7. Contraindications
   I hereby confirm that I am not pregnant or breastfeeding, nor have I taken isotretinoin (Accutane or Roaccutane) in the past year, nor gold therapy. I understand that I should inform my physician of any medical conditions, allergies, medications, smoking history, or recent sun exposure.
8. Photography
   I also agree to having photographs taken. These photographs will be used for educational purposes and may be used for publication.
9. Consent
   I have read the above information regarding the procedure(s)/test(s)/treatment(s), pre- and post-treatment information and instructions, risks and complications, and contraindications. I have asked my physician any questions I may have and am satisfied by the answers to these questions. I accept the risks and potential complications resulting from the procedure(s)/test(s)/treatment(s), deny any contraindications in my medical history, and give hereby give my informed consent to the procedure(s)/test(s)/treatment(s).

_____
Patient/Healthcare Agent/Next-of-Kin Signature   Printed Name   Date

_____
Relationship   Interpreter

Witness
Physician/Practitioner Certification
I hereby certify that the nature, purpose, benefits, risks, and alternatives to (including no treatment and associated risks), the surgical procedure(s)/test(s)/procedure(s), and/or treatments(s) have been explained to the patient And any and all questions answered in full. I believe that the patient/health care agent/guardian/next-of-kin fully understands what has been explained.

_____
Physician Signature   Date
Consent form from M. R. Alexiades-Armenakas, M.D., P.C.*

FIGURE 1 Informed consent form for laser treatment. *Source*: From Macrene R. Alexiades-Armenakas.

Patient Name:

Date:

Treatment #:

Photos: Pre _____ Post _____

Operative Time:

Diagnosis: _____

Anatomic Location: _____

Procedure: _____

The patient was fully informed of the planned procedure, the alternative treatment options, limitations, expected results, risks and complications, both short and long-term. A full disclosure was given. Written informed consent was obtained.

Response to previous treatment was _____

The patient was brought to the procedure room and the area to be treated, was prepared and draped in the usual fashion.

Anesthesia: No _____ Yes _____ Type: Topical _____ Intralesional 1% lidocaine _____

Photosensitizer (5-aminolevulinic acid) applied: No _____ Yes _____ Duration time: _____

Laser therapy was performed using all standard safety precautions. The patient tolerated the procedure well. Wound care was discussed and appropriate dressings were applied. The patient left the procedure room in good condition and was informed concerning postoperative care, both verbally and in writing.

_____ MD _____ Assistant

Laser	Fluence	Spot Size	Pulse Duration	Pulses	Endpoint	Sites

Adapted from: 8. Continuous Wave and Quasi-continuous Wave Lasers, Appendix C. Operative Record, In: Dover, J.S., Arndt, K.A., Geronemus R.G., Alora, M.B.T., eds. Illustrated Cutaneous and Aesthetic Laser Surgery, 2nd Edition., Appleton & Lange, Stamford CT, 2000:184.**

FIGURE 2 Operative record. *Source*: From Ref. 8.

Immediately following laser treatment:
- The treated areas may be red and swollen for hours and, uncommonly, for days.
- Cool compresses are helpful if applied for a ten-minute period per hour for the first several hours.
- For swelling of the face, sleep on your back with your head elevated on pillows. This can be continued over the first few nights.
- Blistering and/or crusting may occur. If so, apply Aquaphor healing ointment twice daily, and healing generally occurs in 7–14 days. If this was not explained to you as an expected event, please call the physician.

In the days and weeks following laser treatment:
- Makeup and sunscreen may be worn *except* over blisters and crusts.
- Avoid excessive sun exposure. If you must go out during midday hours, wear a hat and apply a hypoallergenic sunscreen of SPF 30 or greater except to blisters and crusts.
- Avoid swimming in chlorinated water such as swimming pools for 7–14 days. Ocean or seawater swimming is just acceptable, but also best avoided.
- Do not manipulate the treated areas or undergo any additional procedures for at least 4 weeks following your laser treatment.

Follow-up and ongoing treatments:
- You will be instructed as to the appropriate follow-up interval following your laser treatment. This typically ranges from 3 to 6 weeks, depending upon the laser treatment performed.
- Most laser applications, with some exceptions, require a *series* of ongoing treatments spaced at defined intervals apart. This is necessary to safely and effectively treat the skin condition at hand. It is important to keep your follow-up appointments in order to be properly evaluated and to achieve the best possible results.

Post-laser Instruction Sheet from M. R. Alexiades-Armenakas, M.D., P.C.***

FIGURE 3 Postlaser instruction sheet. *Source*: From Macrene R. Alexiades-Armenakas.

laser specialists should start with the lowest settings on the laser initially, until adequate experience is obtained. Laser test spots may be recommended if the patient is dark-skinned.

SCHEDULING PATIENTS

Patient scheduling in a laser center is complicated and requires that the secretarial, technical, and medical staff all be fully aware of the steps involved in each type of treatment. For example, procedures requiring topical anesthetics require an initial application appointment followed by the treatment. In a center with multiple physicians sharing the same lasers, it is important that the patients not be scheduled for the same laser in the same time slot. Space must also be allocated for the numbing and recovery of patients.

CONCLUSIONS

In summary, setting up a laser center requires a careful selection of lasers by the physician, the implementation of strict and comprehensive laser safety guidelines, careful medical documentation, and the specialized training of office staff. Once these elements are in place, the physician will be able to offer the patients state-of-the-art treatments for a wide variety of dermatologic conditions.

REFERENCES

1. American National Standards Institute (ANSI): Z136.3-2005: Safe Use of Lasers in Health Care Facilities, 2005, The Institute.
2. American National Standards Institute (ANSI): Z136.1-2000, Safe Use of Lasers, 2000, The Institute.
3. American National Standards Institute (ANSI): Z136.5-2000, Safe Use of Lasers in Educational Institutions, 2000, The Institute.
4. Smalley PJ, Goldman MP. Laser safety: regulations, standards, and guidelines for practice. In: Goldman MP, Fitzpatrick RE, eds. Cutaneous Laser Surgery: The Art and Science of Selective Photothermolysis. 2nd edn. St. Louis, Missouri: Mosby, 1999:459–472.
5. Nori S Greene MA, Schrager HM, Falanga V. Infectious occupational exposures in dermatology—review of risks and prevention measures I. For all dermatologists. J Am Acad Dermatol 2005; 53(6):1010–1019.
6. U.S. Department of Labor Occupational Safety and Health Administration, Guidelines for Laser Safety and Hazard Assessment, STD 01-05-001 [PUB 8-1.7], 1991, August 5.
7. Sterling JB, Hanke CW. Office accreditation in dermatology. Semin Cutan Med Surg 2005; 24(3):128–132.
8. Continuous wave and quasi-continuous wave lasers, Appendix C. Operative record. In: Dover JS, Arndt KA, Geronemus RG, Alora MBT, eds. Illustrated Cutaneous and Aesthetic Laser Surgery. 2nd edn. Stamford CT: Appleton & Lange, 2000:184.

Index

AAADP. *See* Aminolevulinic acid dehydratase
    porphyria
Ablative skin rejuvenation
    ethnic skin, 419–421
Absorption spectra, 25
Acid dehydratase porphyria (ADP)
    cutaneous manifestations, 229
    etiology, 229
    laboratory findings and diagnosis, 230
    neurological manifestations, 228–229
Acne, 252
    intense pulsed light, 398
Acne vulgaris
    photodynamic therapy, 380
Actinic keratoses
    photodynamic therapy, 375–376
Actinic keratosis, 127
Actinic prurigo (AP), 149–163,437
    clinical features, 160
    diagnosis, 163
    epidemiology, 159
    etiology and pathogenesis, 159–160
    histopathology, 161–163
    induction, 160
    treatment, 163
Action spectrum, 25–26
    photoaging, 96–97
    photoimmunosuppression, 82
Activated charcoal
    erythropoietic protoporphyria, 235–236
Acute cutaneous lupus erythematosus, 258
Acute intermittent porphyria (AIP), 222–223, 228–230
    cutaneous manifestations, 229
    etiology, 229
    laboratory findings and diagnosis, 230
    neurological manifestations, 228–229
    treatment and prevention, 230
Adenocarcinoma
    sweat gland
        incidence rates, 128
ADP. *See* Acid dehydratase porphyria
Age
    ethnic skin
        cutaneous manifestations, 419–421
    skin cancer, 130
AIP. *See* Acute intermittent porphyria
Airborne contact dermatitis, 209
Alcohol
    PCT, 225–226
Aminolevulinic acid dehydratase porphyria
    (AAADP), 228–230
Amiodarone, 214
Antigen presenting cells
    photoimmunosuppression, 82–84
Antimalarials, 260

Antioxidants, 274–275
    PCT, 226
AP. *See* Actinic prurigo
Apoptosis, 48–49
    TP53, 112–113
Arc lamps, 32–33
Artificial radiation, 31–37
Atopic dermatitis, 255
Autoimmune bullous disease
    photopheresis, 365
Axmann, Hans, 7

Basal cell carcinoma (BCC), 108
    descriptive epidemiology, 125–128
    incidence rates, 127
    photodynamic therapy, 377
BCC. *See* Basal cell carcinoma
Becker's nevus
    ethnic skin
        lasers, 423
Berloque dermatitis, 203
Biomolecules
    excited states, 23–24
Bithionol, 205
    inducing PACD, 208
Blum, Harold, 4
Bowen's disease
    photodynamic therapy, 377
Bowls, Robert, 4
Broadband, 319–334
Broad-spectrum sunscreens, 300–301
Bullous pemphigoid, 261
Butyl methoxydibenzoylmethane, 205, 301

CAD. *See* Chronic actinic dermatitis
Café au lait patch
    ethnic skin
        lasers, 423
Calcium channel antagonists, 215
Candidate chromophores
    photoimmunosuppression, 84
Captan, 209
Cell cycle arrest, 48
Cell responses
    photochemical reactions, 23–24
Cell surface receptor activation, 45
Cellular immunity, 56–59
Characterizing, 38–39
Charcoal
    activated
        erythropoietic protoporphyria, 235
Charcot, Jean Martin, 3
Chlorhexidine diacetate, 205, 208
Chloroquine
    PCT, 226

Chlorpromazine hydrochloride (Thorazine), 208–209
 phototoxicity, 215
Cholestyramine
 erythropoietic protoporphyria, 235
Chronic actinic dermatitis (CAD), 169–183, 438–439
  See also Dermatitis
 clinical aspects, 172–176
 diagnosis, 177–178
 differential diagnosis, 178–179
 histopathology, 176
 management, 179–180
 pathogenesis, 171–172
 phototesting, 177
CIE. *See* Commission Internationale de l'Eclairage
CLE. *See* Cutaneous lupus erythematosus
Coblentz, William, 3
Cockayne syndrome, 245–246
 clinical symptoms, 241
Commission Internationale de
  l'Eclairage (CIE), 25
Congenital erythropoietic porphyria (CWP), 231–233
Congenital melanocytic nevi
 ethnic skin
  lasers, 426
Congenital nevi
 giant pigmented
  skin cancer, 130
Consent forms
 laser center, 458, 460
Contact dermatitis. *See also* Photoallergic contact
  dermatitis (PACD)
 airborne, 209
 photoirritant, 201–204
CPD. *See* Cyclobutyl pyrimidine dimer (CPD)
Cutaneous lupus erythematosus (CLE), 258
Cutaneous photoaging. *See also* Photoaging
 cutaneous hydration, 102–103
 measuring, 100
 photonumeric scales, 101
 properties, 101
 sebum production, 103
 skin structure, 102
 skin surface properties, 101
Cutaneous phototoxicity, 198
Cutaneous porphyrias, 221–238
 diagnosis, 222
 defective enzymes, 223
 mode of inheritance, 143
Cutaneous T cell lymphoma
 incidence rates, 128
 photodynamic therapy, 381
 photopheresis, 360–363
CWP. *See* Congenital erythropoietic porphyria
Cyclobutyl pyrimidine dimer (CPD), 24, 112
Cytochrome P450 enzyme
 PCT, 226
Cytokines, 44–45

Darier's disease, 252
Delayed type hypersensitivity (DTH), 59–61
Dendritic cells, 57–58
Dermatitis. *See also* Chronic actinic
  dermatitis (CAD)
 atopic, 255
 berloque, 203
 contact
  airborne, 209
 hyperpigmented photoirritant, 203

Dermatofibrosarcoma protuberans
 incidence rates, 128
Dermatomyositis, 259–261
Dermatosis
 photoaggravated, 251–266
 photo-induced
  protection against, 303–305
 transient acantholytic, 253–254
Dermatosis papulosa nigra
 laser, 419–421
Dichlorophen, 205
 inducing PACD, 207
Diet. *See* Vitamin D
 skin cancer, 131
Defective enzymes
 cutaneous porphyrias, 223
Diode
 1450 nm, 408–409
Diuretics, 212
DNA
 excision repair enzyme and photolyase, 275
 photochemistry, 24
 photoimmunosuppression, 82
DNA repair
 photoprotection, 282
Documentation
 laser center, 458–459
Dose, 18
 dose rate effects, 20
Drometriazole trisiloxane, 300–301
Drug-induced lupus erythematosus, 209
Drug-induced photosensitivity, 439–440
 systemic, 209–215
Drug-induced pseudoporphyria, 212
Drug photosensitivity, 210
DTH. *See* Delayed type hypersensitivity

Ebermaier, Johan Christoph, 2
Eczema
 PUVA, 354
 solare, 4
Education. *See also* Public education
 skin cancer, 131–132
Electromagnetic spectrum, 30
Ellinger, Friedrich, 6
EM. *See* Erythema multiforme
Emerging sunscreens
 assessment methods and standards, 289–292
Energy
 molecule, 23
 wavelength, 17–18
Epidermal hyperplasia, 81–82
Epstein, Stephen, 5
Equivalent radiometric quantities, 19
Erbium glass, 394
Erythema, 3–4
Erythema multiforme (EM), 254–255
Erythropoietic protoporphyria, 233–236
 activated charcoal, 235
 cholestyramine, 235
Estrogen
 PCT, 223–224
Ethnic skin
 ablative and nonablative skin rejuvenation, 419–423
 aging
  cutaneous manifestations, 418–419
 Becker's nevus
  lasers, 423–424

[Ethnic skin]
 café au lait patch
  lasers, 423
 congenital melanocytic nevi
  lasers, 426–428
 cultural concerns, 419
 facial telangiectasia
  lasers, 428
 Hori's macules
  lasers, 423
 lasers, 417–432
  dermal and mixed lesions, 424–426
  epidermal lesions, 423–424
  hair removal, 426–428
 medical history, 419
 melasma
  lasers, 423
 port wine stain
  lasers, 423
 preoperative considerations, 418
 proliferative hemangioma
  lasers, 428
 special precautions, 418
Extracorporeal photochemotherapy
  (photopheresis), 359–368
Extramammary Paget's disease
 incidence rates, 128

Facial telangiectasia
 ethnic skin
  lasers, 428
Fenticlor, 205
 inducing PACD, 208
Fibroblasts, 47
Filtered solar radiation, 6
Findlay, George, 4
Finsen, Niels, 2, 6, 8
Finsen lamp, 7
Finsen-Reyn lamp, 7
500 Dalton rule, 288
Fluorescence diagnosis, 383
Fluorescent lamps, 33
 phototherapy referral center, 451–452
Fluoroquinolones, 213–214
 phototoxicity index table, 210
Folpet, 209
Foscan (temoporfin), 215
Fractional resurfacing, 421–423
Fragrances, 208
Fraxel
 photorejuvenation, 410
Frequency doubled Nd:YAG, KTP, 403
Furocoumarins
 PICD, 202–204

Giant pigmented congenital nevi
 skin cancer, 130
Goeckerman, William Henry, 8
Gorlin-Goltz syndrome, 108
Graft-vs-host disease
 photopheresis, 363–364
Greiter, Franz, 6
Grover's disease, 253
Günther disease, 231–233

Hammer, Friedrich, 5
Hausser, Karl, 2
HCP. *See* Hereditary coproporphyria
Heinrich, Placidus, 3

Heliotherapy
 leg ulcers, 8
Hemangioma
 proliferative
  ethnic skin, 428
Heme biosynthetic pathway, 220
 intermediates, 221
HEP. *See* Hepatoerythropoietic porphyria
Hepatitis C
 PCT, 225
Hepatoerythropoietic porphyria (HEP), 223, 227–228
 diagnosis, 228
 etiology, 228
 laboratory evaluation, 228
 pathogenesis, 228
 treatment, 228
Hereditary coproporphyria (HCP), 223, 228–230
 cutaneous manifestations, 229
 etiology, 229
 laboratory findings and diagnosis, 230
Hereditary syphilis, 4
Herpes simplex, 254
Herschel, William, 2
Hexachlorophene, 205, 208
High-pressure mercury lamp, 8
High-pressure xenon lamp, 8
Höhensonne lamp, 8
Home, Everard, 2
Homosalate, 205
Hori's macules
 ethnic skin
  lasers, 423, 424
Huldschinsky, Kurt, 8
Humoral immunity, 56–57
Hutchinson, Jonathan, 4
Hydroa vacciniforme (HV), 4, 149–167, 157–159
 clinical features, 160–161
 diagnosis, 163
 epidemiology, 157
 etiology and pathogenesis, 157
 histopathology, 157–158
 treatment, 159
Hydroxychloroquine
 PCT, 226
2-Hydroxy-methoxy methyl benzophenone, 205
Hyperpigmented photoirritant dermatitis, 203

Immediate pigment darkening (IPD), 80
Immune system
 protection factor, 269, 302
Immunity
 humoral, 56–57
 systemic
  UV suppression, 60
Immunomodulators
 intense pulsed light, 397
Incandescent lamps, 32
Infrared lasers
 photorejuvenation, 406–407
Ingram, John, 8
Innate immunity
 photoimmunosuppression, 84
Instruction sheet
 laser center, 461
Intense pulsed light, 35, 389–400
 acne, 398
 clinical indications, 394
 cooling skin, 395–396

[Intense pulsed light]
getting melanin out, 394
getting red out, 393
hair disorders, 396
heating skin, 392–393
immunomodulators, 397
melanin, 394
novel UV light sources, 397
photodynamic therapy, 397
photorejuvenation, 404–406
tattoos, 395
warts, 396
Ionizing radiation
skin cancer, 131
IPD. *See* Immediate pigment darkening
Iron mutations
PCT, 225
Irradiance, 18
vs. exposure time, 21
spectral, 38–39
Irradiation monochromator, 435–437

Kaposi, Moriz, 4
Keratinocytes, 47–48
Keratoacantoma
incidence rates, 128
Ketoprofen, 205
Kromayer lamp, 8
Kuske, Hans, 5

Lamp changes
phototherapy referral center, 452–453
Lamps
Finsen, 6
Finsen-Reyn, 7
fluorescent, 33–34
phototherapy referral center, 449–450
high-pressure mercury, 8
high-pressure xenon, 8
Höhensonne, 7
incandescent, 32
Kromayer, 7
mercury
rachitis, 8
phototherapy referral center, 449–450
Laser(s), 34–35, 389–400
applications, 36
heating skin, 392–393
pigmented lesions, 458
seborrheic keratosis, 419–421
skin epilation, 401–416
skin rejuvenation, 401–416, 459
solar lentigines, 419–420
tattoos, 458
Laser center
consent forms, 458, 460
documentation, 458–459
instruction sheet, 461
laser selection, 457–458
operative report, 459, 461
patient scheduling, 462
physicians, 459–460
postoperative instructions, 459
setting up, 457
LED. *See* Light emitting diodes
Leg ulcers
heliotherapy, 8
phototherapy, 8

Leucotomos
polypodium, 275
Lichen acid mix, 205
Lichen planus actinicus, 256
Light
dosimetry
skin, 39–40
emitting diodes (LED), 36–37
eruption. *See* Polymorphous light eruption
lasers
natural, 31
propagation
through skin, 37–38
sources
photorejuvenation, 402–403
visible
photorejuvenation, 402
Liposarcoma
incidence rates, 128
Local or systemic primary immunity
UV suppression, 59–61
Lomefloxacin, 214
Lupus erythematosus, 256–257, 303
drug-induced, 213
subacute cutaneous, 258
systemic
photopheresis, 366
Lupus vulgaris
phototherapy, 8
Lux1540 fractional 1540nm
photorejuvenation, 410–411
radiofrequency, 411

Malignant melanoma, 108
McLaren, Douglas, 10
MED. *See* Minimal erythema dose
Medical Light Institute, 7
Melanin
intense pulsed light, 392
Melanocytes, 47
tanning responses, 49
Melanocytic nevi
skin cancer, 130
Melanogenesis
mechanism, 80
mediators, 80
Melanoma
descriptive epidemiology, 122–125
malignant, 108
Melasma, 304–305
ethnic skin
lasers, 423, 425–426
Memory or recall immunity
UV suppression, 59–61
Menthylanthranilate, 205
Mercury lamps
rachitis, 6
Merkel cell carcinoma
incidence rates, 128
6-Methycoumarin, 208
Microfine organic particles, 287
Microthermal, fractional resurfacing or
microrejuvenation
photorejuvenation, 402–403
Miescher, Guido, 4
Minimal erythema dose (MED), 3, 6, 19
measuring prior to narrowband or broadband
UVB phototherapy, 433–434

[Minimal erythema dose (MED)]
   measuring with suspected photosensitivity, 435
Minimal phototoxic dose
   measuring prior to psoralen photoche
      motherapy, 435
Mitochondrial damage
   photoaging, 94
Moller, Magnus, 3
8-MOP. *See* Oral 8-methoxypsoralen
Musk ambrette, 205, 206, 208
Mycosis fungoides
   PUVA, 353

Nagelschmidt, Carl Franz, 7
Narrow band, 319–334
Natural light, 31
Natural photoprotection, 3–4
Nd:YAG
   1320 nm, 407
Nevus of Ota
   ethnic skin
      lasers, 423, 424–425
New therapeutic molecules
   photosensitivity testing, 209
Newton, Isaac, 16
Nightingale, Florence, 6
Nonmelanoma skin cancer (NMSCs), 108
Nonsteroidal anti-inflammatory agents (NSAIDs), 209

Octinoxate, 205
Octisalate, 205
Octyl dimethyl PABA, 205
Office-based phototherapy unit, 449–456
   phototherapy referral center
      dosimetry, 454
Olaquindox, 209
Operative report
   laser center, 459, 462
Oppenheim, Moritz, 5
Optical radiation, 18
Oral lichen planus
   photopheresis, 366
Oral 8-methoxypsoralen (8-MOP), 9
Oxidative stress
   photoimmunosuppression, 84
Oxybenzone, 205

PACD. *See* Photoallergic contact dermatitis
Paget's disease
   extramammary
      incidence rates, 128
Papulosa nigra
   laser, 419–421
Para-aminobenzoic acid, 205
Patient scheduling
   laser center, 462
Pellagra, 253–254
Pemphigoid, 261
Pemphigus leprous, 4
Persistent light reactor, 211
Persistent pigment darkening (PPD), 80
Phenergan, 208
Phenothiazines, 208, 214–215
Phenylbenzimidazole, 205
PHisoHex, 208
Phlebotomy
   PCT, 228
Photoaggravated dermatoses, 251–266

Photoaging, 92–106, 305 *See also* Cutaneous
      photoaging
   action spectrum, 96
   clinical changes, 97–99
   histological changes, 100
   mechanisms, 92–96
   mitochondrial damage, 94
   telomeres, 94
   telomeres DNA damage, 94–96
   telomeres shortening, 94
   UV-induced membrane signaling, 93–94
Photoallergen
   solar urticaria, 190–191
Photoallergic agents, 142
Photoallergic contact dermatitis (PACD), 200,
      204–207, 442. *See also* Contact dermatitis
   photopatch testing techniques, 204
   photosensitizing agents, 207–209
Photobiological reaction, 390–392
Photobiology
   history, 1–14
   photopheresis, 366–367
   principles, 15–28
   skin, 37
Photocarcinogenesis, 107–118
Photochemical reactions
   cell responses, 24–25
Photochemotherapy, 9
   extracorporeal, 359–368
   psoralen, 347–358
Photodermatology
   dosimetric terms, 18
Photodermatoses
   classification, 140
   evaluation, 141, 142
   history, 141
   PUVA, 354
Photodynamic therapy, 369–388
   acne vulgaris, 380
   actinic keratoses, 375–376
   adverse effects, 374–375
   basal cell carcinoma, 377–378
   Bowen's disease, 377
   cutaneous T-cell lymphoma, 381
   dysplasia, 359–361
   intense pulsed light, 397
   light sources, 373–374
   mechanism of action, 371
   nonmelanoma skin cancer, 375
   nonmelanoma skin cancer indications, 378–383
   photosensitizers, 371
   poor response, 383
   psoriasis, 380
   reactions, 215
   recalcitrant viral warts, 378–379
Photofrin (porfimer sodium), 215
Photoimmunology, 55–74
Photoimmunosuppression, 82–84
   action spectrum, 83
   antigen presenting cells, 83
   candidate chromophores, 84
   innate immunity, 84
   mechanisms, 83–84
   mediators, 83
   oxidative stress, 84
   Th1/Th2 cytokines, 83
Photo-induced dermatoses
   protection against, 303–304

Photoirritant contact dermatitis (PICD), 200–204
   furocoumarins, 202–203
Photopatch testing, 5, 441–448
   indication, 444
   interpretation, 444–447
   methodology, 444
   PACD, 204
   photosensitive patient, 145
   positive, 443
   relevance, 447
   test substances, 441–444
   ultraviolet dose, 444
Photopheresis, 359–368
   autoimmune bullous disease, 365
   cutaneous T-cell lymphoma, 361–363
   graft-vs-host disease, 363–364
   oral lichen planus, 366
   photobiology, 366–367
   scleroderma, 364–365
   systemic lupus erythematosus, 365
Photoproducts, 112
Photoprotection, 267–278
   assessment, 268–269
   daily, 305
   DNA repair, 282
   natural, 3–4
   novel developments, 279–310
      UVA effects, 299
   public education, 3113–318, 313–317, 316
      community-wide interventions, 315
      health care practitioners and medical students,
         314–315
      programs, 313–316
      recreation areas, 314
      schools, 313–314
      workplace, 315
Photorejuvenation
   affirm, 410
   fraxel, 410
   infrared lasers, 407–409
   intense pulsed light, 404–405
   lasers/lights sources classification, 402–403
   light sources, 404–407
   low energy light emitting diodes, 405–407
   Lux1540 fractional 1540 nm, 410–411
   microthermal, fractional resurfacing or
      microrejuvenation, 409–410
   visible light lasers, 403
Photosensitive patients
   age of onset, 140
   eruption duration, 141–142
   evaluation, 139–148, 141, 146
   family history, 143
   history, 140–141
   laboratory evaluation, 146
   lesion morphology, 144
   photopatch testing, 145
   phototesting, 145
   physical examination, 143–144
   seasonal variation, 141–142
   systemic abnormalities, 143
   window glass, 143
Photosensitivity
   chemical, 199–218
   disorders, 84
   drug-induced, 200–218, 209–210, 439–440
   induced by topical agents, 200–201
   systemic drug-induced, 209–215

[Photosensitivity]
   testing
      new therapeutic molecules, 209
Photosensitization, 24
   protection against, 302–303
Photosensitizers, 7
   exposure, 140–141
   PACD, 207–209
   photodynamic therapy, 371
Photosensitizing drugs, 211
Phototesting, 433–440
   photosensitive patient, 145
Phototherapeutic UVA, 9
Phototherapy, 319–334
   leg ulcers, 8
   lupus vulgaris, 8
   skin diseases, 8–9
Phototherapy referral center, 449–456
   ancillary equipment, 453
   broadband UVB, 451
   canopy units, 451
   dosimetry, 452
   equipment, 451
   fluorescent lamps, 451–452
   forms, 453
   hand and foot units, 451
   lamp changes, 452–453
   localized delivery, 451
   narrowband UVB, 451
   office-based phototherapy unit
      dosimetry, 454
      equipment, 454
      forms, 455
      lamp changes, 454
      procedures, 454–455
      recording treatments, 455
      safety guidelines, 455
      space, 453–454
      staff, 454
      therapy guidelines, 455
      whole-body unit, 454
   procedures, 452–453
   PUVA, 451
   recording treatments, 453
   safety guidelines, 453
   space, 449–450
   staff, 450–451
   standup whole body units, 451
   therapy guidelines, 453
   ultraviolet A-1, 451–452
Phototherapy unit
   office-based, 449–456
Phototoxic agents, 142
Phototoxic drugs, 211–212
Phototoxicity
   cutaneous, 211
   thiazide-induced, 213
Phototoxicity index table
   fluoroquinolones, 210
Physical examination
   photosensitive patient, 143–145
Physicians
   laser center, 459–460
PICD. *See* Photoirritant contact dermatitis
Pigmentation, 3–4
Pigment darkening, 80–81
Pigmented lesions
   lasers, 458

Polymorphous light eruption (PLE), 149–167, 303, 437
  diagnosis, 155
  epidemiology, 150
  etiology, 150–151
  histopathology, 154–155
  induction, 151–152
  pathogenesis, 150–151
  treatment, 155–156
Polypodium leucotomos, 275
Porfimer sodium, 215
Porphyria cutanea tarda, 223–224
  blistering, 224
  hyperpigmentation, 224
  hypertrichosis, 224
Porphyrias. *See also* Acid dehydratase porphyria
    (ADP); Acute intermittent porphyria
    (AIP); Cutaneous porphyrias;
    Hepatoerythropoietic porphyria (HEP);
    Hereditary coproporphyria (HCP);
    Variegate porphyria (VP)
  aminolevulinic acid dehydratase, 228–230
  causing blistering skin lesions, 223
  classification, 221
  congenital erythropoietic, 231–233
  history, 222–223
Port wine stain
  ethnic skin
    lasers, 428
Postoperative instructions
  laser center, 459
PPD. *See* Persistent pigment darkening
Programmed cell death, 48–49
  TP53, 112–113
Proliferative hemangioma
  ethnic skin
    lasers, 428
Promethazine (Phenergan), 208
Protection factor
  immune system, 269, 302
  sun, 268, 289
    evaluation, 299
Protein kinase-mediated signal
    transduction, 45–46
Protoporphyria
  erythropoietic, 227–228
    cholestyramine, 235
Provocation testing, 437
Pseudoporphyria
  drug-induced, 212
Pseudoscleroderma, 223
Psoralen, 348–349
  cellular responses, 350
  cutaneous responses, 349
  maintenance therapy, 351
  pharmacology, 348–349
  photobiology, 349
  precautions, 352
  PUVA
    contraindications, 352–353
    treatment, 350–351
  UVA radiation, 349
Psoralen photochemotherapy, 347–358
Psoralen plus ultraviolet A (PUVA), 9
  bath, 355
  eczema, 354
  mycosis fungoides, 354
  photodermatoses, 354

[Psoralen plus ultraviolet A (PUVA)]
  phototherapy referral center, 449
  psoriasis, 353
  skin cancer, 131
  topical therapy, 355–356
  vitiligo, 354
Psoriasis, 8, 256
  photodynamic therapy, 381
  PUVA, 353–354
Public education. *See also* Education
  photoprotection, 311–318
    recreation arenas, 314
    schools, 313–314
    workplace, 315
Pulsed dye laser, 403–404
Pulsed light. *See* Intense pulsed light
PUVA. *See* Psoralen plus ultraviolet A

Quindoxin, 209
Quinine, 215

Raab, Oscar, 7
Rachitis
  mercury lamps, 8
Radiation. *See also* Ultraviolet radiation
    (UVR)
  artificial, 31–33
  energy form, 30
  ionizing
    skin cancer, 131
  optical, 18
  visible, 16
Radiation sources, 29–40, 31, 38
  skin, 37
  therapeutic, 32
  wavebands, 32
Radiometric calculation, 19
Recalcitrant viral warts
  photodynamic therapy, 379–380
Recall immunity
  UV suppression, 59–61
Red veterinary petrolatum, 6
Rikli, Arnold, 6
Ritter, Johann Wilhelm, 2
Roffo, Angel, 4

Safety
  sunscreens, 283–284
Safety guidelines
  phototherapy referral center, 453
Saidman, Jean, 3
Sandalwood oil, 205, 208
SCC. *See* Squamous cell carcinoma
Scheele, Wilhelm, 2
Schulze, Rudolf, 6
SCLE. *See* Subacute cutaneous lupus
    erythematosus
Scleroderma
  photopheresis, 364–365
Seborrheic keratosis
  lasers, 419–421
Short pulse Q-switched Nd:YAG, 407
Singlet excited state, 23
Skin
  delayed tanning, 80–81
  radical scavenging, 281
Skin barrier
  disturbances, 85

Skin cancer, 108
  age, 130
  analytic epidemiology, 128–131
  classification, 120
  defined, 121
  diet, 129
  epidemiology, 119–138
  gender, 130
  melanocytic nevi, 130
  phenotypic and solar exposure risk factors, 108–110
  prevention and education, 131–132
  PUVA, 131
  risk factors, 130
  smoking, 129
  sunscreens, 133
  tanning devices, 131
  UVR, 110
  world burden, 122
Skin diseases
  phototherapy, 8–9
Skin epilation
  lasers, 401–416
Skin immune system, 56–59
Skin phototypes classification, 20, 109
Skin rejuvenation
  ablative, 421–423
  ablative and nonablative
    ethnic skin, 419–421
  lasers, 401–416, 459
Smoking
  PCT, 226
  skin cancer, 131
Societies, 9
Solar lentigines
  laser, 419–421
Solar radiation
  filtered, 6
Solar ultraviolet
  energy and penetration, 42
  immunosuppression, 61
Solar urticaria, 185–198, 303, 437–438
  augmentation spectrum, 189
  chemical mediators, 192
  clinical course, 193
  clinical manifestations, 186
  coexisting disease, 193
  demography, 186
  drug-induced, 191
  histopathology, 192–193
  inhibition spectrum, 188–189
  passive transfer, 190
  photoallergen, 190–191
  photo-provocation and action spectrum tests, 187–188
  treatment, 193–195
Soluble factors, 44–45
Space
  phototherapy referral center, 449–450
Spectral irradiance, 38–39, 39
Squamous cell carcinoma (SCC), 108
  descriptive epidemiology, 125–128
  incidence rates, 127
Stalled DNA replication and RNA transcription, 46–47
Standard erythema dose, 19
Subacute cutaneous lupus erythematosus (SCLE), 257
Sulisobenzone, 205

Sunburn response, 76–79
  adhesion molecules, 79
  histology, 77
  initiating events, 78
  mechanism, 78
  mediators, 78
  oxidative stress, 78
  proinflammatory cytokines, 79
  time course, 76
  transcription factors, 79
  vasoactive mediators, 79
Sunless tanning agents, 274
Sunlight
  measurement, 56
Sun protection factor, 268, 289
  evaluation, 299
Sunscreen filters photostability, 300
Sunscreens. *See also* Topical sunscreens
  broad-spectrum, 300–301
  chemistry/actives, 284
  children, 269
  efficacy, 283
  emerging
    assessment methods and standards, 289–292
  immune protection, 84
  inducing PACD, 207–208
  new actives, 283–285
  patent freedom, 284
  registration, 283
  safety, 283
  skin cancer, 133
  UVA standards, 290
  UV protection, 281
  vitamin D, 272
Sweat gland
  adenocarcinoma
    incidence rates, 128
Syphilis
  hereditary, 4
Systemic drug-induced photosensitivity, 209–215
Systemic immunity
  UV suppression, 60
Systemic lupus erythematosus
  photopheresis, 365
Systemic primary immunity
  UV suppression, 59–61

Tanning agents
  sunless, 274
Tanning devices
  skin cancer, 131
Tanning response, 80–81
  melanocytes, 49
  time course, 80
Tar products
  PICD, 200–201
Tattoos
  intense pulsed light, 394
  lasers, 458
T cell lymphoma
  cutaneous
    incidence rates, 128
    photodynamic therapy, 381
    photopheresis, 361–363
T-cells, 47
Telangiectasia
  facial
    ethnic skin, 428

Telomeres
  DNA damage
    photoaging, 94–96
  photoaging, 94
  shortening
    photoaging, 94
Temoporfin, 215
Terephtalylidene dicamphor sulfonic acid, 300
Tetrabromosalicylanilide
  inducing PACD, 207
Tetracyclines, 215
Thiazide-induced phototoxicity, 212
Thorazine, 208
  phototoxicity, 215
Th1/Th2 cytokines
  photoimmunosuppression, 84
Tissue optics, 37, 390–392
Topical sunscreens. *See also* Sunscreens
  boosting agents, 283
  formulation improvement, 283
  improvements, 282–283
  micronization, 282
  UV protection, 280
Topical UV filters, 269
TP53
  basal cell carcinoma, 114–115
  programmed cell death, 112
  squamous cell carcinoma, 113–114
Transient acantholytic dermatosis, 253
Tribromosalicylanilide, 205
Trichothiodystrophy, 246–247
  clinical symptoms, 241
Triclosan, 205
  inducing PACD, 207
Tuberculosis
  heliotherapy, 8

UCA. *See* Urocanic acid
Uhlmann, Erich, 8
Ulcers
  leg
    heliotherapy, 8
    phototherapy, 8
Ultraviolet (UV)
  absorbers
    safety, 287–288
  absorption
    skin molecules, 21
  filters
    Europe, 271
    new, 269
    photostability, 271
    topical, 269
    USA approved, 269–271
  induced erythema
    time course, 76
  induced immunosuppression
    biological relevance, 66–68
  protection factor, 268, 269
  radiation
    preventing from reaching skin, 280–281
  transcriptional responses, 47
Ultraviolet A (UVA)
  biological effects, 301
  damage, 42
  filters, 300–301
  immunosuppression, 61
  protection

[Ultraviolet A (UVA)]
  biological effects, 301
  in silico determination, 291
  sunscreen effects, 302–303
  in vivo determination, 290
  and visible light therapy, 335–346
Ultraviolet A1, 335–343
  visible light therapy
    atopic dermatitis, 337–339
    connective tissue disease, 340–342
    cutaneous T-cell lymphoma, 339
    HIV-positive patients, 342–343
    side effects, 342
    T-cell mediated skin disease, 336–337
    urticaria pigmentosa, 339
Ultraviolet B (UVB), 319–334
  damage, 42–43
  filters, 301
  immunosuppression, 61
  induced erythema
    time course, 76
  lamp spectra, 321
  lamp types, 320–321
  phototherapy, 9
    action spectrum, 322
    atopic dermatitis, 330
    combination therapy, 326–328
    cutaneous T cell lymphoma, 330
    home therapy, 328–329
    localized treatment, 325–326
    minimal erythema dose, 322–323
    polymorphous light eruption, 331
    pruritus, 331
    psoriasis, 322–329
    side effects, 326
    treatment regimens, 323–326
    vitiligo, 330
    whole body treatment, 323–326
  sources, 320–321
Ultraviolet damage, 42–43
Ultraviolet-induced signaling and gene regulation,
    44–47
Ultraviolet radiation (UVR), 16. *See also* Radiation
  acute effects, 75–90
  antigen presentation, 61–63
  cellular responses, 47–50
  chronic effects, 91–118
  DNA effects, 42
  immunologic tolerance, 63
  immunosuppressive mediators, 65–66
  lipid effects, 43
  molecular and genetic effects, 41–54
  protein effects, 44
  signature mutations
    DNA photodamage, 111
    tumor suppressor genes, 112–115
  T cells, 63–65
Urocanic acid (UCA)
  photoimmunosuppression, 84
  UV-induced immunosuppression, 66
Uroporphyrinogen decarboxylase (UROD), 223, 225
  mutations
    PCT, 225–226
Urticaria. *See* Solar urticaria
UV. *See* Ultraviolet
UVA. *See* Ultraviolet A
UVB. *See* Ultraviolet B
UVR. *See* Ultraviolet radiation

Variegate porphyria (VP), 223,
        228–231
  cutaneous manifestations, 229
  etiology, 229
  laboratory findings and diagnosis, 230
  neurological manifestations, 228–229
Viral warts
  recalcitrant
    photodynamic therapy, 379–380
Visible light lasers
  photorejuvenation, 403–404
Visible radiation, 16
  skin molecules, 21
  UVR, 17
Vitamin D, 316
  bone health, 82
  controversies, 82
  cutaneous synthesis, 81
  metabolism, 82
  production, 49, 81
  sources, 81
  sunscreens, 272

Vitiligo
  PUVA, 354
VP. *See* Variegate porphyria

Warts
  intense pulsed light, 396
Wavelength
  color, 17
  ranges
    UVR, 16
Willan, Robert, 4
Wound-healing response, 50
Wrinkle reduction
  lasers, 459

Xeroderma pigmentosum (XP), 4, 239–250
  care and management, 244–245
  clinical symptoms, 241–245
  differential diagnosis, 243
  DNA repair genes, 244
  laboratory diagnosis, 243
  nucleotide excision repair, 240–241

9 780367 453190